Encyclopedia of
HEALTH
&
BEHAVIOR

Encyclopedia of
HEALTH
&
BEHAVIOR

2

Editor in Chief
NORMAN B. ANDERSON, PhD
American Psychological Association

A Sage Reference Publication

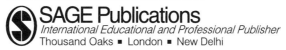

SAGE Publications
International Educational and Professional Publisher
Thousand Oaks ■ London ■ New Delhi

For information:

 Sage Publications, Inc.
2455, Teller Road
Thousand Oaks, California 91320
E-mail: order@sagepub.com

Sage Publications Ltd.
1 Oliver's Yard
55 City Road
London EC1Y 1SP
United Kingdom

Sage Publications India Pvt. Ltd.
B-42, Panchsheel Enclave
Post Box 4109
New Delhi 110 017   India

The following contributors wrote the entries listed while they were employees of the United States federal government. These entries are not copyrighted but exist in the public domain.
Deborah Holtzman and Lawrence W. Green, *Centers for Disease Control and Prevention*
Willo Pequegnat, *Sexually Transmitted Diseases: Prevention*
Edward G. Singleton and Stephen J. Heishman, *Drug Craving*

Printed in the United States of America

Library of Congress Cataloging-in-Publication Data

Encyclopedia of health and behavior/Norman B. Anderson.
    p. cm.
Includes bibliographical references and index.
ISBN 0-7619-2360-8 (Cloth)
  1. Behavioral medicine-Encyclopedias. I. Anderson, Norman B.
R726.5.E53 2004
610′.3—dc22   2003020763

This book is printed on acid-free paper.

04   05   06   07   08   10   9   8   7   6   5   4   3   2   1

Acquisitions Editor:	Jim Brace-Thompson
Editorial Assistant:	Karen Ehrmann
Developmental Editor:	Mary Riso
Project Editor:	Claudia A. Hoffman
Copy Editors:	Kate Peterson, Barbara Coster
Typesetter:	C&M Digitals (P) Ltd.
Indexer:	Molly Hall
Cover Designer:	Ravi Balasuriya

Contents

List of Entries vii

Reader's Guide xi

Entries

 Volume I: A–G 1

 Volume II: H–W 459

Appendix A: Online Resources and
   Health and Behavior Organizations 829

Appendix B: Bibliography 845

Author Index 913

Subject Index 933

List of Entries

Acculturation and Health
Adherence to Treatment Regimens
Adoption of Health Behavior
African American Health and
    Behavior
AIDS and HIV
AIDS and HIV: Adherence to
    Medications in Persons With
    HIV Infection
AIDS and HIV: Prevention of HIV
    Infection
AIDS and HIV: Stress
Alameda County Study
Alcohol Abuse and Dependence
Alcohol Abuse and Dependence:
    Treatment
Allostatis, Allostatic Load, and
    Stress
Alzheimer's Disease: Psychosocial
    Aspects for Caregivers
Anger and Heart Disease
Anger and Hypertension
Anger: Measurement
Anxiety, Heart Disease, and
    Mortality
Anxiety: Its Meaning and
    Measurement
Applied Behavior Analysis
Arthritis: Behavioral Treatment
Arthritis: Psychosocial Aspects
Asian American/Pacific Islander
    Health and Behavior
Asthma: Behavioral Treatment
Asthma and Stress
Autoimmune Diseases:
    Psychosocial Aspects

Behavioral Genetics and Health
Behavioral Risk Factor
    Surveillance System

Bereavement and Health
Binge Drinking in College
    Students
Biofeedback
Blood Pressure and Hypertension:
    Measurement
Blood Pressure and Hypertension:
    Physical Activity
Blood Pressure, Hypertension, and
    Stress
Bogalusa Heart Study
Bulimia Nervosa: Treatment

Cancer and Diet
Cancer and Physical Activity
Cancer Prevention
Cancer: Psychosocial
    Treatment
Cancer Screening
Cancer and Smoking
Cardiac Rehabilitation
Cardiovascular Disease
    Prevention: Community-Level
    Interventions
Cardiovascular Psychophysiology:
    Measures
Cardiovascular Reactivity
Caregiving and Stress
Center for the Advancement of
    Health
Centers for Disease Control and
    Prevention
Cerebrovascular Disease:
    Psychosocial Aspects
Child Abuse, Child Neglect, and
    Health
Chronic Disease Management
Chronic Fatigue Syndrome:
    Psychosocial Aspects

Chronic Illness: Psychological
    Aspects
Chronic Obstructive Pulmonary
    Disease: Psychosocial Aspects
    and Behavioral Treatments
Chronic Pain Management
Church-Based Interventions
Cognitive Function and Health
Community-Based Participatory
    Research
Community Coalitions
Comorbid Mental and Other
    Physical Disorders
Complementary and Alternative
    Medicine
Confounding
Control and Health
Cost-Effectiveness
Crowding and Health
Cultural Factors and Health

Depression: Measurement
Depression: Mortality and Other
    Adverse Outcomes
Depression: Treatment
Diabetes: Behavioral Treatment
Diabetes: Psychosocial Aspects
Diffusion of Innovation
Disasters and Health
Discrimination and Health
Divorce and Health
Doctor-Patient Communication
Drug Abuse: Behavioral Treatment
Drug Abuse: Prevention
Drug Craving

Eating Disorders
Ecological Models: Application to
    Physical Activity

Ecological Momentary Assessment
Ecosocial Theory
Effect Modification
Effort-Reward Imbalance
Emotions: Negative Emotions and
    Health
Emotions: Positive Emotions and
    Health
Endogenous Opioids, Stress, and
    Health
Erectile Dysfunction
Evidence-Based Behavioral
    Medicine
Explanatory Style and Physical
    Health
Expressive Writing and Health

Fibromyalgia Syndrome:
    Biobehavioral Aspects
Fibromyalgia Syndrome:
    Cognitive-Behavioral Treatment
Five a Day—for Better Health!
    Program
Framingham Heart Study
Fundamental Social Causes of
    Disease and Mortality

Gastric Ulcers and Stress
Gate Control Theory of Pain
Gender Differences in Health
General Adaptation Syndrome
Genetic Testing: Ethical, Legal,
    and Social Aspects

Happiness and Health
Hardiness and Health
Harvard Alumni Health Study
Headaches: Psychological
    Management
Health and Behavior Organizations
Health Belief Model
Health Care Costs and Behavior
Health Care Service Utilization:
    Determinants
Health Communication
Health Disparities
Health Literacy
Health Promotion and Disease
    Prevention
Health Psychology

Heart Disease: Anger, Depression,
    and Anxiety
Heart Disease and Diet
Heart Disease and Physical
    Activity
Heart Disease and Reactivity
Heart Disease and Smoking
Heart Disease and Type A
    Behavior
Hopelessness and Health
Hostility and Health
Hostility: Measurement
Hostility: Psychophysiology

Immigrant Populations
    and Health
Immune Responses to Stress
Income Inequality and Health
Infertility and Assisted
    Reproduction: Psychosocial
    Aspects
Injury Prevention in Children
Irritable Bowel Syndrome:
    Psychological Treatment
Irritable Bowel Syndrome:
    Psychosocial Aspects

Job Strain and Health
John Henryism and Health

Key Informants
Kuopio Ischemic Heart Disease
    Risk Factor Study

Latino Health and Behavior
Lipids: Psychosocial Aspects
Loneliness and Health
Low Birth Weight: Psychosocial
    Aspects

Medical Psychology
Metabolic Syndrome and Stress
Minnesota Multiphasic
    Personality Inventory
    (MMPI/MMPI-2)
Motivational Interviewing
Multilevel Methods, Theory, and
    Analysis
Multiple Risk Factor Intervention
    Trial (MRFIT)

Multiple Sclerosis: Psychosocial
    Aspects

National Cholesterol Education
    Program (NCEP)
National Institutes of Health:
    Health and Behavior Research
Neighborhood Effects on Health
    and Behavior

Obesity: Causes and
    Consequences
Obesity in Children: Physical
    Activity and Nutritional
    Approaches
Obesity in Children: Prevention
Obesity: Prevention and Treatment
Occupational Health and Safety
Optimism, Pessimism, and Health
Optimism and Pessimism:
    Measurement

Pain: Psychosocial Aspects
Participatory Research
Peptic Ulcers and Stress
Physical Activity and Health
Physical Activity Interventions
Physical Activity and Mood
Placebos and Health
Pregnancy Outcomes:
    Psychosocial Aspects
Pregnancy Prevention in
    Adolescents
Psychoneuroimmunology
Psychophysiology: Theory and
    Methods

Quality of Life: Measurement

Raynaud's Disease: Behavioral
    Treatment
Repressive Coping and Health
Research to Practice in Health and
    Behavior
Rheumatoid Arthritis:
    Psychosocial Aspects

School-Based Health Promotion
Self-Efficacy
Self-Reported Health

Sexually Transmitted Diseases: Prevention
Sickle Cell Disease: Psychosocial Aspects
Sleep Disorders: Behavioral Treatment
Smoking and Health
Smoking and Nicotine Dependence
Smoking and Nicotine Dependence: Interventions
Smoking Prevention and Tobacco Control Among Youth
Social Capital and Health

Social Integration, Social Networks, and Health
Social Marketing
Social or Status Incongruence
Socioeconomic Status and Health
Spirituality and Health
Stress, Appraisal, and Coping
Stress: Biological Aspects
Stress-Buffering Hypothesis
Stress-Related Growth
Successful Aging
Support Groups and Health

Tailored Communications
Television Viewing and Health

Theory of Planned Behavior
Theory of Reasoned Action
Theory of Triadic Influence
Transtheoretical Model of Behavior Change

Violence Prevention
Vital Exhaustion

Women's Health Issues
Work-Related Stress and Health
Worksite Health Promotion
Wound Healing and Stress

Reader's Guide

ASSESSMENT AND TREATMENT

Adherence to Treatment Regimens
AIDS and HIV: Adherence to Medications in Persons With HIV Infection
Alcohol Abuse and Dependence: Treatment
Anger: Measurement
Anxiety: Its Meaning and Measurement
Applied Behavior Analysis
Arthritis: Behavioral Treatment
Asthma: Behavioral Treatment
Biofeedback
Blood Pressure and Hypertension: Measurement
Blood Pressure and Hypertension: Physical Activity
Bulimia Nervosa: Treatment
Cancer: Psychosocial Treatment
Cancer Screening
Cardiac Rehabilitation
Cardiovascular Psychophysiology: Measures
Cardiovascular Reactivity
Chronic Disease Management
Chronic Obstructive Pulmonary Disease: Psychosocial Aspects and Behavioral Treatments
Chronic Pain Management
Complementary and Alternative Medicine
Depression: Measurement
Depression: Treatment
Diabetes: Behavioral Treatment
Doctor-Patient Communication
Drug Abuse: Behavioral Treatment
Eating Disorders

Ecological Momentary Assessment
Evidence-Based Behavioral Medicine
Expressive Writing and Health
Fibromyalgia Syndrome: Cognitive-Behavioral Treatment
Genetic Testing: Ethical, Legal, and Social Aspects
Headaches: Psychological Management
Health Care Costs and Behavior
Health Care Service Utilization: Determinants
Health Communication
Hostility: Measurement
Irritable Bowel Syndrome: Psychological Treatment
Minnesota Multiphasic Personality Inventory (MMPI/MMPI-2)
Motivational Interviewing
National Cholesterol Education Program (NCEP)
Obesity in Children: Physical Activity and Nutritional Approaches
Obesity: Prevention and Treatment
Optimism and Pessimism: Measurement
Physical Activity Interventions
Psychophysiology: Theory and Methods
Quality of Life: Measurement
Raynaud's Disease: Behavioral Treatment
Sleep Disorders: Behavioral Treatment
Smoking and Nicotine Dependence: Interventions

Smoking Prevention and Tobacco Control Among Youth
Support Groups and Health
Tailored Communications

BASIC PROCESSES, THEORY, AND METHODOLOGY

Adoption of Health Behavior
Alcohol Abuse and Dependence
Allostatis, Allostatic Load, and Stress
Anger: Measurement
Anxiety: Its Meaning and Measurement
Behavioral Genetics and Health
Behavioral Risk Factor Surveillance System
Blood Pressure and Hypertension: Measurement
Cardiovascular Psychophysiology: Measures
Caregiving and Stress
Community-Based Participatory Research
Confounding
Cost-Effectiveness
Crowding and Health
Cultural Factors and Health
Depression: Measurement
Diffusion of Innovation
Discrimination and Health
Doctor-Patient Communication
Ecological Models: Application to Physical Activity
Ecological Momentary Assessment
Ecosocial Theory

Effect Modification
Effort-Reward Imbalance
Endogenous Opioids, Stress, and Health
Erectile Dysfunction
Fibromyalgia Syndrome: Biobehavioral Aspects
Fundamental Social Causes of Disease and Mortality
Gastric Ulcers and Stress
Gate Control Theory of Pain
General Adaptation Syndrome
Genetic Testing: Ethical, Legal, and Social Aspects
Health Belief Model
Health Communication
Hostility: Measurement
Immune Responses to Stress
Income Inequality and Health
Key Informants
Metabolic Syndrome and Stress
Multilevel Methods, Theory, and Analysis
Optimism and Pessimism: Measurement
Participatory Research
Peptic Ulcers and Stress
Psychoneuroimmunology
Psychophysiology: Theory and Methods
Quality of Life: Measurement
Repressive Coping and Health
Self-Efficacy
Smoking and Nicotine Dependence
Social Capital and Health
Social Marketing
Social or Status Incongruence
Stress, Appraisal, and Coping
Stress: Biological Aspects
Stress-Buffering Hypothesis
Successful Aging
Television Viewing and Health
Theory of Planned Behavior
Theory of Reasoned Action
Theory of Triadic Influence
Transtheoretical Model of Behavior Change

Vital Exhaustion
Wound Healing and Stress

BIOPSYCHOSOCIAL INTERACTIONS

AIDS and HIV: Stress
Alcohol Abuse and Dependence
Allostatis, Allostatic Load, and Stress
Anger and Heart Disease
Anger and Hypertension
Anger: Measurement
Anxiety, Heart Disease, and Mortality
Asthma and Stress
Autoimmune Disorders: Psychosocial Aspects
Behavioral Genetics and Health
Blood Pressure, Hypertension, and Stress
Cardiovascular Psychophysiology: Measures
Cardiovascular Reactivity
Caregiving and Stress
Cerebrovascular Disease: Psychosocial Aspects
Chronic Fatigue Syndrome: Psychosocial Aspects
Chronic Illness: Psychological Aspects
Chronic Obstructive Pulmonary Disease: Psychosocial Aspects and Behavioral Treatments
Community-Based Participatory Research
Comorbid Mental and Other Physical Disorders
Control and Health
Depression: Mortality and Other Adverse Outcomes
Diabetes: Psychosocial Aspects
Drug Craving
Emotions: Negative Emotions and Health
Emotions: Positive Emotions and Health
Endogenous Opioids, Stress, and Health
Erectile Dysfunction

Explanatory Style and Physical Health
Fibromyalgia Syndrome: Biobehavioral Aspects
Gastric Ulcers and Stress
General Adaptation Syndrome
Heart Disease: Anger, Depression, and Anxiety
Hostility: Psychophysiology
Immune Responses to Stress
Infertility and Assisted Reproduction: Psychosocial Aspects
Lipids: Psychosocial Aspects
Metabolic Syndrome and Stress
Obesity: Causes and Consequences
Pain: Psychosocial Aspects
Peptic Ulcers and Stress
Placebos and Health
Psychoneuroimmunology
Psychophysiology: Theory and Methods
Stress: Biological Aspects
Vital Exhaustion
Wound Healing and Stress

EPIDEMIOLOGY OF RISK AND PROTECTIVE FACTORS

Acculturation and Health
African American Health and Behavior
AIDS and HIV
Alameda County Study
Alzheimer's Disease: Psychosocial Aspects for Caregivers
Anger and Heart Disease
Anger and Hypertension
Anxiety, Heart Disease, and Mortality
Arthritis: Psychosocial Aspects
Asian American/Pacific Islander Health and Behavior
Asthma and Stress
Autoimmune Disorders: Psychosocial Aspects
Behavioral Risk Factor Surveillance System

Bereavement and Health

Binge Drinking in College Students

Bogalusa Heart Study

Cancer and Diet

Cancer and Physical Activity

Cancer Prevention

Cancer and Smoking

Caregiving and Stress

Cerebrovascular Disease: Psychosocial Aspects

Child Abuse, Child Neglect, and Health

Chronic Fatigue Syndrome: Psychosocial Aspects

Chronic Illness: Psychological Aspects

Cognitive Function and Health

Comorbid Mental and Other Physical Disorders

Control and Health

Crowding and Health

Cultural Factors and Health

Depression: Mortality and Other Adverse Outcomes

Diabetes: Psychosocial Aspects

Disasters and Health

Discrimination and Health

Divorce and Health

Eating Disorders

Effect Modification

Emotions: Negative Emotions and Health

Emotions: Positive Emotions and Health

Endogenous Opioids, Stress, and Health

Explanatory Style and Physical Health

Framingham Heart Study

Fundamental Social Causes of Disease and Mortality

Gastric Ulcers and Stress

Gender Differences in Health

Happiness and Health

Hardiness and Health

Harvard Alumni Health Study

Health Care Costs and Behavior

Health Care Service Utilization: Determinants

Health Disparities

Health Literacy

Heart Disease: Anger, Depression, and Anxiety

Heart Disease and Diet

Heart Disease and Physical Activity

Heart Disease and Reactivity

Heart Disease and Smoking

Heart Disease and Type A Behavior

Hopelessness and Health

Hostility and Health

Immigrant Populations and Health

Income Inequality and Health

Irritable Bowel Syndrome: Psychosocial Aspects

Job Strain and Health

John Henryism and Health

Kuopio Ischemic Heart Disease Risk Factor Study

Latino Health and Behavior

Loneliness and Health

Low Birth Weight: Psychosocial Aspects

Multiple Risk Factor Intervention Trial (MRFIT)

Multiple Sclerosis: Psychosocial Aspects

Neighborhood Effects on Health and Behavior

Obesity: Causes and Consequences

Obesity in Children: Physical Activity and Nutritional Approaches

Obesity in Children: Prevention

Occupational Health and Safety

Optimism, Pessimism, and Health

Physical Activity and Health

Physical Activity and Mood

Placebos and Health

Pregnancy Outcomes: Psychosocial Aspects

Repressive Coping and Health

Rheumatoid Arthritis: Psychosocial Aspects

Self-Reported Health

Sickle Cell Disease: Psychosocial Aspects

Smoking and Health

Social Capital and Health

Social Integration, Social Networks, and Health

Socioeconomic Status and Health

Spirituality and Health

Stress-Related Growth

Successful Aging

Television Viewing and Health

Women's Health Issues

Work-Related Stress and Health

HEALTH PROMOTION AND DISEASE PREVENTION

AIDS and HIV: Prevention of HIV Infection

Blood Pressure, Hypertension, and Stress

Cancer and Diet

Cancer and Physical Activity

Cancer Prevention

Cancer Screening

Cancer and Smoking

Cardiovascular Disease Prevention: Community-Level Interventions

Child Abuse, Child Neglect, and Health

Church-Based Interventions

Community Coalitions

Complementary and Alternative Medicine

Diffusion of Innovation

Drug Abuse: Prevention

Ecological Models: Application to Physical Activity

Evidence-Based Behavioral Medicine

Expressive Writing and Health

Five a Day—for Better Health! Program

Health Care Costs and Behavior

Health Communication

Health Literacy

Health Promotion and Disease Prevention

Heart Disease and Diet
Heart Disease and Physical
    Activity
Heart Disease and Reactivity
Heart Disease and Smoking
Heart Disease and Type A
    Behavior
Hopelessness and Health
Hostility and Health
Injury Prevention in Children
National Cholesterol Education
    Program (NCEP)
Obesity: Causes and
    Consequences
Obesity in Children: Physical
    Activity and Nutritional
    Approaches
Obesity in Children: Prevention
Obesity: Prevention and Treatment
Occupational Health and Safety
Physical Activity and Health
Physical Activity: Interventions
Physical Activity and Mood
Pregnancy Prevention in
    Adolescents
School-Based Health Promotion
Sexually Transmitted Diseases:
    Prevention

Smoking Prevention and Tobacco
    Control Among Youth
Support Groups and Health
Tailored Communications
Violence Prevention
Worksite Health Promotion

POLICY AND
ORGANIZATIONS

Center for the Advancement of
    Health
Centers for Disease Control and
    Prevention
Genetic Testing: Ethical, Legal,
    and Social Aspects
Health and Behavior
    Organizations
Health Care Service Utilization:
    Determinants
Health Literacy
Health Psychology
Medical Psychology
National Institutes of Health:
    Health and Behavior
    Research
Research to Practice in Health and
    Behavior

SOCIAL AND CULTURAL
FACTORS

Acculturation and Health
African American Health and
    Behavior
Asian American/Pacific Islander
    Health and Behavior
Church-Based Interventions
Community Coalitions
Crowding and Health
Cultural Factors and Health
Discrimination and Health
Ecological Models: Application to
    Physical Activity
Ecosocial Theory
Health Disparities
Immigrant Populations and Health
Income Inequality and Health
Latino Health and Behavior
Neighborhood Effects on Health
    and Behavior
Social Marketing
Social Integration, Social
    Networks, and Health
Social or Status Incongruence
Socioeconomic Status and Health
Support Groups and Health

H

HAPPINESS AND HEALTH

Although the relation between psychological processes and health (both mental and physical) is not new, historically there has been a preponderance of research on the negative side—how poor psychological functioning relates to negative health outcomes. Meanwhile, attention has only recently turned toward understanding the antecedents and consequences of positive states. This entry focuses on pleasant emotions and life satisfaction and discusses both mental health and physical health as they relate to subjective well-being.

WHAT IS HAPPINESS?

Understanding the relation between health and happiness naturally raises the question "What is happiness?" Happiness can mean several different things. It can refer to people's overall evaluation of their own lives, or it can refer to momentary feelings of pleasantness. Because of the multiplicity of meanings that happiness holds, researchers sometimes prefer to use the term *subjective well-being* (SWB), although happiness is sometimes used synonymously with SWB. SWB refers to a combination of life satisfaction, pleasant affect, and low negative affect. Life satisfaction is a global cognitive evaluation—how a person feels about his or her life as a whole—although there are specific domain satisfactions as well (e.g., satisfaction with one's marriage). Emotions, on the other hand, specifically reflect on-line evaluations of ongoing events by the affect system. The combination of emotions and life satisfaction is called *subjective well-being* because it emphasizes the individual's own assessment of his or her own life—not the judgment of "experts."

MENTAL HEALTH AND SWB

Some mood states, such as depression, are by definition part of low SWB and ill mental health. After all, depression entails having negative moods and a negative evaluation of one's life. However, mental health includes more than simply the absence of negative moods. In a landmark paper on mental health, Jahoda (1958) called for the inclusion of positive states in conceptions of mental well-being. In other words, to be mentally healthy means to have positive feelings as well as minimal negative feelings. As expected, individuals with a mental illness such as schizophrenia, personality disorder, or depression tend to be less satisfied with their lives and experience greater and more intense negative emotion and less positive emotion than nonclinical populations.

Does mental illness cause a decrease in life satisfaction? For some mental illnesses, the link to SWB is definitional—that is, depression is virtually the same as having low SWB. For other mental illnesses such as schizophrenia, there may be more of a causal link in that having schizophrenia leads to lower SWB. Even so, the causality is not necessarily direct because mental illness is often accompanied by poor social functioning and other problems in living, such as keeping a job, that in turn influence SWB. Medication can improve the SWB of schizophrenics, but again, these effects are complex. Medication can improve the person's moods directly or improve daily functioning, both of which have an impact on SWB. Incidentally, some factors that may mitigate the sufferings of people with mental illness overlap with factors that influence the SWB of nonclinical populations—for example, having close social relationships. Schizophrenics who have a close friend are happier than those with no support network.

Diener and Seligman (2002) examined the relation between mental health and SWB from a different perspective by studying the happiest people. Compared to the very unhappy or moderately happy, not a single person who was identified as very happy scored in the clinical range on scales of psychopathology (e.g., depression, paranoia, schizophrenia), with the exception of some elevated mania scores among a few individuals. Thus, psychopathology seems incompatible with high happiness.

Other mental illnesses such as Alzheimer's disease and dementia are also associated with lower life satisfaction, although the degree depends on several other factors such as social support and level of functioning. Interestingly, the life satisfaction of caregivers of Alzheimer patients, senile family members, or those who had strokes also tends to be low. Caretakers' well-being depends in part on the amount of additional support received. Nevertheless, this suggests an important point—that it is more than one's own health that matters. The health of those around us, particularly close individuals, seems as important as our own health in influencing life satisfaction. These issues become paramount in the changing face of world demographics. The past 300 years has seen an increase in life expectancy, and with it an increase in the proportion of elderly in the population. By 2020, 16% of the U.S. population will be over 65, and by 2050, the average life expectancy for Americans will be 82.6 years. Clearly, longevity is a desirable aim, but research on the SWB of the elderly and their caretakers suggests a further need to consider other aspects of a long life, such as quality of life and level of functioning.

PHYSICAL HEALTH AND SWB

Two-Way Causal Direction

Although there are a variety of ways to examine the relation between physical health and SWB, most researchers and health professionals are interested in determining causal influences. In other words, does happiness lead to better health or are healthy people happier? Unfortunately, the bulk of studies have relied on cross-sectional designs and correlational methods, which do not help us disentangle causal direction. Also, correlational studies are always susceptible to the problem of third variables such as personality factors influencing both the outcome and SWB. Despite these problems, data suggest causality in both directions.

Bad Health Causing Lower SWB

Not surprisingly, bad health is negatively correlated with SWB. Studies of the elderly have shown that more chronic medical conditions are associated with lower life satisfaction. Brickman, Coates, and Janoff-Bulman's (1978) classic study of people with spinal cord injuries showed that, although the accident victims were not abjectly miserable for the rest of their lives, their SWB did decrease and remain lower than preaccident levels. However, as with mental illness, there may be mediational pathways linking health and SWB. For instance, health problems that prevent people from engaging in life's everyday activities or from caring for themselves (e.g., severe heart disease and chronic lung disease) have the greatest impact on lowering life satisfaction. In addition, the chronic fatigue often associated with some illnesses such as multiple sclerosis tends to lower life satisfaction. Studies of chronic pain sufferers such as people with arthritis, chronic headaches, or obesity show that beyond the immediate effects of pain, limitations on daily activities lower SWB.

The few longitudinal studies that exist provide greater insight into the direction of causality. One study of elderly people found that chronic health problems, functional impairment, and somatic complaints predicted lower life satisfaction 3 years later, while self-rated health and good vision were associated with higher life satisfaction. Among individuals with spinal cord injuries, those who attain employment show higher SWB over time, whereas those who are unemployed become less happy. In a 1-year follow-up of patients with chronic health conditions, those who had multiple health problems declined in SWB, while those with only one problem showed improvement after 1 year. In short, people who do not feel well or whose functioning is impaired are not likely to be happy, and more severe or more numerous problems make for even worse outcomes.

If poor health is associated with lower SWB, we might expect the opposite to be true—that good health has positive effects. Unfortunately, it is difficult to determine whether the effects of good and ill health are symmetrical even though we know that health correlates moderately with SWB, especially among the elderly. If good health is considered the default and taken for granted, then the effects of health might fade into the background when health is good, and only surface when health is bad. Clearly, more research is needed to disentangle the effects.

The Issue of Coping/Adaptation

The impact of ill health on SWB is not always intuitive; people can and do often cope with health problems, although they almost always underestimate their ability to do so. For instance, people predict that their SWB will be dramatically lower if they are diagnosed with HIV, but their predictions tend to be worse than reality.

The relation between health and SWB is further complicated by people's expectations, in that some health problems are expected at a certain age. For example, one study found that elderly patients with cancer or chronic ailments did not differ from their healthy peers in terms of SWB. Thus, some illnesses might not produce lower SWB for some people at some points in life. Part of this is due to the strong influence of personality and considerable stability in SWB over time. Many studies now suggest that the best predictor of future SWB is past SWB, not objective life events. In other words, some individuals who endure health problems can still be relatively happy, while others with only minor or no health problems might be unhappy.

Subjective Versus Objective Health

Thus far, we have addressed, "What is happiness?" but the corollary to this question, "What is health?" also warrants scrutiny. Health can be measured subjectively, in terms of people's self-reports of symptoms, or objectively, as the number of doctor visits and doctors' evaluations. This distinction is important because the relation between health and SWB is stronger for subjective health. For objective health measures, the relation is much weaker. This suggests a possible methodological confound in studies using subjective health: Happy people tend to perceive themselves as healthier. However, even number of doctor visits can be influenced by personality by directing our attention (e.g., toward bodily sensations), perceptions (e.g., sensations interpreted as illness), and actions (e.g., seeking medical treatment). Also, doctors' evaluations are naturally influenced by what the patient reports. Highly negative individuals will be more apt to complain. Thus, even objective health measures can be influenced by a patient's happiness.

Some Evidence Suggestive of Causality Going From SWB to Physical Health

The impact of SWB on health outcomes has been examined in four different ways: laboratory experiments, studies of naturally occurring mood, dispositional emotionality, and longitudinal studies.

Immune function. In laboratory experiments, researchers typically induce positive moods and measure the effects on physical markers of immune functioning (e.g., salivary immunoglobulin-A, natural killer cell activity). A consistent finding is that immune function increases after positive mood induction such as watching a humorous video. Similarly, studies of naturally occurring mood have found enhanced immune function on days when positive mood is greater than negative mood, or when positive events outweigh negative ones. When happiness is treated as a dispositional or trait-level construct, dispositionally happy people show better immune function.

Although positive emotion appears to have benefits on the immune system, the evidence is not entirely unequivocal. Some studies have shown that the effects of positive states on physical health are greatest within the context of negative emotions. For example, when humor is used as a coping device or when positive moods buffer negative moods, the effects are particularly salubrious. Similarly, individuals who are instructed to find benefits in a traumatic event often show improved health. Rather than feeling good all the time, healthy people appear to experience a wide range of emotions.

Finally, it is important to note that although low SWB might lead to bad health in terms of getting sick more often, it probably does not enter the causal chain of severe illnesses such as malaria or epilepsy. Happiness might have some additive effects on pre-existing conditions (e.g., making symptoms more or less severe), but probably plays a minimal role in the etiology of serious diseases.

Longevity. As mentioned earlier, subjective health reports can be influenced by personality, thus making it difficult to disentangle the effects of SWB on health. However, one measure that is not confounded with subjective reporting is mortality. Although longitudinal research predicting longevity from SWB is still in its infancy, the existing studies suggest that happiness is associated with increased longevity. First, there is a direct effect in that low life satisfaction predicts an increased risk for suicide. Beyond suicide, however, happiness still predicts longevity. Danner, Snowden, and Friesen (2001) studied a group of nuns and found that the number of positive-emotion words used in autobiographical narratives written in their 20s predicted longevity six decades later. Nuns in the happiest quartile outlived those in the lowest quartile by 9.4 years. These results are particularly convincing because the researchers followed a homogeneous group that was similar in lifestyle. Longevity in this case was not likely confounded by the risky behaviors that often mediate the relationship between happiness and longevity. Similarly, a 2-year longitudinal study examining elderly Hispanics also found that positive emotionality predicted survival even after controlling for health behaviors.

Health behaviors. The relation between SWB and health can operate through health behaviors as well. For instance, happy people tend to pay more attention to health-related information, follow better diets, and exercise more. In addition, there is lower substance abuse among adolescents with high life satisfaction.

Future Research

The past few decades of research on SWB and health have revealed significant and intriguing findings, but many more questions remain. The most definitive statement we can make at this point is that happiness is often associated with better health, but any causal conclusions remain tentative (but promising). Emerging evidence from experimental and longitudinal studies suggests that happiness might lead to better health, although we clearly need more studies of these kinds to tease apart the direction of effects. Meanwhile, third variables that cause both SWB and health continue to present a problem in determining causality.

Future research should examine more complex models of SWB and health, for example, the moderating effects of income and social support. Is the relation between SWB and health more pronounced among those with low income and low social support? Also, greater attention should be paid to separating the effects of positive emotion and negative emotion. Does pleasant affect suppress unpleasant affect? Often researchers measure only the negative (e.g., depression), despite evidence that the two have independent effects. Some evidence now suggests that positive affect has buffering effects on negative affect and that only positive—not negative—emotion leads to health benefits.

GENERAL CONCLUSIONS

The field of SWB and health is an important area, although relatively new. From the research thus far, we can draw three main conclusions: (1) High SWB is inversely related to mental illness; (2) some physical illnesses are associated with lower SWB, but this relation is qualified by functional impairment, personality, and age expectancies; and (3) high SWB is sometimes associated with health benefits. The most compelling evidence is that positive emotion can lead to enhanced immune function, and possibly longevity. However, the data are far from definitive at this point, and many more experimental and longitudinal studies are needed to further disentangle the direction of causality.

—*Ed Diener and Christie Napa Scollon*

See also EMOTIONS: POSITIVE EMOTIONS AND HEALTH

Further Reading

Argyle, M. (2001). *The psychology of happiness*. London: Routledge.

Brickman, P., Coates, D., & Janoff-Bulman, R. (1978). Lottery winners and accident victims: Is happiness relative? *Journal of Personality and Social Psychology, 36*, 917-927.

Danner, D. D., Snowden, D. A., & Friesen, W. V. (2001). Positive emotions in early life and longevity: Findings from the Nun Study. *Journal of Personality and Social Psychology, 80*, 801-813.

Diener, E., & Seligman, M. E. P. (2002). Very happy people. *Psychological Science, 13*, 81-84.

Jahoda, M. (1958). *Current conceptions of positive mental health*. New York: Basic Books.

Kahneman, D., Diener, E., & Schwarz, N. (1999). *Well-being: Foundations of a hedonic psychology*. New York: Russell Sage Foundation.

Lyubomirsky, S., King, L. A., & Diener, E. *A review of the benefits of happiness*. Manuscript in preparation, University of California, Riverside.

HARDINESS AND HEALTH

Hardiness is a set of attitudes and skills that promote resiliency under stressful circumstances by enhancing performance, leadership, morale, and health (e.g., Maddi, 2002). The HardiAttitudes® are the 3Cs of commitment, control, and challenge (Maddi & Kobasa, 1984). Commitment is the conviction that staying involved with people and events, rather than pulling back, is the way to find meaning and value in your life. Control is the inclination to try to influence what is going on around you, rather than sink into powerlessness. Challenge is the belief that, as life is continually changing, you are most fulfilled by continuing to learn from your experiences, whether they are positive or negative, rather than by expecting easy comfort and security. In short, the HardiAttitudes provide the existential courage and motivation to work on transforming stressful circumstances from potential disasters into opportunities instead (Maddi, 2002). This transformation is accomplished through the HardiSkills® (Khoshaba & Maddi, 2001). These skills are for transformational coping (solving problems, rather than denying or avoiding them), activistic social support (giving and getting assistance and encouragement, rather than overprotection or competition), and self-care (relaxation, nutrition, and exercise regimens leading to the moderate arousal that facilitates coping and social support efforts). As the rate of change mounts in our world, the combination of attitudes and skills constituting hardiness is all the more important in preserving and enhancing health and performance.

Hardiness was discovered through a longitudinal study of 450 male and female managers at Illinois Bell Telephone (IBT), from 1975 through 1986, that was designed to precede and follow the federal deregulation of the AT&T monopoly in 1981, so as to make way for a competitive telecommunications industry (Maddi & Kobasa, 1984). Throughout the study, the managers were tested in various psychological and medical ways each year. Still regarded as the largest upheaval in corporate history, the 1981 deregulation led to major downsizing and disruption at IBT.

Indeed, two thirds of the managers in the sample showed marked decreases in health and performance. In contrast, however, the other third not only survived but actually thrived on the upheaval. A determination of how this third of the sample differed from the other two thirds, in the years preceding the deregulation, disclosed the importance of HardiAttitudes and HardiSkills in resilient, as opposed to vulnerable, responses.

Since that time, considerable research on hardiness has been done all around the world. Initial measurement issues concerning an early form of the HardiAttitudes measure have been resolved successfully (Maddi, 1997). Early conceptual issues as to whether HardiAttitudes are anything more than the opposite of negative affectivity or neuroticism have also been successfully resolved (Maddi, 2002). A recent study (Sinclair & Tetrick, 2000) shows that the subscales of commitment, control, and challenge are, as hypothesized, nested under a second-order factor of HardiAttitudes and that this factor is not redundant with negative affectivity.

Ongoing research on the effects of HardiAttitudes has confirmed that they maintain and enhance health and performance under stressful circumstances. In a wide range of stressful contexts, ranging from life-threatening events of military combat, through the culture shock of immigration or work missions abroad, to everyday work or school pressures and demands, the buffering effect of hardiness is shown in decreasing mental and physical illness symptoms, whether these be self-reported or more objectively measured (cf. Maddi, 2002).

Furthermore, research shows that hardiness leads to better performance under stress (cf. Maddi, 2002). Examples are the positive relationship between HardiAttitudes and subsequent (1) basketball performance among varsity players, (2) success rates in officer training school for the Israeli military, (3) leadership behavior among West Point military cadets, (4) retention rate among college students, and (5) speed of recovery of baseline functioning following disruptive culture shock.

There is also research supporting the construct validity of HardiAttitudes (cf. Maddi, 2002). In an experiential sampling study in which participants were paged at random to comment on their ongoing activities, there was a positive relationship between HardiAttitudes and (1) involvement with others and events (commitment), (2) the sense that the activities had been chosen and were influenceable (control), and (3) the positive process of learning from what was going on (challenge). Other findings are consistent with the hypothesis that the mechanism whereby the HardiAttitudes lead to beneficial health and performance effects is by providing the courage and motivation for enacting the HardiSkills. For example, results show that HardiAttitudes are related to the tendency to view life events as less stressful, cope transformationally with these events, avoid excessive physiological arousal, and pursue positive while avoiding negative health practices.

By now, there are hardiness assessment and training techniques useful not only in research but in practice as well. The latest and best HardiAttitudes measure is the Personal Views Survey III-R (Maddi & Khoshaba, 2001b), an 18-item rating scale questionnaire with adequate reliability and validity. The HardiSurvey III-R® (Maddi & Khoshaba, 2001a) is a 65-item rating scale questionnaire, also with adequate reliability and validity, which measures not only HardiAttitudes but also stress, strain, and HardiSkills. This test generates a comprehensive report comparing the person's stress vulnerability and stress resistance. Both tests can be administered on the Internet, or in hard copy form.

HardiTraining® is workbook based and involves the trainee in performing exercises that implement the HardiSkills in dealing with stressful circumstances and use the feedback thus obtained to deepen the HardiAttitudes (Khoshaba & Maddi, 2001). Workbooks are available for adults and for adolescents. One common training format involves several weekly sessions for small groups meeting with a trainer. Also common is an individual format, wherein the person works through the exercises alone, but checks in with a trainer at regular intervals. There is enough flexibility in the approach to permit other training formats as well. There is by now research evidence of the effectiveness of HardiTraining for both working adults and college students.

—*Salvatore R. Maddi and Deborah M. Khoshaba*

Further Reading

Khoshaba, D. M., & Maddi, S. R. (2001). *HardiTraining*. Newport Beach, CA: Hardiness Institute.

Maddi, S. R. (1997). Personal Views Survey II: A measure of dispositional hardiness. In C. P. Zalaquett & R. J. Woods (Eds.), *Evaluating stress: A book of resources*. New York: University Press.

Maddi, S. R. (2002). The story of hardiness: Twenty years of theorizing, research, and practice. *Consulting Psychology Journal, 54*, 173-185.

Maddi, S. R., & Khoshaba, D. M. (2001a). *HardiSurvey III-R®: Test development and Internet instruction manual.* Newport Beach, CA: Hardiness Institute.

Maddi, S. R., & Khoshaba, D. M. (2001b). *Personal Views Survey III-R: Internet instruction manual.* Newport Beach, CA: Hardiness Institute.

Maddi, S. R., & Kobasa, S. C. (1984). *The hardy executive: Health under stress.* Homewood, IL: Dow Jones-Irwin.

Sinclair, R. R., & Tetrick, L. E. (2000). Implications of item wording for hardiness structure, relation with neuroticism, and stress buffering. *Journal of Research in Personality, 34*, 1-25.

HARVARD ALUMNI HEALTH STUDY

The Harvard Alumni Health Study is an ongoing epidemiological study of 36,000 men who matriculated at Harvard University as undergraduates between 1916 and 1950 (no women were admitted during those years). The study was established in the 1960s, when health questionnaires were sent to surviving alumni of these classes. The initial questionnaires, which collected information on sociodemographic characteristics, health habits, and personal and family medical history, were mailed in 1962 or 1966. Follow-up questionnaires collected updated information in 1972, 1977, 1988, 1993, and 1998. The study also obtained information from university archives from a standardized medical anamnesis and physical examination that the men underwent at the time of their entry into Harvard.

These Harvard men were chosen for study for several reasons. First, investigators had hoped to establish a study in which subjects could be followed for many years. For valid results to be obtained from the study, it is crucial that losses to follow-up be minimal. Preliminary work in the 1950s had indicated that the alumni office at Harvard University kept careful records on the whereabouts of students who had graduated, and subsequent research over the years has shown that this continues to be the case.

Second, to conduct a large study at low cost, investigators wanted to collect information by mail and presumed that alumni from an established university would be well educated and interested in their health and thereby able to provide accurate health information on questionnaires. Validation studies subsequently conducted (e.g., that compared alumni self-reports of chronic diseases with their physicians' records) have proved this assumption correct. Finally, at the start of the study in 1962, the investigators could take advantage of information from the standardized medical anamnesis and physical examination done 12 to 46 years previously. This afforded them the opportunity to explore host and environmental data, recorded years in advance of the clinical onset of disease (such as coronary heart disease), as predictors of disease.

The main aims of the Harvard Alumni Health Study were and continue to be to investigate the health effects associated with a physically active way of life. Although the health benefits of physical activity have been extolled since antiquity (e.g., Hippocrates believed that lack of exercise was detrimental to health), this topic had received little scientific study before the 1960s, when the Harvard Alumni Health Study was initiated. In fact, the prevailing belief was that exercise might be harmful. Paul Dudley White (1886-1973), an eminent cardiologist at that time and one of the doctors who attended to President Eisenhower during his heart attack in 1955, was often belittled because he both believed in and practiced a physically active way of life.

Data from the Harvard Alumni Health Study and other studies of physical activity have played a crucial role in changing society's attitude toward physical activity. In the remainder of this entry, we will outline some of the key findings from the Harvard Alumni Health Study regarding the health benefits associated with physical activity.

Beginning in 1966, a series of publications has examined the role of physical activity in preventing coronary heart disease among Harvard alumni. Data from the Harvard Alumni Health Study show that there is a graded, inverse relation between levels of physical activity and rates of coronary heart disease. Men expending 1,000 to 1,999 kilocalories per week in physical activity had rates of coronary heart disease that were about one fifth lower than rates among men who expended less energy. With higher levels of energy expenditure, rates of coronary heart disease declined further.

Activities that were beneficial were those that were at least moderately vigorous in intensity (e.g., brisk walking, jogging or running, swimming laps, playing

tennis, shoveling snow). For men to experience lower rates of heart disease, they had to be presently performing these activities. That is, alumni who had been physically active during their college days but who were sedentary during middle age or later did not fare any better than their counterparts who had been sedentary during both times. However, those who had been sedentary during college but who took up physical activity during middle age or later experienced rates of coronary heart disease similar to those of men who had been active during both times. Even more encouraging, these data show that it is never too late to change: The benefits of taking up a physically active way of life were seen among men in their 40s all the way to those in their 80s.

These data, along with those from other studies, were used as the basis for formulation in 1995 of a new physical activity recommendation for the United States. This recommendation calls for at least 30 minutes of moderate intensity physical activity, such as brisk walking, most days of the week, a level that will generate about 1,000 kilocalories per week. The key role that the Harvard Alumni Health Study has played in elucidating the relation between physical activity and heart disease was acknowledged in 1996 with the joint award of the first International Olympic Committee Medal for work emanating from the Harvard Alumni Health Study, as well as research conducted among British civil servants.

The Harvard Alumni Health Study also examined the relation of physical activity to rates of stroke. As with coronary heart disease, data from the study showed that rates of stroke were lower in physically active men than in less active men. Men who expended 1,000 to 1,999 kilocalories per week had rates of stroke that were about one fourth lower than the rates of stroke among men who expended less than 1,000 kcal/week, and the rate among men who expended 2,000 to 2,999 kilocalories per week was about one half lower than the rate among men who expended less than 1,000 kcal/week. As with coronary heart disease, the activity carried out had to be at least moderately vigorous in intensity to be associated with lower rates of disease.

Because cardiovascular disease is the leading cause of death in men in the United States, preventing coronary heart disease and stroke would be expected to delay premature mortality. The Harvard Alumni Health Study has investigated whether physical activity is associated with increased longevity and was among the earliest studies that attempted to quantify the number of years added. It was estimated that among men aged 35 to 79 years, those who expended at least 2,000 kilocalories per week would enjoy more than 2 years of added life (to age 80) as compared with those who expended less than 500 kilocalories per week.

Beginning in the 1990s, the study expanded its focus to include detailed investigations of the association of physical activity with various cancers. The study observed that physical activity also was associated with lower rates of certain cancers. Men who expended at least 1,000 kilocalories per week in physical activity experienced about half the colon cancer rates of men who were more sedentary. Higher levels of physical activity did not appear to further decrease rates of colon cancer. For lung cancer, there was a graded inverse relation between levels of physical activity and rates of this cancer, after accounting for the effects of cigarette smoking. On the other hand, there was little evidence that physical activity influenced the risk of developing prostate cancer or rectal cancer. Meanwhile, in a parallel study of women alumni from the University of Pennsylvania, physical activity was seen to be associated with lower rates of breast cancer in postmenopausal women.

In addition to the findings described above, data from the Harvard Alumni Health Study, as well as the parallel study of alumni from the University of Pennsylvania, have shown that a physically active way of life is associated with many other health benefits, including lower rates of hypertension, diabetes, and depression. These studies clearly show that physical activity is beneficial for health and that a sedentary way of life is detrimental with regard to many chronic diseases, carrying with it an increase in risk similar in magnitude to that seen with other well-established risk factors, such as cigarette smoking, being overweight, or having high blood pressure.

—*I-Min Lee and Ralph S. Paffenbarger Jr.*

See also Cancer and Physical Activity; Heart Disease and Physical Activity; Physical Activity and Health

Further Reading

Lee, I.-M., Hsieh, C.-c., & Paffenbarger, R. S., Jr. (1995). Exercise intensity and longevity in men: The Harvard Alumni Health Study. *Journal of the American Medical Association, 273,* 1179-1184.

Lee, I.-M., Paffenbarger, R. S., Jr., & Hsieh, C.-c. (1991). Physical activity and risk of developing colorectal cancer among college alumni. *Journal of the National Cancer Institute, 83,* 1324-1329.

Paffenbarger, R. S., Jr., Hyde, R. T., Wing, A. L., Lee, I-M., Jung, D. L., & Kampert, J. B. (1993). The association of changes in physical activity level and other lifestyle characteristics with mortality among men. *New England Journal of Medicine, 328,* 538-545.

Paffenbarger, R. S., Jr., Wing, A. L., & Hyde, R. T. (1978). Physical activity as an index of heart attack risk in college alumni. *American Journal of Epidemiology, 108,* 161-175.

HEADACHES: PSYCHOLOGICAL MANAGEMENT

EPIDEMIOLOGY

Recurrent headaches are prevalent and are associated with substantial individual and societal burden. Approximately 18% of women and 6% of men (e.g., 28 million individuals in the United States; Lipton, Hamelsky, & Stewart, 2001) experience migraine. Approximately 36% of women and 42% of men experienced a tension-type headache in the past year, with 2.8% of women and 1.4% of men experiencing tension-type headaches more than 15 days per month.

Missed workdays and impaired work function resulting from migraine cost employers about $13 billion a year, and direct medical costs run about $1 billion per year. Because tension-type headaches are more prevalent than migraine, they are associated with greater societal costs even though they are associated with less individual disability. As the frequency or severity of either migraine or tension-type headaches increases, the impact of headaches on functioning increases. Consequently, a relatively a small portion (< 50%) of individuals with frequent or severe headaches account for over 80% of the disability and costs associated with these disorders (Lipton et al., 2001).

DIAGNOSIS

The International Headache Society (IHS; Olesen, 1988) classification system for headache disorders employs operational diagnostic criteria modeled after those in the *Diagnostic and Statistical Manual of*

Mental Disorders of the American Psychiatric Association. Primary headache disorders are distinguished from secondary headaches that result from an underlying disease. The two most prevalent primary headache disorders—migraine and tension-type headache—are of great interest in behavioral medicine. Diagnostic criteria are currently under revision, and a draft of these revised diagnostic criteria is available on the IHS Web site (www.i-h-s.org). Of course, the possibility of a secondary cause for headaches must be ruled out by physical and neurological exams and indicated tests before a diagnosis of a primary headache disorder can be made.

PATHOPHYSIOLOGY

Migraine

Migraine is primarily a neuronal disorder (Goadsby, Lipton, & Ferrari, 2002). Imaging studies showing the activation of brain stem regions involved in the control of sensory, nociceptive (pain), and vascular functions during spontaneous migraine provide support for the existence of a brain stem "migraine generator." The sensory disturbances or "aura" that can precede migraine are believed to result from a "spreading depression," or a transient inhibition of neuronal activity, that passes over the cerebral cortex. Pain and other phenomena of migraine are thought to result from activation of trigeminal innervation of the vasculature; it is unclear if it is the spreading depression that induces trigeminal activation or if spreading depression is simply a parallel phenomenon (Goadsby et al., 2002). Nonetheless, activation of trigeminal nerves induces neurogenic inflammation (dilation and leakage of plasma protein) from arteries surrounding the brain, sensitization of nerve endings at these arteries, and sensitization of pain transmission circuits in the trigeminal nucleus. Pain then results when sensitized nerves are stimulated by dilated arteries sending pain signals through highly sensitized pain transmission circuits, but may also be influenced by a dysfunction in supraspinal (limbic) pain modulation systems.

Tension-Type Headache

Frequent tension-type headaches are probably maintained by a central nervous system (CNS) dysfunction (Borkum, in press; Holroyd, 2002). This CNS dysfunction may involve the sensitization of pain transmission circuits in the trigeminal nucleus where input from nerves in the face and head is first integrated and relayed toward the brain. Such sensitization would lower the threshold for the transmission of pain signals, so that little or no input from peripheral nerves (nociceptors) is required for the transmission of pain signals to the brain. A dysfunction in supraspinal (limbic) pain modulation circuits may also maintain pain by permitting, or even facilitating, the transmission of pain signals in the brain.

Headache Precipitants

General population studies indicate that stress, sleep difficulties, and hormonal factors (relevant particularly for migraine) are the triggers most frequently identified by headache sufferers. *Stress* is the most frequently identified headache precipitant for both migraine and tension-type headache (Borkum, in press; Lipchik, Holroyd, & Nash, 2002). Headaches may be triggered by stress or by relaxation following a period of stress ("let-down headaches"). *Sleep* difficulties are commonly identified as a headache trigger, with insufficient sleep, oversleeping, or an irregular sleep schedule identified as most common sleep precipitants. Fluctuations in *reproductive hormones* (menarche, menstruation, pregnancy, menopause, hormone replacement therapy) are associated with headache disorders, particularly migraine. Close to 30% of people with headaches, primarily those with migraine, report that *dietary factors*, such as skipping or delaying meals, or ingesting specific foods (e.g., aged cheeses), beverages (e.g., red wine), or ingredients (nitrites or aspartame) sometimes trigger their headaches. *Environmental stimuli* (e.g., glare, chemical odors) also are commonly identified as headache triggers (Borkum, in press).

Psychosocial Complications

Medication Overuse Headaches

Medication overuse or "rebound" headaches resemble chronic tension-type or chronic migraine headaches; however, it is the frequent use of prescription or nonprescription analgesic medications or abortive medications (combination analgesics, opiates, nonopioid analgesics, barbiturates, ergots, and other abortive agents including triptans) that is worsening the original tension-type or migraine headaches.

Medication overuse headaches can be managed effectively only if the use of the offending medications is reduced or eliminated (Silberstein & Dongmei, 2002).

Comorbid Psychiatric Disorders

Epidemiological studies (Shechter, Lipton, & Silberstein, 2001) confirm that the prevalence of mood and anxiety disorders is elevated in migraine sufferers (relative risk typically between 2 and 3). Longitudinal data further argue that the association between mood disorders and migraine is bidirectional; for example, migraine increased the risk of a *subsequent* episode of major depression (adjusted relative risk = 4.8), but the presence of major depression also increased the risk of *subsequently* developing migraine (adjusted relative risk = 3.3) (Shechter et al., 2001).

The prevalence of both anxiety and mood disorders also appears to be elevated in chronic tension-type headache, at least in clinical samples. Over 40% of chronic tension-type headache patients in primary care settings, and even higher percentages of chronic tension-type headache patients seen in specialty settings, receive either an anxiety or mood disorder diagnosis. The presence of a comorbid anxiety or mood disorder appears to increase the disability associated with either tension or migraine headaches so effective management of psychiatric disorders may improve functioning (Holroyd, 2002).

Medical Management

There are four goals of medication treatment.

Symptomatic. The goal of symptomatic therapy is to reduce pain. Symptomatic medications include analgesics prescribed primarily to reduce pain, such as nonsteroidal anti-inflammatory drugs (NSAIDs, COX-2), mixed analgesics containing barbiturates (e.g., butalbital) or opioids (i.e., codeine), and opioids alone (i.e., oxycodone). The use of opioid and mixed analgesics must be limited because overuse can cause rebound headaches and even addiction. NSAIDs and COX-2 inhibitors may be less likely to induce rebound headaches, but are not free from this problem.

Abortive. If taken early in the migraine episode, the goal of abortive therapy is to interrupt the migraine process, preventing a full-blown migraine from developing; if taken late in the migraine episode, a more realistic goal is to reduce migraine symptoms. Abortive medications include NSAIDs, ergotamine derivatives, and serotonin-receptor agonists (triptans such as sumatriptan, rizatriptan, naratriptan, zolmitriptan, almotriptan, and eletriptan). These agents must be used no more than 2 to 3 days per week to avoid rebound headaches (Goadsby et al., 2002).

Antiemetic. The goal of antiemetic therapy is to reduce nausea and control vomiting. Antiemetics also improve the absorption of some oral medications, including analgesics, and may have antimigraine effects themselves. Antiemetics (e.g., prochlorperazine, metoclopramide) are used to treat the nausea and vomiting associated with migraines. Patients who experience nausea and vomiting are instructed to take an antiemetic before or along with their analgesic.

Preventive. The goal of preventive therapy is to reduce the frequency of headaches. Preventive or prophylactic medications for migraine include beta-blockers, calcium channel blockers, antidepressants (tricyclic, serotonin-reuptake inhibitors, and MAO inhibitors), anticonvulsants, and NSAIDs (Goadsby et al., 2002). Antidepressants (for the most part tricyclics) are the primary preventive medications for tension-type headache.

Psychological Management

Behavioral Interventions

Behavioral interventions emphasize the *prevention* of headaches, although the same headache management skills can be used to influence the severity of headaches as well. The long-term goals of behavior therapy include reduced frequency and severity of headaches, reduced headache-related disability and affective distress, reduced reliance on poorly tolerated or unwanted pharmacotherapy, and enhanced personal control of headaches.

Relaxation training. Relaxation skills presumably enable headache sufferers to exert control over headache-related physiological responses and, more generally, to lower sympathetic arousal. Relaxation also may provide an activity break, as well as help individuals achieve a sense of mastery or self-control over their symptoms. Patients are typically instructed to practice a graduated series of relaxation techniques 20 to 30 minutes per day, and, as they master brief relaxation techniques, to integrate relaxation into their daily activities (Borkum, in press).

Biofeedback training. Thermal (hand warming) feedback—feedback of skin temperature from a finger—and electromyographic (EMG) feedback—feedback of electrical activity from muscles of the scalp, neck, and sometimes the upper body—are the most commonly used biofeedback modalities. However, electroencephalographic (*neurofeedback*) and cephalic vasomotor biofeedback also are used experimentally (Borkum, in press). As with relaxation training, patients practice the self-regulation skills they are learning for about 20-30 minutes per day, and, as they master headache management skills, they are encouraged to integrate use of these skills into their day.

Cognitive-behavioral (stress management) therapy. Cognitive-behavioral therapy (CBT) focuses on the cognitive and affective precipitants and components of headache (Borkum, in press; Holroyd et al., 2001; Lipchik et al., 2002). Cognitive-behavioral interventions attempt to alert patients to the role their thoughts play in generating stress responses and to relationships between stress, coping, and headaches. Patients are encouraged to employ effective strategies for coping with headache-related stresses and headaches themselves.

Integrating treatment techniques. Typically, the above treatment techniques are not used in isolation but are used in the context of therapy that teaches multiple headache management skills and tailors headache management skills to the clinical characteristics of the clients' headaches and to their life situation. In addition to information about the clinical characteristics and pathophysiology of headaches and about behavioral headache management, this might include exercises in identifying headache triggers and early warning signs, exercises to enable patients to effectively use headache medications, strategies for coping with headaches that occur despite self-management efforts, and the development of a migraine management plan including a plan for coping with any reoccurrence of headaches following treatment. An outline of a representative therapy for migraine and for tension-type headache can be found in Lipchik and colleagues (2002).

Treatment Formats

Treatment can be administered either individually or in a group, and can be administered in a clinic-based treatment format or in a home-based treatment format.

Clinic-based treatment format. Clinic-based treatment typically involves 6 to 12 weekly sessions, 45 to 60 minutes in length if treatment is administered individually, and 60 to 120 minutes in length if treatment is administered in a group. This treatment format provides more health care provider time and attention, and allows the provider greater opportunity to directly observe the patient than does a home-based treatment format, but requires the patient to travel more frequently to the clinic, and thus is more costly (Lipchik et al., 2002).

Home-based treatment format. Home-based or minimal-contact treatment involves 3 to 4 monthly treatment sessions 45 to 60 minutes in length for individual sessions, or 60 to 120 minutes in length for group sessions. Clinic visits introduce headache management skills and address problems encountered in acquiring or implementing these skills. Patient manuals and audiotapes guide the actual learning and refinement of headache management skills, which occur at home with phone contacts (Lipchik et al., 2002).

Session structure. With either treatment format, clinic sessions typically involve (1) a review of self-monitoring forms and homework, (2) a discussion of any difficulties encountered in learning and applying headache management skills, (3) the presentation of the rationale for the new headache management skill that will be the focus of the present session, (4) instruction and practice in this new skill, (4) formulation of a homework assignment, and (5) summary.

Efficacy

Migraine. The Agency for Healthcare Research and Quality (AHRQ)[1] sponsored a comprehensive evaluation of evidence for medical, behavioral, and physical treatments for migraine. The AHRQ evidence reports provided the stimulus for the formation of the U.S. Headache Consortium, an affiliation of influential medical organizations[2] created to develop clinical guidelines for the management of migraine. The U.S. Headache Consortium clinical guidelines, published on the American Academy of Neurology Web site (Campbell, Penzien, & Wall, 2000), conclude: "Relaxation training, thermal biofeedback combined with relaxation training, EMG biofeedback, and CBT may be considered as treatment options for the prevention of migraine." The AHRQ meta-analysis of data from available clinical trials found behavioral treatments to yield between 32% and 49% reduction in migraine activity (effect sizes ranging between .37 and .77) compared to 9% reduction in migraine activity with placebo (effect size .15).

Tension-type headache. The evidence report on the management of tension-type (and cervicogenic) headache prepared by the AHRQ (McCrory, Penzien, Hasselblad, & Gray, 2001) similarly concluded: "Behavioral treatments for tension-type headache have a consistent body of research indicating efficacy" (p. 7). The AHRQ meta-analysis of available clinical trials found that relaxation training, EMG biofeedback training, and CBT yielded between 37% and 50% reduction in tension-type headache activity (effect sizes ranging from .64 to .84); in contrast, 17% reduction in headaches has been observed with placebo (effect size of .15).

Integrating Drug and Psychological Therapies

Migraine. Results reported in 25 trials of the preventive drug propranolol HCl and in 35 trials of combined thermal biofeedback plus relaxation (more than 2,400 patients) have been virtually identical: Each treatment yielded, on average, a 55% reduction in migraine activity, and in contrast, (pill) placebo yielded only a 12% reduction in migraine activity. In addition, two trials found that propranolol HCl significantly enhanced the effectiveness of combined relaxation/biofeedback training; however, in one trial propranolol HCl alone proved more effective than combined relaxation/biofeedback training, and about as effective as the combined treatment. Unfortunately, the high dropout rate (38% of patients) from combined relaxation/biofeedback training in that trial raises the possibility that outcomes were compromised by poor patient compliance (Holroyd, 2002).

Tension-type headache. In the AHRQ meta-analysis, results trials of behavioral treatments and trials of the preventive drug amitriptyline HCl yielded comparable outcomes. Two studies also provide information about combining psychological and drug therapy for tension-type headache. In one trial, the combination of amitriptyline HCl and EMG biofeedback training yielded more rapid improvement in tension-type headache activity than EMG biofeedback training alone; however, beginning at Month 8 and continuing through the 24-month evaluation period the combined treatment showed no advantage EMG biofeedback training alone. In fact, at the 20- and 24-month observation periods—after withdrawal from amitriptyline HCl—patients who received EMG biofeedback training alone recorded significantly fewer hours of headache activity than patients who received the combined treatment (Holroyd, 2002).

Holroyd and colleagues (Holroyd et al., 2001) examined the separate and combined effects of CBT and tricyclic antidepressant medication specifically for chronic tension-type headaches. Patients received one of four treatments: tricyclic antidepressant (amitriptyline HCl to 100 mg./day or nortriptyline HCl to 75 mg./day) medication, medication placebo, limited-contact CBT (three clinic sessions) plus antidepressant medication, or CBT plus placebo. Antidepressant medication and CBT each yielded moderate reductions in chronic tension-type headaches, analgesic medication use, and headache-related disability at a 6-month evaluation, but improvements tended to be more rapid in the two-antidepressant medication conditions than with CBT alone. Nonetheless, the combined treatment was more likely (64% of patients) to produce clinically significant ($\geq$ 50%) reductions in chronic tension-type headaches than either antidepressant medication alone (38% of patients) or CBT (35% of patients) alone.

SUMMARY

Recurrent headache disorders are highly prevalent and associated with significant impairments in functioning and health care costs. Although our understanding of headache disorders has progressed significantly in the past decade, the pathophysiology of headache disorders remains incompletely understood. Fortunately, effective medical and behavioral treatments are available and most individuals who suffer with a recurrent headache disorder can benefit from one of the available treatments or combination of treatments.

—Kenneth A. Holroyd

NOTE: Support for this entry was provided in part by a grant from the National Institute of Neurological Disorders and Stroke of the National Institutes of Health (NINDS No. NS32374).

See also CHRONIC PAIN MANAGEMENT; PAIN: PSYCHOSOCIAL ASPECTS

Notes

1. Previously the Agency for Health Care Policy and Research.

2. American Academy of Family Physicians, American Academy of Neurology, American Headache Society, American College of Emergency Physicians, American College of Physicians, American Osteopathic Association, and National Headache Foundation.

Further Reading

Borkum, J. (in press). *Chronic headaches: Biology, psychology and behavioral treatment.* Hillsdale, NJ: Laurence Erlbaum.

Campbell, J. K., Penzien, D. B., & Wall, E. M. (2000). *Evidence-based guidelines for migraine headache: Behavioral and physical treatments.* U.S. Headache Consortium. Retrieved May 15, 2001, from http://www.aan.com/public/practiceguidelines/headache_gl.htm

Goadsby, P. J., Lipton, R. B., & Ferrari, M. D. (2002). Migraine-current understanding and treatment. *New England Journal of Medicine, 346,* 257-270.

Holroyd, K. A. (2002). Assessment and psychological treatment of recurrent headache disorders. *Journal of Consulting and Clinical Psychology, 70,* 656-677.

Holroyd, K. A., O'Donnell, F. J., Stensland, M., Lipchik, G. L., Cordingley, G. E., & Carlson, B. (2001). Management of chronic tension-type headache with tricyclic antidepressant medication, stress-management therapy, and their combination: a randomized controlled trial. *Journal of the American Medical Association, 285,* 2208-2215.

Lipchik, G. L., Holroyd, K. A., & Nash, J. M. (2002). Cognitive-behavioral management of recurrent headache disorders: A minimal-therapist contact approach. In D. C. Turk & R. S. Gatchel (Eds.), *Psychological approaches to pain management* (2nd ed., pp. 356-389). New York: Guilford.

Lipton, R. B., Hamelsky, S. W., & Stewart, W. A. (2001). Epidemiology and impact of headache. In S. D. Silberstein, R. B. Lipton, & D. J. Dalessio (Eds.), *Wolff's headache and other head pain* (7th ed., pp. 85-107). New York: Oxford University Press.

McCrory, D., Penzien, D., Hasselblad, V., & Gray, R. (2001). *Behavioral and physical treatments for tension-type and cervicogenic headache (2085).* Des Moines, IA: Foundation for Chiropractic Education and Research.

Olesen, J. C. (1988). Classification and diagnostic criteria for headache disorders, cranial neuralgias, and facial pain: Headache Classification Committee of the International Headache Society. *Cephalalgia, 8*(Suppl. 7).

Shechter, A. L., Lipton, R. B., & Silberstein, S. D. (2001). Migraine comorbidity. In S. D. Silberstein, R. B. Lipton, & D. J. Dalessio (Eds.), *Wolff's headache and other head pain* (7th ed., pp. 108-118). New York: Oxford University Press.

Silberstein, S. D., & Dongmei, L. (2002). Drug overuse and rebound headache. *Current Pain and Headache Reports, 6,* 240-247.

HEALTH AND BEHAVIOR ORGANIZATIONS

SOCIETY OF BEHAVIORAL MEDICINE

The Society of Behavioral Medicine (SBM) was founded in 1978 as a multidisciplinary, nonprofit organization to advance the science and practice of behavioral medicine. Today, SBM is the nation's premiere multidisciplinary organization dedicated to advancing the service and practice of behavioral medicine. SBM represents more than 2,000 behavioral and biomedical researchers and clinicians from over 18 different disciplines (e.g., psychophysiology, psychology, medicine, epidemiology, genetics, psychoneuroimmunology, nursing, health education, medical sociology, biostatistics, health policy). SBM's membership spans from student members and new investigators to the nation's leading experts in behavioral medicine research, practice, and policy. SBM provides the many disciplines represented with an interactive network for education and collaboration on common research; clinical and public policy concerns related to prevention, diagnosis, and treatment; rehabilitation; and health promotion.

SBM has a two-part mission: (1) to advance the development of scientific knowledge about the behavioral, biological, and social determinants of health and disease, and (2) to promote the application of this knowledge to improve individual and population health outcomes. SBM's goals are to advance this mission through a number of related activities, including sponsoring scientific meetings and publications that promote excellence in behavioral medicine research and practice, and maintaining and fostering the development of multidisciplinary leadership for the field.

SBM holds an annual scientific meeting consisting of invited addresses, debates, symposia, workshops/ seminars, papers, and poster sessions. The first annual meeting was held in 1979. SBM's other major activities include publication of *Annals of Behavioral Medicine*, which aims to foster the exchange of knowledge derived from the disciplines involved in the field of behavioral medicine and the integration of applicable basic and applied research (published by Lawrence Erlbaum Associates); *Outlook*, a quarterly newsletter; and a Web site, www.sbmweb.org.

The organization's structure includes officials elected by the membership, an executive committee, and council and committee chairs appointed by the executive committee. The elected officials include a president, elected to a 1-year term; a secretary-treasurer, elected to a 3-year term; and three member delegates, elected to staggered 3-year terms. The executive committee consists of the elected officials as well as the president-elect and past-president. Councils include Education and Training, Membership, Publications and Communications, and Scientific and Professional Liaison. Committees include Nominating, Finance, Program, Program Oversight, Long Range Planning, and Electronic Communications. There are different levels of membership including student, full, and fellow. In 2002, SBM had 2,100 members.

For further information about SBM, see the Web site, www.sbmweb.org.

INTERNATIONAL SOCIETY OF BEHAVIORAL MEDICINE

The International Society of Behavioral Medicine (ISBM) is a federation of national societies, whose goal is to serve the needs of all health-related disciplines concerned with issues relevant to behavioral medicine. Each national society includes both biomedical and behavioral scientists. Constituent societies of the ISBM presently include Academy of Behavioral Medicine Research (USA); American Psychosomatic Society; Austrasian Society of Behavioral Health and Medicine; Behavioral Medicine Section of the Czech Medical Association; Finnish Section of Behavioral Medicine of the Finnish Association of Social Medicine; Danish Society of Psychosocial Medicine; German Society of Behavioral Medicine and Behavior Modification; Hungarian Society of Behavioural Sciences and Medicine; Japanese Society of Behavioral Medicine; Netherlands Behavioral Medicine Federation; Norwegian Society of Behavioral Medicine; Psychosomatic and Behavioral Medicine Section of the Slovak Medicine Society; Society of Behavioral Medicine (USA); Swedish Society of Behavioral Medicine; and the Venezuelan Interdisciplinary Group of Behavioral Medicine. The Division of Health Psychology of the American Psychological Association and Society of Pediatric Psychology (USA) are affiliate members.

The function of the ISBM is to conduct activities that stimulate research and practice and coordinate communication and interaction within the worldwide behavioral medicine community. One important way to disseminate the concepts and findings of behavioral medicine throughout the world is through the international congresses sponsored by the ISBM. The first international Congress of Behavioral Medicine was held in Uppsala, Sweden, in 1990; the most recent, the seventh, was held in Helsinki, Finland, in 2002, and the eighth will be held in Mainz, Germany, in 2004. A second important way to disseminate the concepts and findings of behavioral medicine throughout the world is through a major scientific journal. The *International Journal of Behavioral Medicine (IJBM)*, published by Lawrence Erlbaum Associates, is the official journal of the ISBM. A third important way to disseminate the concepts and findings throughout the world is through teaching seminars. Seminars have been held in Stockholm, Sweden; Caracas, Venezuela; Bangkok, Thailand; and Vindeln, Sweden.

The ISBM structure includes the Governing Council; elected officials; the Executive Committee; and the Standing Committee. The Governing Council is made up of representatives of each member society, as well as the elected officials and committee chairs. The elected officials include a president, elected to a 2-year term, and a secretary and a treasurer, both elected to 3-year terms. Committees include Communications, Education and Training, International Collaborative Studies, Membership, Organizational Liaison, and Program.

For further information about the ISBM, see the Web site, www.isbm.miami.edu.

DIVISION OF HEALTH PSYCHOLOGY (DIV. 38) OF THE AMERICAN PSYCHOLOGICAL ASSOCIATION

The purpose of the Division of Health Psychology is to advance contributions of psychology as a discipline to the understanding of health and illness through basic and clinical research and by encouraging the integration of biomedical information about health and illness with current psychological knowledge; to promote education and services in the psychology of health and illness; and to inform the psychological and biomedical community, and the general public, on the results of current research and service activities in this area.

Division 38 was established in 1978 to facilitate collaboration among psychologists and other health science and health care professionals interested in the psychological and behavioral aspects of physical and mental health. Division 38 supports the educational, scientific, and professional contributions of psychology to understanding the etiology and promotion and maintenance of health; the prevention, diagnosis, treatment, and rehabilitation of physical and mental illness; the study of psychological, social, emotional, and behavioral factors in physical and mental illness; the improvement of the health care system; and formulation of health policy.

Given its emphasis on behavior and behavioral change, psychology has a unique contribution to make. For example, health psychologists are currently conducting applied research on the development of healthy habits as well as the prevention or reduction of unhealthy behaviors. Psychosocial and physiological linkages in areas such as psychoneuroimmunology, cardiovascular disorders, and other chronic diseases are being defined. Psychologists are in increasing demand in health and medical settings. The single largest area of placement of psychologists in recent years has been in medical centers. Psychologists have become vital members of multidisciplinary clinical and research teams in rehabilitation, cardiology, pediatrics, oncology, anesthesiology, family practice, dentistry, and other medical fields.

The organizational structure of Division 38 includes elected officials (president, secretary, treasurer, and two members-at-large), an executive committee, and standing committees. The standing committees include Convention Program, Education & Training, Research, Health Services, Publications, Finance, Awards, Fellows, Membership, and Nominations and Elections. There are approximately 3,000 members belonging to Division 38. The division holds its annual meeting as part of the American Psychological Association's annual meeting held each August. *Health Psychology* is a scholarly journal, published six times a year, that disseminates scientific investigations examining psychological/behavioral and physical health/illness relationships.

For further information about the Division of Health Psychology, see the Web site, www.health-psych.org.

For additional information about the history of Division 38, see Wallston (1997).

AMERICAN PSYCHOSOMATIC SOCIETY

The mission of the American Psychosomatic Society (APS) is to promote and advance the scientific understanding of the interrelationships among biological, psychological, social, and behavioral factors in human health and disease, and the integration of the fields of science that separately examine each, and to foster the application of this understanding in education and improved health care. The task of psychosomatic medicine is to understand the nature and mechanisms of behavior and psychosocial encounters that may alter the development of the organism, its structure, and its functions. The understanding of these encounters, provided by psychosomatic research and clinical studies, is an essential ingredient for the comprehensive understanding of human disease in order to lessen the burden of human suffering. The study of these factors and their assimilation into medical teaching and practice are central to the mission of the APS.

The APS grew from a desire among several academicians, practitioners, and foundations to link developments in psychology and psychiatry to internal medicine, physiology, and other disciplines. APS was founded in 1943. APS holds its annual meeting in March. The meeting is devoted to the presentation of scientific papers, symposia, workshops, poster sessions, invited lectures, and addresses. As the official organ of the APS, the purpose of the journal, *Psychosomatic Medicine*, is to present experimental and clinical studies dealing with various aspects of the relationships between social, psychological, and behavioral factors and bodily processes in both human and lower animals. The journal is published six times a year. As of 2002, APS has 874 members. There are four categories of membership: regular, associate, emeritus, and corresponding.

The affairs of the APS are governed by a council of 17 members, 7 of whom are ex-officio: 3 elected annually; 13 of whom are elective, serving 3-year terms; and 1 elected for a 2-year term. The ex-officio members are the president, the president-elect, the secretary-treasurer, the outgoing president, the journal's editor-in-chief, the program committee chair, and the newsletter editor. The elected members are chosen to provide appropriate representation to the following fields: internal medicine; psychiatry; pediatrics; neuro-anatomy; physiological sciences, neurophysiology, and psychophysiology; psychology; clinical psychology; sociology; anthropology; and public health.

For further information about the APS, see the Web site, www.psychosomatic.org.

—*Marc Gellman*

See also APPENDIX A

Further Reading

Wallston, K. A. (1997). A history of the Division of Health Psychology: Healthy, wealthy, and Weiss. In D. E. Dewsbury (Ed.), *Unification through division: Histories of the Divisions of the American Psychological Association* (Vol. 2, pp. 239-267). Washington, DC: American Psychological Association.

HEALTH BELIEF MODEL

What does it take for people to act to protect themselves from illness? This is the fundamental question posed by the framers of the health belief model (HBM), and which has continued to be addressed by researchers over the past five decades in the disciplines of public health, health psychology, and health education.

Background. The HBM was originally developed by Godfrey Hochbaum and other research psychologists in the U.S. Public Health Service in the early 1950s as they sought to apply the theories and methods of behavioral science to understanding and predicting health behavior. The original work in this area grew out of an attempt to understand the limited utilization of public health programs for disease prevention and screening (including tuberculosis screening). Hochbaum and his associates, including Irwin Rosenstock, were trained as social psychologists. They drew influences from contemporary learning theory and cognitive theory, particularly the work of Kurt Lewin and others who emphasized the importance of the individual's perceptual and cognitive processes, specifically the perception of the valuation of and expectations regarding particular outcomes in determining a course of action.

The HBM is a value-expectancy theory that attempts to describe the valuation of the desire to avoid illness (or treat it effectively) and the types of expectations about health that are essential in influencing preventive (or self-care) behavior. The HBM has evolved over the years from addressing primarily health-screening behavior to applications covering the full range of health behaviors from lifestyle change for primary prevention to management of chronic illnesses and sick-role behavior.

KEY CONCEPTS OF THE HEALTH BELIEF MODEL

The central variables of the HBM have been redefined over time to incorporate a number of concepts beyond those originally considered (perceived susceptibility to the risk and the perceived benefits of early detection, plus a cue to action) to include the following:

1. *Perceived threat* is a combination of two concepts:

   a. *Susceptibility* is the subjective perception of the individual's risk of developing an illness. In the context of an existing illness, it includes susceptibility to complications of advancing or recurrent disease and acceptance of the diagnosis, as well as more general susceptibility to health problems.

   b. *Perceived severity* is the sense of how serious an illness is and the consequences of leaving it untreated. This concept includes the perception of the possible physical consequences of an illness (e.g., pain, death) and the broader range of social consequences in a person's life (e.g., disability, stigmatization).

2. *Perceived benefits* relate to the anticipated positive effects of taking action. This includes beliefs about

the effectiveness of a course of action in reducing the disease threat, as well as other potential benefits not directly related to health (e.g., quitting smoking might be seen as a way to save money or set a good example for one's children).

3. *Perceived barriers* are the potential negative consequences or costs associated with taking an action to improve health. The factors that could impede a course of action might include concerns about the expense, any possible discomfort or danger associated with the action (e.g., fears about pain or radiation exposure from a mammogram), inconvenience, or competition with other valued activities (e.g., having to miss work to get to an appointment). As noted above, the wide range of potential barriers include logistical barriers such as cost or lack of convenient access to services, and emotional barriers such as fears about physical or emotional harm (including fear of getting a cancer diagnosis). In addition, when addressing changes in lifestyle and personal habits that may be rewarding in their own right (eating high-fat foods or smoking cigarettes), the habit strength or the loss of pleasurable activities (if not addiction) may prove to be potent barriers to health behavior change.

4. *Cues to action* (either internal cues such as thoughts, emotions, or sensations, or external events that act as a prompt) were one of the initial concepts in the HBM. Interestingly, this component of the model has not been as systematically studied as several of the others. Nonetheless, examples clearly exist in effective screening and health maintenance interventions that derive from this concept, such as the success of reminder systems for screening tests. Another example is the phenomenon of having a cancer diagnosis of a relative or friend act to motivate people to obtain a first mammogram or colorectal-screening test.

5. *Other modifying variables* include an array of demographic and sociocultural variables that may greatly influence the performance of health behavior directly, or may interact with the perceptions of susceptibility or seriousness. A particularly powerful example of this variable is a person's level of education, the addition of which has improved the predictive accuracy of the model.

6. *Self-efficacy* as a variable was a relatively late addition to the HBM. The concept of self-efficacy, developed by Albert Bandura in 1977, addresses an additional expectancy that influences the performance of a health behavior. Self-efficacy refers to the level of confidence a person feels regarding his or her ability to perform a behavior. Bandura described a number of processes by which a person's sense of self-efficacy may be influenced, and this issue is particularly important when trying to predict or influence the adoption of new behavior patterns or the changing of lifestyle and habits to improve health outcomes. For example, confidence regarding one's skill at being able to test blood sugar and accurately self-administer insulin is essential to the consistent performance of diabetic self-management.

In summary, the HBM posits that adopting a health behavior change typically requires several beliefs and situations working in concert. First, people must be aware of the health risk and perceive it to be sufficiently serious and likely to affect them to consider taking action. They also need to believe that a particular behavior will be effective in protecting them from a bad outcome in order to overcome whatever possible costs or downside risks they may be concerned about. Moving them toward action may also require the perception of bodily sensations, or events in their physical or social environment to prompt them to act sooner rather than later. In addition, particularly if the required behavior change is the alteration of an element of their lifestyle (rather than a one-shot preventive event), they need to feel that the behavior change will not only be effective but is something they are capable of doing.

EMPIRICAL EVALUATION OF THE HEALTH BELIEF MODEL

A recent MEDLINE search of the HBM found more than 2,300 references, which suggests the scope of the task of summarizing the research influenced by this model. The interested reader is referred to the periodic detailed reviews of the empirical findings and the theoretical advancements in the model. An exhaustive review of the early findings in 1974 by Marshall Becker summarized evidence that there was considerable support for the predictive validity of the variables in the model in several domains of preventive health behavior, screening, and self-care. An updated review by Becker and Nancy Janz in 1984 reflected a burgeoning literature using the model, with extensions of the HBM to the use of inoculations, breast cancer screening, genetic testing, cardiovascular risk factors screening, smoking, and chronic illness management including adherence to asthma, hypertension, and diabetic regimens, including medication, diet, and other health behavior changes. Important theoretical papers have further integrated research findings and advanced the HBM concepts, contributed by Rosenstock and colleagues including Victor Strecher, in the integration of Bandura's social cognitive theory concepts, and in the application of the HBM to chronic illness and sick-role behavior.

Overall, to the extent there are consistent patterns of findings, perceived barriers appear to be the strongest predictor across all kinds of health behavior. Perceived susceptibility appears to be the next strongest predictor of preventive behavior, whereas perceived benefit is a better predictor of self-care behavior in a chronic illness. More recent multivariate modeling has examined the paths by which the variables act in concert to predict health behavior. For example, perceived severity, which frequently is among the weaker predictors of behavior by itself, may exercise its influence on behavior through strengthening the importance of perceived benefits.

Interestingly, the somewhat unwieldy mass of research launched by the HBM has made relatively modest contributions to the theoretical development of the model. The theory itself offers very little specificity regarding the measurement of the variables and relationships between variables. For example, the model implies, but does not specify, that the effects of the variables take place within a sequential process (i.e., barriers are not relevant unless the person perceives some personal susceptibility and seriousness regarding the risk). Also, there are no specific hypotheses about whether the variables affect each other via additive or multiplicative means.

The lack of structure in the model has left researchers free to define the concepts and interpret the relationships as they will. In fact, in some respects the HBM and its variables have served as the root from which most of the health behavior models currently being researched have branched. Other models with similar social and cognitive psychology origins have used the HBM variables in their health behavior applications, but have advanced specific hypotheses regarding the combination principles of the variables and the decision-making process (e.g., the theory of planned behavior

and its successor, the theory of reasoned action by Martin Fishbein and Icek Ajzen). Howard Leventhal's added emphasis on the emotional processing that takes place in parallel to the rational, cognitive cost-benefit decision making of the HBM evolved into his self-regulatory model, and others, such as Suzanne Miller's cognitive-social information processing (C-SHIP) model, which also adds emphasis on social cognitive elements. The insight that behavior change is a process that may unfold over time, rather than an event that happens all at once, has inspired stage models such as the transtheoretical model of James Prochaska and his colleagues, and Neil Weinstein's precaution adoption process model. As the common ancestor, the HBM's conceptual DNA can be found in these models and the research they have inspired.

It has been suggested in several recent reviews by Strecher, Rosenstock, and others that researchers seeking to use the HBM as a conceptual base should (1) pay closer attention to specifying the measurement of the variables; (2) work in more of a hypothesis-testing mode; and (3) examine the relationships between the HBM variables and outcome behaviors in a manner that would yield meaningful information, for example, specifying risk perception with respect to behavioral anchors (e.g., *if you do not quit smoking*, how likely are you to have another heart attack?). The recommendation is that the variables not be tested alone, or tossed into a regression model trying to test for the "strongest swimmers," but rather to elucidate the relationships among variables as they relate to the desired health behavior.

Ultimately, an important goal of the HBM is to inform practice. The HBM has now been applied to populations around the globe to AIDS prevention and treatment, the management of a wide variety of chronic illnesses, cancer prevention and screening, immunization utilization, teen pregnancy, and even examining the influence of the providers' health beliefs as they affect health disparities in minority populations. The HBM and the research inspired by it have already contributed much to the development of effective interventions at the individual and group levels for promoting preventive and self-care health behavior, but much remains to be learned. With greater precision and consistency in measurement and more specific, hypothesis-driven analyses of the interactions and paths by which the variables exert their influence, the blueprints for more precise and effective interventions can be drawn, tailored to the needs of the individual and the demands of the situation.

—*Lynn Clemow*

See also SELF-EFFICACY; THEORY OF PLANNED BEHAVIOR; THEORY OF REASONED ACTION; THEORY OF TRIADIC INFLUENCE; TRANSTHEORETICAL MODEL OF BEHAVIOR CHANGE

Further Reading

Becker, M. H. (1974). The health belief model and personal health behavior. *Health Education Monographs, 2,* 324-473.

Hochbaum, G. M. (1958). *Public participation in medical screening program: A sociopsychological study.* Public Health Service Publication No. 572. Washington, DC: Government Printing Office.

Janz, N. K., & Becker, M. H. (1984). The health belief model: A decade later. *Health Education Quarterly, 11,* 1-47.

Kirscht, J. P. (1974). The health belief model and illness behavior. *Health Education Monographs, 2,* 387-408.

Rosenstock, I. M., Strecher, V. J., & Becker, M. (1988). Social learning theory and the health belief model. *Health Education Quarterly, 15,* 175-183.

Strecher, V., Champion, V., & Rosenstock, I. (1997). The health belief model and health behavior. In D. Gochman (Ed.), *Handbook of health behavior research: Vol. I. Personal and social determinants* (pp. 71-92). New York: Plenum.

Weinstein, N. (1993). Testing four competing theories of health-protective behavior. *Health Psychology, 12,* 324-333.

HEALTH CARE COSTS AND BEHAVIOR

Economic costs are the value of resources consumed in an endeavor. Health care costs are therefore the value of resources used in the provision of health care. These resources include the professional services of health care providers, the facility resources used in providing these services in settings such as hospitals and clinics, pharmaceutical therapy, specialized health services such as radiology and pathology, and health care supplies. A more expansive definition of costs related to health care would include the time required by patients to attend therapy and the support of family caregivers, as well as the true value of pain and suffering related to treatment, less the value of improvements in health.

Resources are valued at their opportunity cost, which is the value of the activity forgone in order to employ the resource. In a competitive market, where suppliers and consumers freely trade their goods and services, opportunity costs may be approximated by market prices. In the health care sector, prices are often distorted by incentives for reimbursement related to health insurance and institutional cost shifting among patient groups including the uninsured. Furthermore, prices are often unobserved, as is the case when services are provided under capitated contracts. Thus, measuring costs often involves a combination of methods including the estimating of costs incurred by facilities, the relative values of physician effort and outpatient procedures, and the average wholesale price of pharmaceuticals.

An important concept when making decisions regarding health care is relative cost. For example, the decision to employ one particular therapy over another may be determined by the relative costs of the two therapies and how they relate to the relative benefits. Often this is conceptualized as incremental costs and benefits. Incremental costs might be the additional costs of one therapy over another. If benefits are valued in monetary terms, one can calculate incremental net benefit, or the incremental benefits less the incremental costs. Incremental costs and benefits are used in economic evaluations of health care programs and include cost-analysis (the economic cost of a program including any cost savings that result), cost-effectiveness analysis (the cost of a program for a given nonmonetary measure of benefit or outcome), and cost-benefit analysis (the total economic value, benefits less costs, when all are valued in monetary terms).

A common form of economic evaluation in health care is cost-effectiveness analysis. Cost-effectiveness analysis is popular in health care evaluation because it allows one to incorporate a measure of the health benefit, the quality of adjusted life year (QALY), but does not require that this benefit be valued in monetary terms. A change in QALYs represents changes in both length of life and quality of life, the latter of which might be approximated by level of functioning. In cost-effectiveness analyses, alternative health care options are presented with respect to their incremental cost-effectiveness, or the difference in costs between a base case and the proposed alternative divided by the difference in outcomes. Sometimes an evaluation will reveal that a proposed change in health care delivery, such as the adoption of a new technology, is cost saving. However, the typical result is that the change would result in additional benefits at an additional cost. It may then be compared to other health care practices currently in use to determine whether it may be considered "cost-effective," a determination that is ultimately subjective, determined in part by the preferences of health care consumers and their willingness to pay for a given level of health benefit.

Cost-effectiveness analysis can be useful not only in deciding between competing health care practices or technologies but also determining at what point to intervene. Resources aimed at reducing morbidity related to a particular disease may be aimed at prevention, screening, or treatment. For example, several health policy options are available to reduce morbidity related to diabetes—ultimately to improve quality of life. These include the intensive treatment and case management of persons with diabetes, with the objective of avoiding future complications; increased screening to reduce the time between onset and initial treatment; and prevention of or lengthening of time until onset among persons who are either glucose intolerant or otherwise at high risk of developing diabetes. Analyses have shown each of these health care practices to be cost-effective. In contrast, some mass screening programs increase treatment without reducing morbidity or mortality. These are generally not cost-effective.

Economic evaluation is a valuable tool that can be used to help determine the efficient allocation of health care resources across alternative health practices. The analysis of aggregate health care expenditures provides a better understanding of how resources are spread across health care sectors and the level of health spending relative to the overall economy. The remainder of this entry reviews the amount and distribution of health care costs as approximated by the federal accounting of health care expenditures: National Health Care Expenditures (NHE) as summarized by the Center for Medicare and Medicaid Services (CMS) in 2000. It then examines the evolution of health care costs over time and relates the apparent increase in costs to the interrelated effects of health insurance and technological change. Following is a discussion of the desirability of allowing health care costs to consume an increasing share of national income. The entry concludes with discussion of probable scenarios for the future of health care costs.

NHE totaled $1.3 trillion in 2000, or $4,637 per U.S. resident, and 13.2% of gross domestic product (GDP). Fifty-five percent of expenditures originated from private sources including health insurance, out-of-pocket payments, and philanthropy; 45% were public expenditures, the largest components of which were federal expenditures on Medicare and expenditures by federal, state, and local governments on Medicaid. Nearly one third of expenditures were for hospital care (31.7%); another third were for professional services including physician, clinic, dentistry, and home health care (32.2%). Pharmacy expenditures were 9.4% of NHE in 2000; nursing home care, 7.1%; administration, 6.2%; and public health activity and research were 5.4%.

Expenditures as a percentage of GDP grew steadily since they were first recorded in 1960 at 5.1% until 1993 when they reached 13.4%. From 1993 to 2000, this ratio has been relatively stable at just over 13%. The distribution of health care expenditures in 2000 is similar to the distribution in 1960, although this masks a large swing in hospital expenditures, which increased as a percentage of NHE from 34% in 1960 to 42% in 1982, with corresponding declines in the percentage of NHE accounted for by professional services and pharmaceuticals. The subsequent decline in hospital expenditures as a percentage of NHE left hospital, professional, and pharmacy ratios in 2000 very close to their ratios in 1960. Notable increases have occurred in administration expenditures, which rose from 3.2% of NHE in 1960 to 6.2% in 2000, and nursing home expenditures, which rose from 4.5% to 7.1%.

It is largely accepted that the rapid increase in NHE that has occurred over the past 40 years is the joint result of advances in technology coupled with the risk-sharing arrangements offered by health insurance. The use of increasingly expensive technologies is evidenced by the inexorable rise in hospital and physician expenditures, and recently in rising expenditures for prescription drugs. Use of these technologies, however, depends both on their availability (supply) and the demand of consumers, which are affected by preferences and price. Traditional fee-for-service health insurance, which allowed widespread access to these technologies through risk spreading, also effectively removed the price sensitivity by consumers that determines efficient outcomes in market equilibrium.

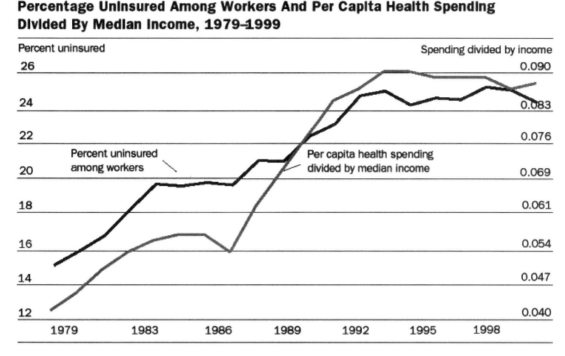

Figure 1   Percentage Uninsured Among Workers and Per Capita Health Spending Divided by Median Income, 1979-1999

SOURCE: Author's analysis of Current Population Survey, March supplements, Annual Demographics Files, 1980-2000, except 1981; and Centers for Medicare and Medicaid Services, National Health Accounts, 1979-1999.

This large increase in health care expenditures as a percentage of GDP is not necessarily detrimental to the U.S. economy. Consumers' spending is driven in large part by their preferences, and it may very well be that consumers prefer to invest an increasing share of their incomes in their health care. There exist, however, at least two fairly convincing pieces of evidence that some health care spending is inefficient and that a reallocation, or possibly even a reduction, in expenditures would make consumers in the United States better off.

The first piece of evidence is the well-documented variation in health care utilization, including hospitalization, and associated costs across the country. The question has been posed as, Which rate is right? In light of comparable mortality rates, it may be that areas of the country with high utilization rates are treating patients too aggressively. There is equally weighty evidence that others do not receive care with potentially high benefits: Those in families with low incomes, as well as those who are African American or Latino, have worse access to medical care and worse health outcomes than those with higher incomes and those who are White. The apparent conclusion is that our health care resources are not distributed such that each dollar is worth what it is buying. Although the overall purchase might be worth it, the value of health insurance would likely increase if some dollars were spent in other areas, and on other consumers.

A second evidentiary item demonstrating decreasing returns to health technology is the decline in the percentage of persons with health insurance. As shown in Figure 1, the percentage of uninsured among workers has increased in direct relation to per capita health spending as a share of income. Economic theory posits that for a given commodity, any increase in its value would increase the likelihood of insuring against its loss, provided that persons are risk adverse. That consumers are not continuing to purchase insurance suggests that increases in health care costs, and the corresponding increases in the price of insurance, are not indicative of increases in value.

It is expected that health expenditures will increase, as will the number of uninsured, until there exists a political consensus to substantially alter the way health care is distributed and financed. Expanding coverage to the uninsured might be accomplished either through the expansion of public programs such as Medicaid or by adoption of universal coverage. Either approach will increase health care expenditures simply by increasing access to care by the uninsured. A more important decision is how to adjust the financing of health care to more efficiently distribute resources.

—Todd Gilmer

See also COST-EFFECTIVENESS; HEALTH CARE SERVICE UTILIZATION: DETERMINANTS; QUALITY OF LIFE: MEASUREMENT

Further Reading

The Dartmouth atlas of health care. (2002). Center for the Evaluative Clinical Sciences, Dartmouth Medical School. Chicago: American Hospital Publishing.

Getzen, T. E. (1997). *Health economics: Fundamentals and flow of funds*. New York: John Wiley.

Newhouse, J. P. (1993). *Free for all? Lessons from the RAND Health Insurance Experiment*. Cambridge, MA: Harvard University Press.

HEALTH CARE SERVICE UTILIZATION: DETERMINANTS

Health care service utilization can be defined as the use of any services provided to a patient in an attempt to improve or maintain health. Such services would include those provided by medical professionals or any allied health care provider (e.g., psychotherapist, home health nurse) and any diagnostic or treatment procedures delivered. Determinants of utilization of services must be clearly distinguished from determinants of health. Often low rates of utilization may reflect poor health due to low access to services, yet at other times low rates of service utilization may be viewed as a measure of health due to a lack of need of services. Two primary issues need to be understood when using health care service utilization as a variable in research: factors that influence utilization and

confounding of these factors, and the methods used to measure service utilization.

One of the first factors used in the study of health care service utilization is how encompassing the term may be. That is, a separation is often used between medical utilization and behavioral health services. Though in part as a result of greater parity between health and mental health services this distinction is lessening, still some researchers have differentiated between these two as tracking systems for these two may be separate.

DETERMINANTS OF UTILIZATION

Several influences on the utilization of health care services have emerged: sociodemographic, behavioral risk factors, and personal and clinical history.

Sociodemographic Factors

Sociodemographic factors include age, gender, and ethnicity. Age is associated with declining health status, greater morbidity of most diseases, and thus utilization of services increases. In fact, many reports have estimated that more than half of one's health care expenditures during one's lifetime are devoted to the final few weeks of life. However, infants and children use services more often than do healthy adults. Gender has also been frequently associated with health and health care utilization. Generally, women are found to access health care more often than men. For example, studies have found that women are referred to further cardiographic testing less frequently when complaining of the same symptom cluster as men; while this difference may show up as greater service utilization for men this is seen as a contributing factor to women's higher fatality rate of first time myocardial infarctions.

Populations that are associated with low social support and poor economic conditions (e.g., divorced, widowed, minorities, low education, low income) tend to use health services more frequently. However, these socioeconomic factors tend to be highly correlated with each other. Numerous studies have reported that non-Hispanic Caucasian patients are more likely to receive primary and secondary preventive services and thus are less likely to need services over time due to improved outcomes in a variety of health domains. For example, after controlling for confounding factors such as age, gender, income, and availability of procedures, African Americans and Latino patients were less likely to receive coronary artery bypass, angioplasty, revascularization, or arteriography than Caucasian patients. Research examining service utilization of millions of elderly Medicare enrollees show that non-Hispanic Caucasian patients received more mammograms, as well as more influenza vaccines, yet racial differences were not apparent for non-elective procedures such as hip replacement surgery. While many of these studies have controlled for the effects of reimbursement to isolate the differences between racial groups, other studies have isolated the impact of reimbursement directly on utilization. That is, physicians tend to avoid the uninsured and underinsured patients due to inadequate reimbursement, difficulty providing "standard of care given financial constraints," and the perception of higher rates of treatment noncompliance associated with these patients. Language-discordant patient-physician pairs have been correlated with increased noncompliance with medications, missed scheduled appointments, and more visits to the emergency room than language-concordant patent-physician dyads. Policy reforms and changes in medical education are often touted as remedies for these systems limitations.

Behavioral Risk Factors

Behaviors that increase risk of chronic illness are often associated with higher service utilization. Such behaviors include smoking, alcohol and substance abuse, a sedentary lifestyle, and overeating. Conditions that result from such behaviors—for example, diabetes, hypertension, and fetal alcohol syndrome—are associated with increased demands on the health care system over a prolonged period of time. Hostility and aggressive behavior have also been associated with coronary artery disease, increased rate of traumatic injuries that require intense medical attention, and increased service utilization.

Personal and Clinical History Factors

One's personal history is associated with increased utilization. Childhood abuse and posttraumatic stress disorder from that and other events are associated with not only increased mental health services, but a higher incidence of such histories is found in those seeking medical services as compared to those who do not use health care services frequently. Specific physiological

markers are often seen as intermediate markers of increased health care service utilization. Blood pressure, HbA1c (diabetes), weight/obesity, and cholesterol are just a few examples of intermediate markers for increased service utilization across the life span.

METHODS OF MEASUREMENT

The method of measurement will be influenced by the focus of what is being measured. That is, if one is assessing overall impact of an intervention then one must also look at costs incurred over time both in the health care system and outside the health care system. Another important issue involved in the measurement of utilization is the time delay of impact expected. That is, preventive services may be offered with little expectation of reduction in service utilization until many years later.

It is very important to understand that health care service utilization can be measured in a multitude of ways. Self-reports of visits to a health care provider are most often used in research. However, several researchers have noted that such self-report strategies are prone to biased recall to varying degrees. Another way to quantify utilization is by assessing costs. One way to avoid such biased reporting is to access actual billing system data (claims data) and count the frequency of services or the costs of such services. The issue in accurately documenting cost is very complex in that regional variations of cost of procedures may make generalization of actual costs nearly impossible. If one is looking at the frequency of visits to providers, there is often differentiation between inpatient and outpatient care, with costs different for each and their accessibility and relevance of the data a question that must be asked prior to resources being devoted to extracting such data. Researchers have also used the number of procedures received by a patient (including laboratory data, radiology assessment technology, or outpatient surgeries), and thus cost is confounded with payor system.

FINAL ISSUES

There are many other issues to be considered when using service utilization in research. One such issue is the time delay of any expected impact of an intervention. That is, if an intervention is to improve one's health it likely is perceived first by the patient, then observed in improved functioning, and perhaps only after a sufficient period of time has passed will it affect the frequency of future health service utilization. That is, preventive services are often promoted as decreasing utilization, yet in some analyses (e.g., cost-utility analyses) it may be difficult to show true effectiveness because of the time delay in benefits.

A controversial issue is determining the "appropriateness" of utilization; whether or not an encounter with the health care system (e.g., preventive health visit, emergency room visit) is appropriate can be very subjective. It is hard to define "appropriate" use of services at a group level when some diagnostic tests may be appropriate for some population at risk but not for others; taking into account the clinical realities of variations in appropriateness between patients is often difficult to incorporate into cross-sectional or cohort research designs.

Another issue is tracking "out of system" costs in that more people are using services from providers not included in the covered systems that use claims databases. Complementary and alternative health care being sought more and more is often not included if one is tracking utilization by electronic systems of data collection.

Cost-offset is another issue to be considered when examining the impact of an intervention on health and utilization outcomes. An important idea with this issue is to account for the cost of an intervention when determining the impact of the intervention; for example, the cost of mental health services often minimizes the medical cost-savings realized from such interventions. Similarly, cost-benefit analyses can be more complicated than may be initially perceived. That is, how one measures benefit—patient quality of life, functioning level, return to work—can lead to very different results.

Cost-effectiveness analyses and cost-utility analyses are just two of many other ways to assess the impact of an intervention on health service utilization. The reader is referred to such topics elsewhere in this volume.

—*William J. Sieber*

See also COST-EFFECTIVENESS; HEALTH CARE COSTS AND BEHAVIOR

Further Reading

Aday, L. A. (2001). *At risk in America: The health and health care needs of vulnerable populations in the United States*. San Francisco: Jossey-Bass.

Fos, P. J., & Fine, D. J. (1998). *Designing health care for populations: Applied epidemiology in health care administration*. San Francisco: Jossey-Bass.

Monheit, A. C., Wilson, R., & Arnett, R. H. (1998). *Informing American health care policy: The dynamics of medical expenditure and insurance surveys, 1977-1996*. New York: John Wiley.

HEALTH COMMUNICATION

Health communication in its broadest definition is any type of communication whose content is concerned with health. As a field, however, health communication is more clearly defined as the process through which one person, group, or governmental or private organization uses various communication strategies and channels to educate, motivate, and perpetuate information, skills, and behaviors that are generally accepted to benefit (improve) the health of individuals and the public. This can occur at the individual, interpersonal, national, and global levels. Health communication is concerned with the strategic use of ethical, persuasive means to craft and deliver campaigns and implement specific strategies designed to promote good health and prevent disease. Ideally, health communication is the *right* information to the *right* people at the *right* time for an intended, beneficial effect.

> Informed opinion and active cooperation on the part of the public are of utmost importance in the improvement of health of the people. (World Health Organization, Preamble to the Constitution)

Many would argue that health communication—through mass media and social marketing campaigns—works best at reinforcing existing attitudes and beliefs to provide people with the skills and resources necessary to make personal behavior changes. Health communication campaigns fail when a message does not reach or is not understood by the target audience. Suffice it to say it is difficult to change strongly held attitudes, which are necessary in changing behavior in the long term. A popular technique in health communication is community centered communication—focusing on the unit of change at the community level, thereby empowering individuals within that body to effect change on multiple levels presenting a variety of points.

In its infancy, health communication efforts primarily focused on reinforcing existing attitudes and beliefs, had unrealistically high expectations for long-term behavior change, and generally did a poor job of reaching the intended audience. This was the "pretelevision era," and most health communication efforts (primarily radio public service announcements and printed materials) were viewed by the public as dry, dull, and boring. In the 1970s, health communication entered into the "era of successes" where specifically targeted media were effective. Today, we are in the 21st century—the "era of moderate effects" or the "communication age," where health communication campaigns have enjoyed more success in being able to change a specified behavior.

The field of health communication is multifaceted and multidisciplinary. People from a variety of disciplinary backgrounds are involved in health communication: professionals in communication, medicine, psychology, public health, sociology, government, and marketing, among others. It is these people who plan, influence, and evaluate health care policy and are involved in the health decision-making process that will enhance the quality of life for individuals and communities across the globe.

Health communication works best when it is a part of a larger public health initiative. Health communication can influence the public agenda, advocate for policies and programs, stimulate debate and dialogue for health as a priority, encourage social norms that benefit health and quality of life, and promote positive changes in the social, economic, and physical environment. Communication can facilitate better health care at the individual, community, family, and system levels, but it alone cannot deliver facility-based clinical or technical services, counseling, and supplies. For this reason, health communication efforts should be coordinated with other programs to improve quality and access to services, strengthen institutions, and formulate effective policies for the betterment of the public's health.

Health professionals and communication experts concur that the power of health communication lies not just in its ability to raise awareness and educate the public, but rather in its ability to change behavior. True health behavior change is much more complex than simply "getting the message out there." The first step for any effective health communication effort is to understand the target audience(s)—the motives and environmental influences on individuals and groups.

It is crucial to understand that health communication takes place within a particular context. Public policy, the community and culture, interpersonal factors, societal norms and values, intrapersonal factors, and organizational/institutional factors all play a role in the overall effectiveness of health communication efforts.

An example of the growing interest in health communication is witnessed by the establishment of academic programs at colleges and universities. The first such program that combined the communication expertise of a college with a medical school was the Emerson-Tufts Health Communication Program, which in its initial years offered a joint degree to its students. Programs at Michigan State, Illinois, and Rutgers universities followed. Specific academic publications also added to the credibility of health communication as an accepted academic discipline. *Health Communication* and the *Journal of Health Communication* are two of the premier journals in this area.

The increasing complexity of health communication, including new definitions of health, evolution of new media, and the needs of diverse global audiences, demands broad, interdisciplinary, multisectoral approaches to the health communication field. An Institute of Medicine (IOM) report (*Bridging Disciplines in the Brain: Behavioral and Clinical Sciences*) states that "solutions to existing and future health problems will likely require drawing on a variety of disciplines and approaches in which interdisciplinary efforts characterized not only the cutting edge of research but also the utilization of knowledge." Other studies have suggested the need for health communication professionals to apply more recent and innovative communication theories, as well as continued efforts to strengthen the links between outreach activities and community-based support groups to ensure sustainable impact.

Better planning, more applicable design frameworks, and state-of-the-art expertise are required to manage these complex, interdisciplinary health communication interventions. Past experience suggests the necessity for integration of communication at the strategic framework and planning level as the best way to maximize the successful use and impact of communication interventions. Unfortunately, a lack of formal training and limited resources often limit the ability to design and to properly manage communication activities in the field. What is called for, given this situation, are partnerships with universities, training institutions, private sector media, and nongovernmental organizations in meeting the health communication objectives.

Communication has become a mature discipline in the United States, consisting of theories, interventions, processes, competencies, and techniques. Thirty years of investment in organizations and partners who have focused on many facets of communication has helped in the development. Furthermore, behavior change has produced many successes in terms of clients' and consumers' understanding of a variety of health conditions. This includes the use of contraceptives, oral rehydration therapy (ORT), hand and food washing, and condoms to prevent HIV/AIDS and sexually transmitted infections (STIs) as well as improved counseling from family planning/reproductive health (FP/RH) providers.

Much of the success of these programs can be attributed to communication science methodologies, which include formative research (client needs and preferences, political/social/family context), as well as mechanisms for incorporating these into the design, development, and implementation of program design and execution. Health communication activities may be organized into a formal program to share local experiences, provide specialized technical support, and manage resources. We have outlined a few of these ideas in the following sections.

COMMUNICATION CAMPAIGN FRAMEWORK

When designing health promotion campaigns or materials, health communicators will often use strategic planning tools, which include problem analysis, strategic choices, target audience, behavioral objectives, message development, communication channels, stakeholders, and evaluation. Problem analysis involves detailing what you know about the problem; defining its epidemiology and physiology; understanding the environmental, political, and historical influences; and knowing what resources and additional information are necessary for a successful health communication effort. Formative research—such as surveys, focus groups, and interviews—is often done to gain a better understanding of the target audience for a health message and give insight into areas where positive change can be encouraged.

Many health communication activities are designed with a variety of incentives and disincentives for individuals, providers, institutions, and policymakers. Research

is necessary at every stage of the communication process to support and sustain the desired outcome for health competence. Appropriate communication research can identify ideal strategies for performance incentives at the system or individual level, and also identify the necessary environmental (and in some cases economic) structures that can be enhanced.

Ideally, this research and subsequent application will optimize communication effects and can help to drive message development that will appeal to the target audience and promote positive behavior change. The communication channel(s) used (television, radio, print media, etc.) and stakeholders can also be determined through an exploration of this formative research.

Finally, an evaluation component is an essential part of any health communication strategy. Though the effects on behavior may be difficult to gauge in the short term, intermediate outcomes and analysis of the process are important tools in determining how a health communication intervention is performing, and adjustments can be made accordingly. In addition, this type of accountability can help in securing future funding to sustain and further promote and expand these projects.

Types of Health Communication

A contaminated food or drug being pulled off the shelf; a chemical spill that threatens a local water source; or the potential health effects of impending biological, chemical, or nuclear terrorism are all examples of times when effective health crisis/risk communication are essential for the public. Preparing for a crisis demands careful planning and an attention to detail for an acute event. Before a crisis occurs, it is recommended that leaders develop a theme or potential goals to be accomplished. This type of communication differs from health education and promotion, which tend to focus on more long-term chronic health problems such as vaccination programs and fortification of foods with folic acid to prevent birth defects. Antismoking and antidrug campaigns are examples of campaigns that might try to focus on behavior change.

Media Strategies for the Health Professional

Communication is the process of sending and receiving information by mean of a shared language or other symbol system. Decisions made about the source, audience, message, and communication channels all play a role in health communication. Professionals working in this field will also work out how these various factors interact.

The source of the health communication information is one fundamental determinant of a successful effort. The audience receiving a message will assess the source of information according to its character, trustworthiness, knowledge and expertise, use of goodwill, and charisma. Decisions about character and trustworthiness are made based on a speaker's intent, reliability, and sincerity. A speaker's employment, job title, education, and experience can also influence how the source of a message is perceived. By building and nurturing relationships, effective health communication efforts can also develop goodwill and charisma within an audience. Determination of the target audience is essential when developing health messages and deciding on the sources and communication channels to use. These three components of a health communication effort will be different for different audiences.

Knowledge accumulated about certain populations can help to establish the demographics and characteristics of that population that are important for developing and delivering health messages for behavior change. Finally, feedback from the target audience and evaluation of the communication message and delivery can be invaluable for improving the existing effort, as well as designing and executing future health communication efforts.

Knowledge Gap Hypothesis

This hypothesis states that as information increases, those with a high socioeconomic status and more education will learn faster and easier than those without education and a high socioeconomic status. This hypothesis predicts that, over time, educated people learn faster, highly publicized topics are learned faster, and knowledge gaps decrease when issues have a high degree of conflict and information is repeated. This knowledge gap does not need to be perpetual, for the following reasons:

- As repetition and conflict increase, the knowledge gap gets smaller (e.g., the idea that safe sex and using condoms can prevent the spread of HIV).
- As more people reach an increased state of literacy, the knowledge gap will also decrease.
- At some point there may also be a ceiling effect where most or all of the people are brought up to a certain level of understanding (e.g., knowledge of the

importance of sanitary conditions and good hygiene in keeping people healthy).

When designing health communication campaigns, organizers will often seek to reduce this gap by paying particular attention to literacy and education levels and addressing language and other barriers to receiving messages. Health communication information also becomes more accessible when messages are designed with social and cultural sensitivity and an idea of the types of technologies that may be necessary for message delivery.

NEW TECHNOLOGIES AND THE FUTURE OF HEALTH COMMUNICATION

New technologies now facilitate two-way horizontal exchange of information and dialogue through the creation of portals and development gateways. These gateways create platforms for users with the same interests to talk to each other. While not the solution for all those that seek improved access to information, one approach for the creation of "knowledge communities" can be effective. In these communities, program planners, research, policymakers, communicators, and others can acquire information, resources, and tools; contribute their knowledge and experience on specific topics; and share materials, dialogue, and solve problems with those working in the same areas. The result is improved communication, learning, and building of networks and communities of practice around significant development challenges.

Improved communication infrastructure and the development of the Internet and other technologies give local institutions the opportunity to create, publish, and disseminate local information and knowledge, and the ability to access information produced in other countries more quickly and more affordably. The Office of Population has already contributed to improving the capacity of select developing country institutions to use some of the new technologies for information and dissemination. For example, Office of Population programs (e.g., the Population Information Program) began to use and train local institutions in the use of CD-ROM technology more than 8 years ago. As a result, CD-ROMs containing up-to-date information on the latest developments, information practices, and research in the family planning/reproductive health field are produced and currently used by more than 500 organizations in 95 countries.

Institutions' capacity to produce their own CD-ROMs, develop Web sites, and improve their ability to work with new and traditional technologies needs strengthening. In collaboration with missions and regional bureaus, this subresult will provide technical assistance and training to select regional and local institutions and programs to create strategies for information dissemination; develop Web sites and list servs; use search engines; and improve dissemination efforts. Small grants could also be provided to pilot test innovative ways to create, publish, disseminate, and exchange information among an organization's affiliates or between knowledge communities within or across countries.

The public physical and political environments are constantly in a state of flux. There will always be a demand to educate new target audiences about new developments related to health in novel and contemporary ways. Future health communicators can work to maintain and increase the level of knowledge and understanding on both the individual and community levels. Programs that address low-income status and literacy will help to close the knowledge and communication gaps that exist, and future research should give us more insight on the links between knowledge and behavior change. Social marketing and entertainment education are expanding subfields of health communication that borrow concepts from the commercial business sector and the entertainment industry to develop campaigns that advance social causes.

As health communication professionals delve further into the potential of interactive health communication, the capacity of people to access and use health information and support will increase. In addition, there will be a heightened understanding of issues related to health communication and a continuance of high-quality, effective, and responsive information. New futures for the field will emerge as communication professionals and the public embrace new technologies. Improved ways of delivering information and technologies, the use of more interactive and personalized health messages and information, and tie-ins to existing products, programs, and frames of reference also promise to advance the field.

—*Scott Ratzan,*
J. Gregory Payne, and Skye K. Schulte

See also HEALTH BELIEF MODEL; THEORY OF PLANNED BEHAVIOR; TRANSTHEORETICAL MODEL OF BEHAVIOR CHANGE

Further Reading

Glanz, K., Lewis, F. M., & Rimer, B. K. (Eds.). (1997). *Health behavior and health education.* San Francisco: Jossey-Bass.

Maibach, E., & Parrott, R. L. (1995). *Designing health messages: Approaches from communication theory and public health practice.* Thousand Oaks, CA: Sage.

Payne, J. G. (2002). Principles of oral communication for health professionals. In D. Nelson (Ed.), *Health communication.* Washington, DC: American Public Health Association.

Payne, J. G., & Ratzan, S. C. (1993). A thinking globally, acting locally AIDS Action 2000 Plan: The COAST model—Health communication as negotiation. In S. C. Ratzan (Ed.), *AIDS: Effective health communication for the 1990s* (pp. 233-254). Washington, DC: Taylor & Francis.

Ratzan, S., Payne, J. G., & Masset, H. (1994, November). Effective health message design: The America Responds to AIDS Campaign. *American Behavioral Scientist, 38*(2), 294-311.

Ratzan, S., Sterans, N., Payne, J. G., Amato, P., & Madoff, M. (1994, November). Education for the health communication professional: A collaborative curricular partnership. *American Behavioral Scientist, 38*(2), 361-380.

Ratzan, S. C. (Ed.). (1993). *AIDS: Effective health communication for the 1990s.* Washington, DC: Taylor & Francis.

Ratzan, S. C. (Ed.). (1994, November). Health communication: Challenges for the 21st century. *American Behavioral Scientist, 38*(2). [Special issue]

Ratzan, S. C., Payne, J. G., & Bishop, C. (1996, Spring). Status and scope of health communication. *Journal of Health Communication, 1*(1).

Rice, R. E., & Katz, J. E. (2001). *The Internet and health communication: Experiences and expectations.* Thousand Oaks, CA: Sage.

Science Panel on Interactive Communication and Health. (1999). *Wired for health and well-being: The emergence of interactive health communication* (T. R. Eng & D. H. Gustafson, Eds.). Washington, DC: U.S. Department of Health and Human Services, Government Printing Office.

HEALTH DISPARITIES

In 1985, Margaret Heckler, the U.S. Secretary of Health and Human Services at the time, released the *Report of the Secretary's Task Force on Black and*

Minority Health, which documented striking disparities in mortality rates for cardiovascular diseases, cancer, diabetes, unintentional injury, liver diseases, and infant mortality for ethnic minority populations. Thirteen years later in 1998, then President Bill Clinton issued an ambitious challenge in a radio address to the nation when he suggested that disparities in health status should be eliminated by the year 2010. The president's call to action was motivated by the frequent finding of persistent ethnic disparities in rates of mortality and morbidity among nearly all of the leading causes of death and disability in the United States.

In its response, the National Institutes of Health (NIH) undertook development of a strategic plan designed to guide research that would address the problem. Disparities were defined as "differences in the incidence, prevalence, mortality, and burden of diseases and other adverse health conditions that exist among specific population groups in the United States." The six key areas identified in which American ethnic minority populations consistently experience disparities in health outcomes and access to care were cardiovascular disease, infant mortality, cancer screening and management, diabetes, HIV/AIDS infection, and immunizations.

Since 1999, research investigating the determinants of disparities in these conditions has increased considerably. However, group differences in health outcomes persist, and in some cases disparities are progressively widening. Many experts now suggest that complete remediation of the disparities dilemma by the year 2010 is impossible. Rather, without substantial intervention, the available evidence suggests that some groups of Americans may experience disproportionately high rates of disease morbidity and mortality for an indefinite period of time.

This entry describes the nature of ethnic disparities in key health outcomes and discusses selected determinants (primarily social) of disparities in health.

CARDIOVASCULAR DISEASES

Diseases of the cardiovascular system (CVD) constitute the leading causes of death for American men and women, irrespective of ethnicity. In 1995, CVD resulted in approximately one third of the deaths among Asian Americans/Pacific Islanders, 25% among Hispanic men, 33% among Hispanic women, and one quarter of the deaths among

American Indians/Alaskan Natives. There are marked disparities in CVD in African Americans when compared to Whites. For example, in 1995, mortality rates from CVD were 49% higher among African American men and 67% higher among African American women compared to their White counterparts. African Americans have higher mortality than Whites for coronary heart disease (CHD), the major form of CVD. For other ethnic groups, CVD and CHD mortality rates are similar to or lower than for the White population. Newer, more effective treatments and prevention efforts have led to an overall decrease in CHD mortality. However, while the total CHD death rate declined by 20% (from 1987 to 1995), the decrease was only 13% among Blacks. Compared to Whites in 1995, CHD mortality was 40% lower for Asian Americans but 40% higher for Blacks.

CEREBROVASCULAR DISEASE

Stroke, one of the leading causes of disability in the United States, disproportionately affects African Americans. Compared to Whites, mortality rates from stroke are almost 100% higher among Black men and 70% higher among Black women. Ethnic disparities are even more pronounced at younger ages; among Blacks and Hispanics ages 20-44, stroke incidence is almost 2.5 times higher compared to Whites. Stroke is the only major cause of death for which Asian American males have higher morality rates compared to Whites.

HYPERTENSION

One of the most consistent epidemiological findings is the disproportionately high rate of hypertension prevalence among African Americans, which contributes to the high rates of stroke. While the rate of hypertension is 25% in the overall population, it is almost 40% for African Americans. Among Hispanics, Mexican American men and women are at particularly high risk for hypertension—a finding that has been attributed to the high rates of obesity in this population. Birthplace and location of current residence also both exert a strong effect on hypertension status. Compared to those in other regions, residence in the Southeast is associated with a higher prevalence of hypertension, particularly among ethnic minorities.

INFANT MORTALITY

Although infant mortality rates have dropped for all groups over the past few decades, ethnic disparities remain. For example, in 1950, the mortality rate of Black infants was almost twice that of White children. In 1995, rates of infant death among Blacks were twice those of Whites as well as Hispanics and Asians. This widening disparity in infant mortality is a trend that has persisted over the past 20 years. The rates of infant mortality among Hispanics are roughly equal to those of Whites, despite the lower overall socioeconomic position of Hispanic Americans. The overall infant mortality rate tends to be higher for children born to teenage mothers, but this is not the case for African Americans. The higher rates of teenage pregnancy in African Americans do not account for the higher than average infant mortality rate.

CANCER

African Americans have the highest rates of cancer incidence and mortality (approximately 35% higher than for Whites), but disparities extend to other groups as well. Compared to other minority groups, American Indians/Alaskan Natives have the lowest levels of survival from all cancers. From 1993 to 1997, breast cancer rates among Asian American women over age 50 increased approximately 6% each year, while the increase among White women averaged only 1.5% each year. African American women had the slightest increase during this period. Black women are disproportionately more likely to die from breast cancer than are women of any other ethnic group. There are also wide disparities in cervical cancer incidence and mortality. While both Black and Hispanic women are at elevated risk for the condition, Vietnamese American women have a fivefold greater rate of cervical cancer incidence compared to Whites.

African American men have both the highest rates of prostate cancer in the world and the lowest levels of survival. Compared to White men, Blacks are 2 to 3 times as likely to die of prostate cancer, explained partly by diagnosis at a later stage of the disease. Black men are also almost 50% more likely to develop lung cancer, a condition that also affects Native Hawaiian men at higher levels.

Ethnic minorities are less likely to be routinely screened for nearly all cancers. For example, only an estimated 38% of Hispanic women age 40 years and older have had regular mammogram screening.

DIABETES

An estimated 2.8 million African Americans are currently diagnosed with diabetes, making them about twice as likely as Whites to be diabetic. This Black-White disparity extends to diabetes mortality, which is approximately 27% higher among African Americans. Compared to Whites, the diabetes prevalence is 2.8 times higher among American Indians and 2 times higher among Hispanics. Interestingly, the Pima population of Native Americans in Arizona has the highest prevalence of diabetes anywhere in the world. Among Hispanics, both Puerto Ricans and those living in the Southwest have the highest rates of diabetes, while Cubans have much lower levels. Almost all groups making up the Asian American/Pacific Islander population have higher rates of diabetes compared to Whites.

HIV/AIDS INFECTION

Although African Americans and Hispanics comprise only a quarter of the total U.S. population, together the groups accounted for approximately 55% of adult HIV/AIDS cases and fully 82% of pediatric HIV/AIDS cases in 1999.

The disparities are most pressing for women; almost 80% of HIV/AIDS-infected women are ethnic minorities. Most individuals affected by HIV/AIDS contract the condition through heterosexual interaction. However, in 1995, half of all HIV/AIDS cases among African Americans and nearly a quarter of cases among Hispanics resulted from injection drug use. By 1999, HIV/AIDS accounted for almost half of the deaths among African Americans and nearly 20% among Hispanics. HIV/AIDS remains the leading cause of death among African American men ages 25-44.

IMMUNIZATIONS

Routine vaccinations are important tools in preventing the emergence of more serious health outcomes. Although mandatory requirements for most schools virtually ensure vaccination by age 5, a large proportion of American children receive vaccinations much earlier. Whether a child ages 19 to 35 months has received the recommended vaccinations can be used as a proxy for access to and utilization of medical care. There are relatively small differences between ethnic groups in immunization rates after controlling for socioeconomic position. However, poor children in all groups are less likely to be current on recommended vaccinations when compared to children in higher socioeconomic strata. Disparities in immunization rates do not exist solely among the young; in 1999, both African Americans and Hispanics over age 65 were significantly less likely to report having received influenza and pneumococcal vaccines.

SOCIAL AND BEHAVIORAL DETERMINANTS OF DISPARITIES IN HEALTH

Over the past decade, increasing research attention has attempted to elucidate specific determinants and causal pathways linking ethnicity with disparities in health outcomes. It is generally accepted that disparities are not caused by any single factor; rather, a complex set of etiological factors likely promote group differences in health. Because of the consistent strength of ethnic differences in health and the burgeoning rise in genetic research over the past two decades, some have suggested that genetic factors may be a primary underlying cause of health disparities. A purely deterministic genetic explanation, however, has been rejected by a majority of researchers. Although variation in gene expression likely results in increased susceptibility to certain risk factors, it is unlikely that group differences have a sole genetic cause.

Biological factors, however, should not be dismissed as determinants of ethnic disparities. For example, a number of biological variables are believed to be associated with the high incidence of hypertension and diabetes among African Americans. These potential determinants include African Americans' greater salt sensitivity, increased vascular resistance, higher prevalence of left ventricular hypertrophy, increased prevalence of insulin resistance, and hyperinsulinemia.

Most integrative models of disease etiology stress the importance of social, psychosocial, and behavioral factors in disease development, progression, and mortality. That many of the leading causes of death are socially and behaviorally based may be of considerable importance to ethnic minorities, who overwhelmingly experience the most deleterious social conditions.

Factors studied most frequently as possible determinants of health disparities include socioeconomic position, health behaviors, obesity, and

social/psychosocial determinants such as stress, social support, discrimination, and access to health care. Although much of this research has focused on Black-White differences, the number of studies of other groups (particularly Hispanic Americans) is increasing.

Socioeconomic Position

Socioeconomic position (SEP) reflects an individual's relative and absolute standing in society and may be composed of factors such as income, wealth, educational attainment, occupational status, and neighborhood-level factors (e.g., concentration of poverty, violence, access to resources). The strong inverse association between SEP and health is likely the most robust and consistent finding in epidemiology. In disparities research, a frequent practice is to statistically adjust for SEP and examine whether any residual ethnic group differences remain. This is problematic in part because typical measures of SEP do not adequately capture the complexity of SEP or changes in social standing. Also, ethnicity and SEP may exert both independent and interactive effects on health outcomes. In any case, many ethnic differences in health outcomes persist after controlling for SEP variables. Ethnic minorities of low SEP have poorer health outcomes (in nearly all conditions) when compared to those in higher socioeconomic strata.

Some evidence suggests that among African Americans, ethnicity may be more powerful than SEP in predicting prevalence and mortality from specific conditions (e.g., all-cause mortality, hypertension, infant mortality, and diabetes), but this may not apply to other ethnic minority populations. For example, Hispanic Americans are sometimes found to have better overall health than other ethnic groups, despite their lower SEP. This finding has been termed the "Hispanic paradox" and some have suggested that strong social networks, acculturation, dietary practices, immigration policy, and cultural factors may all buffer the effects of low SEP among Hispanic Americans. This highlights the complex interaction of socioeconomic factors and ethnicity in the prediction of health outcomes.

Health Behaviors

Health behaviors identified as contributors to group differences in health outcomes include cigarette smoking, alcohol consumption, dietary practices, and physical activity. Obesity, which is closely linked to dietary practices and physical activity, is also very relevant to ethnic disparities in health. Individual behavioral risk factors are potentially modifiable, and their reduction through primary or secondary prevention efforts is widely considered an important approach to reducing health disparities.

Cigarette Smoking

Rates of cigarette smoking have declined since 1965 when more that half of all Americans were active smokers. In 1997, adult smoking prevalence was highest among American Indians/Alaskan Natives (34.1%) followed by African Americans (26.7%), Whites (25.3%), Hispanics (20.4%), and Asian Americans and Pacific Islanders (16.9%). Gender differences are also apparent in the smoking rates of ethnic minorities. White women have higher smoking rates compared to African American, Hispanic, and Asian American/Pacific Islander women. Although ethnic minorities generally have lower smoking rates relative to Whites, they incur significantly higher rates of mortality from tobacco-related disorders. In addition, there is some evidence that Blacks and Hispanics may respond less effectively to smoking cessation treatments.

A great deal of research has focused on smoking reduction during adolescence, when smoking prevalence is higher among Whites than among Hispanic and African American youth. Although smoking rates have declined significantly among African American youth over the past three decades, recent data suggest that the group's smoking prevalence is rising.

Alcohol Consumption

In addition to the adverse psychosocial effects of heavy drinking, excessive alcohol consumption is a primary risk factor for liver cirrhosis and has been identified as a risk factor for hypertension and other cardiovascular conditions. The data surrounding alcohol intake and CVD are somewhat more complicated, as evidence suggests that moderate alcohol intake actually protects against CVD incidence.

Compared to Whites, Hispanics have higher average levels of alcohol consumption. Men in certain Hispanic subgroups, including Puerto Ricans and Mexicans, have vastly higher rates of alcohol consumption compared to non-Hispanic males. There has

been much popular attention directed to the high proportion of alcoholism among Native Americans, who on average are more likely to engage in heavy drinking compared to other populations. Because biological evidence suggests similar alcohol metabolic rates between Native Americans and other groups, research is increasingly focusing on socioeconomic pressures and cultural practices to explain the association.

Dietary Practices, Physical Activity, Overweight, and Obesity

Overweight and obesity, which result from an excess of calorie intake and insufficient caloric expenditure from physical activity, are important risk factors for many of the leading causes of death in the United States including CVD, diabetes, and some cancers. Recent trends of increasing obesity in both adults and children have led to designation of an "obesity epidemic." African American and Mexican American women have substantially higher rates of obesity than White women. There is also a high prevalence of obesity among Hispanic populations (particularly among second- and third-generation immigrants), American Indians/Alaskan Natives, Native Hawaiians, and Samoans. Regional differences are also present such that southern African Americans and Hispanic Americans in border states have higher rates of obesity than those in other geographic locations. Among women, low SEP predisposes to obesity although this does not account for the ethnic differences.

Although excess weight serves as an overall risk factor for disease, the association of obesity with mortality varies by ethnicity. Several groups, including Asian Americans, may have a greater tendency than Whites toward abdominal obesity, a risk factor for diabetes and some cardiovascular conditions independent of the overall level of obesity.

There may be a genetic contribution to the development of obesity among some groups, though this has been difficult to establish. In any event, environmental factors such as unhealthy nutritional practices and sedentary lifestyles are believed largely responsible for the expression of obesity. Fast food and junk food are cheap, time-effective dietary choices that are far more accessible to many low-SEP minorities than are fruits and vegetables. Similarly, regular physical activity requires time, flexibility, safe neighborhoods, parks and recreational facilities, child care resources—all of which are less common among ethnic minority communities, particularly those characterized by low SEP.

Dietary factors other than excess calorie intake that have been associated with chronic health conditions include high intakes of saturated fat and cholesterol and sodium and low intakes of fruits and vegetables and dietary fiber. Very little empirical research exists to describe the relation between these nutritional factors and health disparities. Data based on an overall score of dietary quality indicate higher-risk dietary patterns in ethnic minority populations than in Whites, except for Asian Americans. Dietary quality also varies by SEP, improving with education or income. However, ethnic differences in dietary quality may be influenced by cultural practices that are partly independent of SEP.

Low levels of physical activity are a risk factor for chronic disease incidence and recurrence of a number of conditions, independent of their association with obesity. Regular exercise is least common among African Americans, followed by Hispanics and Whites. Asian Americans/Pacific Islanders also have been reported to be more sedentary in comparison to Whites. The only exception to this pattern occurs in Black males ages 18-29, among whom regular exercise is more common, compared to Whites. There is a positive relation between SEP and physical activity among most groups, with the exception of Asian Americans/Pacific Islanders.

Stress

The notion that chronic stress may exert a deleterious effect on health is not a new one, but the investigation of stress has been complicated by its numerous conceptualizations. Practically, stress has been used as a general descriptor of a latent (or unobservable) force that mediates the relation between more specific determinants (i.e., low SEP, discrimination) and biological and/or behavioral outcomes. Stress has been shown to affect a variety of biological functions. In most cases, ethnic minorities (particularly African Americans) have been shown to be more likely to encounter the most deleterious stress-induced biological outcomes.

Stress has been studied in numerous domains relevant to health disparities. However, much of this work either has not explicitly addressed ethnic differences or has not been designed to test health as an outcome variable. Many suggest that there is a social class gradient in exposure to chronic stress, such that individuals of lower status are (1) more likely to encounter adverse stressors and (2) less likely to be adequately prepared to manage these demands. Because of their lower relative social standing, ethnic minorities are believed to be at significant risk for suffering from their encounters with chronic stressors. In addition, disadvantaged social status has consistently been shown to moderate the effect of stress on physiological outcomes. However, there has been very little work investigating physiological reactions to stress in groups other than African Americans.

Social Support

The health benefits of social connectedness with individuals, groups, or communities have been investigated in myriad academic disciplines for many decades. As a result, the terminology used to describe the concept varies widely. Most investigators, however, posit a buffering effect of social support against the negative impact of stress and other determinants of disease. While elevated social support is generally believed to be positive for most groups, it is unclear whether the absence of support is uniformly negative.

There is mounting evidence to suggest that significant ethnic differences in social support exist. Collectively, ethnic minority groups are believed to have higher levels of social support in comparison to Whites. However, the structure and function of these support systems vary widely between groups. While most Hispanic Americans are believed to rely heavily on their familial networks, African Americans have similarly functional systems that are comprised of wide networks of immediate and extended family members, as well as friends and institutions (particularly churches and local community). Among Native Americans/Alaskan Natives, social support is derived primarily from family and community.

There is good evidence to suggest that cardiovascular health risk is lowered among African Americans with high levels of perceived social support. Less is known about the health benefits of social support among Hispanics, although early studies suggest that social support operates in the expected protective direction. The social support benefit on health appears not to be as strong for Asian Americans, although the reasons for these findings are unclear.

Discrimination

There has been increasing recent interest in investigating discrimination as a determinant of health outcomes among historically marginalized American ethnic groups. The interest in studying racial discrimination emerges from the frequent finding that members of ethnic minority groups (particularly African Americans) and those of low SEP are likely to encounter situations throughout their lives that limit their access to the resources necessary for the maintenance of good health. There has been some debate as to the taxonomical classification of discrimination, but there are at least two broad categories currently under study: institutional and interpersonal discrimination.

Studies examining the impact on minority health of biased institutional practices have only recently emerged. Many of these studies examine how such policies promote residential segregation, particularly in locations characterized by lower SEP and multiple exposures to toxic agents. Other work has examined bias in medical treatment practices, often showing systemic bias against African Americans and other groups.

Most studies have examined the impact of interpersonal discrimination on a variety of health outcomes. It should be noted, however, that studies in this area are concerned with perceptions of discrimination, and generally do not seek to objectively investigate the validity of subjects' claims. The overwhelming majority of these studies have been conducted among African Americans, primarily because of the group's historical exposure to discriminatory acts.

Reports of racial discrimination at work and in everyday life have been associated with increased blood pressure and cardiovascular reactivity. The same has been shown in controlled laboratory experiments examining cardiovascular reactions to vignettes depicting racial provocation. Krieger's seminal study showed that Black-White differences in blood pressure were reduced substantially when encounters with discrimination were adjusted for. Although this work provides preliminary evidence that discrimination may be associated with health outcomes, nearly all authors suggest that more work must be done.

Access to Health Care Resources

The concept of access refers both to entry to and entry within the system of care. Many investigations have documented ethnic differences in access to health care. For example, compared to only 14% of Whites, fully one third of ethnic minorities over age 18 do not have adequate health insurance coverage. These ethnic disparities are closely tied to SEP and are often found to decrease significantly after adjustment for socioeconomic factors. Irrespective of ethnic group membership, those of low SEP spend considerably more of their income on medical expenses.

Investigators are increasingly recognizing that myriad factors, comprising political, social, occupational, and individual sources, interact to affect health care access and quality.

Disparities in health care remain even when access is held constant. The 2002 Institute of Medicine publication *Unequal Treatment: Confronting Racial and Ethnic Disparities in Health Care* reported ethnic differences in the treatment of nearly every major health concern. Relative to Whites, Blacks and Hispanics are less likely to receive advanced cardiac procedures and medication, even at the same level of CVD severity.

Ethnic and socioeconomic minority group membership affects the provision of quality care in numerous ways, including communication with providers. In addition to more conventional language barriers, many minorities report feeling as though their providers do not listen to and respond to their unique concerns. Other factors include perceived discrimination, patient's mistrust and refusal of services, diagnostic errors, lack of insurance coverage, and many others.

In summary, there are widespread and persistent ethnic disparities in many major health outcomes. The etiology of these group differences is likely comprised of myriad social, psychosocial, behavioral, and biological factors. Given the multifaceted nature of ethnic disparities, a similarly complex approach to intervention is necessary to remediate their deleterious effects.

—*Gary G. Bennett*

See also AFRICAN AMERICAN HEALTH AND BEHAVIOR; ALLOSTATIS, ALLOSTATIC LOAD, AND STRESS; ASIAN AMERICAN/PACIFIC ISLANDER HEALTH AND BEHAVIOR; BLOOD PRESSURE, HYPERTENSION, AND STRESS; CULTURAL FACTORS AND HEALTH; DISCRIMINATION AND HEALTH; GENDER DIFFERENCES IN HEALTH; JOHN HENRYISM AND HEALTH; LATINO HEALTH AND BEHAVIOR; SOCIOECONOMIC STATUS AND HEALTH

Further Reading

Byrd, W. M., & Clayton, L. A. (2000). *An American health dilemma: The medical history of African Americans and the problem of race*. New York: Routledge.

Clark, R., Anderson, N., Clark, V., & Williams, D. (1999). Racism as a stressor for African Americans: A biopsychosocial model. *American Psychologist, 54*, 805-816.

Cooper-Patrick, L., et al. (1999). Race, gender, and partnership in the patient-physician relationship. *Journal of the American Medical Association, 282*, 583-589.

Franzini, L., Ribble, J., & Keddie, A. (2001). Understanding the Hispanic paradox. *Ethnicity and Disease, 11*, 496-518.

Institute of Medicine. (2002). Assessing potential sources of racial and ethnic disparities in care: The clinical encounter. In *Unequal treatment: Confronting racial and ethnic disparities in health care*. Washington, DC: National Academy Press.

Kaufman, J., Cooper, R., & McGee, D. (1997). Socioeconomic status and health in Backs and Whites: The problem of residual confounding and the resiliency of race. *Epidemiology, 8*, 621-628.

Kington, R. S., & Nickens, H. W. (2001). Racial and ethnic differences in health: Recent trends, current patterns, future directions. In N. J. Smelser, W. J. Wilson, & F. Mitchell (Eds.), *America becoming: Racial trends and their consequences* (Vol. 2, pp. 253-310). Washington, DC: National Academy Press.

Krieger, N., Sidney, S., & Coakley, E. (1998). Racial discrimination and skin color in the CARDIA Study: Implications for public health research. *American Journal of Public Health, 88*, 1308-1313.

Schulman, K., et al. (1999). The effect of race and sex on physicians' recommendations for cardiac catheterization. *New England Journal of Medicine, 244*, 1392-1393.

Singh, G., & Siahpush, M. (2001). All-cause and cause-specific mortality of immigrants and native born in the United States. *American Journal of Public Health, 91*, 392-399.

Williams, D. R. (2001). Racial variations in adult health status: Patterns, paradoxes, and prospects. In N. J. Smelser, W. J. Wilson, & F. Mitchell (Eds.), *America becoming: Racial trends and their consequences* (Vol. 2, pp. 371-410). Washington, DC: National Academy Press.

HEALTH LITERACY

Health literacy is a relatively new term that emerged in the 1990s; however, consensus has not yet been reached about its definition. For some, health literacy means the ability to function within health care settings and in relation to health materials. For others, the scope of the term *health literacy* is broader than a focus on the spoken or written word and includes background knowledge, scientific understanding, and/or knowledge of the human body. Still others highlight the ability to access information and to navigate institutions and services. In 1995, the Joint Committee on National Health Education Standards provided a definition that encompassed a broad range of contexts: "the capacity of individuals to obtain, interpret and understand basic health information and services and the competence to use such information and services in ways which enhance health." Healthy People 2010, the U.S. Department of Health and Human Services document establishing health goals and objectives for the nation, defined health literacy as "the degree to which individuals have the capacity to obtain, process, and understand basic health information and services needed to make appropriate health decisions."

Health literacy, though still variously defined, has emerged as an item of interest on the national agenda. Practitioners and researchers in a variety of health fields (including public health, medicine, oral health, mental health, occupational health and safety, environmental health) have a stake in the careful examination and delineation of health literacy skills of the public. The increased attention that health literacy garnered at the turn of the century had, in part, been driven by the findings from the first national assessment of adult literacy in the United States. The National Adult Literacy Survey, conducted in 1992, measured the ability of adults to use the written word for everyday tasks and found that half of U.S. adults have limited functional literacy skills.

FUNCTIONAL LITERACY

Functional literacy was defined by the National Literacy Act of 1991 as "the ability to read, write, and speak in English, and compute and solve problems at levels of proficiency necessary to function on the job and in society, to achieve one's goals, and develop one's knowledge and potential." The National Adult Literacy Survey (NALS) was conducted with a sample of more than 26,000 adults and used materials drawn from everyday life, including health-related items. Both the materials used in the survey and the tasks the adults were asked to perform were carefully measured for levels of difficulty and complexity. Materials included newspaper articles and editorials, signs and advertisements, and commonly used forms.

Tasks ranged in difficulty as well. Participants were asked to locate a piece of information, match two pieces of information, integrate different pieces of information and derive a finding, formulate an answer by finding needed information, and analyze or interpret statements such as those found in an editorial. The functional literacy test was scored on a 500-point scale. The average adult in the United States scores between 267 and 273 on tests of the ability to use information in prose format, document format, and for basic arithmetic calculations. Thus, the average U.S. adult reader can generally locate and match information but has difficulty integrating or analyzing information with accuracy and consistency. Educational and economic analysts note that the average adult does not quite have the literacy skills required for tasks needed in the workplace and for full participation in the activities of everyday civic life. Fully 47% to 51% of adults have low or limited literacy skills, and a disproportionate percentage of these adults are poor or elderly.

Educators note that reading is part of a complex phenomenon. As people develop literacy, they develop a number of other skills, including reading for meaning as opposed to decoding individual words. They learn to describe with accuracy, to give and understand instructions without relying on face-to-face interactions and a shared context. Furthermore, they develop a working vocabulary and an ability to understand categories and abstract concepts. Linguists and reading experts indicate that literacy influences one's ability to access information and navigate in literate environments. Literacy has an impact on cognitive and linguistic abilities and incorporates a variety of skills such as reading, oral presentation, and oral comprehension. Literacy skills are considered to be essential for accessing information and building knowledge.

LITERACY AND HEALTH

Links between education and health have been well established, but educational status was gathered routinely in health research as a marker of socioeconomic status and had not been examined in terms of key components. For many in public health, the NALS

findings and an expanded understanding of functional literacy had implications for their mandate to inform and, when necessary, alert the public. Those in medicine, needing to engage patients as partners in care and in recovery, were concerned with interpersonal communication and with the consequences of errors. Health practitioners, researchers, and policymakers were troubled by the legal and ethical implications for adequate protection of human subjects, patient autonomy in informed consent procedures, and equal access to care and services. In addition, health literacy's impact on health disparities and on costs was of increasing concern.

RESEARCH TO DATE

Since the 1970s, most of the studies published in public health and medical journals that mention literacy or health literacy have focused on assessments of the reading grade level of materials used for health purposes such as patient education materials and instructions. Some researchers assessed the readability of materials targeted at specific diseases such as cancer or diabetes; others focused on specific types of materials such as patient package inserts or materials used in institutional settings for emergency department discharge instructions or informed consent. Despite the many kinds of health-related materials analyzed for readability, a clear trend emerges from the literature: The reading level or literacy demands of health materials including educational brochures, directives, forms, documents, and Web postings have been assessed at grade levels calculated beyond high school level and inappropriate for the average adult.

A number of studies, examining both the reading level of materials and the reading ability of the intended audience, found that the literacy demands of the materials exceeded the literacy skills of the readers for whom they were developed. There is growing recognition that a mismatch between the skills of the average person and the reading demands of the written materials developed for the public presents a violation of basic communication principles.

Methodological strides made in the early 1990s, particularly in the development of new tools for rapid literacy measurement in clinical settings, had enabled researchers to move beyond a focus on written materials and explore links between the literacy level of patients and a variety of health outcomes. Although research on the relationship between literacy levels and poor health status is relatively sparse, examples include inquiries related to the link between literacy and screening behaviors, hospitalization, chronic disease management, and outcomes. For example, studies to date indicate that among people managing a chronic disease, those with limited literacy skills are less informed about the basic elements of their care plan and are less likely to understand and follow the recommended regime than are those with stronger literacy skills. Some studies have shown this disparity through markers such as blood glucose levels in studies of patients with diabetes.

At the same time, people accessing medical, dental, and mental health settings need oral language skills to describe symptoms so that a practitioner can complete a diagnosis. An individual's oral skills and oral comprehension abilities can curtail his or her dialogue with providers. Literacy skills can be further compromised by health-related factors such as illness, pain, stress, and a power differential between patients and providers. Researchers are just beginning to explore these issues.

In addition, all literacy skills are context specific. Health contexts tend to be inundated with scientific terms and the specialized jargon of various specialties. While the literacy skills of individuals are of critical importance, so too are the communication skills of those in the health fields. People's ability to understand print and oral health discussions is related to the clarity of the communication.

Researchers have not yet adequately studied everyday encounters in all of the health-related contexts. Adults are engaged in a wide variety of activities related to health promotion, health protection, disease prevention, and care. As such, they read labels for foods, household goods, and over-the-counter medicines and supplements. They are expected to follow instructions for the use of household and work chemicals and equipment. They monitor their own health and the well-being of others. They are expected to follow directions for minor illnesses, follow-up care, and chronic disease management. They are engaged in civic activities and make decisions related to community and national safety issues, to the environment, and for policy options. Increased health literacy would logically support these activities.

Health literacy represents a new area of inquiry and offers potentials for new discoveries. The exploration of those mechanisms through which literacy may affect health behaviors, health status, service utilization, and health disparities is vital to the development of effective and appropriate strategies for improving the health of the nation.

—Rima E. Rudd

Further Reading

Kirsch, I. S., Jungeblut, A., Jenkins, L., & Kolstad, A. (1993). *Adult literacy in America.* Washington, DC: Office of Educational Research and Improvement.

Office of Disease Prevention and Health Promotion. (2002). *Health communication objectives for Healthy People 2010.* Washington, DC: U.S. Department of Health and Human Services.

Purcell-Gates, V. (1995). *Other people's words: The cycle of low literacy.* Cambridge, MA: Harvard University Press.

Rudd, R. E. (2002). Health Literacy Action Plan. In Office of Disease Prevention and Health Promotion, *Health communication objectives for Healthy People 2010.* Washington, DC: U.S. Department of Health and Human Services.

Rudd, R. E., Moeykens, B. A., & Colton, T. (2000). Health and literacy: A review of the medical and public health literature. In J. P. Comings, C. Smith, & B. Garner (Eds.), *Annual review of adult learning and literacy* (pp. 158-199). San Francisco: Jossey-Bass.

HEALTH PROMOTION AND DISEASE PREVENTION

The field of health promotion and disease prevention emerged out of the recognition that many illnesses and diseases such as cancer, cardiovascular disease, and diabetes are related to lifestyle or environmental factors, for example, dietary intake, physical activity, tobacco use, sunscreen use, and drug and alcohol use. With the discovery that approximately 70% of all premature deaths before the age of 65 could be accounted for by lifestyle and environmental factors, researchers, educators, and clinicians began to investigate behavioral factors in order to improve health and prevent illness. Thus, the field of health promotion and disease prevention emerged as a discipline focused on improving health and preventing illnesses through the investigation of lifestyle or behavioral factors.

The field of health promotion and disease prevention has grown steadily since the publication of the 1974 *Lalonde Report*, which was the first government report to highlight the notion that biology, environment, lifestyle, and health care all affect health status. International efforts that facilitated the development of the field of health promotion include the 1986 International Conference on Health Promotion in Ottawa, Ontario, Canada; the 1992 International Conference on Health Promotion in Santafé de Bogotá, Colombia; and the 1993 First Caribbean Conference of Health Promotion in Port of Spain, Trinidad and Tobago. The subsequent publication of several documents also described international and national initiatives to promote health and prevent disease (i.e., *The Lalonde Report, The Ottawa Charter for Health Promotion,* Latin America's *Health Promotion and Equity, Caribbean Charter for Health Promotion,* and *Healthy People 2010*). There are numerous objectives to these initiatives, including increasing life span, reducing health disparities, and providing access to preventive services.

Scholars have proposed numerous ways to define the field of health promotion and disease prevention. Definitions of *health promotion* tend to emphasize a combination of educational, political, regulatory, and organizational interventions aimed at improving personal and/or public health and well-being. Whereas the field of health promotion tends to focus on promoting health and increasing well-being, the field of *disease prevention* tends to focus on halting illnesses or diseases, and identifying methods to change risk factors in order to avoid illnesses or diseases. Numerous disease prevention interventions, for example, target smoking as a risk factor for lung cancer.

The field of health promotion and disease prevention grew out of the multidisciplinary field of health education, which tends to use educational principles to improve health and prevent illnesses. However, in addition to using educational principles, health promotion and disease prevention experts also use a number of additional strategies to promote health and prevent illnesses. These strategies include individual or group therapy or counseling, communication and media campaigns aimed at health education, health program development and organizational change, and health policy development and advocacy.

Researchers, educators, and clinicians from various disciplines are committed to improving health and preventing disease through lifestyle or behavioral modification. *Health educators* study methods and theories to change health behaviors. *Health psychologists* study behavior change and mental processes to understand health and illnesses. *Public health experts*, on the other hand, focus on a broader field than health promotion and disease prevention and tend to conduct population-based health studies (vs. studies on individuals). Public health interventions may also include health assessment and surveillance methods, environment and health policy protection, and health care services.

Health promotion and disease prevention interventions may be developed at the individual, community, organizational, or governmental level. Interventions that focus on individuals tend to target personal knowledge, attitudes, and/or behaviors. Interventions that focus on organizations, communities, or the environment tend to target policies, practices, programs, facilities, or resources. Finally, interventions at the government level tend to target legislation, regulation, and enforcement of health policies. For example, at the individual level, obesity prevention interventions may focus on healthful eating; at the community level, obesity prevention interventions may focus on increasing the accessibility of parks as a strategy for increasing physical activity; at the organizational level, the interventions may focus on increasing healthful eating options and on developing weight control programs; and finally, at the government level, obesity prevention interventions may focus on supporting obesity research and regulating the fast food industry.

Health promotion and disease prevention interventions may be classified into three broad areas: primary prevention, secondary prevention, and tertiary prevention interventions. Primary prevention interventions, such as tobacco awareness and sunscreen use campaigns, are designed to prevent an illness from occurring in healthy people. Secondary prevention interventions, such as mammography screening in women at risk for breast cancer, are designed to identify or treat an emerging illness or disease. Finally, tertiary prevention interventions, such as drug and alcohol abuse treatments, are designed to treat current diseases or illnesses or prevent them from recurring. Regardless of the specific classification of health promotion and disease prevention interventions, it is important to develop assessments and treatments that are effective and culturally appropriate for diverse ethnic, cultural, and socioeconomic status groups.

—*Lisa A. Pualani Sánchez-Johnsen*

Further Reading

Glanz, K., Rimer, L., & Lewis, F. M. (2002). *Health behavior and health education.* San Francisco: Jossey-Bass.

Joint Committee on Health Education Terminology. (1991). Report of the Joint Committee on Health Education Terminology. *Journal of Health Education, 22*(2), 97-108.

Pan American Health Organization. (1996). *Health promotion: An anthology.* Scientific Publication No. 557. Washington, DC: PAHO, World Health Organization.

Simons-Morton, B. G., Greene, W. H., & Gottlieb, N. H. (1995). *Introduction to health education and health promotion.* Prospect Heights, IL: Waveland.

U.S. Department of Health and Human Services. (2000). *Healthy People 2010* (2nd ed.). *With understanding and improving health and objectives for improving health* (2 vols.). Washington, DC: Government Printing Office.

HEALTH PSYCHOLOGY

Health psychology is a relatively new subfield of psychology that relates knowledge from all subdomains of psychology to health. A widely accepted definition has been provided by Matarazzo (1982) and was endorsed by the then newly established Division of Health Psychology of the American Psychological Association. Matarazzo stated:

> Health Psychology is the aggregate of the specific educational, scientific, and professional contributions of the discipline of psychology to the promotion and maintenance of health, the prevention and treatment of illness, the identification of etiologic and diagnostic correlates of health, illness and related dysfunction, and the analysis and improvement of the health care system and health policy formation. (p. 4)

CONTENT OF THE FIELD

The broad and rather dry-sounding definition above may come alive by considering a few examples of the work that health psychologists engage in:

- A researcher is interested in the unique compliance problems that diabetic teenagers have, and uses developmental stage knowledge to differentiate compliance issues in teenagers from those of older diabetics.

- A psychologist employed by a general hospital consults with hospital administrators and nursing staff on which surgery patients to place together in a room; this effort stems from observations that patients who are presurgery recover most quickly with the least complications when they share a room with a postsurgery patient who is recovering well (Kulik & Mahler, 1987).

- Psychologists are advising health department officials on how to create effective antismoking advertising that uses knowledge from basic attitude formation research conducted by social psychologists.

- Clinical psychologists with extensive training in psychotherapy apply knowledge of stress reduction techniques to help hypertensive patients bring their blood pressure under control (Linden, Lenz, & Con, 2001).

It may also help to define health psychology by highlighting its definitional overlap and its uniqueness relative to the terms *psychosomatics, medical psychology,* and *behavioral medicine.* A quick review of scientific journals that have these terms in their title reveals that many health- and psychology-related topics are equally covered in all these journals. High-profile journals in the field are *Health Psychology, Psychosomatic Medicine, Psychological Medicine,* and *Annals of Behavioral Medicine,* to name a few. What differentiates the term and the field of health psychology from these others, however, is first, the emphasis on it being unmistakably delineated and labeled as a subfield of psychology rather than another discipline, and second, the stress is on health rather than illness, which, in turn, is more readily linked to medicine (it would be unfair to say that medicine is inherently not interested in health, but tradition has made it a more reactive discipline that is expected to solve existing problems rather than focus on various types of prevention). A third distinction is that the term health psychology sends a broad invitation to contribute to all subspecialties of psychology, whereas the more medically sounding labels tend to presume that "health psychologists" have clinical training and know their way around hospitals.

Finally, one needs to recognize that undergraduate courses and the accompanying textbooks usually represent the first organized exposure to a new field and as such define the field simply by what topics they include and how they are organized. A survey of popular textbooks indicates that almost all of them have chapters on these topics:

History of and models in health psychology

Research methods in health psychology

A review of relevant physiological systems

Prevention

Stress and health

Effectiveness of psychological interventions for health problems

Health behavior

Illness behavior

Patient-practitioner interaction

The patient in the hospital

Adherence to prescribed treatment regimes

Psychology and nutrition and exercise

Pain

Coping with chronic disease

Death and dying

HISTORY AND PREVAILING MODELS

The most elementary and oldest concept that marks health psychology is that of a holistic understanding of mind and body that can be traced back to Oriental physicians around 2600 B.C. and Greek philosophers, particularly Hippocrates. More modern thinkers have criticized the traditional medical model that has evolved since Hippocrates as being overly narrow and organ-focused. Particularly influential has been Engel's (1977) critique of the medical model and the proposition of a model that considers the joint and interacting roles of biological, environmental, social, and psychological influences on health and disease. Additional landmarks in the history of health psychology have been (1) the establishment of Division 38 of the American Psychological Association; (2) the creation of the division's "house journal," *Health Psychology*; and (3) the publication of the first undergraduate textbook in health psychology (Feuerstein, Labbe, & Kuczmierczyk, 1986).

—*Wolfgang Linden*

Further Reading

Andersen, B. J., Auslander, W. F., Jung, K. C., Miller, J. P., & Santiago, J. V. (1990). Assessing family sharing of diabetes responsibilities. *Journal of Pediatric Psychology, 15*, 477-492.

Engel, G. L. (1977). The need for a new medical model: A challenge for biomedicine. *Science, 196*, 129-136.

Feuerstein, M., Labbe, E. E., & Kuczmierczyk, A. R. (1986). *Health psychology: A psychobiological perspective*. New York: Plenum.

Kulik, J. A., & Mahler, H. I. M. (1987). Effects of pre-operative roommate assignment on pre-operative anxiety and recovery from coronary bypass surgery. *Health Psychology, 6*, 525-543.

Linden, W., Lenz, J. W., & Con, A. (2001). Individualized stress management for primary hypertension: A controlled trial. *Archives of Internal Medicine, 161*, 1071-1080.

Matarazzo, J. D. (1982). Behavioral health's challenge to academic, scientific, and professional psychology. *American Psychologist, 37*, 1-14.

HEART DISEASE: ANGER, DEPRESSION, AND ANXIETY

EPIDEMIOLOGY

It has long been assumed that the emotional distress (depression/anxiety/irritability) commonly observed in coronary heart disease (CHD) patients is a "natural" reaction to the diagnosis. This is an erroneous, harmful, and expensive assumption. It is now clear that, for large numbers of patients, emotional distress predates and predicts the onset of CHD. For those who do not have premorbid emotional distress, reactive depression/anxiety (and anger) will still adversely affect the progression of atherosclerosis, ischemic episodes, myocardial infarction (MI)/death, noncompliance, symptoms, and utilization.

Major depression occurs in 18% to 20% of CHD patients (a fivefold increase over general population levels), and "minor" depression (dysthymia or adjustment disorder with depressed mood) occurs in another 10% to 15% (also a fivefold increase over general population levels). The distinction between major (per *DSM-IV* criteria) and minor depression (Beck scores of 10 or greater) has not been found to be useful in terms of predicting MI and death over the first 6 months post-MI, and minor depression is actually superior at predicting mortality over the first 18 months post-MI, in part because it captures all major depressive patients as well. In the available studies, depression appears to be the most potent predictor of mortality over the first 6 to 18 months post-MI, and anxiety appears to be the most potent predictor of CHD mortality in initially healthy populations. However, when patient denial/minimization is circumvented, anger appears to be the best predictor of early onset CHD, particularly in males.

Noncardiac chest pain may occur in up to 50% of CHD patients, betokening widespread panic-like events. Beitman has, in fact, proposed the term "non-fear panic attacks" to describe those events where patients have many of the physical symptoms of panic but deny subjective anxiety/fear. Anger, depression, and anxiety are very strong predictors of morbidity/mortality, with risk ratios often larger than those observed for traditional risk factors such as hypercholesterolemia, hypertension, and smoking. Other outcomes of clinical interest have also been found to be affected by, or associated with, one or more of these three emotions. These include chest pain, coronary artery disease (CAD), fatigue, utilization, hypertension, and noncompliance with smoking cessation, diabetic, and exercise regimens.

MECHANISMS

Emotional distress may affect the development and aggravation of CHD via psychophysiological or psychobehavioral pathways. These pathways are not mutually exclusive, and there is, at present, no reason to assume that one pathway is the sole culprit. In fact, available evidence suggests that each pathway is plausible. The behaviorally mediated pathways are so well established that they require little discussion. Evidence is available demonstrating that emotional distress (particularly anger and depression) is a predictor of failure to stop smoking, and both cognitive-behavioral therapy and psychopharmacotherapy increase cessation/maintenance rates. Compliance to pill taking, diabetic regimens, and exercise has also been found to be influenced adversely by emotional distress, although no intervention trials have yet demonstrated improvement results from treatment.

The psychophysiological pathways are also multiple and not mutually exclusive. The acute induction of ischemia by acute mental stress in patients with documented CAD is well established. These observations are complemented by the increase in sudden death seen during natural experiments such as earthquakes and bombings. These psychologically induced events may be due to induced vasoconstriction, vasomotoric-induced plaque rupture, and/or enhanced platelet aggregability superimposed on a plaque.

Distress-related immunocompetance may be impaired as a result of depression, leading to chronic smoldering infection, and/or chronic, subclinical inflammation may promote plaque growth and/or instability.

The acute induction of ischemia may also help account for the increased chest pain seen in patients with emotional distress (particularly anxiety and depression) and the reduction of chest pain associated with treatment of emotional distress. On the other hand, diminished beta endorphins associated with anxiety and depression may simply make patients hypersensitive to ischemic events.

DIAGNOSIS

As Appels and others have shown, emotional distress in CHD patients often manifests as "fatigue" or "vital exhaustion" (prolonged sleep onset or nocturnal awakening, chronic tiredness, and/or irritability) rather than classic depression. Because these symptoms are almost always misconstrued as a result of the CHD rather than primary psychological phenomena, they result in more aggressive cardiac treatment rather than referral for psychosocial or psychopharmacological intervention. For example, depression has been found to strongly contaminate New York Heart Association (NYHA) ratings in heart failure.

Screening of CHD patients should take place at the time of initial diagnosis and then periodically as suspected by noncompliance, resting chest pain, chronic difficulties falling asleep, staying asleep, or awakening tired, and chronic fatigue. We recommend the use of the Hospital Anxiety and Depression Scale (HADS) completed by the patient because of its brevity, innocuous content, and easy scoring. Because cardiac patients (particularly males) are prone to denial of emotional distress, self-report alone is inadequate in screening patients. Spouse/friend ratings have been found to be superior to self-report at correlating with CAD severity, age at initial diagnosis, and chest pain at 5-year follow-up. Furthermore, discrepancies between self and spouse/friend ratings, with the spouse/friend reporting higher levels of distress, is an even stronger correlate of CAD severity and mortality. We use the Ketterer Stress Symptom Frequency Checklist–Revised (KSSFCR) to circumvent denial. By asking the patient to select "someone who knows you well" to complete and return (by mail) a separate screening questionnaire, patient denial is minimized. To date, the KSSFCR is the only normed, standardized, and validated means of achieving this end.

The first task in diagnosis and treatment is to rule out organic causes of "depression." In CHD populations, this means screening for common comorbid conditions such as sleep apnea, cocaine abuse, and dementia. Because these conditions cause, or mimic, some of the symptoms of depression, they are often misconstrued by patients, families, and physicians alike. Assuming these conditions have been ruled out, several other considerations are important.

Depression is, more often than not, comorbid with elevations in anger/hostility ("irritability") and/or anxiety (panic attacks, generalized anxiety disorder [GAD], or "worry"). In every single-sample test of the uniqueness or confounding of the negative emotions as predictors of clinical status or outcomes of which we are aware, only one measure emerges as necessary to capture all relevant variance in the outcome variable. Thus, screening for multiple measures is almost certainly unnecessary and, from a cost-effectiveness standpoint, wasteful. As in most medical populations, formal *DSM-IV* criteria are rarely useful. Most cardiac patients present with atypical depression/anxiety manifested as chest pain, disturbed sleep, fatigue, or irritability rather than the usual symptoms of sad mood, crying, hopelessness, guilt, or suicidality. This is most likely due to denial or minimization, as discussed below.

TREATMENT

Treatment of emotional distress has been found to decrease MI and death, chest pain, continued smoking or relapse, ischemic episodes, and utilization. Although not yet tested in intervention trials, there is reason to believe that treatment will improve compliance to pill taking, diabetic regimens, and exercise.

Obviously, the presence of cocaine abuse or sleep apnea requires referral for treatment focused on these conditions. For drug abuse, it is rarely helpful to

attempt treatment of emotional distress before abstinence is achieved, since much of the patient's emotionality is attributable to fluctuating levels of psychoactives in the central nervous system (CNS) and will only confuse the cognitive-behavioral treatment. For sleep apnea, idiosyncratic drug reactions can occur.

Exercise is known to reduce both cardiac events and emotional distress. Any patient not already engaged in a regular exercise program should be considered for cardiac rehabilitation.

At the present time, cognitive-behavioral stress management is the best established means of improving cardiac outcomes. Risk reductions for MI and death average about 34%. The use of selective serotonin reuptake inhibitors (SSRIs) is relatively new, but well established as safe. Because the older tricyclic antidepressants caused various anticholinergic side effects (dry mouth, blurred vision, orthostatic hypotension, and lengthening of the QT), clinicians have generally shied away from their use in cardiac populations. More important, the newer SSRIs not only have none of these concerns but have shown exceptional promise in reducing cardiac events. In a case-control comparison, Sauer et al. found MI rates to be reduced by 55% to 65%. This is the same magnitude risk reduction observed for coronary artery bypass surgery in left main CAD. In a small safety and efficacy trial of sertraline (Zoloft), originally unintended to measure cardiac outcomes, these findings appear to be supported. Because of drug-drug interactions for many of the SSRIs, the preferred agents are sertraline (Zoloft) and citalopram (Celexa). Generally low doses (25-50 mg of Zoloft or 10-20 mg of Celexa) are adequate.

In two large trials of cognitive-behavioral treatment, women experienced adverse outcomes as a result of treatment. It may be that sex-specific cognitive-behavioral treatment will prove necessary. But the benefits of SSRIs need to be studied for females.

—*Mark W. Ketterer*

See also HEART DISEASE AND DIET; HEART DISEASE AND PHYSICAL ACTIVITY; HEART DISEASE AND SMOKING; HEART DISEASE AND REACTIVITY; HEART DISEASE AND TYPE A BEHAVIOR

Further Reading

Allison, T. G., Williams, D. E., Miller, T. D., Patten, C. A., Bailey, K. R., Squires, R. W., et al. (1995). Medical and economic costs of psychologic distress in patients with coronary artery disease. *Mayo Clinic Proceedings, 70,* 734-742.

Dusseldorp, E., Van Elderen, T., Maes, S., Meulman, J., & Kraaij, V. (1999). A meta-analysis of psychoeducational programs for coronary heart disease. *Health Psychology, 18,* 506-519.

Ketterer, M. W., Denollet, J., Goldberg, A. D., McCullough, P. A., Farha, A. J., Clark, V., et al. (2002). The big mush: Psychometric measures are confounded and nonindependent in their association with age at initial diagnosis of ICHD. *Journal of Cardiovascular Risk, 9,* 41-48.

Ketterer, M. W., Freedland, K. E., Krantz, D. S., Kaufman, P., Forman, S., Greene, A., et al. (2000). Psychological correlates of mental stress-induced ischemia in the laboratory: The psychophysiological investigations of myocardial ischemia (PIMI) study. *Journal of Health Psychology, 5,* 75-85.

Ketterer, M. W., Kenyon, L., Folet, B. A., Brymer, J., Rhoads, K., Kraft, P., et al. (1996). Denial of depression as an independent correlate of coronary artery disease. *Journal of Health Psychology, 1,* 93-105.

Ketterer, M. W., Mahr, G., & Goldberg, A. D. (2000). Psychological factors affecting a medical condition: Ischemic coronary heart disease. *Journal of Psychosomatic Research, 48,* 357-367.

Lewin, B. (1997). The psychological and behavioral management of angina. *Journal of Psychosomatic Research, 43,* 453-462.

O'Connor Sauer, W. H., Berlin, J. A., & Kimmel, S. E. (2001). Selective serotonin reuptake inhibitors and myocardial infarction. *Circulation, 104,* 1894-1898.

HEART DISEASE AND DIET

The relationship between diet and coronary heart disease (CHD) has been a topic of extensive research in clinical and epidemiological studies. In the past two decades, at least 20 prospective cohort studies have examined the relationship between dietary factors and risk of CHD. This entry briefly reviews epidemiological and clinical trial evidence regarding the role of specific dietary factors in the cause and prevention of CHD.

TYPES OF DIETARY FATS

The classic "diet-heart" hypothesis postulates that high intake of saturated fats and cholesterol and low intake of polyunsaturated fat increase the level of serum cholesterol, which leads to development of atheromatous plaques and eventually to myocardial infarction. In the seminal Seven Countries Study conducted by Ancel Keys and colleagues (1980), intake of saturated fat as a percentage of calories had strong correlation with coronary death rates across 16 defined populations in seven countries ($r = .84$). Interestingly, the correlation between the percentage of energy from total fat and CHD incidence was only modest ($r = .39$). Indeed, the regions with the highest CHD rate (Finland) and the lowest rate (Crete) had the same amount of total fat intake, at about 40% of energy, which was the highest among the 16 populations. Migration studies have also linked dietary factors and CHD.

In 1973, Kato and colleagues compared CHD incidence rates among three defined Japanese populations living in Japan, Hawaii, and San Francisco. Age-adjusted CHD incidence rates were 1.6 per 1,000 person-years in Japan, 3.0 in Hawaii, and 3.7 in San Francisco. With transition to the United States, mean saturated fat intake as percentage of total energy increased, with the highest intake in San Francisco. These data indicate that the substantial differences in CHD rates among the three areas were probably attributed to changes in diet (especially increase in saturated fat intake) and lifestyle, rather than to genetic factors. However, because multiple factors changed simultaneously, it is not possible to pinpoint specific causal factors.

A number of prospective cohort studies have directly addressed associations between diet fat and risk of CHD, but the results from these studies have been inconsistent due to small size and inadequate dietary measurements. In 1997, Hu and colleagues conducted a detailed prospective analysis of dietary fat and CHD among 80,082 women ages 34 to 59 in the Nurses' Health Study. The study was particularly powerful because of large sample sizes and repeated assessments of diet. In multivariate analyses, a higher intake of trans fatty acids and saturated fat, to a lesser extent, was positively associated with CHD risk, whereas a higher intake of mono- and polyunsaturated fat was associated with a lower risk. Total fat was not significantly related to CHD risk. This study concludes that replacing saturated (found in animal products) and trans fats (found in stick margarine, vegetable shortening, and commercial bakery and deep-fried products) with nonhydrogenated mono- and polyunsaturated fats (natural liquid vegetable oils) is more effective in preventing CHD than reducing overall fat intake.

Controlled metabolic studies have established that exchanging saturated fat for carbohydrate increases low-density lipoprotein (LDL) as well as high-density lipoprotein (HDL) cholesterol, whereas exchanging mono- or polyunsaturated fat for carbohydrate lowers LDL cholesterol and triglycerides and raises HDL cholesterol. Metabolic studies have also consistently indicated adverse effects of trans fat intake on blood lipids. Trans fatty acids raise LDL cholesterol levels and lower HDL cholesterol relative to natural unsaturated fatty acids. As such, the increase in the ratio of total to HDL cholesterol for trans fat is approximately double that for the same amount of saturated fat.

CHOLESTEROL AND EGGS

In controlled metabolic studies conducted in humans, dietary cholesterol raises levels of total and LDL cholesterol in blood, but the effects are relatively small compared with saturated and trans fatty acids, and individuals vary widely in the response to dietary cholesterol on plasma levels. Although several studies have found a modest association between dietary cholesterol and risk of CHD, there is little direct evidence linking higher egg consumption, a main source of dietary cholesterol, and increased risk of CHD. The Nurses' Health Study and Health Professionals' Follow-Up Study found no evidence of an overall positive association between moderate egg consumption (up to 1 egg/day) and risk of CHD in either men or women.

N-3 FATTY ACIDS

A low rate of cardiovascular disease in populations with very high intake of fish, such as Alaskan Native Americans, Greenland Eskimos, and Japanese living in fishing villages, suggests that fish oil may be protective against atherosclerosis. Kromhout and colleagues (Kromhout, Bosschieter, & Coulander, 1985) found in the Dutch component of the Seven Countries Study that men who consumed 30 g of fish per day had a 50% lower CHD mortality than men who rarely ate fish during 20 years of follow-up. The Western Electric Study found that men who consume 35 g or more of fish per day had a 40% lower risk of fatal CHD. In the U.S. Physicians' Health Study, weekly fish consumption was associated with a 50% lower risk of sudden cardiac death, but in the same cohort, no significant association was observed between fish consumption and overall cardiovascular endpoints. The Nurses' Health Study found about a 30% lower risk of CHD associated with two to four servings of fish per week. The Health Professionals' Follow-Up Study found no overall association between dietary intake of n-3 fatty acids or fish intake and the risk of coronary disease, but there was a nonsignificant trend for a reduction in risk for fatal CHD with increasing fish consumption. Two interventional studies, the Diet and Reinfarction Trial (DART) and the GISSI-Prevenzione trial, have found that increased fish consumption or fish oil supplementation reduces coronary mortality among postmyocardial infarction patients.

TYPES OF CARBOHYDRATES

That different carbohydrate-containing foods lead to different glycemic responses has led to the development of the concept *glycemic index* (GI), a term first coined by Jenkins and colleagues (1981). GI is a ranking of foods based on the extent that blood glucose rises (the area under the curve for blood glucose levels) after ingesting a test food as compared to a standard weight (50 g) of reference carbohydrate (glucose or white bread).

The GI depends largely on the rate of digestion and rapidity of absorption of carbohydrate. Typically, foods with low degree of starch gelatinization (more compact granules) such as spaghetti and oatmeal and high level of viscose soluble fiber such as barley, oats, and rye have a slower rate of digestion and lower GI values. Physical form of the foods is another important determinant of GI. Whole-grain products with intact bran and germ typically have lower GI values. In contrast, refined carbohydrate-containing foods such as white bread tend to have higher GI values because grinding or milling of cereals removes most of the bran and much of the germ and reduces the particle size, allowing for more rapid attack by digestive enzymes.

The ratio of amylose (straight chain of 50 to 300 glucose molecules) to amylopectin (branched chain of 300 to 5,000 glucose molecules) in food is also an important factor influencing GI values. Foods with a higher ratio of amylose to amylopectin such as legumes and parboiled rice tend to have lower GI values. This is because the tight compact structure of amylose renders it physically less accessible to enzyme attack and therefore harder to digest, and amylopectin molecules, on the other hand, are larger and more open to digestive enzymatic attack.

The concept of glycemic load (GL; the product of the GI value of a food and its carbohydrate content) has been developed to represent both the quality and quantity of the carbohydrates consumed. Using white bread as the reference, each unit of dietary GL represents the equivalent glycemic effect of 1 g of carbohydrate from white bread. Several large population-based studies have documented an inverse association between dietary GI or GL values and HDL levels and a positive association with triglycerides. Epidemiological studies have found that a higher dietary GL, especially combined with low intake of cereal fiber, significantly elevated long-term risk of Type 2 diabetes. A higher dietary GL has also been associated with elevated risk of CHD in the Nurses' Health Study.

Whole-grain products such as whole wheat breads, brown rice, oats, and barley tend to produce slower glycemic and insulinemic responses than highly processed refined grains. Whole grains are also rich in fiber, antioxidant vitamins, magnesium, and phytochemicals. Epidemiological studies have consistently found an inverse association between whole grain consumption and risk of diabetes and CHD. The Nurses' Health Study observed a 25% lower risk of CHD (nonfatal myocardial infarction and CHD death) among women who ate nearly three servings of whole grains a day compared with those who ate less than a serving per week.

FIBER

Dietary fiber includes the cell walls of plants and other indigestible components of plants. Soluble fibers (pectins, gums, mucilages, and psyllium) lower total and LDL cholesterol through increased bile acid excretion and decreased hepatic synthesis of cholesterol and fatty acids. Based on a recent meta-analysis of 67 controlled trials, the magnitude of cholesterol-lowering effects of soluble fiber is only modest. For example, ingesting 3 g soluble fiber form oats (three servings of oatmeal) decreases cholesterol by only 2%. However, fiber may have other benefits, including improving glycemic control and reducing hyperinsulinemia. Numerous prospective cohort studies examined the relationship between fiber intake and risk of CHD and virtually all found an inverse association. In the Nurses' Health Study, for each 10-g increase in total fiber intake, there was about 20% reduction in CHD risk. The strongest association was found for cereal fiber, as opposed to fruit and vegetable fiber.

ANTIOXIDANTS

A body of epidemiological evidence links intake of vitamin E and reduced risk of CHD. The Nurses' Health Study and the Health Professional's Follow-Up Study demonstrated a lower risk for CHD in the men and women who had higher daily consumption of vitamin E, particularly in those subjects that took vitamin E supplements. The Iowa Women's Study found that dietary vitamin E intake, as opposed to supplement vitamin E, was inversely associated with the risk of death from CHD, but in that study, data on duration of vitamin E supplement use were not available.

Results from clinical trials regarding the effects of vitamin E supplementation on the risk of CVD have been largely disappointing; most of the trials did not find protective effects of vitamin E supplements on CHD among patients with existing heart disease. On the other hand, large prospective cohort studies continue to supply strong evidence that high intakes of carotenoid-rich foods such as fruits and vegetables lower risk of cardiovascular disease. In the most recent analysis of the Nurses' Health Study, each 1-serving/d increase in intake of fruits or vegetables was associated with a 4% lower risk for CHD and a 6% lower risk for ischemic stroke. The discrepancy between observational studies and supplementation trials raises the question whether the antioxidants coming from supplements, in high dose and not part of a balanced mix of antioxidants, function in the same way as those from diet.

FOLATE

Folic acid and other B vitamins are the primary determinants of plasma homocysteine concentrations, a recognized independent risk factor for CHD. Epidemiological studies have found that higher plasma levels of folate or increased consumption of folate was associated with significantly lower risk of CHD. In 1998, the recommended dietary allowance (RDA) for folic acid was raised to 400 micrograms per day, more than doubling the previous RDA set in 1989. A multivitamin supplement typically contains 400 mcg of folic acid. Beginning in 1997, flour has been fortified with folate, adding about 100 mcg per day of folate to the average American's diet. Most cold breakfast cereals are also fortified to provide 100 mcg of folate per day. Other good dietary sources of folate include orange juice, spinach, and lentils.

ALCOHOL

Numerous epidemiological studies have documented an inverse association between alcohol consumption and risk of CHD, in both men and women. In general, consumption of one or two drinks per day has corresponded to a reduction in risk of approximately 20% to 40%. Light to moderate alcohol consumption has also been associated with a lower risk of stroke.

DIETARY PATTERNS

Instead of looking at individual nutrients or foods, dietary pattern analysis examines the effects of overall diet. Since dietary patterns cannot be measured directly, statistical methods have been used to characterize dietary patterns using collected dietary information. Three approaches have been used in the literature: factor analysis, cluster analysis, and dietary indices.

Factor analysis is a multivariate statistical technique, which, in a dietary context, uses information reported on food frequency questionnaires or in dietary records to identify common underlying dimensions (factors or patterns) of food consumption. It aggregates specific food items or food groups based on the degree to which food items in the dataset are correlated with one another.

In contrast to factor analysis, cluster analysis aggregates individuals into relatively homogeneous subgroups (clusters) with similar diets. When the cluster procedure is completed, further analyses (e.g., comparing dietary profiles across clusters) are necessary to interpret the identified patterns.

A variety of dietary indices have been proposed to assess overall diet quality. These indices are typically constructed on the basis of dietary recommendations. For example, the healthy eating index (HEI) is a single, summary measure of the degree to which a person's diet conforms to the serving recommendations of the

U.S. Department of Agriculture (USDA) Food Guide Pyramid for five major food groups and to specific recommendations in the Dietary Guidelines for Americans. The diet quality index (DQI) is a summary score of the degree to which a person's diet conforms to specific dietary recommendations from Diet and Health.

In 1999, Hu and colleagues conducted the first validation study to test the reproducibility and validity of dietary patterns assessed by a food frequency questionnaire (FFQ). Using factor analysis, they identified two major patterns. The first pattern (labeled the "prudent pattern") was characterized by higher intake of vegetables, fruits, legumes, whole grains, fish, and poultry, while the second pattern (labeled the "Western pattern") was characterized by higher intake of red meat, processed meat, refined grains, sweets/desserts, French fries, and high-fat dairy products. The reliability correlations for the factor scores between the two FFQs were 0.70 for the prudent pattern and 0.67 for the Western pattern. The correlations (corrected for week-to-week variation in diet records) between the FFQ and diet records were 0.52 for the prudent pattern and 0.74 for the Western pattern. In subsequent analyses, they found that the major dietary patterns derived from factor analysis predicted long-term risk of CHD. Specifically, the higher prudent pattern score was associated with a lower risk, whereas the higher Western pattern score was associated with an elevated risk.

SUMMARY

Cumulative evidence from multiple lines of research indicates that types of fats and carbohydrates are more important than total amounts of fats and carbohydrates in determining risk of CHD. Evidence is now clear that replacing saturated and trans fats with unsaturated fats (including sources of n-3 fatty acids) and substituting whole-grain forms of carbohydrate for refined grains will reduce risk of coronary heart disease. In addition, available evidence strongly supports that a dietary pattern rich in these nutrients is likely to reduce risk of CHD.

—*Frank B. Hu*

See also HEART DISEASE: ANGER, DEPRESSION, AND ANXIETY; HEART DISEASE AND PHYSICAL ACTIVITY; HEART DISEASE AND REACTIVITY; HEART DISEASE AND SMOKING; HEART DISEASE AND TYPE A BEHAVIOR

Further Reading

Ascherio, A., Katan, M. B., Zock, P. L., Stampfer, M. J., & Willett, W. C. (1999). Trans fatty acids and coronary heart disease. *New England Journal of Medicine, 340,* 1994-1998.

Hu, F. B., Manson, J. E., & Willett, W. C. (2001). Types of dietary fat and risk of coronary heart disease: A critical review. *Journal of the American College of Nutrition, 20,* 5-19.

Hu, F. B., Rimm, E., Smith-Warner, S. A., Feskanich, D., Stampfer, M. J., Ascherio, A., Sampson, L., & Willett, W. C. (1999). Reproducibility and validity of dietary patterns assessed by a food frequency questionnaire. *American Journal of Clinical Nutrition, 69,* 243-249.

Hu, F. B., Stampfer, M. J., Manson, J. E., Rimm, E., Colditz, G. A., Rosner, B. A., Hennekens, C. H., & Willett, W. C. (1997). Dietary fat intake and risk of coronary heart disease in women. *New England Journal of Medicine, 337,* 1491-1499.

Hu, F. B., Stampfer, M. J., Rimm, E. B., Manson, J. E., Ascherio, A., Colditz, G. A., Rosner, B. A., Spiegelman, D., Speizer, F. E., Sacks, F. M., Hennekens, C. H., & Willett, W. C. (1999). A prospective study of egg consumption and risk of cardiovascular disease in men and women. *Journal of the American Medical Association, 281,* 1387-1394.

Hu, F. B., & Willett, W. C. (2002). Diet and coronary heart disease in women. In P. S. Douglas (Ed.), *Cardiovascular health and disease in women* (2nd ed.). Philadelphia: W. B. Saunders.

Jenkins, D. J., Wolever, T. M., Taylor, R. H., Barker, H., Fielden, H., Baldwin, J. M., Bowling, A. C., Newman, H. C., Jenkins, A. L., & Goff, D. V. (1981). Glycemic index of foods: A physiological basis for carbohydrate exchange. *American Journal of Clinical Nutrition, 34,* 362-366.

Keys, A. (1980). *Seven countries: A multivariate analysis of death and coronary heart disease.* Cambridge, MA: Harvard University Press.

Kromhout, D., Bosschieter, E. B., & Coulander, C. (1985). The inverse relation between fish consumption and 20-year mortality from coronary heart disease. *New England Journal of Medicine, 312*(19), 1205-1209.

Willett, W. C. (1998). *Nutritional epidemiology* (2nd ed.). New York: Oxford University Press.

HEART DISEASE AND PHYSICAL ACTIVITY

Coronary heart disease (CHD) is the leading cause of death in the United States, accounting for over half of all deaths, with an estimated economic cost of more than $320 billion per year. Physical inactivity is a risk factor that may be modifiable and could result in significant reductions in the incidence of CHD. Although it was not until 1992 that the American Heart Association declared physical inactivity to be an independent risk factor for the development of CHD, a number of epidemiological studies conducted over the past four decades have demonstrated an inverse relationship between the level of physical activity and the risk of developing CHD. Moreover, it has been consistently reported that approximately 80% of American adults undertake insufficient amounts of physical activity to gain any health benefit. Physical inactivity may also be disproportionately high in women, minorities, and individuals with lower socioeconomic status.

PRIMARY PREVENTION

Systematic increases in physical activity, which can be performed both in the workplace and during leisure time, consistently improve cardiorespiratory fitness in healthy younger and older individuals. Physical training, that is, dedicated efforts to perform aerobic exercise such as walking, jogging, biking, and swimming, can improve fitness by 15% to 30% after 3 months and may rise by as much as 50% over a 2-year period.

A 1990 meta-analysis of 27 prospective studies in healthy participants showed that sedentary individuals have nearly twice the risk of future CHD as those who are physically active. In addition, it has been shown that active people are not only less likely to have CHD, but compared to their sedentary counterparts, they are also likely to develop less severe heart disease with a delayed onset. Some studies have even found that when compared to those individuals who engage in very high levels of physical activity and who have high levels of fitness, a sedentary or low-activity lifestyle with low fitness levels is associated with up to a sixfold increase in both all-cause and CHD mortality. The reduction in risk associated with physical activity has been observed for both leisure time and work-related physical activity.

Physical activity also is associated with a reduction in CHD risk factors such as hypertension, hyperlipidemia, and diabetes. Other non-CHD benefits include reduced risk of gallbladder disease, increased bone density, and improved psychological functioning. Maintenance of exercise is required to sustain or improve cardiorespiratory fitness; for example, in healthy physically active individuals, 3 weeks of inactivity results in a 10% reduction in fitness, and 3-12 weeks of sedentary behavior can reduce fitness by about 20%.

Recent data from the Health Professionals' Follow-Up Study (44,452 men ages 40 to 75 years), the Nurses' Health Study (72,488 female nurses ages 40 to 65 years), and the Women's Health Initiative (73,743 postmenopausal women ages 50 to 79 years) all have found an inverse dose-response relationship between self-reported energy expenditure from weekly physical activity (average amount of energy expended per hour per week) and risk of developing CHD in initially healthy individuals. After adjusting for multiple risk factors there was a reduction in CHD of 30% to 50% for those in the highest activity quintile when compared to the lowest activity group. All three of these studies found both the intensity (rate of energy expenditure during an activity) and duration of physical activity to be important determinants in the reduction of CHD risk. Studies that have used objective measures of cardiorespiratory fitness (e.g., assessed maximal oxygen uptake) have tended to show an even stronger association with reductions in CHD events than self-report global measures of physical activity, with 70% reduction in CHD risk for those with the highest physical fitness compared to participants who have the lowest levels of fitness.

The majority of the early epidemiological studies involved primarily middle-aged male participants. However, more recent evidence suggests that older men and women also benefit from increased physical activity. For example, reduced levels of walking in 2,678 men, ages 71 to 93 years from the Honolulu Heart Study, were associated with a twofold increase in CHD, and the Iowa Women's Health Study found, in 40,417 women mean age 62 years, an inverse relationship between physical activity and all-cause mortality measured at 7-year follow-up. The Longitudinal Study of Aging found that in 5,901 individuals age 70 or older, high self-reported levels of physical activity were associated with a 54% reduction in all-cause mortality. In addition, studies have generally shown that even moderate-intensity activity is sufficient to obtain significant health benefits, with those that engage in high-intensity activities showing only modest additional reductions in CHD risk. Research has shown that 30 minutes of exercise every day is associated with a 40% to 50% reduction in risk.

There have been several randomized clinical trials that have shown exercise to improve standard CHD risk factors, such as blood pressure and cholesterol levels, and surrogate markers of disease, endothelial function and left ventricular structure, for example. However, to our knowledge, there have been no trials that have assessed the effects of primary prevention physical activity on mortality or other hard clinical CHD end points.

SECONDARY PREVENTION

Chronic exercise training is associated with improvements in cardiorespiratory fitness and functional capacity in patients with established CHD. Twelve weeks of aerobic exercise 30 minutes, three times a week at a moderate intensity (60-85% maximal capacity) is usually sufficient to improve aerobic fitness, enhance functional capacity, and increase the aerobic threshold, which are usually what limit patients' ability to perform the normal activities of daily life.

There have been more than a dozen randomized controlled trials of exercise in CHD patients. In a 1988 meta-analysis of trials involving nearly 4,500 post-myocardial infarction (MI) patients, 6 weeks of moderate-intensity exercise (30-40 minutes at 65-75% of maximum VO_2) was found to reduce 3-year all-cause and CHD mortality by 25%, when compared to control groups of patients who did not exercise. However, when considered individually, the majority of intervention trials fail to find a significant reduction in long-term outcome for those that participated in exercise compared to a nonexercising control group. These data are further complicated by the lack of trials that focus only on exercise and not on multifactorial cardiac rehabilitation, the high prevalence of men (80%), and the relatively young age of the population (< 65 years old). These studies also were conducted before thrombolytic therapy, coronary-stenting, and treatment with angiotensin-converting-enzyme inhibitors, β-blockers, and statins were widely used. A recent report from the British Regional Heart Study, however, supports the findings of the meta-analysis in that walking at least 4 hours per week, in an elderly (age = 63 years old) sample of 772 men with CHD, was associated with a 5-year reduction in all-cause and cardiovascular mortality of 55% and 59%, respectively.

Despite the exercise-related reductions in all-cause and cardiovascular mortality, there is no definitive evidence that exercise is associated with reduced cardiovascular morbidity in CHD patients. None of the reported meta-analyses, controlled trials, or non-randomized trials of exercise have found a significant reduction in nonfatal MI of exercisers compared to nonexercisers.

Increased physical activity in patients with more severe CHD, for example, patients with congestive heart failure (CHF), also appears beneficial. For example, preliminary cross-sectional data in patients with CHF estimated a 100-fold increased risk for MI and a 50-fold increased risk of sudden death in sedentary patients compared to habitual exercisers. Exercise training studies also demonstrate that patients with more severe CHD benefit from exercise. However, sample sizes are limited and there is no conclusive evidence that exercise will reduce long-term mortality in these patients. The ACTION trial is an ongoing multicenter clinical trial of exercise in CHF patients that will address this issue.

In addition to the physical benefits of increased physical activity, improvements in psychological well-being and stress reduction have been seen following participation in an exercise program. Measures of depression, anxiety, emotional distress, self-confidence, social isolation, and quality of life have generally been shown to improve after exercise.

Although exercise appears effective in the reduction of fatal CHD events, a multi-intervention approach including behavioral cardiac risk modification, education, and counseling has been shown to enhance the improvements reported in exercise-only interventions. These other intensive additions also provide added benefit by aiding in the long-term adherence of an exercise program.

RESISTANCE EXERCISE

In studies of low-risk coronary patients, mild to moderate resistance exercise has been shown to improve both muscular strength and cardiovascular endurance. Resistance training, that is, weight lifting or strength exercises, also maintains or increases muscle mass (which helps with exercise-induced carbohydrate metabolism), improves basal metabolism, and has beneficial effects on bone mineral density and flexibility. Apart from providing variety to an exercise regimen, resistance training can improve performance in a variety of tasks encountered in daily life. As such, resistance exercise provides a valuable complement to cardiorespiratory exercise.

RECOMMENDED LEVELS OF EXERCISE

There is still much debate regarding the type, frequency, intensity, and duration of physical activity that confers the greatest health benefits. However, there is no question that being sedentary confers a significant increase in risk in both healthy and cardiac populations. Current guidelines recommend 30-60 minutes of moderate-intensity aerobic exercise (60-75% of maximal capacity) on most, and preferably all, days of the week. This minimum level of physical activity should significantly reduce CHD risk for both healthy individuals and CHD patients. Examples of activities considered to be of moderate intensity include brisk walking (3-4 mph), general calisthenics, home repair work, gardening, and heavy cleaning in the home.

Higher-intensity exercise (70-85% maximal capacity) will result in faster, and potentially larger, improvements in cardiorespiratory fitness. However, the greater tolerance of moderate exercise by patients, and the reduced risk of injury, will likely lead to better long-term adherence. Recommended levels of resistance training are 10-15 repetitions, at a moderate to high intensity, for each of 8-10 different exercise sets covering the whole body (arms, shoulders, chest, trunk, back, hip, and legs). These exercises should be carried out at least twice per week.

RISK OF EXERCISE

For most persons, exercise is a relatively safe activity, but as with the majority of therapies in cardiovascular medicine, there is a small degree of risk associated with exercise. Surveys of supervised exercise programs have found the risk of cardiac arrest to be 1 per 112,000 patient hours of aerobic exercise, nonfatal MI to be 1 per 294,000 patient hours, and sudden cardiac death to be 1 per 784,000 patient hours. In addition, an increased risk of musculoskeletal injury (falls and joint injuries) is associated with increased physical activity; however, these are normally not serious and rarely require medical treatment. These potential risks can be reduced by medical evaluation prior to the onset of a program, an appropriately devised and supervised exercise program, the use of correct equipment, and education about risk management.

POSSIBLE MECHANISMS OF BENEFIT

Increased physical activity sustained over time results in a reduction of myocardial oxygen demand for any given amount of physical work. This change is due to improvements in oxygen delivery to the muscles (higher maximal cardiac output) and oxygen extraction by the muscles, with the net result being an overall increase in an individual's ability to utilize oxygen. This change has a specific benefit for symptomatic CHD patients, as improved fitness will allow them to achieve a higher level of activity before reaching the level of myocardial oxygen demand that results in myocardial ischemia and angina (chest pain). Other direct benefits of exercise on the heart include increased myocardial function, with some studies showing improvements in cardiac performance following sustained exercise, and increased electrical stability of the myocardium, which is thought to occur due to reductions in sympathetic tone and catecholamine release. In addition to the direct effects that exercise has on the heart, it also modulates many biological domains, and by doing so confers enhanced cardioprotection.

Regular exercise is associated with lower levels of blood pressure and heart rate at rest and submaximal workloads. On average, exercise training can reduce resting systolic and diastolic blood pressure, in cardiac patients, by at least 5 mm Hg. Reduced heart rate and lower blood pressure may be accounted for by reductions in peripheral resistance and a drop in resting catecholamine levels, indicative of reduced sympathetic nervous system activity, following chronic exercise training. This phenomenon also has been reported in healthy individuals and patients with essential hypertension.

Improvements in lipid profile and carbohydrate metabolism have been seen following exercise training. Decreases in plasma triglycerides and low-density lipoproteins, increases in high-density lipoproteins, improved adipose tissue distribution, and beneficial changes in insulin sensitivity all have been observed following increases in physical activity.

The endothelium, the layer of vascular cells that are in direct contact with the blood, has many endocrine, autocrine, and paracrine regulatory functions. Endothelial dysfunction is a key component in the development of atherosclerosis and is prevalent in patients with coronary risk factors (e.g., hypertension, hyperlipidemia, and diabetes mellitus). Emerging research suggests that endothelial function is improved following participation in aerobic exercise. Recent evidence also suggests that increases in physical activity reduce thrombogenesis, the process of clot formation in the blood. Plasma levels of fibrinogen, the final substrate of coagulation, the clotting process, have been inversely related to activity levels, and beneficial changes in the fibrinolytic (clot dissolution) system and platelet activation, a prothrombotic process, have been observed following chronic exercise. For example, in a study of post-coronary bypass patients, 4 weeks of exercise was associated with improved endothelium-mediated vasodilation, reduced platelet activation, enhanced fibrinolysis, and beneficial changes in plasma viscosity.

Improved autonomic nervous system functioning, as measured by heart rate variability, is associated with higher levels of physical activity and has been shown to improve following exercise training. An imbalance between sympathetic and parasympathetic activity has been shown to increase the risk of cardiac events. Exercise-induced increases in the high-frequency component of the power spectral analysis, which is thought to reflect improved parasympathetic activity, may correct this imbalance and reduce CHD risk.

Exercise also may be associated with other health benefits that may reduce the risk for CHD events including smoking cessation and improvements in clinical depression. This latter finding is important because depression also is a risk factor for CHD events and has been associated with decreased compliance to prescribed medical therapies.

ADHERENCE

Despite the important health benefits of exercise, long-term adherence to exercise is low. Over 50% of those people who start an exercise program are estimated to stop after 6 months. The issue of adherence is critical because exercise must be maintained for extended periods of time for the health benefits to be realized. Indeed, those who could obtain the greatest benefits from exercise tend to be those individuals who fail to continue exercising.

A number of studies have characterized persons most likely to be nonadherent including demographic, physiological, and psychological characteristics. Demographic variables, such as age, gender, and education, generally fail to distinguish between those who stop exercising and those who continue to exercise. Physical condition has been found to be an important predictor of continued participation in exercise. Those individuals with greater cardiorespiratory fitness and/or increased muscular strength are more likely to maintain exercise both during and after an exercise intervention. A recent review of behavioral medicine interventions found that higher levels of psychological morbidity and more severe symptoms tended to be related to a higher dropout rate in participants. Social introversion and depression have also been related to premature dropout from cardiac rehabilitation programs. It should be noted, however, that there is limited research in this area, especially among elderly populations.

A number of psychological theories have been used to explain exercise behavior. The transtheoretical model of behavior change recently has been applied to the study of exercise behavior. This model postulates that changes in behavior occur in the following stages: precontemplation, contemplation, preparation, action, and maintenance. The stages of change model is both dynamic and stable, as individuals can move back and forth between the stages before developing a stable behavior pattern. This model allows for potential barriers and causes to differ in relative importance within each stage, which means that particular interventions can be tailored to match the corresponding causes of behavior at a specific stage.

For those individuals who participate in structured exercise programs, simple strategies, such as printed reminders, phones calls, involvement of family and/or friends, logistical assistance (e.g., transport and child care), and added incentives (e.g., reward system where participants can obtain T-shirts, pens, or other such goods), may be sufficient to sustain participation. However, in some cases more intensive methods may need to be employed. One potential way in which adherence can be improved is by using motivational interviewing. Motivational interviewing is an approach to the assessment and intervention based on the stages of change model that is designed to identify and reinforce individuals' personal self-motivating statements and reasons to change behavior. This approach to health promotion interventions emphasizes the use of individualized risk appraisal, identification of potential risk reduction strategies, techniques to increase self-efficacy for behavior change, and strategies to prevent relapse and promote retention.

SUMMARY

Despite the large diversity in populations studied, methodologies employed, and measures of physical activity used, exercise has consistently been shown to be inversely related to CHD risk. Being physically active is associated with approximately a 50% reduction in the incidence of CHD. This beneficial effect of activity is seen in those individuals with and without preexisting CHD and in younger and older men and women. The reductions are independent of exercise-induced changes in known cardiovascular risk factors (e.g., blood pressure, lipid profile, and insulin sensitivity).

Finally, of the nearly 14 million Americans who have CHD, it has been estimated that more than 8.5 million would benefit from exercise. Fewer than 20% of CHD patients who could benefit from cardiac rehabilitation actually participate in such programs. Also, despite the important advantages of exercise, long-term adherence to exercise is low. It has been estimated that more than half of the people who start an exercise program will stop after 6 months. Because exercise must be maintained for extended periods of time for the health benefits to be realized, strategies to increase exercise adoption and retention are needed.

—*Simon L. Bacon and James A. Blumenthal*

See also HEART DISEASE: ANGER, DEPRESSION, AND ANXIETY; HEART DISEASE AND DIET; HEART DISEASE AND REACTIVITY; HEART DISEASE AND SMOKING; HEART DISEASE AND TYPE A BEHAVIOR; PHYSICAL ACTIVITY AND HEALTH; PHYSICAL ACTIVITY INTERVENTIONS; PHYSICAL ACTIVITY AND MOOD

Further Reading

Ades, P. A. (2001). Cardiac rehabilitation and secondary prevention of coronary heart disease. *New England Journal of Medicine, 345*, 892-902.

Berlin, J. A., & Colditz, G. A. (1990). A meta-analysis of physical activity in the prevention of coronary heart disease. *American Journal of Epidemiology, 1332*, 612-628.

Fletcher, G. F., Balady, G. J., Amsterdam, E. A., Chaitman, B., et al. (2001). Exercise standards for testing and training. A statement for healthcare professionals from the American Heart Association. *Circulation, 104*, 1694-1740.

Fletcher, G. F., Blalady, G., Blair, S. N., Blumenthal, J., et al. (1996). Statement on exercise: Benefits and recommendations for physical activity programs for all Americans. *Circulation, 94*, 857-862.

Miller, W. R., & Rollnick, S. (1991). *Motivational interviewing: Preparing people for change*. New York: Guilford.

Oldridge, N. B., Guyatt, G. H., Fisher, M. E., & Rimm, A. A. (1988). Cardiac rehabilitation after myocardial infarction: Combined experience of randomized clinical trials. *Journal of the American Medical Association, 260*, 945-990.

Wenger, N. K., Froehlicher, E. S., Smith, L. K., Ades, P. A., et al. (1995). *Cardiac rehabilitation: Clinical practice guidelines*. Rockville, MD: Agency for Health Care Policy and Research and the National Heart, Lung, and Blood Institute.

HEART DISEASE AND REACTIVITY

Longitudinal research indicates that excessive cardiovascular reactivity to stress is an important independent risk factor for the development of heart disease. Cardiovascular reactivity to stress refers to changes in cardiovascular activity (e.g., heart rate, blood pressure) in response to environmental demands, either physical or psychological, challenging or threatening. The term *heart disease* encompasses a variety of cardiovascular diseases, including essential hypertension (high blood pressure), coronary heart disease (coronary atherosclerosis), myocardial infarction (heart attack), and stroke.

Despite significant advances in prevention and treatment, heart disease remains the leading cause of death in the United States. Traditional risk factors for heart disease, such as family history, smoking, obesity, high cholesterol, and diabetes mellitus, predict only a portion of the new cases of cardiovascular disease that develop each year, so there is considerable room for improvement in prediction through the discovery of new risk factors. Psychosocial factors such as environmental stress and certain personality traits (e.g., anger, hostility, competitiveness, dominance, and Type A behavior) have emerged as significant predictors of heart disease. Numerous studies suggest that the pathophysiological link between these psychosocial risk factors and cardiovascular disease may involve excessive sympathetically mediated cardiovascular responses to stress. Going a step further, the "reactivity hypothesis" postulates that excessive cardiovascular reactivity to stress (i.e., cardiovascular hyperreactivity) is an independent marker or mechanism for the development of cardiovascular disease. This hypothesis has generated considerable research over the past 25 years on individual differences in cardiovascular reactivity to stress and risk for cardiovascular disease, using both clinical and preclinical indicators of disease in populations ranging from children to adults.

CARDIOVASCULAR REACTIVITY TO STRESS

Just as exercise stress testing provides important information about cardiac function that is not available from a resting electrocardiogram, the assessment of cardiovascular reactivity to stress provides unique information about hemodynamic function that cannot be gleaned from resting measures of blood pressure (BP) and heart rate (HR). Different laboratory stress tasks tend to elicit different patterns of cardiovascular reactivity, a phenomenon known as stimulus specificity. For example, tasks that involve effortful *active coping* (e.g., mental arithmetic, competitive video games, and active avoidance tasks) elicit primarily a *cardiac* response pattern mediated by the sympathetic nervous system (SNS), including increases in HR, myocardial contractile force (the strength of the heartbeat), cardiac output (CO; the amount of blood pumped by the heart in liters per minute), and systolic BP (SBP). In contrast, tasks that involve inhibitory or *passive coping* (e.g., cold stress, mirror tracing, and passive avoidance tasks) elicit primarily a *vascular* response pattern mediated by the SNS, including increases in total peripheral vascular resistance (TPR; the systemic resistance to blood flow through the arteries) and diastolic BP (DBP), along with HR responses mediated by the parasympathetic nervous system (PNS).

Paul A. Obrist, a pioneer in theory and research on cardiovascular reactivity, was perhaps the first psychophysiologist to distinguish between patterns of cardiovascular and autonomic reactivity elicited by active versus passive coping tasks. Nevertheless, as Obrist noted early on, there are substantial individual differences in the magnitude and pattern of cardiovascular responses to stress that cut across different types of tasks. Such individual differences are an important prerequisite in establishing cardiovascular reactivity to stress as a risk factor for cardiovascular disease because heart disease develops only in some individuals.

Stability and Heritability
of Cardiovascular Reactivity to Stress

Given that heart disease develops over a protracted period of time in the context of varying environmental demands, most researchers posit that cardiovascular reactivity to stress must be a relatively stable trait of individuals over time and across various laboratory challenges in order to qualify as a marker or mechanism of cardiovascular disease. Moreover, given that most forms of heart disease have a substantial genetic component, it seems reasonable to posit that individual differences in cardiovascular reactivity to stress must show a substantial degree of heritability.

Numerous studies have documented the stability of individual differences in cardiovascular reactivity to stress over time and different stressors in both children and adults. Estimates of intertask consistency range from $r = .15$ to $r = .82$ for various measures of reactivity, with greater consistency occurring across tasks that elicit similar hemodynamic response patterns (e.g., mental arithmetic and video game challenges). Average estimates of the temporal stability for reactivity to various tasks over retest intervals ranging from 2 days to 10 years are $r = .61$ for HR, $r = .51$ for SBP, and $r = .34$ for DBP. In general, the temporal stability of cardiovascular reactivity improves when (a) measures are aggregated across comparable tasks, (b) data are acquired and scored using standardized procedures, and (c) steps are taken to counteract response habituation over repeated testing sessions. Under these conditions, estimates of the stability of cardiovascular reactivity range from $r = .60$ to .85. Thus, measures of cardiovascular reactivity to stress are sufficiently stable over time to serve as potential markers or mechanisms of cardiovascular disease.

Twin studies have documented substantial heritability for measures of cardiovascular reactivity to stress, with heritability estimates (h^2) ranging from .22 to .81 for HR and BP reactivity to mental arithmetic, video game, and cold stress. In an emerging trend, recent studies have reported associations between cardiovascular reactivity to stress and variations in specific genes that regulate relevant neurotransmitters, hormones, and their receptors.

Technological Advances
in Hemodynamic Assessment

Most research on cardiovascular reactivity to stress has relied on traditional noninvasive measures of cardiovascular function such as SBP, DBP, and HR. Nonetheless, consistent with Ohm's law, BP responses to stress arise from interactive changes in CO and TPR ($BP = CO \times TPR$). Moreover, HR responses to stress arise from complex interactions between the SNS (accelerative effects) and the PNS (decelerative effects). Fortunately, technological innovations such as impedance cardiography offer reliable and valid noninvasive measures of CO and TPR, as well as valid measures of myocardial contractile force such as the cardiac preejection period (PEP; the time it takes the heart to contract strongly enough to pump blood out to the body during each heartbeat).

Impedance cardiography works by applying a safe amount of radio frequency electrical current across the chest and then sensing the decrease in electrical resistance or impedance that occurs as the heart pumps blood to the body. Impedance cardiographic measures of cardiovascular reactivity to stress exhibit satisfactory temporal stability in children and adults, with retest reliability coefficients ranging from $r = .49$ to .65 for CO, $r = .38$ to .58 for TPR, and $r = .43$ to .69 for PEP. In addition to providing information about cardiac and vascular contributions to BP reactivity, impedance cardiographic measures such as PEP and CO are particularly sensitive to SNS stimulation of β-adrenergic receptors on the heart, which are the primary cardiac receptors for the SNS neurotransmitter norepinephrine and the related adrenal hormone epinephrine. Thus, while the study of BP and HR can be extremely informative, the added dimension of cardiovascular assessment provided by impedance cardiographic measures of CO, TPR, and PEP offers great promise for investigating specific mechanisms of BP control and heart disease risk.

Cardiovascular Reactivity
to Stress and Heart Disease

Studies of the association between cardiovascular reactivity to stress and heart disease have involved both animal models and human populations. Despite some conflicting reports, the evidence shows by and large that excessive cardiovascular reactivity to stress is associated with a number of established risk factors for cardiovascular disease, including sex, race, socioeconomic status, and family history of heart disease, as well as psychological predictors of heart disease such as anger, hostility, competitiveness, dominance, Type A behavior, and depression. Much of this evidence has come from cross-sectional studies that cannot establish whether cardiovascular reactivity is a marker or mechanism of disease, but these findings have encouraged a remarkable number of prospective studies designed to determine whether cardiovascular reactivity to stress is predictive of future heart disease.

Much of the prospective research on cardiovascular reactivity as a risk factor for heart disease has involved longitudinal studies of children and young adults who are healthy at the time of initial assessment. A focus on children and young adults, rather than cardiac patients and older adults, is an important and appropriate research strategy because heart disease has its origins in childhood and adolescence, but healthy individuals in this age range should have minimal end-organ damage resulting from disease processes. Thus, this strategy permits the identification of factors that are potential causes as opposed to consequences of cardiovascular disease. Moreover, identifying early markers and etiological factors may help identify individuals at risk for heart disease, thereby enhancing early prevention and treatment efforts. Nevertheless, longitudinal studies of heart disease risk in children and young adults require lengthy periods of study before significant numbers of individuals develop clinical disease end points such as established hypertension, coronary heart disease, myocardial infarction, or stroke.

In the meantime, many researchers have resorted to a method of successive approximation by studying the association between cardiovascular reactivity to stress and preclinical indictors of heart disease that are strong predictors of cardiovascular morbidity and mortality, such as pre-hypertensive elevations in blood pressure over a span of a few years, and ultrasound measures of left ventricular mass (a measure of heart size) and carotid atherosclerosis (a measure of clogging in the carotid arteries). Although the study of these intermediate preclinical indicators is an efficient stopgap, it is nonetheless a step removed from establishing a definitive link between cardiovascular reactivity and heart disease.

Cardiovascular Reactivity to Stress and Essential Hypertension

Several important animal models of hypertension have been developed, using primarily genetically vulnerable strains of mice and rats (e.g., spontaneously hypertensive and borderline hypertensive rats).

Animal studies using these models have generally shown that environmental stress can trigger elevations in BP and the development of hypertension, and that SNS activation and cardiovascular reactivity contribute significantly to the etiological process.

A number of human case-control studies have shown that cardiovascular reactivity to stress is exaggerated in patients with essential hypertension and in normotensive people at risk for hypertension, including individuals with a family history of hypertension, individuals with borderline hypertension, and African Americans. This research has focused primarily on cardiovascular responses mediated by the SNS, but recent evidence suggests that additional vasoconstrictive substances such as endothelin-1 and vasodilatory substances such as nitric oxide may contribute to cardiovascular reactivity as well.

Although elevated TPR is the prevailing hemodynamic characteristic of established hypertension, early stages in the development of hypertension may involve increased TPR, increased CO, or a combination of the two. Moreover, these different hemodynamic profiles may occur to different degrees in different subgroups of people at risk for hypertension, such as young African Americans and borderline hypertensives. For example, research suggests that young African Americans tend to show heightened vascular reactivity to stress, whereas young borderline hypertensives (especially males) tend to show heightened cardiac reactivity to stress. The fact that these early hemodynamic profiles somehow shift eventually to sustained elevations in TPR during the development of hypertension reinforces the importance of studying young individuals at early stages of risk in longitudinal investigations.

Over a dozen different laboratories have published more than two dozen longitudinal studies evaluating the association between cardiovascular reactivity to stress in children and adults and the subsequent development of elevated resting BP. Despite some notable failures, more than 75% of these studies have found supportive evidence indicating that excessive cardiovascular reactivity to stress is a significant predictor of later elevated BP and essential hypertension.

Three studies have reported that BP reactivity to the cold pressor test, involving the immersion of a hand or a foot in ice water, predicts the development of essential hypertension in adulthood over a period of 20 years or longer. Using preclinical elevations in resting BP as an intermediate indicator, several studies have shown that excessive cardiovascular responses to various forms of cold stress (the cold pressor test, cold stress with an icepack on the forehead, and whole-body cold exposure) predict BP elevations in children and adolescents over periods ranging from 1 to 5 years.

Over a dozen studies have shown that cardiovascular hyperreactivity to psychological stress predicts later elevations in resting BP and the development of hypertension. Most of these studies used mental arithmetic tasks or challenging video games to elicit psychological stress. Several studies have found that cardiovascular responses during a competitive video game task predict elevations in resting BP in children and young adults over a period of 1 to 5 years, and one of these studies found that BP hyperreactivity predicted the early development of hypertension in young adults. Likewise, several studies have shown that cardiovascular responses to mental arithmetic stress predict subsequent elevations in resting BP in children and adults, including the development of established hypertension in young borderline hypertensives, over periods ranging from 5 months to 10 years. Other studies have reported positive associations between cardiovascular reactivity and later elevated BP and hypertension using other psychological stressors, such as active shock-avoidance, mirror tracing, and anticipation of bicycle exercise.

In most of these studies, the relationship between measures of cardiovascular reactivity to stress and subsequent BP elevations and hypertension remained significant after controlling for other risk factors for high blood pressure, including initial resting BP, age, sex, race, socioeconomic status, body mass, and family history of heart disease. Thus, measures of cardiovascular reactivity to cold and psychological stress are apparently unique and independent predictors of future elevations in resting BP and the development of essential hypertension.

Studies of cardiovascular reactivity to stress and hypertensive risk have relied almost exclusively on measures of BP reactivity. However, even studies that have included more sophisticated hemodynamic measures of cardiac and vascular reactivity, such as impedance cardiographic measures of CO and TPR, have generally found that measures of BP reactivity were the best predictors of preclinical and clinical elevations in BP. Given that BP responses result from the interactive effects of cardiac and vascular responses (BP = CO × TPR), these findings may signify

that hypertensive risk is greatest when the normal homeostatic balance between cardiac performance and vascular resistance breaks down, so that both CO and TPR increase during stress, thereby generating heightened BP responses.

Cardiovascular Reactivity to Stress and Coronary Heart Disease

Perhaps the best evidence for the role of behavioral factors in the pathophysiology of coronary heart disease comes from an animal model developed by Jay R. Kaplan, Stephen B. Manuck, and colleagues, using the cynomolgus macaque. This species of monkey engages in complex patterns of social interaction resembling aspects of human social behavior, including the establishment of social status hierarchies. Like humans, these monkeys also develop coronary atherosclerosis, cardiovascular abnormalities, and high rates of myocardial infarction when fed a diet high in saturated fat and cholesterol. Kaplan, Manuck, and colleagues have used threat of capture and disruption of social hierarchies, sometimes in combination with dietary manipulations of saturated fat and cholesterol, to study the impact of psychosocial stress on the development of coronary atherosclerosis in these monkeys.

Several key findings from this elegant work support an association between cardiovascular reactivity to stress and the development of coronary heart disease. First, psychosocial stress, involving exposure to a new social group or the threat of capture by an experimenter, elicited significant increases in HR in most monkeys. Second, there were substantial individual differences in the magnitude of these HR responses to stress. Third, the monkeys that showed the largest HR reactions to threat developed enlarged hearts and the largest atherosclerotic lesions in coronary arteries. Fourth, pharmacological treatment with β-adrenergic antagonists (β-blockers) blocked the HR response to social stress and prevented coronary endothelial injury, particularly at branching sites in the coronary arteries where the greatest degree of hemodynamic stress occurs. Thus, this research demonstrated a positive association between cardiac reactivity to stress and key clinical features of coronary heart disease, and provided important evidence suggesting that β-adrenergic SNS activation and hemodynamic stress in critical arterial segments may contribute to the pathophysiological process.

A substantial number of studies have evaluated the relationship between cardiovascular reactivity to stress and clinical indicators of coronary heart disease in cardiac patients. The clinical indicators have included cardiac events such as myocardial infarction, measures of arterial occlusion determined by coronary angiography, and measures of myocardial ischemia (measures of deficient blood flow and oxygen delivery to the heart) determined by radionuclide ventriculography, echocardiography, or electrocardiography during exercise stress testing. Although some of these studies have failed to find any association between cardiovascular reactivity and clinical indications of coronary heart disease, several studies have reported positive results. For the most part, the positive findings have involved significant associations between clinical outcomes and increases in DBP and TPR during cold or psychological stress.

The Psychophysiological Investigations of Myocardial Ischemia (PIMI) study is an excellent example of a large-scale investigation of cardiovascular reactivity to stress and clinical events in cardiac patients. The PIMI study found that a substantial number of patients with coronary artery disease experienced myocardial ischemia during psychological stress in the laboratory, involving public speaking and the Stroop color-word conflict test, and that these ischemic episodes were associated with increases in TPR. Ischemic episodes in the laboratory also were associated with increases in HR and BP during public speaking, which was generally more provocative than the Stroop test. In contrast, episodes of myocardial ischemia in daily life, as determined by ambulatory electrocardiography, were associated with a different profile of cardiovascular reactivity during public speaking in the laboratory, consisting of increases in myocardial contractile force and CO, but *decreases* in TPR. Although these findings are promising, further research is needed to resolve the discrepancies and elucidate the underlying mechanisms of ischemia in different environments.

Compared to the work on elevated BP and hypertension, there has been relatively little longitudinal research on cardiovascular reactivity to stress and the development of coronary heart disease. Half a dozen longitudinal studies have evaluated the relationship between cardiovascular reactivity to stress in adults and later indices of cardiovascular morbidity and mortality over periods ranging from 3 to 27 years. Various forms of stress have been used in these studies,

including the cold pressor test and a variety of psychological stressors (e.g., mental arithmetic, public speaking, the Stroop test), but all of the studies have relied solely on measures of BP and HR reactivity. The results have been mixed, with about half of the studies reporting that BP reactivity predicted later cardiac events after controlling for other cardiovascular risk factors.

A number of studies have investigated the relationship between cardiovascular reactivity to stress and preclinical indicators of coronary heart disease. The principal preclinical indicators used so far have been ultrasound measures of left ventricular mass (LVM) and carotid atherosclerosis. Increased LVM is strongly predictive of cardiovascular morbidity and mortality, whereas carotid atherosclerosis is moderately associated with coronary atherosclerosis.

Several cross-sectional studies have investigated the relationship between cardiovascular reactivity to stress and LVM in children and adults. The studies with children were conducted in Karen A. Matthews's laboratory at the University of Pittsburgh and Frank A. Treiber's laboratory at the Medical College of Georgia. Both laboratories have included impedance cardiographic measures of cardiac and vascular reactivity as well as measures of BP reactivity. These studies have found fairly consistent evidence of a positive relationship between heightened cardiovascular reactivity to stress, especially vasoconstrictive reactivity, and increased LVM in children. All of the adult studies were conducted in different laboratories and were limited to measures of BP reactivity. The results of these studies were less consistent, although each study reported at least some evidence of an association between BP reactivity and cardiac structure.

In addition to these cross-sectional studies, longitudinal studies of children conducted in Treiber's laboratory have found that cardiovascular hyperreactivity to various forms of physical and psychological stress predicted increases in LVM between 2 and 4 years later. An additional longitudinal study of middle-aged Swedish men found that BP hyperreactivity to physical and psychological stress predicted increases in LVM over a 3-year period. For the most part, the association between cardiovascular reactivity and later LVM in these longitudinal studies remained significant after controlling for factors such as sex, race, body mass, and initial baseline measures.

Two cross-sectional studies and four longitudinal studies of middle-aged adults have examined the relationship between cardiovascular reactivity to psychological stress and extent of carotid atherosclerosis. One of the cross-sectional studies examined BP reactivity in anticipation of bicycle exercise, using data from the Kuopio Ischemic Heart Disease (KIHD) Study, a population-based epidemiological study of middle-aged men in Finland. The other cross-sectional study investigated BP reactivity to a battery of behavioral challenges in middle-aged, untreated hypertensive men. Both studies found positive associations between BP reactivity and extent of carotid atherosclerosis.

Likewise, all four longitudinal studies found that BP hyperreactivity to psychological stress predicted the development of carotid atherosclerosis in middle-aged men and women over periods ranging from 2 to 4 years. Two of these studies reported longitudinal data from the KIHD study, and found that the progression of carotid atherosclerosis in men over a 4-year period was predicted by a combination of anticipatory BP reactivity and chronic life stress, as measured by job stress in one study and socio-economic disadvantage in the other. The associations between BP reactivity and carotid atherosclerosis in these studies generally remained significant after controlling for various risk factors and confounds, suggesting that excessive BP reactivity to stress is an independent predictor of this preclinical indicator of coronary heart disease.

Finally, further prospective data from the KIHD study has shown that SBP hyperreactivity in anticipation of bicycle exercise predicted the incidence of stroke in middle-aged Finnish men over 11 years later. The relationship was strongest for ischemic strokes. Adjusting for other risk factors did not alter the predictive relationship, suggesting that SBP reactivity to stress is a promising independent risk factor for stroke and cerebrovascular disease.

LINGERING QUESTIONS AND FUTURE DIRECTIONS

The available evidence indicates that excessive cardiovascular reactivity to stress is a useful predictor of heart disease, but several issues remain unresolved. Although these issues are relevant to considerations of cardiovascular reactivity as a marker or risk factor, they are especially relevant to considerations of cardiovascular reactivity as a possible casual mechanism of heart disease.

Many of the longitudinal studies of cardiovascular reactivity to stress and risk for heart disease have used a single stressor to elicit cardiovascular responses, and many studies have assessed reactivity by using a single BP measurement during stress. As already noted, measurement reliability and accuracy generally improve when multiple measurements are obtained over multiple tasks, so many of these studies probably suffered from poor measurement reliability, thereby hampering attempts at replication and generalization in new studies. A thorough evaluation of individual differences in cardiovascular reactivity to stress is likely to require more sophisticated approaches involving multiple cardiac, vascular, and BP measurements obtained repeatedly during a battery of stressors that "covers the waterfront" of stressful experiences that occur regularly in real life.

As noted earlier, heart disease develops over a protracted period of time in the context of varying environmental demands. Therefore, many investigators posit that cardiovascular reactivity to stress in the laboratory should generalize to reactivity in daily life where the disease process unfolds. However, relatively few studies have evaluated the relationship between laboratory assessments of cardiovascular reactivity during standardized tests and ambulatory assessments of cardiovascular reactivity during daily life.

Some of these studies have yielded disappointing results, which some investigators have ascribed to shortcomings in laboratory research. However, there are considerable difficulties and shortcomings in ambulatory research that require attention. Methodological advancements in ambulatory cardiovascular assessment are clearly needed, as are theoretical advancements in the conceptualization of cardiovascular reactivity as a potential mechanism in the development of heart disease. For example, some ambulatory studies have used rather gross or arbitrary distinctions to characterize daily events and situations as stressful or nonstressful (e.g., work vs. home environments). A better characterization of stressful events and situations in daily life, along with development of parallel stressors for use in the laboratory, would likely improve the correlation between ambulatory and laboratory measures of cardiovascular reactivity.

Researchers have used a variety of methods to define cardiovascular responses to stress, including simple gain or change scores (i.e., the difference between stress and baseline periods), baseline-adjusted gain scores, absolute response levels, peak responses, and average responses. The inconsistent use of such different approaches across studies is problematic. It is unclear whether peak or sustained cardiovascular responses are most significant, or whether the amount of change or the absolute response level is most critical, in the development of cardiovascular disease. Additional research on the topography of cardiovascular responses to stress may be crucial for understanding the association between cardiovascular reactivity and heart disease.

It also is increasingly clear that the "reactivity hypothesis" requires revision and elaboration. For example, there is considerable evidence indicating that repeated exposure to stress attenuates cardiovascular reactivity. It is difficult to reconcile this habituation of cardiovascular reactivity with the strong form of the reactivity hypothesis, which postulates that recurrent activation of excessive cardiovascular responses to stress leads to the development of heart disease. Further research on factors that promote or disrupt cardiovascular reactivity and adaptation to recurrent stress may clarify the role of cardiovascular reactivity in the development of heart disease.

Based on recent longitudinal findings, Kathleen C. Light and colleagues at the University of North Carolina have proposed a "gene and environment modulated reactivity hypothesis." Briefly stated, they have hypothesized that heightened cardiovascular reactivity to stress is primarily associated with an increased risk of cardiovascular disease in individuals with a genetic vulnerability for heart disease and/or high exposure to chronic or recurrent environmental stress (e.g., socioeconomic disadvantage, high job stress). Some of the findings from the KIHD study, reviewed earlier, are consistent with this hypothesis. Personality is also a potential moderator of the association between cardiovascular reactivity to stress and heart disease, as personality plays an important role in determining an individual's perceptions of and responses to environmental stress. Of course, this revised hypothesis is considerably more complicated than the original version of the reactivity hypothesis, particularly since cardiovascular reactivity itself is influenced by both genetic and environmental factors.

In summary, a proper evaluation of the potential etiological significance of cardiovascular reactivity to stress in the development of heart disease awaits important theoretical and methodological advancements. Fortunately, a number of investigators are pursuing innovative solutions to these problems. In the meantime, it seems safest to view cardiovascular reactivity to stress as a promising risk factor that may provide useful independent information for the prediction of various forms of heart disease.

—*Robert M. Kelsey*

See also BLOOD PRESSURE AND HYPERTENSION: MEASUREMENT; BLOOD PRESSURE, HYPERTENSION, AND STRESS; CARDIOVASCULAR PSYCHOPHYSIOLOGY: MEASURES; CARDIOVASCULAR REACTIVITY; HEART DISEASE: ANGER, DEPRESSION, AND ANXIETY; HEART DISEASE AND TYPE A BEHAVIOR

Further Reading

Allen, M. T., Matthews, K. A., & Sherman, F. S. (1997). Cardiovascular reactivity to stress and left ventricular mass in youth. *Hypertension, 30,* 782-787.

Blascovich, J., & Katkin, E. S. (1993). *Cardiovascular reactivity to psychological stress and disease.* Washington, DC: American Psychological Association.

Goldberg, A. D., Becker, L. C., Bonsall, R., Cohen, J. D., Ketterer, M. W., Kaufman, P. G., Krantz, D. S., Light, K. C., McMahon, R. P., Noreuil, T., Pepine, C. J., Raczynski, J., Stone, P. H., Strother, D., Taylor, H., & Sheps, D. S. (1996). Ischemic, hemodynamic, and neurohormonal responses to mental and exercise stress: Experience from the Psychophysiological Investigations of Myocardial Ischemia Study (PIMI). *Circulation, 94,* 2402-2409.

Krantz, D. S., & Manuck, S. B. (1984). Acute psychophysiologic reactivity and risk for cardiovascular disease: A review and methodologic critique. *Psychological Bulletin, 96,* 435-464.

Light, K. C., Girdler, S. S., Sherwood, A., Bragdon, E. E., Brownley, K. A., West, S. G., & Hinderleiter, A. L. (1999). High stress responsivity predicts later blood pressure only in combination with positive family history and high life stress. *Hypertension, 33,* 1458-1464.

Manuck, S. B., Kaplan, J. R., Adams, M. R., & Clarkson, T. B. (1988). Effects of stress and the sympathetic nervous system on coronary artery atherosclerosis in the cynomolgus macaque. *American Heart Journal, 116,* 328-333.

Obrist, P. A. (1981). *Cardiovascular psychophysiology: A perspective.* New York: Plenum.

Sherwood, A., Allen, M. T., Fahrenberg, J., Kelsey, R. M., Lovallo, W. R., & van Doornen, L. J. P. (1990). Committee report: Methodological guidelines for impedance cardiography. *Psychophysiology, 27,* 1-23.

Treiber, F. A., Kamarck, T., Schneiderman, N., Sheffield, D., Kapuku, G., & Taylor, T. (2003). Cardiovascular reactivity and development of preclinical and clinical disease states. *Psychosomatic Medicine, 65*, 46-62.

HEART DISEASE AND SMOKING

THE BURDEN OF HEART DISEASE ASSOCIATED WITH SMOKING

Coronary heart disease (CHD) is the leading cause of death among women (42.3%) and men (38.1%) in the United States. An estimated 1.1 million Americans develop a new or recurrent heart attack each year. Cigarette smoking is one of the most important modifiable risk factors for heart disease. Epidemiological studies indicate that smoking increases the risk of CHD incidence and mortality by a factor of 2 to 3. According to the Office of the Surgeon General, 41% and 45% of CHD deaths among women and men aged less than 65 years, respectively, are attributable to cigarette smoking (U.S. Department of Health and Human Services [DHHS], 1989). The attributable risks for CHD deaths among women and men over the age of 65 are 12% and 21%, respectively. These attributable risks translate into 115,000 CHD deaths each year caused by cigarette smoking.

The risk for CHD rises with the number of cigarettes smoked daily, the total number of years of smoking, the degree of inhalation, and early age at initiation of smoking (DHHS, 2001). There is no discernable threshold of smoking intensity below which increased risk of CHD is not apparent. Regular smokers of as few as 1 to 4 cigarettes per day have been shown to experience a near doubling in the risk of CHD compared with never smokers (Kawachi et al., 1994). Cigarette smoking also has been shown to interact with other risk factors, particularly hypertension, elevated serum cholesterol, and diabetes mellitus, to greatly increase the risk of CHD.

Epidemiological and experimental studies have yielded little or no evidence supporting harm reduction for CHD stemming from the use of filtered or "low yield" cigarettes. It is well known that users of these products behaviorally compensate for the reduced yield of nicotine and tar by increasing the amount of cigarettes smoked, by inhaling more frequently and more deeply, or by blocking the air dilution vents on cigarette filters. Consequently, the intake of toxic tobacco constituents remains unchanged among smokers who switch from "conventional" yield to low-yield cigarettes. Epidemiological studies have indicated no material difference in the risk of CHD among users of conventional cigarettes compared with users of brands advertised as yielding lower levels of nicotine, tar, or carbon monoxide.

Besides CHD, active smoking has been linked to other cardiovascular diseases, including stroke, peripheral vascular disease, and ruptured aortic aneurysms (DHHS, 2001).

CAUSAL MECHANISMS LINKING SMOKING TO CHD RISK

Cigarette smoking increases the risk of CHD through a combination of acute and long-term pathophysiological mechanisms. In the short term, exposure to cigarette smoke can cause an imbalance between myocardial oxygen supply and demand, coronary artery spasm, increased platelet adhesiveness and aggregation, and a decreased ventricular fibrillation threshold. These acute effects can manifest as coronary ischemia and symptoms of angina, blockage of compromised coronary blood vessels (the most common cause of acute myocardial infarction), and cardiac arrhythmias and sudden cardiac death. In the long term, cigarette smoking contributes to the development and progression of coronary atherosclerosis, which is the pathological thickening and occlusion of the lumen of the coronary blood vessels that predispose them to blood clots (thrombosis) and "heart attack." The likely mechanisms underlying these chronic effects of cigarette smoking on atherosclerosis progression include repetitive injury to the lining of the coronary blood vessels (the endothelium) caused by the toxic constituents of tobacco smoke, as well as long-term metabolic disturbances such as a decreased high-density lipoprotein (HDL)/low-density lipoprotein (LDL) ratio, and abnormalities in the synthesis of thromboxane A_2 and prostacyclin.

Observational evidence has established a link between smoking and the progression of subclinical atherosclerosis, as assessed by noninvasive, B-mode ultrasound measurement of plaque size, vessel wall thickness, and degree of narrowing (stenosis) of the carotid arteries (DHHS, 2001). Furthermore, a dose-response relationship has been demonstrated between pack-years of smoking and carotid arterial wall thickness. Cessation of smoking appears to slow the progression of atherosclerosis. In turn, subclinical carotid atherosclerosis has been shown to be a marker of future risk of CHD as well as stroke and transient ischemic attacks.

THE BENEFITS OF SMOKING CESSATION

Longitudinal studies of smoking cessation indicate a substantial (25-45%) reduction in the excess risk of CHD within 1 to 2 years of quitting. However, due to the cumulative, long-term damage wrought by smoking, it takes longer than 2 years for the excess risk of CHD among former smokers to completely revert to the level of never smokers. Current evidence suggests that it takes at least 5 years, and perhaps as long as 10 to 15 years of cessation, for the risk of CHD to completely dissipate. On the other hand, the benefits of smoking cessation for reduced CHD risk appear to be available to smokers regardless of their age at initiation of smoking, age at quitting, intensity of smoking prior to cessation, and overall duration of smoking, as well as the presence of established CHD (Kawachi et al., 1994).

PASSIVE SMOKING AND CHD RISK

Passive smoking (also referred to as involuntary smoking) refers to the second-hand exposure to side-stream tobacco smoke emitted from the burning end of a lit cigarette. Side-stream tobacco smoke contains the same mixture of toxic compounds as mainstream smoke (the cigarette smoke inhaled by the smoker), but often in higher concentrations due to the incomplete combustion of tobacco. Given that there is no demonstrable lower limit for the toxic effects of cigarette smoke, it is biologically plausible that individuals exposed to side-stream smoke would experience a similar range of adverse effects as active smokers, albeit in smaller doses.

Nearly two dozen cohort studies and case-control studies have now examined the association between passive smoking and CHD risk (DHHS, 2001). Although few of the risk estimates in individual studies were statistically significant, pooled estimates from meta-analyses indicate a significant 30% increase in the risk for CHD with passive smoking. Based on these findings, as well as supporting experimental

evidence on pathological mechanisms, the Office of the Surgeon General has concluded that the association between passive smoking and CHD in smokers is causal (DHHS, 2001). Passive smoking has been estimated to be responsible for an additional 30,000 excess cases of CHD deaths each year in the United States.

—*Ichiro Kawachi*

See also HEART DISEASE: ANGER, DEPRESSION, AND ANXIETY; HEART DISEASE AND DIET; HEART DISEASE AND PHYSICAL ACTIVITY; HEART DISEASE AND TYPE A BEHAVIOR; SMOKING AND HEALTH; SMOKING AND NICOTINE DEPENDENCE: INTERVENTIONS; SMOKING PREVENTION AND TOBACCO CONTROL AMONG YOUTH

Further Reading

Kawachi, I., Colditz, G. A., Stampfer, M. J., Willett, W. C., Manson, J. E., Rosner, B., Speizer, F. E., & Hennekens, C. H. (1994). Smoking cessation and time course of decreased risk of coronary heart disease in women. *Archives of Internal Medicine, 154,* 169-175.

U.S. Department of Health and Human Services. (1989). *Reducing the health consequences of smoking: 25 years of progress. A report of the surgeon general.* DHHS Publication No. (CDC) 89-8411. Rockville, MD: U.S. Department of Health and Human Services, Public Health Service, Centers for Disease Control, Center for Chronic Disease Prevention and Health Promotion, Office on Smoking and Health.

U.S. Department of Health and Human Services. (2001). *Women and smoking: A report of the surgeon general.* Rockville, MD: U.S. Department of Health and Human Services, Public Health Service, Office of the Surgeon General.

HEART DISEASE AND TYPE A BEHAVIOR

CHARACTERISTICS AND ASSESSMENT

In the 1950s, cardiologists Meyer Friedman and Ray Rosenman observed that their cardiac patients were more likely to display a specific combination of behaviors called the Type A behavior pattern (TABP) in comparison to individuals without heart disease.

TABP was defined as an action-emotion complex stimulated by certain environmental events, and is characterized by impatience, a tendency toward hostility and aggressiveness, and a heightened sense of time urgency. TABP was also often manifested by facial tension, rapid and impatient speech, tongue and teeth clicking, and expressed or suppressed hostility. A contrasting Type B behavior pattern was characterized by the relative lack of these behavioral characteristics and the tendency toward more relaxed behavior.

Two general methods have been used to assess the presence or absence of TABP: structured interviews and self-report questionnaires. The Structured Interview (SI) method developed by Rosenman and Friedman, and a subsequent videotaped Structured Interview (VSI), are considered the best means of TABP assessment. During the SI, individuals are asked a series of questions such as how they react to waiting in lines, driving in slow traffic, and facing deadlines at work and home. The interviewer evaluates the degree to which feelings of impatience, hostility, and/or competitiveness are expressed, as well as the style of response. Stylistic indications of TABP would include explosive, loud, and rapid speech, and indications of a potential for hostility. The VSI is videotaped so that Type A indicators such as head nodding, rapid eye blinking, hostile facial expressions, and vigorous gestures can be seen. Disadvantages of using the SI and the VSI are the intensive interviewer training that is required, variability due to the interviewer's behavior while interviewing subjects, and the variability in scoring taped interviews.

Several self-report questionnaires have been used in studying TABP, such as the Bortner Rating Scale Type, the Framingham Type A Scale, and the Jenkins Activity Survey (JAS). The disadvantage of such measures, however, is that they rely on self-perceptions, which may not be accurate. Furthermore, individuals may be influenced by the desire to endorse socially admired characteristics. Nevertheless, self-report methods have the distinct advantages of being less expensive and easier to administer than structured interviews, and have proven to predict coronary disease in some studies (see below). Structured interviews are generally preferred over questionnaires because they directly evaluate behavior and have the strongest association with coronary heart disease (CHD).

EARLY RESEARCH ON TABP ASSOCIATIONS WITH HEART DISEASE

Large-scale epidemiological studies on TABP as a risk factor for heart disease began in the early 1960s. The Western Collaborative Group Study (WCGS) followed 3,524 men, ages 39 to 59 years, with annual follow-ups for approximately 8 to 9 years (Rosenman et al., 1975). Information such as medical history, socioeconomic factors, physical activity, diet, and cigarette smoking was collected, but the particular focus of the study was the measurement of coronary-prone behavior. TABP was assessed using the SI, with the final behavioral rating being made without knowledge of standard risk factors. Three key findings of the WCGS supported the TABP-heart disease association: (1) TABP was an independent risk factor for heart disease, (2) men characterized as Type A had roughly twice the risk of developing heart disease as their Type B counterparts, and (3) the pattern was a good predictor of a second heart attack in men who had already suffered one.

Similar results were found in another large, prospective study, the Framingham Heart Study, which has followed more than 5,209 healthy residents of the town of Framingham, Massachusetts, since 1948 (Haynes, Feinleib, & Kannel, 1980). Participants were between 30 and 60 years of age at the time of enrollment, and included both men and women. Type A behavior in Framingham participants was significantly correlated with the risk of CHD in both men and women. These and subsequent studies offered enough evidence for the National Heart, Lung, and Blood Institute to publish a critical review in 1981 in which a consensus of psychologists and cardiologists concluded that TABP was an independent risk factor for coronary heart disease in middle-aged U.S. citizens in industrialized geographic areas (Review Panel on Coronary-Prone Behavior and Coronary Heart Disease, 1981).

CONTRADICTORY FINDINGS

Despite these promising early results, the majority of studies conducted since 1979 have not reported a positive relationship between TABP and coronary heart disease. For example, an 8.5-year follow-up of the WCGS revealed that among patients who survived the 24-hour period following a coronary event, Type A patients had a significantly lower mortality rate than Type B patients. Furthermore, a 22-year follow-up of the WCGS study found that Type A behavior was not predictive of disease progression and that Type A behavior was found to be associated with longer survival in the WCGS cohort. Other studies such as the Multiple Risk Factor Intervention Trial (MRFIT) have also called the cardiovascular significance of TABP into question. From 1973 to 1976, the MRFIT study enrolled 12,866 men between the ages of 35 and 57. The men were free of heart disease at the time of enrollment, but were selected because of their high risk factors, such as smoking status, high blood pressure, and high cholesterol. Type A behavior was also of interest, and was classified by using the JAS and SI methods. Half of the participants received counseling in smoking cessation and diet; all were monitored for heart disease for up to 17 years. No difference in the rates of heart disease development was found as a function of Type A behavior assessed by either the JAS or SI (Shekelle et al., 1985).

It has been suggested that the discrepancy among study outcomes may be due to the methods used to assess Type A in these studies. Friedman and Ghandour (1993) have argued that the detection of TABP, similar to other diseases, cannot be made by either a written or orally administered questionnaire. Nevertheless, TABP investigations have generally employed some type of questionnaire to assess Type A behavior. Other proposed methodological problems are sample bias due to the obvious exclusion of patients with fatal myocardial infarctions, restriction of range when using high-risk groups, and inconsistency in scoring methods to evaluate disease.

Attempting to reconcile contradictory results, some researchers have broken the Type A behavior construct into subcomponents. What most studies have found is that the hostility and anger dimensions of TABP appear to be the most predictive of CHD.

DISEASE MECHANISMS

Assuming an association between TABP and coronary disease, individuals with TABP may be more vulnerable to heart disease than Type B persons because they have a substantially greater sympathetic nervous system response to stressful or demanding circumstances. This response is characterized by increases in heart rate and blood pressure, and a surge in adrenal hormones. Because Type A people tend to overrespond to challenges, no matter how large or small, and because they place themselves in a greater number of demanding circumstances, they experience these heightened physiological responses for longer periods of time each day. It has been suggested that the frequent surges of epinephrine and other adrenal hormones, which increase stress in the cardiovascular system, may injure the inner layer (endothelium) of the coronary artery walls, making them more susceptible to atherosclerosis. Studies have also found that Type A individuals tend to maintain high levels of stress hormones throughout the daytime hours—levels that do not decrease until after they have gone to sleep. The deleterious effects of stress hormones on the heart and the arteries are therefore greater in Type A persons.

TABP MODIFICATION

Modifying Type A behavior can be difficult, particularly in a success-oriented culture that rewards competition and ambition. Behavior modification, relaxation techniques, and biofeedback training have also been successfully used in altering TABP. A multifactor approach, however, may be most beneficial, as demonstrated by the Recurrent Coronary Prevention Project (RCPP; Friedman, Thoresen, & Gill, 1986).

In this study, approximately 900 TABP patients who had suffered a myocardial infarction (i.e., heart attack) were randomly assigned to either a control group or a treatment group. The control group received standard counseling, in the form of group discussions about the importance of diet, exercise, and medication adherence to avoid future cardiac events. In addition to this standard counseling, patients in the treatment group also received counseling designed to modify the beliefs and expectations underlying Type A behavior. More specifically, beliefs about material achievement, being in control, and striving for the approval of others were challenged. Behavioral changes such as talking more slowly and interrupting less were also promoted. After 4 years, there was a 45% lower occurrence of a second myocardial infarction or sudden cardiac death in the group given TABP modification. The RCPP was initially designed to continue for at least 6 years; however, the National Heart, Lung, and Blood Institute insisted that because the researchers had been able to demonstrate that TABP modification significantly prevented coronary recurrences, the TABP modification should be given to the control groups. After 1 year, the percentage of recurrence dropped dramatically in the original control group.

The occupational stress and organizational psychology literature also suggests that in order to reduce Type A behavior and/or hostility, factors such as job demands, time urgency, hostility, job insecurity, and a punitive climate in the work environment need to be modified.

CONTRIBUTIONS OF TABP RESEARCH

Although the anger and hostility subcomponents of Type A behavior are now largely considered the "toxic" elements of the construct, the original TABP studies contributed to a new and growing field called behavioral medicine, dealing with the influence of psychological and behavioral factors on health. TABP research resulted in the recognition of the fact that behavioral characteristics can be as influential on the disease process as such traditional factors as high cholesterol and high blood pressure. This subsequently led to decades of fruitful behavioral research, as well as attention to the role of stress and hostility in coronary heart disease.

—*David Krantz and Carolyn Phan Kao*

See also ANGER: MEASUREMENT; ANGER AND HEART DISEASE; ANGER AND HYPERTENSION; HEART DISEASE: ANGER, DEPRESSION, AND ANXIETY; HOSTILITY AND HEALTH; HOSTILITY: MEASUREMENT; HOSTILITY: PSYCHOPHYSIOLOGY

Further Reading

Friedman, M., & Ghandour, G. (1993). Medical diagnosis of Type A behavior. *American Heart Journal, 126*, 607-618.

Friedman, M., Thoresen, C. E., & Gill, J. J. (1986). Alteration of Type A behavior and its effect on cardiac recurrences in post-myocardial infarction patients: Summary results of the Recurrent Coronary Prevention Project. *American Heart Journal, 112*, 653-662.

Haynes, S. G., Feinleib, M., & Kannel, W. B. (1980). Hispanic Health and Behavior. See Latino Health and Behavior. The relationship of psychosocial factors to coronary heart disease in the Framingham Study: Eight-year incidence of coronary heart disease. *American Journal of Epidemiology, 111*, 37-58.

Review Panel on Coronary-Prone Behavior and Coronary Heart Disease. (1981). Coronary-prone behavior and coronary heart disease: A critical review. *Circulation, 63*, 1199-1215.

Rosenman, R. H., Brand, J. H., Jenkins, C. D., Friedman, M., Straus, R., & Wurm, M. (1975). Coronary heart disease in the Western Collaborative Group Study: Final follow-up experience of 8.5 years. *Journal of the American Medical Association, 233*, 872-877.

Shekelle, R. B., Hulley, S. B., Neaton, J., Billings, J., Borhani, N., Gerace, T., Jacobs, D., Lassser, N., Mittlemark, M., & Stamler, J. (1985). The MRFIT behavioral pattern study II: Type A behavior pattern and risk of coronary death in MRFIT. *American Journal of Epidemiology, 112*, 559-570.

HISPANIC HEALTH AND BEHAVIOR.
See LATINO HEALTH AND BEHAVIOR

HOPELESSNESS AND HEALTH

The accumulating scientific evidence regarding the connections between hope, well-being, and physical health is reviewed briefly in the subsequent sections.

HOPELESSNESS AND HOPE

Although there are numerous ways of conceptualizing hopelessness, there is a common underlying theme: Being hopeless means expecting an undesirable future. This negative expectation, which stems from the perception that any further effort is futile, depletes people of the necessary energy to strive toward their life goals. Over the past decades, science has started to uncover the dire consequences of such hopelessness.

In contrast, researchers also have begun to study the positive roles of hope in human functioning. By examining both hopelessness and hope, a clearer picture may be attained as to how these variables influence our mental well-being and physical health. On this point, physician Leonard Sagan (1987) concluded that the recent improvements in overall world health are due to more than just advances in technology: Specifically, he stated that the decline of hopelessness and the rise in hope were the reasons for the declines in worldwide despair and death.

HOPE AND HEALTH MAINTENANCE

Research has shown that hopelessness is related significantly to a number of important health markers. It has been implicated in the development of breast cancer, cervical cancer, myocardial infarction, and shorter overall life span. For example, in studies of women predisposed to cervical cancer, Arthur Schmale and Howard Iker (1971) discovered that hopelessness predicted the presence of cancer in 82% of the participants. There also is compelling evidence that hope has long-term consequences for physical health. In this regard, Susan Everson and her colleagues (1996) found that higher levels of hope were related to fewer biological and behavioral risk factors.

One reason that hope is important in maintaining health is that it leads to more healthy behaviors such as physical exercise; conversely, higher hope is related to the decreased likelihood of unhealthy behaviors such as high-risk sexual activities. C. R. Snyder and his colleagues (Irving, Snyder, & Crowson, 1998) have found that women with higher levels of hope scored higher on a cancer facts test, they were more knowledgeable about their health, and these woman reported a greater willingness to do things to improve their health. In addition, if people believe they have the power to influence their health status, they are more likely to take the steps to remain healthy. For example, women who believe in the effectiveness of breast cancer screening procedures are more likely to get screening for themselves. Hence, having hope results in people taking responsibility for their own well-being.

Hopelessness also appears to affect the immune system. The experience of hopelessness has been shown to decrease cortisol levels in the body, thereby impairing the immune system functioning. Thus, with hopelessness compromising their immune systems, people are increasingly likely to develop a host of illnesses.

HOPE AND HEALTH RECOVERY

Once a person succumbs to illness, hopelessness plays an important part in the recovery process. This relationship has long been known to practicing health care professionals, and the field is replete with stories of how hope made all the difference in the recovery of particular patients. For example, William M. Buchholz (1988) recounted the story of how an oncologist increased the effectiveness of a treatment for metastatic lung cancer merely by arranging the acronym for the drug cocktail to spell H-O-P-E. One possible interpretation for this and other placebo effects in medicine is that they give people hope.

Recently, empirical research has supported what physicians and nurses have long understood regarding hopelessness and health recovery. Susan Swindells and her colleagues (1999) found that hopelessness

correlated with poorer physical functioning in HIV-positive patients. Because it reduces the desire to live, hopelessness can make disease treatment nearly impossible as it leads to a desire for a quick death, especially in terminally ill patients. This lack of will to survive also results in patients being less likely to follow their treatment regimens. In a study of 295 ill patients, for example, A. Srikumar Menon and colleagues (Menon, Campbell, Ruskin, & Hebel, 2000) found that patients with greater levels of hopelessness were less likely to desire life-saving treatments for their illness—hopeless patients being 5 times more likely to refuse required CPR procedures.

In addition, there seems to be a direct link between hopelessness and the ability to survive. For example, in a study of 74 men diagnosed with AIDS, Geoffrey Reed and his colleagues (1994) discovered that the men who realistically accepted the imminence of their deaths lived significantly shorter lives than those who did not have such a realistic view of their condition. Thus, the realistically hopeless men were less likely to survive their illnesses. Furthermore, hopelessness consistently emerges as the strongest predictor of suicide in both children and adults (e.g., Beck & Steer, 1989).

With their positive expectations for the future, higher-hope people are more likely to engage in active coping behaviors, including the adherence to their treatment regimens. Moreover, hope has been beneficial to patients who were being treated for a wide variety of illnesses and injuries such as burns, spinal cord injuries, blindness, and fibromyalgia. In addition, arthritis patients with higher levels of hope have manifested better upper and lower extremity functioning; moreover, higher levels of hope enable people to handle higher levels of distress, including physical pain.

What are the mechanisms by which hopelessness and hope affect the recovery process? One answer to this question pertains to the fact that more hopeful people are more willing to deal directly with their problems. Thus, the belief that one can improve the situation leads to more healthy behaviors. This type of active coping leads to a fighting spirit that, in turn, is related to better adjustment and longer survival periods when dealing with illness.

ETIOLOGY OF HOPELESSNESS

Given that hope is such a crucial part of our lives, how is it that some people come to lose it? According to C. R. Snyder (1994), hopelessness is a psychological state in which people arrive at an enduring sense of apathy toward their life goals. Snyder posited that people regress from being hopeful to being hopeless in a series of steps. The catalysts for this demise of hope are profound goal blockages. In other words, when important goals are unattainable for prolonged periods of time, this undermines hope. These goal blockages lead from thoughts of hope to feelings of rage. With time, the rage degenerates into despair, which eventually turns into apathy. Once people no longer care about achieving their life goals, they have reached a state of hopelessness. This hopelessness may appear as depression in some individuals, or as a total lack of emotion in others. Although Snyder argued that hopelessness can occur at any stage in life, from infancy through adulthood, little research has been conducted on this aspect of his theory. Most of the evidence for the various avenues of hopelessness comes from case studies. More research on a wider range of populations is needed.

INSTILLING HOPE

There is a long history in the medical field of attempting to give hope to patients. Health care providers have used many strategies to elevate the hopes of their patients, ranging from framing things in the best possible light to outright deception. Having hope is considered to be so important that physicians sometimes use deception in order to increase the levels of this powerful motive in their patients. For example, physicians may perform unnecessary procedures to provide the patient with hope for improvement.

Based on his theory of hope, Snyder and his colleagues have developed specific measures to tap the levels of hope in people (see Snyder, 1994), as well as treatment interventions that are aimed at improving the level of hope. This hope therapy is intended to help people to develop clearer goals, to generate many strategies for reaching these goals, to muster the requisite energy to pursue goals, and to interpret goal barriers as challenges rather than threats. Although the theoretical foundation for such interventions is strong, more research is warranted to understand the role of hope in improving physical health.

—*C. R. Snyder and Kevin L. Rand*

See also DEPRESSION: MEASUREMENT; DEPRESSION:
   MORTALITY AND OTHER ADVERSE OUTCOMES; DEPRESSION:
   TREATMENT

Further Reading

Beck, A. T., & Steer, R. A. (1989). Clinical predictors of eventual suicide: A five- to ten-year study of suicide attempters. *Journal of Addictive Disorders, 17*, 203-209.

Buchholz, W. M. (1988). The medical uses of hope. *Western Journal of Medicine, 148*, 69.

Everson, S. A., Goldberg, D. E., Kaplan, G. A., Cohen, R. D., Pukkala, E., Tuomilehto, J., & Salonen, J. T. (1996). Hopelessness and risk of mortality and incidence of myocardial infarction and cancer. *Psychosomatic Medicine, 58*, 113-121.

Irving, L. M., Snyder, C. R., & Crowson, J. J., Jr. (1998). Hope and the negotiation of cancer facts by college women. *Journal of Personality, 66*, 195-214.

Menon, A. S., Campbell, D., Ruskin, P., & Hebel, J. R. (2000). Depression, hopelessness, and the desire for life-saving treatments among elderly medically ill veterans. *American Journal of Geriatric Psychiatry, 8*, 333-342.

Reed, G. M., Kemeny, M. E., Taylor, S. E., Wang, H. Y. J., et al. (1994). Realistic acceptance as a predictor of decreased survival time in gay men with AIDS. *Health Psychology, 13*, 299-307.

Sagan, L. A. (1987). *The health of nations: True causes of sickness and well-being.* New York: Basic Books.

Schmale, A. H., & Iker, H. P. (1971). Hopelessness as a predictor of cervical cancer. *Social Science Medicine, 5*, 95-100.

Snyder, C. R. (1994). *The psychology of hope: You can get there from here.* New York: Free Press.

Swindells, S., Mohr, J., Justis, J. C., Berman, S., Squier, C., Wagener, M. M., & Singh, N. (1999). Quality of life in patients with human immunodeficiency virus infection: Impact of social support, coping style and hopelessness. *International Journal of STD and AIDS, 10*, 383-391.

HOSTILITY AND HEALTH

HISTORICAL OVERVIEW OF HOSTILITY AND HEALTH

The link between emotions and health, commonly conceptualized as the "mind-body connection," has been known since ancient times. Perhaps the first ever recorded heart attack is described in the Old Testament (1 Sam. 25), circa 1050 B.C. The victim, an important and very rich man called Nabal, was renowned for being "churlish and evil in his doings."

In 1882, Sir William Osler postulated that personality was a risk factor for coronary heart disease. In the late 1950s, Friedman and Rosenman described the Type A behavior pattern, characterized by competition, aggression, and sense of time urgency. The Western Collaborative Group Study team was among the first to report an association between Type A behavior pattern and coronary heart disease in the United States. However, the Type A behavior hypothesis was not confirmed by subsequent investigations, and evidence emerged indicating that particular ingredients of Type A behavior, namely, hostility and unexpressed anger, were the real culprits.

DEFINITION AND MEASUREMENT

Hostility is a broad multidimensional personality and character trait having attitudinal (cynicism and mistrust of others), emotional (anger), and behavioral (aggression) components. Cynicism refers to a generally negative view of humankind, depicting others as unworthy, deceitful, and selfish.

Hostility has traditionally being measured by the Cook-Medley scale, which contains 50 true-false items. As an example, the Cook-Medley includes the following items: "I think most people would lie to get ahead"; "It is safer to trust nobody"; "No one cares much what happens to you"; "Most people will use somewhat unfair means to gain profit or an advantage rather than lose it"; "I tend to be on my guard with people who are somewhat more friendly than I had expected"; "I have at times had to be rough with people who were rude to me." This instrument was first developed to identify teachers having difficulty with their students and was empirically derived using preexisting items from the Minnesota Multiphasic Personality Inventory (MMPI). Other validated instruments to measure hostility include the Buss-Durkee Hostility Inventory, the Novaco Anger Inventory, and the Multidimensional Anger Inventory.

HOSTILITY AS A PREDICTOR OF HEART DISEASE AND POTENTIAL PHYSIOLOGICAL MECHANISMS

There are numerous studies examining hostility as a predictor of coronary heart disease outcomes. In particular, high hostility scores have been found to be related to increased risk of angiographically documented coronary atherosclerosis, essential hypertension, coronary heart disease incidence, and all-cause mortality. It has also been shown that hostility is a predictor of re-stenosis after coronary angioplasty, of carotid intimal media thickness among healthy postmenopausal women, and of carotid atherosclerosis progression in middle-aged men. In a recent study among young adults in four U.S. metropolitan areas, there was a positive, graded association between hostility measured at baseline (using the Cook-Medley scale) and coronary artery calcification measured using electron-beam computed tomography 10 years later. However, there are also studies reporting no relationship between hostility and coronary heart disease outcomes or between hostility and subclinical coronary artery disease.

To elucidate mechanisms whereby hostility might contribute to coronary heart disease risk, numerous studies have evaluated associations between hostility and social, behavioral, and physiological coronary risk factors in children and adolescents, young adults, and middle-aged persons. Hostility might contribute to the development of coronary atherosclerosis through concomitant unhealthy lifestyle behaviors (i.e., tobacco use, diet, or poor compliance with medications), but also via multiple physiological pathways. For example, a number of recent investigations have found relationships between hostility and casual blood pressure readings, cardiovascular reactivity, blood pressure morning surge, increased platelet activation, and reduced beta-adrenergic receptor responsiveness. Epinephrine is a recognized platelet activator, and hostile individuals tend to show a marked increase of catecholamine during psychological stress. Furthermore, down regulation of the adrenergic receptor has been linked to prolonged neuroendocrine responses to either psychological stressors or chronic stress associated with frequent and prolonged bouts of anger.

Therapy directed at reducing hostility has been shown to reduce the risk of nonfatal re-infarction by more than 50%. Recent evidence suggests that formal cardiac rehabilitation and exercise training programs can reduce hostility and improve quality of life after major coronary events.

ANGER, A DIMENSION OF HOSTILITY, AND ITS ASSOCIATION WITH HEART DISEASE

Anger is the affective state most commonly associated with myocardial ischemia and life-threatening arrhythmias. The scope of the problem is sizable: It has been estimated that at least 36,000 (2.4% of 1.5 million) heart attacks are precipitated annually in the United States by anger.

Specific instruments designed to measure anger include the Spielberger Trait Anger Scale, which measures the frequency of feeling of anger, and the Anger Expression Scale, which measures the extent to which feelings of anger are suppressed (anger-in) or expressed (anger-out).

There are numerous studies documenting an association between anger and manifestations of coronary disease, in particular triggering of myocardial infarction. In the Normative Aging Study, a dose-response relation was found between level of anger and overall risk of coronary heart disease. In the Caerphilly study among 2,890 men ages 49 to 65 years living in South Wales, both anger-out and suppressed anger showed associations with incident coronary heart disease that were independent of physiological, psychosocial, and behavioral risk factors. Researchers from the Stockholm Heart Epidemiology Program showed that, during a period of 1 hour after an episode of anger, the risk of myocardial infarction was 9 times higher compared to a control period free of anger. These results were confirmed by the Determinants of Myocardial Infarction Onset Study in the United States, but the investigators showed that the risk of having a myocardial infarction triggered by isolated episodes of anger depended on the level of educational attainment: The risk of myocardial infarction associated with anger was twice as high among those with less than high school education compared with patients with at least some college education.

HOSTILITY AND NON-CORONARY HEART DISEASE HEALTH OUTCOMES

Most research on hostility and health has focused on the development and course of coronary heart disease; thus, the epidemiological data relating hostility and other aspects of health are scarce. There are a few published studies on the relation of hostility with glucose metabolism and insulin sensitivity, breast cancer, and elderly suicide.

In a biracial sample, hostility was found differentially related to measures of glucose metabolism in African Americans and Caucasians: It was significantly related to fasting glucose in African Americans and to insulin sensitivity and fasting insulin in Caucasian subjects. Furthermore, while the relationship of hostility to insulin sensitivity and fasting insulin was partially dependent on body mass index in Caucasians, the relationship of hostility to fasting glucose was unrelated to body mass index in African Americans. A team of Finnish researchers examined the relationship between personality characteristics and the risk of breast cancer among women age 18 years or more, including Type A behavior and an author-constructed measure of hostility. These results indicated no increase in breast cancer risk in relation to Type A behavior and hostility. Elderly suicide is an increasing public health problem. In a recent study, the psychopathological profile of elderly suicidal ideators was characterized by the presence of hostility. The authors speculated that hostility is often accompanied by failure to control impulses, which is an essential characteristic in suicidal behavior.

AREAS FOR FURTHER RESEARCH

Since anger and hostility often correlate with other psychosocial factors involving depressive disorder, anxiety, social isolation, interpersonal conflict, job stress, self-control skills, and sense of coherence, an important area for future studies is to assess the degree to which anger and hostility confer increased risk independently of these other psychosocial variables, as well as the potential interactions or synergistic effects between them.

Another area that deserves attention is the possible influence of diet on hostility, particularly n-3 polyunsaturated fatty acids, which are preferentially contained in fatty fish (salmon, tuna, mackerel), n-3 enriched eggs, green leafy vegetables, flaxseed, rapeseed, walnuts, and vegetable oils, principally soybean and canola. In a trial among young adults in Japan, docosahexaenoic acid (DHA, 22:6 n-3) supplementation with fish oil capsules prevented extra-aggression at times of mental stress and lowered resting plasma norepinephrine concentrations by 31%. In another trial, a high fish diet intervention as part of a cholesterol-lowering program resulted in a reduction of aggressive hostility. In an observational study of subjects with a history of impulsive behaviors, plasma DHA was negatively correlated with serotonin and dopamine metabolites in cerebrospinal fluid, suggesting that the dietary intake of DHA may influence neurotransmitter concentrations.

Additional research is warranted to elucidate the effectiveness and anger-reducing interventions in both the secondary prevention setting (i.e., persons with known coronary disease) and in the primary prevention setting (i.e., persons without known coronary disease).

—*Carlos Iribarren*

See also ANGER AND HEART DISEASE; ANGER AND HYPERTENSION; ANGER: MEASUREMENT; HEART DISEASE: ANGER, DEPRESSION, AND ANXIETY; HEART DISEASE AND DIET; HEART DISEASE AND PHYSICAL ACTIVITY; HEART DISEASE AND REACTIVITY; HEART DISEASE AND SMOKING; HEART DISEASE AND TYPE A BEHAVIOR

Further Reading

Barefoot, J. C., Dodge, K. A., Peterson, B. L., Dahlstrom, W. G., & Williams, R. B., Jr. (1989). The Cook-Medley Hostility Scale: Item content and ability to predict survival. *Psychosomatic Medicine, 51*, 46-57.

Cook, W. W., & Medley, D. M. (1954). Proposed hostility and pharisaic-virtue scales for the MMPI. *Journal of Applied Psychology, 38*, 414-418.

Friedman, M., & Rosenman, R. H. (1971). Type A behavior pattern: Its association with coronary heart disease. *Annals of Clinical Research, 3,* 300-312.

Hamazaki, T., Sawazaki, S., Itomura, M., Asaoka, E., Nagao, Y., Nishimura, N., Yazawa, K., Kuwamori, T., & Kobayashi, M. (1996). The effect of docosahexaenoic acid on aggression in young adults: A placebo-controlled double-blind study. *Journal of Clinical Investigation, 97*, 1129-1133.

Iribarren, C., Sidney, S., Liu, K., Markovitz, J. H., Bild, D. E., Roseman, J. M., & Mathews, K. (2000). Association of hostility with coronary artery calcification in young adults: The CARDIA Study. *Journal of the American Medical Association, 283*, 2546-2551.

Kawachi, I., Sparrow, D., Spiro, A., Vokonas, P., & Weiss, S. T. (1996). A prospective study of anger and coronary heart disease: The Normative Aging Study. *Circulation, 94*, 2090-2095.

Lavie, C. J., & Milani, R. V. (1999). Effects of cardiac rehabilitation and exercise training programs on coronary patients with high levels of hostility. *Mayo Clinic Proceedings, 74*, 959-966.

Matthews, K. A., & Haynes, S. G. (1986). Type A behavior pattern and coronary disease risk: Update and critical evaluation. *American Journal of Epidemiology, 123*, 923-960.

Miller, T. Q., Smith, T. W., Turner, C. W., Guijarro, M. L., & Hallet, A. J. (1996). A meta-analytic review of research on hostility and physical health. *Psychological Bulletin, 119*, 322-348.

Musante, L., Treiber, F. A., Davis, H., Strong, W. B., & Levy, M. (1992). Hostility: Relationship to lifestyle behaviors and physical risk factors. *Behavioral Medicine, 18*, 21-26.

Myrtek, M. (2001). Meta-analyses of prospective studies on coronary heart disease, Type A personality, and hostility. *International Journal of Cardiology, 79*, 245-251.

Rozanski, A., Blumenthal, J. A., & Kaplan, J. (1999). Impact of psychological factors on the pathogenesis of cardiovascular disease and implications for therapy. *Circulation, 99*, 2192-2217.

Schrijvers, C. T., Bosma, H., & Mackenbach, J. P. (2002). Hostility and the educational gradient in health: The mediating role of health-related behaviours. *European Journal of Public Health, 12*, 110-116.

HOSTILITY: MEASUREMENT

The measurement of hostility is an important issue for behavioral medicine researchers and health care practitioners because some studies have found that hostile people are at increased risk of developing physical disorders such as heart disease and high blood pressure. (For a review, see Miller, Smith, Turner, Guijarro, & Hallet, 1996.) Researchers have defined hostility in a variety of ways, but most definitions describe the hostile person as someone who is consistently cynical toward others, expecting them to be untrustworthy, self-interested, and potentially threatening. This perspective emphasizes cognitive aspects of the self by focusing on attitudes and beliefs. However, because hostile attitudes often are accompanied by anger and aggression, researchers frequently conceptualize and measure hostility as a multidimensional pattern of cognitive, affective, and behavioral characteristics. For example, a cynical person who expects to be taken advantage of by others may feel irritated or resentful about the situation. Along similar lines, a hostile, angry person may express those negative attitudes and emotions by yelling or displaying physically violent behavior. Nonetheless, hostile cognitions or attitudes do not necessarily translate into angry affect or behavioral aggression in every setting and the three constructs can be thought of as describing related but distinct domains.

Caution is in order when interpreting studies about hostility and health, because the terms *hostility, anger*, and *aggression* sometimes are used interchangeably.

Researchers have taken two main approaches in measuring hostility: behavioral assessments and self-report questionnaires. Both strategies attempt to identify individual differences in the propensity for hostility and the related dimensions of anger and aggression.

THE BEHAVIORAL MEASUREMENT OF HOSTILITY

One major strategy for the measurement of hostility involves assessing speech behaviors during a laboratory procedure called the Structured Interview (SI). The SI (which initially was developed as a tool for evaluating Type A behavior) involves presenting the participant with a series of planned provocations in an attempt to elicit relevant behaviors. For example, the interviewer rushes and interrupts the participant, abruptly changes topics, and challenges some of the participant's responses. Interviewers are carefully trained so that all interviewees encounter equivalent levels of challenge during the procedure. The SI requires approximately 10 minutes to administer and interviews are audiotaped for later scoring. Two behavioral techniques for scoring hostility from the SI are particularly important: Potential for Hostility (PH) and the Interview Hostility Assessment Technique (IHAT).

Theodore Dembroski and colleagues conceptualized PH as the stable tendency to experience anger across a variety of social situations. PH scores reflected the auditor's impression of the participant's behavior during the SI on three dimensions: hostile content, intensity of response, and interaction style. Someone who showed marked hostile content would report frequent feelings of frustration or irritation during daily activities. The intensity of response category tapped the emphasis and extremity of hostile statements, as well as the use of obscenities, emotionally laden language, and changes in voice volume and tone. Finally, the interaction style dimension captured condescending, arrogant, or uncooperative behaviors displayed during the SI. In samples of patients, people with high PH scores were found to have more advanced coronary artery disease (e.g., Dembroski, MacDougall, Williams, Haney, & Blumenthal, 1985).

John Barefoot, Thomas Haney, and their colleagues and Duke University refined the behavioral assessment of hostility by developing the IHAT. The IHAT combines Dembroski's emphasis on hostile interaction style with a carefully defined behavioral scoring system. The IHAT focuses primarily on vocal behaviors and tends to disregard the content of the participant's statements, unless that content is communicated in a hostile fashion. IHAT auditors evaluate SI audiotapes one speaking turn at a time. Each speaking turn (or statement uttered by the interviewee) is scored for the presence and intensity of four behaviors: indirect challenge, direct challenge, hostile withhold/evasion, and irritation. An indirect challenge is scored if the participant subtly deprecates the interviewer, often with an annoyed tone. For example, an interviewee might respond by saying, "Of course!" in a manner that suggests that the interviewer's question was foolish. Overtly antagonistic responses (e.g., sarcastically saying, "Haven't we been over that already?") are scored as direct challenges. A hostile withhold/evade is counted if the interviewee is purposefully uncooperative or refuses to answer a question. Vocal behaviors such as rapid speech, sighs, harsh tone, and explosive emphasis typically are scored in the irritation category. Patients with high IHAT scores have been found to have more severe coronary artery disease than those with lower IHAT scores and this pattern persists even after accounting for the role of traditional heart disease risk factors such as elevated blood lipids and smoking (Haney et al., 1996).

The major advantage associated with measurement systems such as PH and the IHAT is that researchers are evaluating ratings of behavior made by trained observers, rather than people's personal descriptions of whether they consider themselves to be hostile. This is important because hostile individuals may deny or simply be unaware of their interaction style. In other words, a hostile person might not admit to being hostile if asked directly. However, administering and scoring the SI is an expensive and labor-intensive process. In addition, it can be challenging to train auditors to agree with each other in the consistent scoring of hostile vocal characteristics.

SELF-REPORT HOSTILITY MEASURES

Self-report questionnaires designed to assess individual differences in hostility began to appear in the 1950s. Hostility questionnaires present people with a series of written statements that reflect hostile, angry, and aggressive themes. Respondents record whether they find each item to be self-descriptive, either by circling "true" or "false" or by selecting a number from a rating scale. Responses then are scored as a numerical index that can be used to study the associations among self-reports of hostility and related behaviors and health outcomes.

Self-report measures always are potentially problematic in that respondents may not rate themselves accurately or honestly. As described previously, this can be troublesome for the measurement of hostility because people may not be able or willing to acknowledge possessing a trait that is socially undesirable. However, the tendency for people to present themselves in unrealistically positive terms can be reduced by assuring respondents that their confidentiality will be protected. Self-report hostility questionnaires are attractive for clinicians and researchers because they are efficient and inexpensive to administer. There are many self-report measures of hostility and related constructs available. (For a review, see Martin, Watson, & Wan, 2000.) Two of the most commonly used questionnaires are the Cook-Medley Hostility (Ho) Scale and the Buss Durkee Hostility Inventory (BDHI).

Historically, the Ho Scale was developed by Walter Cook and Donald Medley (1954), who were attempting to create a questionnaire that would identify people likely to have good rapport with others. The items were drawn from the Minnesota Multiphasic Personality Inventory (MMPI), which is a broad personality scale commonly used by clinical psychologists. The Ho Scale currently is viewed as a measure of hostile interpersonal attitudes, such as cynicism, antagonism, and manipulativeness. The Ho Scale became popular among behavioral medicine researchers because some studies found that Ho Scale scores were associated with heart disease and mortality (for a review, see Miller et al., 1996).

The Ho Scale is composed of 50 true or false items and respondents' answers usually are reported as a single composite score. Sample items include, "When someone does me a wrong I feel I should pay him back if I can, just for the principle of the thing" and "I have often met people who were supposed to be experts who were no better than I." Although the Ho Scale has been widely used, questions have been raised about the structure of the measure. Respondents seem to answer Ho Scale items erratically and are inconsistent in endorsing items that appear to be logically related. Nonetheless, Ho Scale scores show meaningful relationships with a variety of health-related variables. People with high Ho Scale scores report high levels of daily stress and negative mood and low levels of social support; in addition, high Ho Scale scores are related to increases in blood pressure and cortisol (Smith, 1992).

Arnold Buss and Ann Durkee (1957) designed the BDHI to distinguish among several aspects of hostility commonly observed by clinicians conducting psychological assessment and therapy. The 75 true or false items were written to represent seven types of hostility (assault, indirect hostility, irritability, negativism, resentment, suspicion, and verbal hostility); several items also were included that pertained to feelings of guilt. BDHI responses typically are represented as a composite score; subscale scores reflecting the various dimensions also may be reported.

Studies of patterns in the way people answer BDHI items show that responses generally can be grouped into two broad categories: an emotional and attitudinal dimension that reflects the personal experience of angry emotions and thoughts and a motor component that represents overt physical and verbal expressions of anger. Aron Siegman and colleagues (Siegman, Dembroski, & Ringel, 1987) found that people with high scores on the expressive dimensions of the BDHI tended to have more severe coronary artery disease than respondents who described themselves as less likely to express their anger.

Although the BDHI had been widely used by psychologists, Buss eventually came to feel that its items were troublesome for at least two reasons. First, many people have difficulty describing their behavior in simple true versus false terms. Second, several BDHI items seemed to blur the intended distinctions among different facets of hostility. As a consequence, Buss and Mark Perry (1992) refined and extended the BDHI items in a new measure called the Aggression Questionnaire (AQ). The AQ includes four subscales: physical aggression, verbal aggression, anger, and hostility, and careful efforts were made during the construction of the items to avoid overlap among these categories. Consistent with its name, the AQ Hostility subscale relates to attitudinal elements of cynicism and mistrust, with items such as "I am sometimes eaten up with jealousy" and "At times I feel like I have gotten a raw deal out of life." Because the AQ is a fairly new measure, the associations among AQ scores and health outcomes are unexplored.

—*René Martin and S. Beth Bellman*

See also ANGER: MEASUREMENT; HOSTILITY AND HEALTH

Further Reading

Barefoot, J. C. (1992). Developments in the measurement of hostility. In H. Friedman (Ed.), *Hostility, coping, and health* (pp. 13-31). Washington, DC: American Psychological Association.

Buss, A. H., & Durkee, A. (1957). An inventory for assessing different kinds of hostility. *Journal of Consulting Psychology, 21,* 343-349.

Buss, A. H., & Perry, M. (1992). The aggression question- naire. *Journal of Personality and Social Psychology, 63,* 452-459.

Cook, W. W., & Medley, D. M. (1954). Proposed hostility and pharisaic-virtue scales for the MMPI. *Journal of Applied Psychology, 38,* 414-418.

Dembroski, T. M., MacDougall, J. M., Williams, R. B., Haney, T. L., & Blumenthal, J. (1985). Components of Type A, hostility, and anger-in: Relationship to angio- graphic findings. *Psychosomatic Medicine, 47,* 219-233.

Haney, T. L., Maynard, K. E., Houseworth, S. J., Scherwitz, L. W., Williams, R. B., & Barefoot, J. C. (1996). Interpersonal hostility assessment technique: Description and validation against the criterion of coro- nary artery disease. *Journal of Personality Assessment, 66,* 386-401.

Martin, R., Watson, D., & Wan, C. K. (2000). A three-fac- tor model of trait anger: Dimensions of affect, behavior, and cognition. *Journal of Personality, 86,* 869-897.

Miller, T. Q., Smith, T. W., Turner, C. W., Guijarro, M. L., & Hallet, A. J. (1996). A meta-analytic review of research on hostility and physical health. *Psychological Bulletin, 119,* 322-348.

Siegman, A. W., Dembroski, T. M., & Ringel, N. (1987). Components of hostility and severity of coronary artery disease. *Psychosomatic Medicine, 49,* 127-135.

Smith, T. W. (1992). Hostility and health: Current status of a psychosomatic hypothesis. *Health Psychology, 11,* 139-150.

HOSTILITY: PSYCHOPHYSIOLOGY

DEFINITION OF HOSTILITY

Hostility is a multidimensional construct consist- ing of cognitive, affective, and behavioral dimensions. The cognitive dimension consists of cynicism and mistrust of others. The affective dimension includes feelings of anger, irritation, rage, contempt, resentment, and bitterness. The behavioral dimension includes various acts of physical and verbal aggression. Researchers are interested in the physiological corre- lates of hostility because several studies have shown that hostility is a significant risk factor for coronary heart disease (CHD). We will consider evidence regarding the associations of cognitive, affective, and behavioral components to physiology in turn.

MECHANISMS LINKING HOSTILITY TO CHD

The precise mechanisms through which hostility confers risk for CHD are not known. One hypothesis suggests that repeated, exaggerated, and prolonged activation of the sympathetic nervous system and neu- roendocrine components of the human stress response mediates the hostility-CHD relationship. This con- tributes to poor health in at least two ways. First, over time stress-induced hemodynamic changes (e.g., increased blood pressure, sheer stress, and turbulence) and the increases in catecholamines (i.e., epinephrine and norepinephrine) and other stress-related hor- mones, such as cortisol, may act to initiate and/or has- ten the atherosclerotic process. This is supported by studies that have found stress-induced changes in blood pressure and/or heart rate to be associated with coronary artery disease in cynomolgus monkeys and the progression of carotid atherosclerosis in humans. Second, the acute physiological changes associated with the human stress response may lead to arrhyth- mias, myocardial ischemia, thrombus formation, and plaque rupture and thus serve as a trigger of heart attacks and sudden death in vulnerable individuals.

HOSTILITY AND PHYSIOLOGY: CHRONIC EFFECTS

The Cook-Medley Hostility Scale and Physiological Reactivity

Blood pressure and heart rate (laboratory studies). One of the most commonly used measures of trait hostility is the Cook-Medley Hostility Scale (CMHS). Although the scale contains items that reflect the affective and behavioral dimensions of hostility, a large portion of the items reflect cynicism and mistrust. This scale has been widely used in studies investigating the relation between hostility and physio- logical reactivity in response to mental and social stress. Physiological reactivity refers to stress-induced changes in physiological measures (e.g., blood pressure, heart rate, norepinephrine level) from some baseline or resting state. One important finding in this literature is that the relation between hostility and physiological reactivity depends on the characteristics of the task used to elicit mental stress. This was demonstrated by an early study in which male subjects engaged in a challenging anagram task. One half of the subjects were provoked by verbal harassment while they completed the task and the other half were not. The results demonstrated that high CMHS scores were associated with heightened and prolonged diastolic blood pressure, but only for subjects who were provoked and angered. Subsequent studies using samples of both and males and females have reported similar findings, although there have been a small number of studies that have failed to find that the CMHS is associated with higher levels of blood pressure and/or heart rate.

Blood pressure and heart rate (ambulatory studies). Hostile people not only have greater physiological reactivity in response to interpersonal stress, they also report the experience of interpersonal stress more frequently in their daily lives. It has been hypothesized that hostile people, who are mistrustful and attribute hostile intent to others' behavior, approach or respond to interpersonal situations in ways that create conflict. A limitation to laboratory paradigms is that they do not take into account the frequency in which people experience interpersonal stress during the day. Ambulatory monitoring techniques provide a way to evaluate hostility as a predictor of blood pressure and heart rate during normal daily activities. Because these techniques monitor physiology multiple times over the course of the day, they have the potential to capture subjects' exposure to stressful situations throughout the day.

Several studies using this methodology have provided evidence that high hostile subjects show elevated levels of blood pressure and/or heart rate during waking hours or while asleep. One study found that the CMHS was associated with high systolic blood pressure levels and the perceptions of interpersonal stress partially accounted for the relationship between hostility and systolic blood pressure. Another study found that high hostile men showed higher levels of diastolic blood pressure and heart rate during the day. Furthermore, high hostile subjects showed higher systolic blood pressure, but only in situations in which they were interacting with someone else. Results from

other studies provide further support for the association between the CMHS and ambulatory blood pressure and heart rate.

However, there are some indications that these phenomena may be stronger in men than in women. The use of this methodology can provide compelling evidence for the negative impact of hostility during daily interpersonal stressors.

Stress hormones. The focus on blood pressure and heart rate has expanded to include other important indices of the stress response. The CMHS has been associated with heightened levels of norepinephrine and cortisol and poorer recovery in response to laboratory paradigms. It also has been associated with higher urinary cortisol excretion, but only during daytime hours. In addition, there is evidence that hostile people have chronically elevated levels of epinephrine during their daily lives.

Heart rate variability. Heart rate variability, an index of parasympathetic nervous system (PNS) function, is another important variable that has received some attention in this literature. High-frequency heart rate variability is thought to reflect PNS modulation of cardiac function and is believed to be an indicator of cardiac health. Lower levels of high-frequency heart rate variability have predicted the development of coronary artery disease and cardiac events. One study found that CMHS is associated with lower levels of high-frequency heart rate variability in the laboratory. In a study using ambulatory monitoring techniques, there was an inverse relationship between hostility and heart rate variability, but only during the day in men younger than 40.

Anger and Physiological Reactivity

The emotion of anger is associated with a number of physiological changes that may have implications for the development of CHD. Anger is associated with increases in blood pressure and heart rate during laboratory procedures and daily life. Levels of the stress hormones norepinephrine, epinephrine, and cortisol become elevated in response to laboratory procedures that engender feelings of anger. In some cases, these changes can be very dramatic, such as when people are experiencing intense feelings of anger or when they lose their temper. For example, a series of studies have found that having people talk about anger-arousing events in a loud and fast voice (i.e., an angry voice) resulted in increases of blood pressure and heart rate as high as 44 mm Hg for systolic blood pressure, 56 mm Hg for diastolic blood pressure, and 53 beats per minute for heart rate. These studies involved the discussion of past experiences, which likely underestimate the levels of blood pressure and heart rate that occurred at the time of the event. Such extreme physiological reactions may potentially be damaging to one's cardiovascular health. More frequently occurring lower-intensity feelings of anger with its associated physiological changes may also have a negative impact on health.

Anger-Out, Anger-In, and Physiological Reactivity

Blood pressure and heart rate (laboratory studies). The way in which anger is managed or expressed is thought to play a role in the development of coronary artery disease and CHD. A major distinction in that respect is between the outward expression of anger (*anger-out*) and the experience of anger (*anger-in*). Anger-out and anger-in were originally conceptualized as existing on a continuum in which behavior ranged from the strong inhibition of angry feelings to the strong outward expression of angry feelings. However, a more contemporary view describes them as independent modes of anger expression. Trait anger-out has been defined as reflecting individual differences in the frequency in which angry feelings are expressed in verbally or physically aggressive behavior. In contrast, trait anger-in refers to the frequency with which angry feelings are experienced, but held in or suppressed. One early study examined dimensions of anger expression as predictors of physiological reactivity during a challenging anagram task. It was found that the outward expression of anger was associated with heightened levels of systolic blood pressure and forearm blood flow, but only during a task in which subjects were provoked and angered. Anger-in was not associated with changes in blood pressure in either condition, but was associated with greater forearm blood flow in the harassment condition. Other investigations, using anger induction paradigms, have consistently reported similar findings for measures of anger-out. In contrast, there has been little evidence suggesting that anger-in is associated with physiological reactivity.

Although subjects may become very angry in response to these paradigms, they typically do not express their anger. Furthermore, it has been hypothesized that the relation between these two modes of anger expression and reactivity may depend on whether subjects are given the opportunity to express their anger. At least three studies have evaluated the relation between measures of trait anger expression and reactivity using anger induction techniques, such as anger recall and role-playing of interpersonal conflicts, which encourage the free expression of anger. In all three studies, measures of the outward expression of anger were associated with higher levels of diastolic blood pressure reactivity. In contrast, there was no evidence suggesting that individuals scoring high on measures of anger-in responded with elevated levels of physiological reactivity. Thus, across a variety of laboratory paradigms that engender feelings of anger, it appears that it is primarily anger-out and not anger-in that is associated with elevated levels of physiological reactivity.

Blood pressure and heart rate (ambulatory studies). Relatively few studies have investigated the relation between anger expression and ambulatory measures of blood pressure and heart rate. In one study, it was found that neither anger-out nor anger-in were related to ambulatory blood pressure in young male and female college students. Another study found that anger-out was not associated with ambulatory blood pressure or heart rate in a group of college students. The results for anger-in are mixed. One study reported that anger-in was not associated with blood pressure or heart rate in male and female college students, and the other reported that high levels of anger-in were related to higher levels of systolic blood pressure in a sample of hypertensive women. Thus, ambulatory studies do not yield the type of evidence observed in laboratory settings.

Stress hormones. The relationship between anger expression and stress hormones has also received some attention. Ratings by family members of subjects' propensity for aggression were associated with morning plasma concentrations of norepinephrine. Three studies have evaluated the relation between the outward expression of anger and physiological reactivity to an interpersonally stressful task.

In the first study, individuals scoring high on a measure of the outward expression of anger exhibited elevated levels of norepinephrine, cortisol, systolic blood pressure, and heart rate, relative to individuals who scored low on the measure. In the second study, a behavioral measure of aggressive responding, which correlates highly with other measures of anger-out, was positively associated with elevated levels of norepinephrine, epinephrine, and cortisol in response to stress. Another study found a positive relation between anger-out and norepinephrine in response to a task in which subjects were provoked and angered. Furthermore, a measure of anger-in was not related to changes in norepinephrine. Finally, one study found that the relation between anger-out and early-morning levels of cortisol depended on level of work stress. Specifically, anger-out was associated with higher elevations of cortisol in individuals who reported high levels of work stress. This relation was not apparent at other times in the day. Thus, the evidence from these studies appears to parallel the findings from studies examining anger-out as a predictor of changes in blood pressure in response to interpersonal stress. At the present time, too few studies have examined the relation between anger-in and stress hormones to draw any firm conclusions.

HOSTILITY AND PHYSIOLOGY: ACUTE EFFECTS

Another way in which anger may play a role in cardiovascular health is by triggering coronary events in vulnerable individuals. Indeed, anecdotal reports have long linked strong feelings of anger with coronary events. More recently, evidence from two studies suggests that intense outbursts of anger are potent triggers of heart attacks. Anger-induced myocardial ischemia and ventricular arrhythmias via alterations in autonomic tone are potential physiological mechanisms accounting for these findings. The effect of anger on the physiology of patients with heart disease has been the focus of some research because these individuals are prone to such events. Therefore, these studies provide a unique opportunity to better understand how anger plays a role in triggering coronary events. The evidence of studies of these kinds indicates that anger is capable of inducing myocardial ischemia and ventricular arrhythmias during daily activities as well as during laboratory tasks designed to engender such feelings.

Hostile traits that are associated with heightened physiological reactivity in response to anger-induced stress may play a role in triggering coronary events. As described in previous sections, traits such as cynical mistrust and anger-out are associated with a wide range of stress-induced physiological changes that may trigger heart attacks in vulnerable individuals. Thus, hostility may play an important role in cardiovascular health across all phases of the disease process.

CONCLUSIONS

There is ample evidence that the cognitive, affective, and behavioral components of this psychological complex are associated with a variety of physiological responses. These are plausible mechanisms accounting for the association between hostility and CHD.

—*Stephen H. Boyle,*
John C. Barefoot, and Redford B. Williams

See also ANGER AND HEART DISEASE; ANGER AND HYPERTENSION; ANGER: MEASUREMENT; CARDIOVASCULAR PSYCHOPHYSIOLOGY: MEASURES; CARDIOVASCULAR REACTIVITY; HEART DISEASE: ANGER, DEPRESSION, AND ANXIETY; HOSTILITY AND HEALTH; HOSTILITY: MEASUREMENT

Further Reading

Houston, B. K. (1994). Anger, hostility, and psychophysiological reactivity. In A. W. Siegman & T. W. Smith (Eds.), *Anger, hostility, and the heart* (pp. 97-115). Hillsdale, NJ: Lawrence Erlbaum.

Kop, W. J. (1999). Chronic and acute psychological risk factors for clinical manifestations of coronary artery disease. *Psychosomatic Medicine, 61*(4), 476-487.

Siegman, A. W. (1994). Cardiovascular consequences of expressing and repressing anger. In A. W. Siegman & T. W. Smith (Eds.), *Anger, hostility, and the heart* (pp. 173-197). Hillsdale, NJ: Lawrence Erlbaum.

Smith, T. W. (1994). Concepts and methods in the study of anger, hostility, and health. In A. W. Siegman & T. W. Smith (Eds.), *Anger, hostility, and the heart* (pp. 23-42). Hillsdale, NJ: Lawrence Erlbaum.

I

IMMIGRANT POPULATIONS AND HEALTH

According to the 2000 census, approximately 1 out of every 10 people in the United States (11% of the total population) is an immigrant. Therefore, it is important to understand the unique profiles of immigrants, as well as the contextual factors that affect immigrant health. This entry presents a brief outline of the current demographics of immigrant populations and discusses a number of issues relevant to immigrant health. In order to develop a framework from which to consider the health of immigrants in the United States, emphasis is placed on acculturation, tuberculosis, access to health care, policy, and psychosocial factors.

DEMOGRAPHICS

Patterns of immigration have shifted considerably during the course of American history. Throughout most of the 1800s, Europeans accounted for the majority of the immigrant population. Reasons for immigrating ranged from poor economic conditions to fear of religious or political persecution. According to the 2000 census, European immigrants comprise only 15% of the total foreign-born population; the majority is composed of Latino and Asian immigrants. Fifty-one percent of the total foreign-born population is composed of Latino immigrants. Mexicans (54%) comprise the highest proportion of Latino immigrants, followed by Cubans (7%), El Salvadorans (5%), and Dominicans (5%). Immigrants from Asian countries represent 26% of the foreign-born population. China (19%), the Philippines (17%), India (14%), Vietnam (12%), and Korea (10%) are the largest contributors to the Asian foreign-born population.

The first significant waves of immigration from Latin American and Asian countries began in the late 1800s. Immigration policies during specific historical points, including some that targeted inclusion or exclusion of specific groups, influenced the rates and patterns of immigration. For instance, in the late 1800s, Chinese immigration was promoted by the recruitment of laborers to work on the Central Pacific Railroad Company's transcontinental railroad. A period of economic decline following the completion of the project led to the Chinese Exclusionary Act of 1882, which prohibited admission of Chinese laborers into the United States. Two years later, the law was revised to exclude all Chinese, and was in force until 1943. The Quota Law (1921) and National Origins Act (1924) established a quota system that discriminated against Eastern and Southern European and Japanese immigrants, respectively. During the Great Depression, a repatriation campaign forced large numbers of Mexicans to leave the country. But later, a labor shortage led to the bracero agreement, which encouraged Mexican farm workers to enter the United States.

The amendments to the Immigration and Nationality Act in 1965 removed many of the barriers for immigrants from Latin America, Asia, and Africa. After that time, however, the economic, cultural, and political climate in the United States has continued to influence migration patterns.

DEFINING IMMIGRANT

The definition of immigrant varies across social science and legal domains. Social science definitions encompass life transitions, displacement from social settings, and adjustment to cultural values and norms—sometimes without regard to legal status. In contrast, legal definitions often capture the temporality and policy aspects of immigration but do not address psychosocial adjustment issues. For instance, U.S. immigration law categorizes individuals as either citizens or aliens. Citizen designation includes individuals born in the United States or those who derive citizenship from parents, or are naturalized. Aliens are further classified as (a) immigrants, who are lawfully admitted into the United States for permanent or conditional residence, and (b) nonimmigrants, individuals who enter the country for a temporary period. Therefore, some individuals classified as "immigrants" according to social science definitions would be considered citizens under immigration law (e.g., individuals who were naturalized). Defining immigrant according to Public Benefit Law determines eligibility for federal programs by classifying immigrant status into a "qualified" category, including legal immigrants, refugees, asylees, legalized aliens, and parolees. However, individuals considered immigrants for federal programs are not necessarily considered immigrants under immigration law. Because social and legal definitions do not overlap, precise classification of immigrants is critical for designing research on health, policy, and health care utilization of immigrant populations.

HEALTH AND ACCULTURATION

Foreign-born individuals have better health on global indicators (e.g., self-reported health, activity limitation, and bed days) than their U.S.-born counterparts. This becomes particularly salient in the case of the epidemiological paradox of mortality among Latinos. Latinos are disproportionately represented among the poor, but the all-cause mortality rate is lower among Latinos than non-Latino Whites. Several explanations for the paradox have been proposed, including the *healthy migrant hypothesis* that selection of Latino migrants in good health results in lower mortality. Another migratory explanation, the *salmon bias hypothesis,* proposes that the desire to die in one's birthplace leads many Latinos to engage in return migration, resulting in an artificially low Latino mortality rate because out-of-country deaths are not tabulated in U.S. mortality statistics. In contrast to migratory artifact explanations, the *health behaviors hypothesis* proposes that the lower mortality is genuine and is due to favorable health behaviors and risk factor profiles among Latinos, which contribute to their lower mortality. Tests of these hypotheses present numerous methodological issues and challenges. Nevertheless, the salmon and healthy migrant hypotheses have not been supported in recent research. Whether favorable health behaviors account for the epidemiological paradox remains a question for future research.

In light of the relatively good health of immigrants and the epidemiological paradox, it is interesting to note that positive health behaviors worsen with acculturation. Acculturation refers to the process by which immigrants adopt the attitudes, values, customs, beliefs, and behavior of a new culture. Alcohol consumption, smoking, and a number of other risky behaviors increase with acculturation. The mechanisms accounting for these findings are not clear, but may include loss of protective cultural health beliefs, behavioral practices, identity and values, and responses to continued discrimination.

Cancer rates, infant mortality, and other physical and mental health indicators, in addition to health behaviors, worsen with acculturation. For example, the incidence and mortality rates of various cancers (e.g., lung, colon, breast, ovary) among Latino immigrants are lower than those of their U.S.-born counterparts and U.S.-born non-Latino Whites. Furthermore, trends over time indicate that, for forms of cancer that are responsive to lifestyle and environmental factors (e.g., colon but not stomach cancer), the mortality rates of immigrant Latino groups increase toward those of the United States and are higher than rates found in their country of origin. Acculturation, therefore, presents some interesting challenges as it concerns the health of immigrants.

TUBERCULOSIS

Tuberculosis (TB) has received a great deal of attention as an immigrant health issue. The migration of individuals from high prevalence to industrialized countries is a major factor sustaining TB prevalence. The proportion of immigrants among persons reported having TB exceeds 50% in some states

(California, New York, Texas, Florida, New Jersey, and Illinois). One of the most common hypotheses concerning the high rate of TB among the foreign-born is latent infection due to previous residence in a high prevalence country. Another frequently cited factor is the number of years elapsed since arrival in the low prevalence country. Some studies suggest that the rate of developing TB is higher in the first 2 to 5 years after arrival. Although some researchers attribute this increase to the stress of migration and resettlement, others cite lack of access to health care.

ACCESS TO HEALTH CARE

Access to health care is a primary determinant of health status. Due to an increasing rise in the cost of health services, affordability (the ability to pay for care or health insurance) is a fundamental barrier to health care access for many Americans. Studies reveal that noncitizen immigrants are more likely to lack health insurance coverage than the native born and immigrants who have become citizens. Employment characteristics, legal status, and length of residency in the United States impact the uninsurance rates of immigrants. Among full-time workers, immigrants are more likely than nonimmigrants to obtain low-wage jobs that do not provide employer-sponsored health insurance.

Although access to health care is often conceptualized simply as affordability, it is important to consider other dimensions. For example, two other components of access—availability and accessibility—influence utilization of health and social services. Availability is defined by the location, concentration, and capacity of health care services in a given community. Accessibility describes the ease of obtaining services in the community, such as distance, transportation, and travel. Studies indicate that more physicians tend to practice in middle- and high-income rather than low-income neighborhoods in which immigrants are more likely to live, which results in a lack of choice and services available for obtaining medical care.

Accommodation, another component of access to health care, describes the tailoring of health services to fit the needs of a community. A large proportion of immigrants are classified as Limited English Proficient (LEP), which refers to the inability to speak, read, write, or understand English at a level that permits effective interaction. Therefore, bilingual or multilingual staff, translated materials, and interpreter services are critical elements facilitating access to care for immigrants. A deficiency in such services can lead to miscommunication, misdiagnosis, patient dissatisfaction, and errors in and less adherence to medical treatment. Federal law mandates linguistically appropriate health care. Title VI of the Civil Rights Act of 1964 states, "No person in the United States shall, on the ground of race, color, or national origin, be excluded from participation in, be denied the benefits of, or be subjected to discrimination under any program or activity receiving Federal assistance." Health institutions receiving federal funds are required to post policies regarding language access. Failure to accommodate programs to meet the needs of linguistically diverse populations creates access barriers.

Another component of access to health care, acceptability, refers to the actual and perceived value of care by the patient. Because culture influences how individuals define illness, suffering, and dying, the lack of cross-cultural skills among health care providers or their failure to understand cultural values may lead to poor patient outcomes and inappropriate interactions in clinical settings. For instance, Latino cultural values include the expectation that individuals be treated with *respeto* (respect) and *cortesía* (courtesy). These values take particular significance in the health care setting. Cultural incompatibility with mainstream health providers has been identified as a major obstacle against seeking health care, particularly in regard to mental health services. The importance of understanding cultural beliefs and values has led to a growing movement in cultural competence education in the health professions.

POLICY ISSUES

Anti-immigrant sentiment and policy also affect health care access and utilization. Prior to the passage of any federal or state policy regarding public welfare programs, legal immigrants, like U.S. citizens, were entitled to and eligible for federal programs. But the passage of the Personal Responsibility and Work Opportunity Reconciliation Act of 1996 (PRWORA) rendered immigrants ineligible for immediate access to federal programs. A new system of classification was developed creating a "qualified immigrant category," which included, among other groups, lawful permanent residents. Some qualified immigrants must wait 5 years from the legal date of entry into the

United States to obtain federal benefits. Those immigrants who are not qualified are ineligible for benefits regardless of entry date. However, they are granted access to emergency services, emergency Medicaid, immunizations, and screenings for communicable diseases (e.g., HIV/AIDS and tuberculosis). States have the authority to create Medicaid and Child Health Insurance Plan (CHIP) programs, which provide benefits during the 5-year period to particular postenactment immigrants, providing another alternative to health care.

In addition, the Illegal Immigration Reform and Immigrant Responsibility Act of 1996 and California's Proposition 187 (passed in 1993 but not enacted) discourage immigrants and their children from accessing health care because of fears of becoming a "public charge" (i.e., dependent upon public benefits). Whether an immigrant is likely to become a public charge is one of the criteria used to determine entrance or immigrant status in the United States. Despite the Department of Justice's statement that Medicaid and CHIP recipients are independent of the public charge status, some immigrants have responded to these policies by not seeking health care from government resources, further exacerbating health problems. In addition, many families do not apply for public benefits to which they are entitled because of limited awareness of eligibility requirements, particularly for children. Because more immigrants delay care, there is an overreliance upon safety net facilities.

PSYCHOSOCIAL ISSUES

In addition to anti-immigrant programs and policies, and barriers to health care that foster significant hardships, immigrants encounter a multitude of other stressors. Migration leads to profound changes in social networks, socioeconomic status and culture, and exposure to ethnic and racial discrimination. Among various immigrant groups, the cultural orientation to family offers an important social resource for dealing with these multiple stressors. The family provides strong social networks and multigenerational reciprocal support systems that promote physical and psychological well-being.

Upon settlement in the United States, contextual factors, such as neighborhood characteristics, serve as both resources and barriers to health. Settlement in ethnic enclaves (e.g., Little Havana in Miami, Chinatown

in New York City) creates mutual, supportive environments with a shared culture. Simultaneously, poverty, underemployment and unemployment, congested and substandard housing, and high rates of communicable diseases (e.g., TB), infant mortality, and crime characterize many of these communities.

The issue of ethnic enclaves bears directly on immigrant health. But there is a paucity of research in behavioral medicine on the role of broad contextual factors, such as ethnic enclaves, in promoting health. Much research in behavioral medicine is based on individual-level theories that ignore social factors. Furthermore, a deficit model often underlies research on the health of immigrants, in that assumptions are made about social forces *acting upon* individuals and groups, with little consideration of the cultural strengths and other social resources that enable individuals to act upon their environments and social circumstances. Research on social capital provides a framework from which to identify the social structures in ethnic enclaves that may enhance health. Social capital is defined broadly as the aspects of social structures that provide resources to individuals. Measures of social capital include membership and engagement in civic associations, levels of interpersonal trust, and perceptions of reciprocity. There is a growing body of evidence that social capital is an important resource for promoting health. Social capital may operate via several mechanisms, including the mobilization of social support, promotion of healthy behaviors, and other psychosocial processes. Interestingly, the communal (versus individual) cultural orientation that is characteristic of various immigrant groups suggests a major role for social capital in promoting health in ethnic enclaves. For example, the communal orientation of immigrant groups has led to the development of mutual aid organizations that provide legal, social, and other services to community residents and recent immigrants.

In conclusion, the goal of Health Care for All, promulgated by many government agencies, must extend to and encompass all individuals in the United States. The variety of cultural, structural, psychosocial, and policy barriers to health that are unique to immigrant groups must continue to be studied and addressed. It is important, therefore, to avoid attributing adverse health outcomes to cultural variables in lieu of a thorough exploration of the broader social and policy factors that may be involved. Furthermore, these broad contextual factors should also be considered when developing programs of research and service aimed at improving the health of immigrants.

—Ana F. Abraído-Lanza, Kellee White, and Elizabeth Vásquez

See also ACCULTURATION AND HEALTH; CULTURAL FACTORS AND HEALTH; HEALTH DISPARITIES; SOCIAL CAPITAL AND HEALTH; SOCIAL INTEGRATION, SOCIAL NETWORKS, AND HEALTH

Further Reading

Abraído-Lanza, A. F., Dohrenwend, B. P., Ng-Mak, D. S., & Turner, J. B. (1999). The Latino mortality paradox: A test of the "salmon bias" and healthy migrant hypotheses. *American Journal of Public Health, 89,* 1543-1548.

Angel, J. L., & Angel, R. J. (1992). Age at migration, social connections, and well-being among elderly Hispanics. *Journal of Aging and Health, 4,* 480-499.

Bagley, S. P., Angel, R., Dilworth-Anderson, P., Liu, W., & Schinke, S. (1995). Panel V: Adaptive health behaviors among ethnic minorities. *Health Psychology, 14,* 632-640.

Carrasquillo, O., Carrasquillo, A. I., & Shea, S. (2000). Health insurance coverage of immigrants living in the United States: Differences by citizenship status and country of origin. *American Journal of Public Health, 90,* 917-923.

Cornelius, L. J. (2000). Limited choices for medical care among minority populations. In C. J. R. Hogue, M. A. Hargraves, & K. S. Collins (Eds.), *Minority health in America: Findings and policy implications from the Commonwealth Fund minority survey* (pp. 176-193). Baltimore: Johns Hopkins University Press.

Cheung, F. K., & Snowden, L. R. (1990). Community mental health and ethnic minority populations. *Community Mental Health Journal, 26,* 277-291.

Chun, K. M., Balls Organista, P., & Marín, G. (Eds.). (2003). *Acculturation: Advances in theory, measurement and applied research.* Washington, DC: American Psychological Association.

Cromley, E. K. (2002). *GIS and Public Health.* New York: Guilford.

Kawachi, I., & Berkman, L. (2000). Social cohesion, social capital and health. In L. F. Berkman & I. Kawachi (Eds.), *Social epidemiology.* New York: Oxford University Press.

Loue, S. (Ed.). (1998). *Handbook of immigrant health.* New York: Plenum.

Mallin, K., & Anderson, K. (1988). Cancer mortality in Illinois Mexican and Puerto Rican immigrants, 1979-1984. *International Journal of Cancer, 41,* 670-676.

Marín, G., & Marín, B. V. (1991). *Research with Hispanic populations.* Newbury Park, CA: Sage.

Markides, K. S., & Coreil, J. (1986). The health of Hispanics in the southwestern United States: An epidemiologic paradox. *Public Health Reports, 101,* 253-265.

Markides, K. S., Boldt, J. S., & Ray, L. A. (1986). Sources of helping and intergenerational solidarity: A three-generation study of Mexican Americans. *Journal of Gerontology, 41,* 506-511.

Pablos-Méndez, A. (1994). Letter to the editor. *Journal of the American Medical Association, 271,* 1237-1238.

Rogler, L. H. (1994). International migrations: A framework for directing research. *American Psychologist, 49,* 701-708.

Rosenwaike, I., & Shai, D. (1986). Trends in cancer mortality among Puerto Rican-born migrants to New York City. *International Journal of Epidemiology, 15,* 30-35.

Schlosberg, C. (1999-2000). *Immigrant access to health benefits: A resource manual.* Washington, DC: Access Project and the National Health Law Program.

Scribner, R. (1996). Paradox as paradigm: The health outcomes of Mexican Americans [Editorial]. *American Journal of Public Health, 86,* 303-305.

Sorlie, P. D., Backlund, E., Johnson, N. J., & Rogot, E. (1993). Mortality by Hispanic status in the United States. *Journal of the American Medical Association, 270,* 2464-2468.

Talbot, E. A., Moore, M., McCray, E., & Binkin, N. J. (2000). Tuberculosis among foreign-born persons in the United States, 1993-1998. *Journal of the American Medical Association, 284,* 2894-2900.

Tornieporth, N. G., Ptachewich, Y., Poltoraskaia, N., Ravi, B. S., Katapadi, M., Berger, J. J., et al. (1997). Tuberculosis among foreign-born persons in New York City, 1992-1994: Implications for tuberculosis control. *International Journal of Tuberculosis and Lung Disease, 1,* 528-535.

Warshauer, M. E., Silverman, D. T., Schottenfeld, D., & Pollack, E. S. (1986). Stomach and colorectal cancers in Puerto Rican-born residents of New York City. *Journal of the National Cancer Institute, 76,* 591-595.

IMMUNE RESPONSES TO STRESS

Stress is "a physical, chemical, or emotional factor that causes bodily or mental tension and may be a factor in disease causation" (*Merriam-Webster's* 1998).

Stress has been described as harmful to one's health. The field of psychoneuroimmunology focuses on the influence of behavior on the interactions between the central nervous system, the endocrine system, and the immune system, and the impact on health. Effects on the immune system by one's behavior are mediated by a complex network of signals functioning in the bidirectional communication between the nervous, endocrine, and immune systems.

It was initially observed that the experience of stress has suppressive effects on the immune system. Recent data, however, have suggested that the magnitude and direction of this effect may be dependent on the characteristics and timing of the stressor. In general, acute stressors (lasting from minutes to hours) tend to stimulate the activity of the immune system, while chronic stressors (lasting from days to months or years) suppress the immune response. The fact that acute stressors up-regulate certain components of the immune response does not necessarily mean that the outcome is beneficial. For example, an acute stressor may produce or exacerbate skin allergies. Aside from the duration of the stressor, the nature of the stressor itself tends to have differing effects on various aspects of the immune system.

Two mechanisms by which the immune system can be affected by stress include the hypothalamic-pituitary-adrenal (HPA) axis and the sympathetic-adrenal medullary (SAM) axis. The term *axis* in this context is used to describe the physiological interactions that take place between the hypothalamus, pituitary gland, and adrenal gland. These mechanisms operate by producing biological mediators, including cytokines (a class of small proteins produced by immune and other types of cells that control the immune response) and neuroendocrine hormones, which interact with and affect cellular components of the immune system. For example, stress-induced activation of the HPA axis influences the immune system by the release of neuroendocrine hormones from the pituitary gland. Mediated by receptors for neuroendocrine hormones and neuropeptides, white blood cells in the lymph nodes and bone marrow (lymphoid and myeloid cells respectively) are able to respond to signals from the HPA axis and modify their functions.

In addition, the sympathetic nervous system plays a role in stress-induced changes in immune response through the SAM axis. For example, lymphoid and myeloid cells also have receptors for the catecholamines epinephrine and norepinephrine, which

enable them to respond to signals from the SAM axis. Immune cells can be stimulated to release cytokines, which in turn stimulate the increased production of corticotropin-releasing hormone (CRH) by the hypothalamus. CRH promotes the release of adrenocorticotropic hormone (ACTH) and corticosterone by the pituitary gland and the adrenal cortex respectively. It has also been demonstrated that various aspects of the immune response, such as proliferation of B- and T-lymphocytes, cytokine production, antibody responses to "nonself" molecules, migration of monocytes and neutrophils, and natural killer (NK) cell activity, can be affected by glucocorticoid hormones, such as cortisol, as well as peptides, such as ACTH, endorphins, substance P, and somatostatin.

In addition to cytokine production, it has been shown that white blood cells are themselves capable of synthesizing hormones, including ACTH, growth hormone, and prolactin. Furthermore, primary and secondary lymphoid organs, including bone marrow, thymus, spleen, and lymph nodes, are innervated by nerve fibers of the autonomic nervous system. The close association of these nerve terminals with immune cells allows direct neural-immune interaction through the formation of neuroeffector junctions. Norepinephrine, substance P, and other neurotransmitters are released at these junctions and can subsequently affect immune cells in the microenvironment of a lymph node, thereby affecting their function. The implications of these interactions are not yet understood.

White blood cells such as lymphocytes, monocytes/macrophages, and granulocytes have been shown to exhibit receptors for many neurotransmitters. It has been described that catecholamines can cause changes in immune function such as migration and multiplication of lymphocytes, B-lymphocyte antibody production, and cell destruction through the regulation of cyclic AMP (cAMP) levels. In addition, it has been shown that the treatment of leukocytes with catecholamines in tissue culture results in the suppression of interleukin (IL)-12 synthesis and an increase in IL-10 production. This can cause a shift in the T-helper (Th) lymphocyte population from Th1, which function in cell-mediated immune activities, to Th2 functions, which are involved in antibody responses.

Examples of stress-associated immune changes are provided in studies involving medical students taking examinations. The effect of examination stress on healthy medical students can cause a decrease in NK cell activity, a decrease in the response of leukocytes to plant products that induce cell division (mitogens), a decrease in production of interferon-gamma (IFN-γ) by leukocytes, a decrease in the antibody and virus specific T-lymphocyte responses to a hepatitis B vaccination, and changes in the ability of the immune system to control the expression of dormant herpes viruses such as Epstein-Barr virus (EBV) and herpes simplex virus type 1 (HSV-1). These medical students also reported an increased incidence of upper respiratory tract infections.

A stress-induced Th1/Th2 shift has also been observed in animal models. A restraint stress model used in studies with mice suggests that stress drives a shift in the Th1/Th2 balance toward Th2 dominance. A significant decrease in NK cell activity and in IFN-γ production by mitogen-stimulated cells isolated from spleens, and a concomitant increase in serum corticosterone levels, were observed after restraint stress. Another study showed that restraint stress inhibited migration of leukocytes and Th1 cytokine production during *Listeria monocytogenes* infection.

The chronic stress of caregiving for a spouse with dementia was associated with the down-regulation of cellular immune responses. For example, leukocytes from the caregivers exhibited an inhibition of T-lymphocyte responses to mitogens and a monoclonal antibody to the T-cell receptor, a poorer memory immune response to HSV-1, and an inhibition of the ability of NK cells to respond to genetically engineered IL-2 and IFN-γ. Caregivers also had a higher incidence of respiratory infections.

One of the factors implicated in the dysregulation of the immune response is the cytokine IL-6. Elevated levels of serum IL-6 are associated with stress and depression in humans. These results are consistent with those seen in rats exhibiting increased levels of plasma IL-6 after exposure to various stressors. This observed elevation in plasma IL-6 paralleled the increase in plasma cortisol. Together, these results support the idea that IL-6, along with other proinflammatory cytokines, plays a role in mediating effects of stress on the immune system and a role in increasing the possibility of extending inflammatory responses that can have important health outcomes such as risk for cardiovascular disease.

These studies suggest that psychological stress can affect immune responses to a degree that is large enough to put individuals at risk for the development and severity of infectious disease. This is of medical concern, since the aging process results in a dampening of some components of the immune system, making older individuals at risk for stress-associated decreases in cellular immunity.

—*Eric V. Yang and Ronald Glaser*

See also AIDS AND HIV: STRESS; ALLOSTATIS, ALLOSTATIC LOAD, AND STRESS; BEREAVEMENT AND HEALTH; CAREGIVING AND STRESS; STRESS: BIOLOGICAL ASPECTS; WOUND HEALING AND STRESS; PSYCHONEUROIMMUNOLOGY

Further Reading

Ader, R., Felten, D. L., & Cohen, N. (2001). *Psychoneuroimmunology*. San Diego, CA: Academic Press.

Glaser, R., & Kiecolt-Glaser, J. K. (1994). *Handbook of human stress and immunity*. San Diego, CA: Academic Press.

Merriam-Webster's collegiate dictionary. (1998). Springfield, MA: Merriam-Webster.

Rabin, B. S. (1999). *Stress, immune function, and health: The connection*. New York: Wiley-Liss.

INCOME INEQUALITY AND HEALTH

RELATIONSHIPS BETWEEN INCOME AND HEALTH

It is widely accepted that income is related to an individual's level of health. Higher incomes enable individuals to afford the goods and services necessary to promote health. It is equally recognized that poor health leads to loss of income, for example, because of extra expenditures on medical care, or because of loss of employment. This entry does not dwell further on the reverse causal pathway from poor health to lower income (for a detailed discussion of this pathway, see Subramanian, Belli, & Kawachi, 2002). Instead, we begin by discussing the various alternative hypotheses linking income to health outcomes. To summarize, four possible hypotheses have been put forward to explain the association between income and health.

Absolute Income Hypothesis

The absolute income hypothesis posits that individuals' health is determined solely by their own level

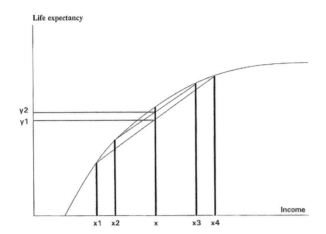

Figure 1   The Concave Relationship Between Income and Life Expectancy

of income (and not anyone else's income). The relationship of individual income to health outcomes (such as risk of mortality) is sometimes described as a "gradient," that is, at each level of income, individuals experience better health than those immediately below them. Stated another way, worse health status is not confined to those individuals who live below some predefined poverty threshold (compared with those who are above it). Higher incomes appear to be associated with better health outcomes even within the middle-class range of incomes. On the other hand, to describe the association between income and health as a gradient is possibly misleading, since the relationship is not strictly linear, but rather concave (Figure 1), that is, there are diminishing returns to health improvement with additional rises in income (up to a point where the theoretical maximum life span is attained). We return later to the concave relationship between income and health.

Relative Income Hypothesis

A second hypothesis linking income to health is the so-called relative income hypothesis, which posits that an individual's level of health is determined not just by the person's own level of income but also by the incomes of others in his or her community. In other words, the gap (or relative distance) between a person's income and the community average level of income may matter for health, in addition to a person's own (absolute) level of income. For example, a person earning $10,000 per year might experience a different level of health, depending on whether others

in the community also earn $10,000, or $1 million. If the gap between a person's income and his or her community average income is large, this may result in invidious social comparisons and stress from efforts to catch up with the community standard of living. Sociologists have referred to this process as "relative deprivation." Relative deprivation may be harmful to health for reasons other than psychosocial processes. For example, rising community living standards are often associated with an enlargement of the range of consumer goods that are necessary to function as a member of that community. Many consumer goods, such as the telephone, the automobile, and access to the Internet, have followed the trajectory, starting out as luxury goods and eventually ending up as necessities. It follows that the income gap between the middle and bottom of the income distribution must be kept small in order to minimize the degree of social exclusion and relative deprivation.

Relative Rank Hypothesis

A third hypothesis concerning the relationship between income and health is the relative rank hypothesis. According to this hypothesis, it is not the goods and services that money can purchase that are relevant for improving health but rather the rank (or status) that extra income confers to the individual within the socioeconomic hierarchy. The theoretical basis for this hypothesis stems from repeated observations of the importance of rank in nonhuman primates (e.g., troops of baboons and macaque monkeys). In nonhuman primate societies, it has been observed that the lower the rank of the animal within a troop, the worse its health status. This finding is so robust that dominant animals that are experimentally assigned to a subordinate status develop depression, coronary disease, and other ailments.

Income Inequality Hypothesis

The fourth and last hypothesis linking income to health is the income inequality hypothesis, which posits that an individual's level of health is determined not just by his or her own level of income but also by the extent of inequality in the distribution of income within his or her community.

In empirical terms, the absolute income hypothesis has been corroborated numerous times and appears quite robust. Much less empirical evidence exists to

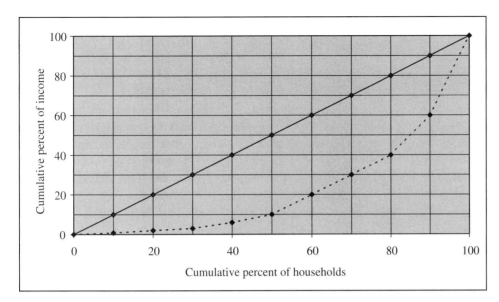

Figure 2   Lorenz Curve

aggregate income within that community accruing to each group. Under conditions of perfect equality in the distribution of income (Gini = 0), each decile group would account for exactly 10% of the aggregate income, such that the Lorenz curve would follow the 45-degree line of equality. In reality, the Lorenz curve falls below the 45-degree line of equality, because the bottom groups in the income distribution earn considerably less than their equal shares. (In Figure 2, it takes the bottom half of households to account for just 10% of the aggregate income.) The degree to which the Lorenz curve departs from the 45-degree line of equality is a measure of income inequality. As it turns out, the Gini coefficient is the ratio of the area between the Lorenz curve and the 45-degree line of equality, to the area of the triangle below the 45-degree line of equality.

support the relative income hypothesis, in part because of the difficulties of determining the relevant *reference group* against which individuals compare their incomes. Similarly, little work has been undertaken on the relative rank hypothesis, owing to the difficulty of isolating a pure rank effect from the simultaneous effects of income (i.e., rank and income are highly confounded). In contrast to the relative income and relative rank hypotheses, a growing number of studies have examined the effects of income inequality on population and individual health outcomes.

THE MEASUREMENT OF INCOME INEQUALITY

Various measures are available to quantify the extent of income inequality within a given community or society. Of these, the Gini coefficient is frequently used. Algebraically, the Gini coefficient is defined as half of the arithmetic average of the absolute differences between all pairs of incomes in a population, the total then being normalized on mean income. If incomes in a population are distributed completely equally, the Gini value is zero; and if one person has all the income (the condition of maximum inequality), the Gini is 1.0. The Gini coefficient can also be illustrated through the use of the *Lorenz curve* (Figure 2). On the horizontal axis, the population (in this case, households) is sorted and ranked according to income, from the lowest decile group to the top decile group. The vertical axis then plots the proportion of the

INCOME INEQUALITY AND HEALTH THEORY

There is a straightforward relationship between the degree of income inequality in society and its average level of health achievement. The relationship is illustrated in Figure 1. As mentioned earlier, the relationship between individual income and life expectancy is concave, such that each additional dollar of income raises individual health by a decreasing amount. In a hypothetical community consisting of just two individuals—a rich one (with income $x4$) and a poor one (with income $x1$)—transferring a given amount of money (amount $x4$ minus $x3$) from the rich to the poor will result in an improvement in the average life expectancy of that community (from $y1$ to $y2$), because the improvement in the health of the poor person will more than offset the loss in health of the rich person. Indeed, it is possible that by transferring incomes from the relatively flat part of the income/health curve, there would be no loss in health for the wealthy.

By extending this argument, one can see that, given two communities with the same average income level, the community with the narrower distribution of income will have better average health status, all other things being equal. The basic reasoning behind this argument applies equally to the distribution of income within a society as well as between countries of the world.

Besides the above argument, income inequality may also have an additional effect on health by causing a downward *shift* in the income/health curve. In other words, at each level of income, individuals living in a less egalitarian community might experience worse health status. Testing this hypothesis requires hierarchical data, with information gathered on both individual incomes, as well as the extent of income inequality in the community within which he or she resides (see below).

Mechanisms Linking Income Inequality and Health

Four mechanisms have been put forward to explain the link between income inequality and worse health status.

The first mechanism is through adverse patterns of social spending, accompanying the widening of income differentials consequently leading to reduced access to life opportunities. When the income distance widens between the rich and the poor, their interests begin to diverge, and groups find that they have less in common with each other. For instance, in more unequal societies, the pooling of resources that could finance public services such as health care systems and education is difficult to achieve. Because the rich tend to rely more on privately financed services, this translates into pressure to cut social spending, which in turn affects the access to social services for the poor.

A second set of processes is linked to diminished social cohesion that manifests through increased social tensions, erosion of social trust and mutual aid, and intergroup conflict. The wider the gap between the rich and poor, the greater is the strain on the social fabric and vice versa. For instance, during World War II in Britain, narrowing income differentials were accompanied by a greater sense of solidarity and social cohesion, besides an improvement in life expectancy. It is postulated that certain features of social relations—such as the level of trust between citizens, norms of reciprocity and mutual aid, and the ability to cooperate—represent resources for achieving collective ends (see entry on Social Capital and Health).

A third potential pathway involves psychosocial pathways through which income inequality may result in invidious social comparisons, frustration, and stress, accompanied by negative emotions, hostility, and downstream physiological consequences. According to this view, income inequality results in direct physiological damage (through the repeated stress-triggered activation of the neuroendocrine and other systems), as well as more adverse patterns of coping behaviors, such as smoking or excessive drinking.

The above pathways are not mutually exclusive, though most empirical studies have focused on the first two mechanisms linking income inequality to health. Occasionally, the "access to life opportunities" and "psychosocial" interpretation of the income inequality-health link have been cast as if they were competing mechanisms. In reality, it is usually not possible to disentangle their unique effects from one another. In principle, all material resources of some relevance to daily life have some psychosocial meaning attached to them. For example, home or car ownership has both a material interpretation as well as a psychosocial one (as in the symbolic sense of security that home or car ownership affords). An Internet or telephone connection enables subscribers to find jobs or keep their jobs (calling in sick), as well as fulfill their sense of social connectedness. Even employment or money fosters a sense of control.

Income Inequality and Health—Empirical Evidence

A growing body of literature has found that income inequality, over and above the effects of poverty and individual income, is detrimental to population health. Cross-sectional ecological studies have suggested that income inequality is associated with lower life expectancy, higher infant mortality, higher homicide rates, depressive symptoms, and lower self-rated health, in both developing countries and developed ones. An inverse relationship between economic inequality and lower health achievement has been reported *within* countries as diverse as the United States, the United Kingdom, Taiwan, and Brazil, as well as *between* different countries.

However, in order to address the potential confounding of income inequality by individual income, studies must collect information on both income at the individual level and income distribution at the aggregate level, that is, they must be multilevel. Three trends emerge from the published multilevel analyses of income inequality and health. First, studies supporting a link between income inequality and health outcomes have been almost exclusively carried out within the United States, one of the most unequal societies in the ranks of the highly industrialized countries. In contrast, over half of the null studies have been carried out in societies that are more egalitarian than the United States, and moreover have welfare state protections that are more far-reaching than in the United States (e.g., Japan, Sweden, Denmark, New Zealand, and even the United Kingdom). Second, studies with positive findings generally tended to have larger sample sizes, especially comparing the positive and negative studies carried out on data within the United States. Third, studies with positive findings for income inequality have largely conceptualized income-inequality as a U.S. state-level covariate. By contrast, the majority of studies with null results have been carried out at units of aggregation that are smaller than the U.S. states (e.g., municipalities in Sweden, parishes within a single city, regions within New Zealand, constituency and regions in the United Kingdom, or U.S. counties and metropolitan areas).

Summarizing the existing data to date, there is a strong suggestion that studies need to be sufficiently powered to find an effect of income inequality on individual health outcomes. In other words, there must be a sufficient number of individuals within a sufficient number of areas to make the multilevel analysis meaningful. Furthermore, the studies suggest a more consistent effect of income inequality at larger units of aggregation (states) than at smaller units (such as census tracts, wards, or parishes). Although this pattern is largely driven by the U.S. state-level analyses, it provides a clue that the mechanisms underlying the observed association between income inequality and health likely involve political decisions at the state level regarding patterns of social spending that affect health. It must be noted that most studies on income inequality and health have paid less attention to other substantive issues such as the potential lag period between exposure to income inequality and health outcomes; the potential for a threshold effect of income inequality on population health; as well as the potential for cross-level interactions whereby state

income-inequality may affect the health of different population groups differently.

—*S. V. Subramanian and Ichiro Kawachi*

See also Ecosocial Theory; Health Disparities; Neighborhood Effects on Health and Behavior; Socioeconomic Status and Health

Further Reading

Kawachi, I., & Kennedy, B. P. (1999). Income inequality and health: Pathways and mechanisms. *Health Services Research, 34*, 215-227.

Kawachi, I., & Kennedy, B. P. (2002). *The health of nations.* New York: New Press.

Kawachi, I., Kennedy, B. P., & Wilkinson, R. G. (Eds.). (1999). *Income inequality and health: A reader.* New York: New Press.

Subramanian, S. V., Belli, P., & Kawachi, I. (2002). The macroeconomic determinants of health. *Annual Reviews of Public Health, 23*, 287-302.

Subramanian, S.V., Blakely, T., & Kawachi, I. (2003). Income inequality as a public health concern: Where do we stand? *Health Services Research, 38*(1), 153-167.

Wagstaff, A., & van Doorslaer, E. (2000). Income inequality and health: what does the literature tell us? *Annual Reviews of Public Health, 21*, 543-567.

INFERTILITY AND ASSISTED REPRODUCTION: PSYCHOSOCIAL ASPECTS

CAUSES OF INFERTILITY

A medical diagnosis of infertility is made when a pregnancy does not occur after one year of unprotected sexual intercourse. It is estimated that one in every six couples of childbearing age experience medically diagnosable infertility problems. For many years there was a belief in a diagnosis of psychogenic infertility, where infertility was seen to have psychological causes. However, extensive psychological research over many years has found no evidence to support this diagnosis. Furthermore, advancements in scientific analysis of the biological aspects of reproduction, namely eggs, sperm, and the male and female reproductive systems, have enabled the identification of medical causes of infertility in cases that were previously determined to be "idiopathic infertility," or infertility of unknown cause. In general, male factor problems relating to sperm numbers, morphology (shape), or motility account for 40% of infertility diagnoses; female factor problems such as ovulation disorders, fallopian tube blockages, endometriosis, or age-related egg problems account for another 40% of diagnoses; and combined male/female subfertility accounts for the remaining 20% of infertility cases.

Behavioral medicine research in infertility has focused primarily on the psychosocial consequences of infertility and its treatment, psychosocial factors associated with in vitro fertilization (IVF) outcome, and the development of psychosocial interventions to enhance coping with IVF treatment. We now briefly review types of infertility treatment available and the role of psychosocial factors in infertility and its treatment.

INFERTILITY TREATMENT: ASSISTED REPRODUCTION

Medical treatment for infertility has changed significantly following the development of IVF-assisted reproduction techniques. IVF is a process involving the fertilization of eggs from sperm outside the woman's body. The resultant fertilized egg, or zygote, is incubated for several days and replaced several days later in the woman's uterus. Although pregnancy rates worldwide have improved with IVF, implantation rates (i.e., the pregnancy rate per transferred embryo) currently range from 10% to 30%, depending on the IVF clinic and the age of the woman. However, there is significant variability in the reporting of treatment results as well as differences in the number of embryos transferred in any one cycle. Prior to the development of IVF, assisted reproductive treatment was limited to hormonal treatment for ovulatory problems, microsurgery for repair of tubal damage or vas deferens blockage, or insemination with sperm from either the male partner or an anonymous sperm donor. These treatments continue to be offered, but the assisted reproductive technologies of IVF, including recent variations such as intracytoplasmic sperm injection (ICSI), are utilized in more complex or difficult situations. While a medical diagnosis of infertility strictly relates to heterosexual couples practicing regular intercourse, infertility treatment may also be offered to the so-called social infertility of single women, lesbian couples, and heterosexual couples who do not have regular sexual intercourse.

Psychosocial Impact of Infertility and Assisted Reproduction

Negative Affect

Despite there being no evidence to support the commonly held belief that infertility is caused by stress, there is considerable evidence that infertility and its treatment is the cause of significant stress and distress among infertile couples. Infertile women express higher levels of distress than fertile women, with the greatest distress peaking between the second and third year postinfertility diagnosis (Domar et al., 2000). Furthermore, research by Suzanne Miller and colleagues (1998) has found that infertile women report levels of infertility-related intrusive thoughts comparable with psychiatric outpatients being treated for stress reactions to traumatic events. Infertility-related distress appears to fluctuate throughout the infertility treatment cycle. A number of studies have found increased anxiety and depression in women both before treatment (but after diagnosis) and after unsuccessful treatment or neonatal loss. The grief reactions of the infertility experience have been likened to the loss of a loved one or of a longed for baby. Women frequently describe experiencing feelings of loss at each monthly menstrual period and particularly after an unsuccessful assisted reproductive cycle. Very little infertility research has included male partners; however, the limited research available consistently shows that at all points in the IVF cycle, women experience far greater infertility-related distress than do their male partners.

Coping Responses

For most couples, the diagnosis of infertility typically involves appraisals of threat and loss in relation to their expectations of parenthood. Less frequently, couples appraise an infertility diagnosis positively, perceiving this as an opportunity to enhance their personal relationship and to foster closer bonds. Coping responses to infertility vary according to the duration of infertility and within each member of the infertile couple. A perception of being out of control is a common response to infertility diagnosis. Problem-focused coping (e.g., seeking information) has been found to increase levels of well-being and reduce anxiety and depression, particularly in coping with initial diagnosis and the commencement of IVF treatment. However, over time, if IVF treatment continues to be unsuccessful, emotion-focused coping or blunting strategies (e.g., emotional discharge and venting) become more adaptive in coping with the uncontrollable aspects of treatment. Moreover, the availability of social support has been found to facilitate adjustment to infertility over the long term. The coping strategies adopted by infertile women differ from those used by their partners. In general, women report utilizing a greater range of infertility-related coping strategies than men. This difference may be a reflection of the greater level of distress experienced by women. Furthermore, while women have been found to openly discuss their infertility among their wider support network of family and friends, men are more likely to discuss their infertility with only their spouse.

Interpersonal Relationships

Infertility additionally exerts considerable influence on the self-image and interpersonal relationships of infertile couples. In particular, spousal and other family relationships appear to be most affected by the experience of infertility. For a man, a diagnosis of sperm problems can affect his view of himself as a sexual and masculine being. In the case of an infertile woman, finding that she may not be able to conceive a child challenges her perceptions of herself as a mother, and for a family, an assumed next generation and an expected continuity may not occur. Infertility is an isolating experience, with loneliness particularly evident among women undergoing assisted reproduction. The impact of infertility can be seen as a long-term process, rather than a sequence of distinct events. Over time, the effects of infertility have been found to permeate through personal, work, and family relationships. Research by Boivin and colleagues suggests that the relationship between treatment failure and personal and marital distress appears to be curvilinear. Infertile couples with a moderate amount of treatment failure experience the most distress, whereas distress is lower for couples with low or high treatment failure rates, irrespective of age, years infertile, or years in treatment. These findings suggest that the experience of infertility-related distress is a necessary part of the process toward long-term adjustment.

Another aspect of the impact of infertility on interpersonal relationships is the effect of assisted reproduction on the experience of pregnancy and parenting following successful treatment. Women conceiving through IVF report greater pregnancy-related anxiety, anticipate more difficult infants upon birth, and undergo less preparation for childbirth and parenthood than naturally conceiving women. However, as parents, mothers of children conceived using assisted reproduction experience less parenting stress and more positive mother-child and father-child relationships than mothers of naturally conceived children. Furthermore, in contrast to the greater parenting difficulties anticipated in IVF-conceived pregnancies, at 12 months postpartum, no differences have been found in child functioning in terms of attachment and parental responsiveness. Thus, while conception and pregnancy for couples utilizing assisted reproduction is characterized by increased anxiety and distress, the experience of parenting appears to be positive, with the children indistinguishable from their naturally conceived counterparts. The long-term effects of assisted reproduction conception on parental and child functioning are yet to be determined.

Psychosocial Factors Associated With IVF Outcome

There is some evidence that psychological factors, such as stress and anxiety, influence the outcome of assisted reproductive treatment. In general, women experiencing greater levels of infertility-related stress have poorer IVF treatment outcomes, in terms of number of eggs retrieved, number of eggs fertilized, and successful implantation/pregnancy. The results of a large, prospective multicenter trial in the Netherlands suggest that high levels of pretreatment anxiety and depression are associated with fewer pregnancies. Moreover, stress experienced prior to the commencement of IVF treatment appears to have the greatest negative impact on pregnancy outcome, compared with stress experienced throughout the IVF treatment cycle. A prolonged or chronic condition of stress also appears to be linked with lower IVF implantation rates. Moreover, recent research by Sherman, Montrone, and Miller (2002) suggests that other psychological factors may impact IVF pregnancy outcome. It was found that for women, the use of humor as a coping response, and for men, high levels of infertility-related distress, were associated with greater IVF pregnancy rates. Taken together, these findings suggest that psychosocial interventions may impact fertility status and the outcome of infertility treatment. To date, very few studies have evaluated this hypothesis by developing psychophysiological interventions designed to minimize stress. There is some evidence that group-based psychological interventions designed to reduce stress among infertile women may lead to increased pregnancy rates. However, a lack of appropriate controls in these studies throws into question this apparent effect. Moreover, the underlying mechanisms by which such an effect could occur have still not been delineated, and remain open to investigation.

Interventions

Worldwide there is acceptance of the importance of psychosocial support as a necessary component of assisted reproductive treatment for infertility. Psychosocial support entails patient education, implications counseling, decision-making counseling, and psychotherapeutic interventions. A variety of support approaches may be used depending on the stage of diagnosis and/or treatment, the degree of patient distress, and whether or not third party reproductive assistance is required. Counseling approaches entailing implications, decision making, and assessment are most often used when there is consideration of the use of third party-assisted reproduction. Consideration is given to the use of donated gametes (sperm or eggs) and embryos, or when it is proposed that a woman act as a surrogate to carry a pregnancy for an infertile couple. Complex social and psychological issues exist for all involved in third-party infertility treatment, as well as for any resultant offspring of this form of infertility treatment. In addition, counseling deals with issues related to privacy and disclosure of the identity of the biological parents of the child. Despite the general acceptance of the need for infertility counseling, few counseling approaches are theory guided, and there has been little effort to systematically evaluate the efficacy of counseling for couples undergoing IVF treatment.

The acknowledgment that infertility and its treatment is associated with psychological distress has led to the development of a small number of theoretically guided psychotherapeutic interventions targeted at infertile couples undergoing assisted reproduction. Patient education, cognitive-behavioral, and psychophysiological interventions are most often used in an infertility context. Pretreatment information sessions are frequently conducted in either couple or group

settings to assist patients to cope with understanding the technology and complexities of the treatment process. The rationale behind this approach is that by informing couples of what to expect when undergoing infertility treatment, they will be empowered, feel a greater sense of control, and be able to make informed decisions regarding treatment. The provision of pretreatment information has been found to assist infertile couples in mobilizing coping resources, in turn, assisting them in enhancing adjustment during treatment. However, patient education alone has limited usefulness, since its effectiveness varies as a function of the type of information provided (e.g., procedural, sensory, suggested coping strategies), the controllability of the stressor, and individual differences in response style (e.g., preference for information).

Cognitive-behavioral interventions involve techniques designed to instruct the infertile couple in effective coping strategies and problem solving, reappraising dysfunctional cognitions, and "preliving" through role-play and behavioral rehearsal. In a related vein, psychophysiological interventions are designed specifically to minimize the physiological (i.e., hormonal, neurochemical, and neuroanatomical) reaction to the stress of infertility and its treatment, by incorporating techniques such as relaxation training. Support strategies to assist with management of distress, anxiety, and depression include individual, couple, and group interventions. Strategies include stress management, relaxation techniques, cognitive reframing, and family therapy. Alice Domar utilized a multimodal cognitive group therapy approach (i.e., relaxation training, stress management, cognitive restructuring, gentle stretching exercise, and general health and nutrition education) to derive a reduction in anxiety and depression among infertile women. There is some evidence to suggest that both cognitive-behavioral and psychophysiological intervention approaches have their merits for reducing anxiety and depression among infertile women. However, a lack of adequate controls for these studies draws into question the validity of these findings.

Another factor that needs to be taken into account when designing intervention protocols is individual differences in response style. Specifically, according to Miller's C-SHIP model, individuals are characterized by a distinctive profile of cognitive-affective response styles (high vs. low monitors). High monitors (who typically focus on and scan for health-related messages) are more likely to seek health-related information, whereas low monitors (who distract from and ignore health-related messages) fare better when provided with minimal information. Therefore, high monitors should benefit most from psychosocial interventions designed to reduce excessive risk-related distress and to facilitate deeper processing, and fuller anticipation, of the personal consequences of infertility treatment. In contrast, low monitors should benefit most from psychosocial interventions that increase awareness of infertility and its treatment while at the same time providing a means of managing any infertility-related distress.

In summary, the experience of infertility is associated with psychological distress for both women and men. However, individual coping responses differ within infertile couples and as a function of the specific nature and duration of the infertility experience. A lack of theory-guided counseling interventions, and the dearth of appropriately controlled evaluation studies, precludes any definitive judgment of the efficacy of counseling interventions for infertile couples. To date, cognitive-behavioral approaches appear to hold the greatest promise, perhaps combined with the use of relaxation training. Despite the evidence that both the male partner and female partner responses may influence pregnancy outcome, psychosocial interventions have primarily targeted infertile women and have failed to address the unique needs of male partners. The differences in responses to infertility between men and women highlight the need for theory-guided psychosocial interventions tailored to the unique needs of each member of the infertile couple.

—Kerry Sherman, Miranda Montrone, and Suzanne M. Miller

See also Low Birth Weight: Psychosocial Aspects; Pregnancy Outcomes: Psychosocial Aspects; Stress, Appraisal, and Coping

Further Reading

Connolly, K. J., Edelmann, R. J., Bartlett, H., Cooke, I. D., Lenton, E., & Pike, S. (1993). An evaluation of counselling for couples undergoing treatment for in-vitro fertilization. *Human Reproduction, 8*, 1332-1338.

Domar, A. D., Clapp, D., Slawsby, E., Kessel, B., Orav, J., & Freizinger, M. (2000). The impact of group psychological interventions on distress in infertile women. *Health Psychology, 19*, 568-575.

Gallinelli, A., Roncaglia, R., Matteo, M. L., Ciaccio, I., Volpe, A., & Facchinetti, F. (2001). Immunological changes and stress are associated with different implantation rates in patients undergoing in vitro fertilization embryo transfer. *Fertility & Sterility, 76*, 85-91.

Hammer Burns, L., & Covington, S. N. (1998). *Infertility counselling: A comprehensive handbook for clinicians.* New York: Parthenon.

Leiblum, S. R. (1997). *Infertility: Psychological issues and counseling strategies.* New York: John Wiley.

Miller, S. M., Mischel, W., Schroeder, C. M., Buzaglo, J. S., Hurley, K., Schreiber, P., et al. (1998). *Psychology and Health, 13*, 847-858.

Sherman, K. A., Montrone, M., & Miller, S. M. (2002, March). *Coping strategies and pregnancy outcome among couples undergoing in-vitro fertilisation* [Abstracts]. Sixtieth Annual Scientific Meeting, American Psychosomatic Society, Barcelona, Spain.

Slade, P., Emery, J., & Lieberman, B. A. (1997). A prospective, longitudinal study of emotions and relationships in in vitro fertilization treatment. *Human Reproduction, 12*, 183-190.

INJURY PREVENTION IN CHILDREN

THE PROBLEM OF INJURIES TO CHILDREN

Understanding Injury

The safety of children is one of the most pressing public health issues of our time. Injuries are responsible for more deaths in children over age 1 than any other health threat, and for every death from an injury, there are many more hospitalizations, emergency department visits, and outpatient treatment. Injuries occur when energy is transferred in ways, amounts, and rates that damage body structures and tissues. This can occur when a soccer player collides with a goal post, when an infant falls down the stairs, when a toddler swallows a household cleaner, or when two vehicles collide. While injuries are sometimes thought of as "accidents" or chance events of nature, it becomes clear that many injuries could have been prevented when the situations in which they happen are examined. For example, we know that teenage drivers demonstrate a higher rate of crashes and injuries than do adult drivers. However, the majority of these crashes and injuries occur in certain higher-risk situations, such as driving at night and with friends, and so could be prevented by restricting the conditions of driving. To emphasize the preventable nature of injuries, most health professionals prefer to call these events "unintentional injuries" rather than "accidents." Injuries may also be intentional, caused by acts of violence or abuse. Although important, the prevention of intentional injuries is quite different from the prevention of unintentional injuries, and so is not addressed in this entry.

Just as scientific advances such as immunizations and antibiotics led to improvements in the health of children, science also provides the public health community with tools for reducing the burden of childhood injuries. This entry addresses the problem of childhood injuries, what types of interventions have been developed to target this problem, and how individuals, organizations, and communities can help.

Epidemiology of Childhood Injuries

The public health burden attributable to injury can be examined both in terms of morbidity and mortality. Data from the National Center for Health Statistics indicate that 8,913 children died due to an unintentional injury in the year 2000, and more children over the age of 1 die from an injury than from any disease. In addition, according to the National Center for Injury Prevention and Control, for every childhood death caused by injury, there are an estimated 34 hospitalizations, 1,000 emergency department visits, and many more visits to health care providers. Each year, between 20% and 25% of all children sustain an injury severe enough to require medical attention, missed school, or bed rest. These injuries not only result in costs to life and health, but in financial costs as well. For example, in 1996, childhood unintentional injuries resulted in $14 billion in lifetime medical spending, $1 billion in other resource costs, and $66 billion in present and future work losses, imposing quality-of-life losses equivalent to 92,400 child deaths (Miller, Romano, & Spicer, 2000). While considerable progress has been made in decreasing injuries to children in the United States, it is estimated that almost one third of those injuries to children could be prevented using existing technology and strategies (Rivara & Grossman, 1996).

Prevalence of injury is not evenly distributed across demographic groups, further evidence of the nonrandom nature of unintentional injuries. The most common risk factors include male gender and low socioeconomic status (Grossman, 2000). These differences are likely attributable to both behavioral and environmental factors. For example, males tend to engage in more high-risk behaviors using fewer protective measures than females. Parents of lower socioeconomic status likely have fewer resources to devote to injury prevention measures, and their children may experience greater environmental exposure to risk for injury.

The most prevalent causes of childhood unintentional injuries vary by age, as children grow out of some kinds of risks and into others. For example, injuries common in young children include falls and burns, while sports-related injuries are common among adolescents. However, other injuries are important across ages. From infancy to young adulthood, motor vehicle crashes are a leading cause of death; drowning and house fires are also prevalent causes.

HISTORY OF INJURY PREVENTION EFFORTS

During the middle of the 20th century, infectious diseases and birth defects were among the most serious and widespread health problems, affecting many more people than injury events. As a result, injuries, thought then to be largely unavoidable, received little attention from the medical community. However, as progress was made in addressing the most widespread medical conditions, it became clear that injury events were responsible for a disproportionate number of deaths and suffering. Unintentional injuries are now the leading cause of death in the United States from ages 1 to 34.

Important work in addressing injuries began with a seminal work by DeHaven in 1942 (as cited in National Committee for Injury Prevention and Control, 1989). He was the first to study the biomechanics of injury and to recognize that individuals could be protected more effectively or "crash-packaged" when injury events occurred. Gordon followed this work and in 1949 (as cited in National Committee for Injury Prevention and Control, 1989) proposed that injuries could be studied like infectious diseases. He offered that injuries happen when the host (the person injured), the agent (the cause of the injury), and the environment in which the injury occurs interact to produce the injury event. Then Haddon defined the agent as the "energy" that caused the injury and the "vector" as the source that delivers the energy. The result of this work was the development of the Haddon matrix (Haddon, 1972), a table that classifies injury prevention strategies according to how they address the injury problem. Based on this matrix, injury prevention strategies may target the agent, the host, or the environment; they can also target different points in time relative to the injury. Pre-event strategies are those that prevent injuries from happening in the first place, while strategies targeting the event itself are designed to prevent injuries from being as serious when they do happen. Post-event strategies address the consequences of injury. For example, sports injuries can be addressed in the pre-event phase by targeting the individual or host through appropriate preseason conditioning. The agent of sports injuries can also be addressed in the event phase through the design and use of protective equipment, and the environment can be addressed in the post-event phase by providing certified athletic trainers at sporting events. The work of Haddon and others led to a shift in the public health community away from individual responsibility and the "accident-proneness" of individuals to the redesign of environments and products (Haddon, 1970).

INJURY PREVENTION STRATEGIES

Classification of Approaches

Strategies for any target and time point within Haddon's matrix may involve either active or passive approaches. Active approaches rely on changing the behavior of individuals to prevent injury, while passive approaches work automatically, without active participation on the part of the individual. Once implemented, passive approaches do not require repeated behavior change from the individual. An example of the difference between these strategies is illustrated in approaches to prevent injury from automobile collisions. Seat belts are an active approach. In order for individuals to be protected, they must buckle the seat belt every time they are in the car. Air bags, on the other hand, provide protection without the individual having to initiate any action, as do car design modifications such as manufacturing cars with a crumple zone and environmental changes such as modifying median spaces. Because passive approaches do not rely on obtaining repeated protective behavior from individuals, they are more effective and reliable in preventing injury than active approaches. As such, the public health community typically favors passive

approaches, except when they are not available or feasible. When passive approaches are not available or feasible, active strategies that require only one-time action on the part of the individual (such as turning down the temperature on one's hot water heater to prevent scalding of children) are the next most effective approach.

The majority of injury prevention strategies can be classified as educational, environmental, or legislative. Educational approaches are typically active; that is, they are designed to encourage individuals to adopt or continue prevention behaviors by increasing knowledge about a particular hazard or changing attitudes about the hazard. Environmental approaches, on the other hand, are typically passive, involving the modification of the environment in some way to prevent injury to individuals. Legislative approaches may be either active or passive, since either individual behavior or environmental modifications may be legislated. Educational, environmental, and legislative approaches are all important in reducing unintentional injury.

Educational Approaches

Educational approaches to injury prevention are based on the premise that, given sufficient information, people will generally act to protect and promote their health. For example, we may assume that knowledge about the risks of baby walkers will discourage parents from using them. However, it is now well known that human behavior is much more complex than this. An individual's behavior is influenced by numerous factors, including attitudes, norms, environmental facilitators and barriers, and the characteristics of one's social groups or organizations. To be effective, then, educational approaches need to address relevant determinants of children's or parents' behavior. There are several theories of behavior that identify the most relevant determinants of behavior and are useful in guiding the development of behavioral interventions to prevent injury. Among these are the health belief model (Rosenstock, 1974), theory of reasoned action (Ajzen, 1988), social cognitive theory (Bandura, 1986), precede-proceed model (Green & Kreuter, 1999), and precaution adoption process model (Weinstein & Sandman, 2002).

Educational strategies have been used extensively in both clinical and community settings. In clinical settings, efforts often target parents when they obtain health care services for their children. Because information received from health care providers typically has high credibility, this approach can be successful in persuading parents to adopt injury prevention practices. A review of injury prevention strategies in clinical settings (DiGuiseppi & Roberts, 2000) found that these types of efforts could be effective in promoting the use of safety behaviors by parents but only when guided by theories of behavior and behavior-change strategies.

Community-based educational strategies target a group of individuals or a geographic area, such as a school, neighborhood, or city. As with educational strategies in the clinical setting, the effectiveness of community-based approaches varies depending on the quality and comprehensiveness of the program. Community-based educational approaches that are successful use an array of strategies to target a series of factors influencing health behaviors; are based on theories of behavior change; are integrated into the community and tailored according to community needs; and involve community stakeholders in the development of strategies (Klassen, MacKay, Moher, Walker, & Jones, 2000). An example of such a program is the Seattle Bike Helmet campaign, which included strategies for increasing parents' awareness of the effectiveness of bicycle helmets, changing peer norms to make helmets "cool," and subsidizing helmet costs. The program resulted in an increase in bicycle helmet use among children and adolescents from 2% to 60% in 10 years (DiGuiseppi, Rivara, Koepsell, & Polissar, 1989).

Environmental and Policy Approaches

It is often possible to modify some aspect of the environment to decrease the risk for injury. When injury can be prevented through changing the environment rather than individual behavior, benefits are likely to be greater and more evenly distributed in the population. These types of approaches are especially useful for vulnerable populations such as children. For example, a review of community-based injury prevention interventions (Klassen et al., 2000) found limited support for the effectiveness of community-based education for improving pedestrian safety among young children. The author concluded that young children are not developmentally prepared to learn and react appropriately to traffic. As such, environmental modifications that limit the speed of

traffic and its proximity to children, such as speed limits, speed bumps, traffic signs, routing heavy traffic away from neighborhoods, and narrowing roads, are likely to demonstrate greater effectiveness.

Environmental approaches to injury prevention may include product modifications as well as changes in the physical environment. Changes in the environment include strategies such as the above-mentioned traffic safety measures, the installation of air bags in cars, the use of fences with self-latching gates around pools, and the use of breakaway bases in baseball. Product modifications that have become standard in the United States include the use of child-resistant caps for medications, flame-retardant sleepwear, presetting of home hot water heaters to prevent excessively high hot water temperatures, and the replacement of traditional infant walkers with devices that allow infants to play in an upright position but that do not roll. Environmental changes such as these may occur through community efforts or legislation. In either case, the principles of individual and community behavior change addressed earlier remain important, as such changes may require individual and community support. As such, it can be particularly effective to combine educational and environmental approaches. For example, the Safe Kids/Healthy Neighborhoods Coalition in the Harlem neighborhood of New York City focused on renovating playgrounds, providing safe, supervised activities, providing injury and violence prevention education, and providing safety equipment at a reasonable cost. This program was effective in reducing targeted injuries, decreasing them by 44% over target injuries (Davidson et al., 1994).

Perhaps the most powerful approach to injury prevention is the use of legislative authority. Legislation may address the behavior of individuals, such as requiring the use of seat belts, car seats, and motorcycle helmets; environmental or product modifications, such as mandating child-resistant caps on medications, fences around pools, or the installation of universal child restraint attachment systems; or legal processes, as in the enactment of graduated drivers licensing. The effectiveness of a legislative approach is illustrated in the history of efforts to promote car seat use. Despite educational efforts, car seats were not extensively used in the United States until required by law. Similar processes have been observed with bicycle helmet usage. In a study comparing bicycle helmet use in three adjoining Maryland counties, children in the county implementing combined education and legislative strategies showed a substantial increase in helmet use, while little change was observed in two neighboring counties using educational efforts only or no intervention (Dannenberg, Gielen, Beilenson, Wilson, & Joffe, 1993). When undertaken, then, legislation typically has a substantial impact on reducing injuries. For example, enactment of laws regarding childproof packaging of medications resulted in a 45% reduction from projected levels in childhood deaths due to unintentional ingestion of drugs (Rodgers, 1996). Analysis of motor vehicle crash data in New Zealand and the United States suggests that graduated driver licensing reduces crash injuries among adolescents (Ferguson, Leaf, Williams, & Preusser, 1996; Langley, Wagenaar, & Begg, 1996).

The use of legislation to reduce injury, while effective, requires that consideration be given to the inherent restriction of personal freedom for the promotion of societal health and welfare. When injury prevention behaviors or product specifications are mandated by law, the freedom of the individual is reduced. This trade-off between personal choice and societal protection has prompted long-standing debate, which is not often given adequate acknowledgment by either those favoring or those opposing a given legislation. Public health professionals recognize that legislation inherently restricts personal freedom, but also that society as a whole bears at least some of the costs associated with harm to its members. As such, restriction of individual freedom may be warranted for greater societal benefit.

Prior to the passage of legislation for injury prevention, then, a number of questions must be answered. What is the societal burden of the injury? To what degree does the legislation restrict individual freedom? How effective in reducing injury do we anticipate the legislation to be? Is the legislation enforceable? What other means are available to achieve a comparable reduction in injury? If it is determined that legislation is an appropriate approach, a number of other considerations are important. In general, one must consider the level of public support for the legislation and whether educational approaches are also needed to increase acceptance of and compliance with the legislation. If use of a particular product is to be required, certain factors need to be present. For example, before legislation regarding child safety seats was enacted, public support for their importance needed to be widespread, regulations for the manufacture of child safety seats according to a prescribed set of safety and performance standards needed to be in place, and the seats needed to be widely available and affordable. In addition to these considerations, any potential adverse effects of legislation must also be addressed. For example, in Australia, after the passage of a law mandating bicycle helmet use, there was a 36% decrease in bicycle riding among children (Centers for Disease Control and Prevention, 1993), which was believed to be attributable to the law. It is unlikely that proponents of the law expected it to result in a decrease in physical activity, a critically important health behavior. Perhaps this adverse effect could have been prevented through prelegislation education and efforts toward influencing social norms regarding helmet use.

Decision Making Regarding Injury Prevention Strategies

An important issue, then, is determining the most appropriate strategy or set of strategies to use to address a given problem area. In general, legislative approaches are most appropriate for injuries with a high cost to society (i.e., morbidity, mortality, financial) and for which other approaches are insufficient, or for protection of vulnerable populations such as children. Similarly, environmental approaches should be used whenever possible for the protection of children and other high-risk groups, for whom educational interventions may not be realistic. Because of their greater effectiveness, environmental approaches should also be considered for any injury with high prevalence and/or high cost to society. Finally, educational approaches are important for areas that cannot be adequately or appropriately addressed through environmental or legislative approaches, or for those that don't yet have the popular support necessary to address through environmental or legislative approaches. Educational approaches are most effective when they are theoretically driven and directed toward changing concrete behaviors that prevent specific injuries and have few environmental or attitudinal barriers. Overall, the most effective approaches use multiple strategies, and combine education with environmental or legislative change.

A comprehensive overview of issues involved in decision making regarding injury prevention strategies is provided by Runyan (1998). She contends that determining which injury prevention strategies to use

Table 1   Value Criteria for Evaluating Injury Prevention Strategies

Effectiveness

How well a given strategy actually reduces the problem should be a primary consideration. Unfortunately, this criterion may be ignored by well-meaning persons who observe a health threat and simply attempt to do "something" to address it.

Cost

The cost of implementing the strategy should be determined and then considered with the first criteria to provide an estimate of cost-effectiveness. It is useful to consider the cost of the strategy as compared to the costs of not implementing it.

Freedom

Strategies, especially legislation, may involve restricting the freedom of some persons. Consideration must be given to the benefits to society obtained by the strategy compared to the restriction in freedom imposed.

Equity

Equity may be either horizontal or vertical. Horizontal equity involves treating all people equally, as in regulations regarding car seat use or medication packaging. Vertical equity, on the other hand, involves unequal treatment that results in greater equity. An example of a strategy promoting vertical equity would be providing smoke detectors to low-income persons.

Stigmatization

A program or policy should not stigmatize persons or groups in the process of preventing injury. A strategy to which a population is opposed is unlikely to be effective. As such, one must take into account the sociocultural context in which a strategy is implemented.

Feasibility

The strategy under consideration must be feasible to implement. The resources required must be available, and the strategy must be both technologically and politically feasible.

for a given problem requires the delineation and weighting of relevant value criteria, and conceptualizes this as the "3rd dimension" of the Haddon matrix. Relevant value criteria must be determined for any particular issue, but typically include the following: effectiveness, cost, freedom, equity, stigmatization, preferences of the affected community or individuals, and feasibility (see Table 1).

MAKING IT HAPPEN

Preventing injuries to children requires efforts throughout the community and within the larger social context. Parents and other adults act as the most direct protectors of children, implementing injury protection measures in the home and acting as child advocates to keep their environments free from hazards. School personnel play a key role in promoting safety in the school environment and often in providing basic safety education to children. Health care providers also have an important role in counseling parents on injury prevention as part of regular preventive health care, providing specific advice relevant to the age and developmental stage of the child. Moreover, given their credibility and presence in the community, they are an important voice for the promotion of environmental changes and legislation that address injury prevention. Support for injury prevention measures is also needed from community leaders and coalitions, who may advocate for environmental change and legislative measures in their community.

Such efforts from individuals and groups are critical, but to be fully effective, they require an infrastructure to work in. Promoting and sustaining injury prevention activities requires organizational and structural support. This includes the collection and maintenance of reliable data on injuries, the training of clinical and research professionals in injury prevention, the availability of funding for injury research and practice, and the coordination of injury prevention efforts across local, state, federal, and nonprofit sectors. Much progress has been made in preventing injuries among children, but much more can be done. Coordinated efforts at the individual and community level, combined with organizational and structural support, are needed to reduce the public health burden of injury to children. By building on our history of addressing pressing public health issues and by drawing upon existing public health tools, we can ensure that children have safer environments and minimized risk of injury.

—*Tonja R. Nansel and Nancy L. Weaver*

See also ADOPTION OF HEALTH BEHAVIOR; HEALTH BELIEF MODEL; HEALTH PROMOTION AND DISEASE PREVENTION; THEORY OF PLANNED BEHAVIOR; THEORY OF REASONED ACTION

Further Reading

Ajzen, I. (1988). *Attitudes, personality, and behavior.* Chicago: Dorsey.

Bandura, A. (1986). *Social foundations of thought and action: A social cognitive theory.* Englewood Cliffs, NJ: Prentice Hall.

Centers for Disease Control and Prevention. (1993). Mandatory bicycle helmet use: Victoria, Australia. *Morbidity and Mortality Weekly Report, 42,* 359-363.

Dannenberg, A. L., Gielen, A. C., Beilenson, P. L., Wilson, M. H., & Joffe, A. (1993). Bicycle helmet laws and educational campaigns: An evaluation of strategies to increase children's helmet use. *American Journal of Public Health, 83,* 667-674.

Davidson, L. L., Durkin, M. S., Kuhn, L., O'Connor, P., Barlow, B., & Heagarty, M. C. (1994). The impact of the Safe Kids/Healthy Neighborhoods Injury Prevention Program in Harlem, 1988 through 1991. *American Journal of Public Health, 84,* 580-586.

DiGuiseppi, C. G., Rivara, F. P., Koepsell, T. D., & Polissar, L. (1989). Bicycle helmet use by children: Evaluation of a community-wide helmet campaign. *Journal of the American Medical Association, 262,* 2256-2261.

DiGuiseppi, C., & Roberts, I. G. (2000). Individual-level injury prevention strategies in the clinical setting. *Future of Children, 10*(1), 53-82.

Ferguson, S. A., Leaf, W. A., Williams, A. F., & Preusser, D. F. (1996). Differences in young driver crash involvement in states with varying licensure practices. *Accident Analysis and Prevention, 28,* 171-180.

Green, L. W., & Kreuter, M. W. (1999). *Health promotion planning: An educational and ecological approach.* Mountain View, CA: Mayfield.

Grossman, D. C. (2000). The history of injury control and the epidemiology of child and adolescent injuries. *Future of Children, 10*(1), 23-52.

Haddon, W., Jr. (1970). On the escape of tigers: An ecologic note. *American Journal of Public Health, 60,* 2229-2234.

Haddon, W., Jr. (1972). A logical framework for categorizing highway safety phenomena and activity. *Journal of Trauma, 12,* 193-207.

Klassen, T. P., MacKay, J. M., Moher, D., Walker, A., & Jones, A. L. (2000). Community-based injury prevention interventions. *Future of Children, 10*(1), 83-110.

Langley, J. D., Wagenaar, A. C., & Begg, D. J. (1996). An evaluation of the New Zealand graduated driver licensing system. *Accident Analysis and Prevention, 28,* 139-146.

Miller, T. R., Romano, E. O., & Spicer, R. S. (2000). The cost of childhood unintentional injuries and the value of prevention. *Future of Children, 10*(1), 137-163.

National Center for Health Statistics Vital Statistics System. (2003). *Web-based injury statistics query and reporting system.* Retrieved from http://www.cdc.gov/ncipc/wisqars/

National Center for Injury Prevention and Control. (2001). *Injury fact book 2001-2002.* Atlanta, GA: Centers for Disease Control and Prevention.

National Center for Injury Prevention and Control. (2003). *Childhood injury fact sheet.* Retrieved from http://www.cdc.gov/ncipc/factsheets/childh.htm

National Committee for Injury Prevention and Control. (1989). Injury prevention: Meeting the challenge. *American Journal of Preventive Medicine, 5*(3 Suppl.), 1-303.

Rivara, F. P., & Grossman, D. C. (1996). Prevention of traumatic deaths to children in the United States: How far have we come and where do we need to go? *Pediatrics, 97,* 791-797.

Rodgers, G. B. (1996). The safety effects of child-resistant packaging for oral prescription drugs: Two decades of experience. *Journal of the American Medical Association, 275,* 1661-1665.

Rosenstock, I. M. (1974). The health belief model and preventive health behavior. *Health Education Monographs, 2,* 354-386.

Runyan, C. W. (1998). Using the Haddon matrix: Introducing the third dimension. *Injury Prevention, 4,* 302-307.

Weinstein, N. D., & Sandman, P. M. (2002). The precaution adoption process model and its application. In R. J. DiClementi, R. A. Crosby, & M. C. Kegler (Eds.), *Emerging theories in health promotion practice and research: Strategies for improving public health* (pp. 16-39). San Francisco: Jossey-Bass.

IRRITABLE BOWEL SYNDROME: PSYCHOLOGICAL TREATMENT

Irritable bowel syndrome (IBS) is a widespread functional disorder of the lower gastrointestinal (GI) tract. A sizable proportion of IBS patients have noticeable psychological distress as measured by standardized psychological tests and as shown by a high occurrence of comorbid psychiatric disorders. Despite these situations, initial treatment of IBS tends to be with drugs and/or dietary interventions such as adding bran fiber to the diet. Recent meta-analytic reviews have not supported the efficacy of any particular class of drugs for IBS nor the efficacy of adding bran to diet.

Over the last 20 years, a large number of controlled studies have appeared supporting the efficacy of various psychological treatments for IBS. A detailed summary of this research appears in a recent book, *Irritable Bowel Syndrome: Psychosocial Assessment and Treatment* (Blanchard, 2001). Moreover, detailed assessment and treatment protocols for two of the three primary treatment approaches, hypnotherapy and cognitive-behavioral therapy, are also available in that book.

At this point there is strong research support for three separate psychological approaches to the treatment of IBS: hypnotherapy, brief psychodynamic psychotherapy, and cognitive-behavioral therapy. The latter term is used to encompass a variety of cognitive and behavioral techniques that have been used separately as treatments as well as in various combinations. The remainder of this entry briefly describes these three approaches, summarizes a prototypic research report illustrating the approach, and summarizes the research support behind the approach.

HYPNOTHERAPY

The initial description of hypnotherapy for IBS was by Whorwell, Prior, and Faragher (1984) in England. Thirty patients with refractory IBS (they had failed various drug and dietary treatments) were randomly assigned to either seven hypnotherapy sessions over 3 months or to seven sessions of psychological support plus a drug placebo.

The hypnotherapy began with an arm levitation induction. The hypnotherapy aimed at general relaxation, gaining control of intestinal motility, and some ego strengthening. An audiotape to guide daily autohypnosis practice was given to the patients. Evaluation was by means of a daily GI symptom diary and an independent assessor. All treatments, both hypnosis and supportive psychotherapy, were by the same therapist.

Results showed significantly greater reductions in bowel habit disturbance, abdominal pain, and bloating for those receiving hypnotherapy in comparison to the control group. The hypnotherapy also led to a greater increase in ratings of general well-being. A very impressive part of the results was that all 15 patients receiving hypnotherapy were either symptom free or suffering from only mild symptoms at the end of the 3-month treatment.

In later reports from this group, at an 18-month follow-up, 2 of 15 hypnotherapy recipients had relapses and were successfully treated with a single booster session. Results from a total of 50 IBS patients were positive for 42 cases (84% success rate). Patients who were possibly suffering from psychiatric disorders or who had primarily intractable abdominal pain were less likely to respond. The treatment protocol was evidently lengthened from 7 sessions to 10 or 12 sessions over 3 months. In a second randomized, controlled trial by this research team, hypnotherapy was superior to a wait list condition on reduction of abdominal pain, bowel habit dysfunction, and bloating.

A very important independent replication of these results was also completed in England in 1989. Individually administered hypnotherapy and group-administered hypnotherapy did equally well, leading to 61% of 33 total patients being symptom free or improved at the 3-month point.

Last, a study from my laboratory, utilizing Whorwell's protocols, replicated Whorwell's hypnotherapy treatment in the United States with 11 patients. Those initially receiving treatment were significantly superior to a symptom monitoring, wait list control. The latter were crossed over to treatment. Overall, 55% of patients were improved, based on a reduction in a composite GI symptom score from the diary, and 18% were somewhat improved. There were also significant reductions in state and trait anxiety. Results held up well at a 2-month follow-up. Success in GI symptom relief was not related to hypnotic susceptibility.

Conclusions

Hypnotherapy has been shown in four separate controlled trials to be of noticeable benefit in comparison to control conditions. Most important, the positive results have been replicated in two independent centers with different therapists. Results have held up well for at least 18 months. From 55% to 100% of patients benefit from treatment.

BRIEF PSYCHODYNAMIC PSYCHOTHERAPY

The strongest trial evaluating brief psychodynamic psychotherapy was conducted in England by Guthrie, Creed, Dawson, and Tomenson (1991) and involved 102 IBS patients who had failed to respond to standard medical care over the previous 6 months. Fifty-three patients were randomized to psychotherapy, while 49 were on a 3-month wait list. Thirty-three of the latter were crossed over and received the treatment. Evaluation was by patient symptom diary, independent medical assessor ratings, and a psychiatrist's structured ratings of anxiety and depression.

All treatments were conducted by a single therapist. Treatment consisted of a long (2- to 4-hour) initial interview in which bowel symptoms and psychological problems were explored in depth. There followed six additional interviews over 3 months during which there was an attempt to help the patient adopt a positive attitude and to change beliefs and attitudes in small steps. Patients were given a relaxation tape for regular home practice.

The psychotherapy patients showed greater improvement in anxiety and depression than the controls. Global ratings by both physicians and patients showed greater change on a composite of all GI symptoms than found for the controls. Sixty-seven percent of the 46 treatment completers were improved. At the 6- to 9-month follow-up using global patient ratings, 73% of the treated patients rated themselves as improved.

The other psychotherapy trial is from Sweden and is the earliest (1983) controlled evaluation of psychological treatment for IBS. Fifty chronic IBS patients received 10 sessions over 3 months of psychotherapy, while 51 additional IBS patients were randomized to routine medical care using the full array of medications. The psychotherapy was described as aimed at modifying maladaptive behaviors and finding new solutions to problems. However, therapy was described as dynamically oriented and supportive, with most work on a conscious level. The number of therapists is not specified. Five patients dropped out but were reevaluated.

Evaluations at the end of treatment and a 12-month follow-up were by independent evaluators using global ratings of several symptom clusters. The results showed significantly greater improvement for psychotherapy in comparison to routine medical care on abdominal pain and total somatic symptoms at post-treatment. At the 12-month follow-up, the treated group continued to show greater improvement on these two ratings plus greater improvement in bowel dysfunction. There was comparable improvement in both groups on ratings of mental symptoms. No data were available on the fraction of the sample that improved.

Conclusions

Brief psychodynamic psychotherapy has been shown to be superior to routine medical care in two large-scale, controlled trials; the results appear to hold up well over follow-ups of 6 to 12 months. The therapies seem quite different in details and thus are not replications like those available in the hypnotherapy literature. However, conceptually, the two treatments are similar and certainly support the efficacy of this approach.

COGNITIVE AND BEHAVIORAL THERAPIES

Combinations of CBT

Combinations of cognitive and behavioral techniques have been evaluated in nine studies conducted in England, Canada, the Netherlands, and the United States. Most have been relatively small trials with fewer than 20 patients in the active treatment condition. At least two of these controlled trials, however, had 30 or more patients per condition. Most ($n = 7$) of the studies have used individually administered treatments; however, two of the controlled trials, and one quasi-controlled trial from our center, have used CBT in small groups. The controlled trials have all used some form of relaxation training and its application, usually abbreviated progressive muscle relaxation (PMR). Almost all provide some education about IBS, normal bowel functioning, and the possible relation of stress to bowel symptoms. Some have included assertiveness training. The cognitive therapy components usually are modeled after the work of Meichenbaum or Beck. In this they usually are trying to address and change potentially negative, or self-defeating, self-dialogue (Meichenbaum) or identifying and correcting cognitive fallacies and negative schema (Beck). Emphasis is placed in both approaches on having participants keep a diary of their self-dialogue and thoughts surrounding stressful events and onset of pain and other bowel symptoms. In some trials from our center we have added thermal biofeedback for hand warming as an additional relaxation technique. Others have focused on operant approaches to pain management.

Evaluation has usually been by patient symptom diary, psychological tests, and patient global ratings. Control conditions have usually been waiting list, symptom monitoring controls, or routine medical care. Two studies also used sophisticated psychological attention-placebo controls in addition to symptom monitoring, while another used a psychoeducation group in addition to routine medical care.

Results have been mixed. In all studies there has been some differential improvement of CBT versus one of the control conditions. However, in some studies the difference was only on a psychological test (reduction of anxiety or depressive symptoms) or on global ratings. However, in several studies there was differential improvement on GI symptoms from a patient diary favoring active treatment. Follow-ups of up to 4 years have shown reasonably good maintenance of symptom reduction as validated by the GI symptom diary. Interestingly, in the large-scale studies comparing CBT to a psychological control and symptom monitoring or routine medical care, there were no significant advantages for CBT over the active psychological control.

A prototypical report by Blanchard et al. (1992) described two studies identical in treatment conditions and measurement. In the first, there was only one therapist and 10 patients per condition. In the second, there were 6 therapists and 30 patients per condition. In each instance, patients were seen for 12 individual sessions over 8 weeks with evaluation by patient symptom diary and psychological tests.

The CBT condition contained patient education, PMR, thermal biofeedback, and cognitive therapy modeled after the work of Meichenbaum. The active psychological control condition combined pseudo-meditation and biofeedback for alpha suppression. A symptom monitoring control was the third condition.

In both instances, the CBT showed arithmetically greater reductions in a composite GI symptom measure from the diary than the attention placebo control or the symptom monitoring control. Fractions of the samples improved were 60% in the small study but only 47% in the larger study. Three-month follow-up data showed better maintenance for CBT than the attention placebo condition.

Conclusion

When combinations of behavioral and cognitive procedures have been subjected to rigorous tests by comparing them to active psychological control conditions as well as symptom monitoring controls, even in moderate-sized trials with 30 or more patients per condition, the CBT treatment has not been superior to the active psychological control. Nevertheless, 50% or more of patients have been improved, and the average within group decrease in GI symptoms, and in measures of psychological distress, are significant. These combination treatments seem to work.

INDIVIDUAL BEHAVIORAL AND COGNITIVE TREATMENTS

Our inability at my center to successfully replicate the positive results from the CBT combination treatments has led us to evaluate individual components of the treatment package. In two studies we have found a pure relaxation condition superior to a symptom monitoring control on a composite measure of GI symptoms from a daily diary. Thus, both PMR and a more passive form of relaxation, meditation based on Benson's relaxation response, were superior to symptom monitoring. We did find the PMR condition had a high dropout rate (about 40%).

Pure Cognitive Therapy

There have been three controlled studies evaluating a purely cognitive therapy approach to IBS. In all three, individually administered cognitive therapy, 10 sessions over 8 to 10 weeks, has been superior to a symptom-monitoring control. In one it was superior to a psychoeducational support group (described in more detail below); in another it was equivalent to cognitive therapy administered in small groups. Each trial had a different single therapist (an advanced doctoral student in clinical psychology). Evaluation was by means of GI symptom diaries and psychological tests.

At my center we have obtained our most consistent results with this approach: 70% of patients improved based on the composite GI symptom score derived from the daily diaries; the average GI symptom score was reduced by 60%. There was also significant improvement in standardized psychological tests measuring anxiety and depression. In probably the strongest study testing individual cognitive therapy, Payne and Blanchard (1995) randomly assigned 12 IBS patients to individual cognitive therapy, 12 to psychoeducational support groups, and 10 to a symptom monitoring, wait list control. The sample was 85% female, of average age 40.1 years, who had been suffering from IBS for 16.1 years. Eighty-five percent met criteria for one or more Axis I psychiatric disorders.

In the cognitive therapy, the patient was given a model of the relation of thoughts to stress and to IBS symptoms and asked to begin monitoring stressful situations and surrounding thoughts. After systematically working to correct self-talk, treatment began to focus on logical fallacies and cognitive schema as they related to IBS symptoms and stress.

In the psychoeducational condition, participants met in small groups of three to five and dealt with a number of topics such as diet and symptoms. The emphasis was on teaching participants to be able to talk about IBS issues with peers and derive support from the experience.

Results showed an average reduction in GI symptoms of 67% for cognitive therapy, 31% for the support group, and 10% for those in symptom monitoring. Three quarters of those in cognitive therapy were improved based on symptom diaries. There was differential benefit for those in cognitive therapy on most individual GI symptoms in comparison to each control group. Moreover, there was a differential reduction of symptoms of anxiety and depression. Most important, the level of expectation of benefit from pretreatment questionnaires was equivalent for the two treated groups. The symptomatic reduction results held up well at a 3-month follow-up.

To the best of my knowledge, this is the only CBT study for which a cognitive or behavioral treatment has been superior to a highly credible psychological placebo condition.

Conclusions

Our results from my center with cognitive therapy are impressive and consistent. Across three separate replications, we have seen strong results, leading me to conclude that it is the best treatment among the cognitive and behavioral therapies that have been applied to IBS.

OVERALL SUMMARY

The strongest evidence to support the efficacy of a psychological treatment for IBS is for hypnotherapy. The independent replications in randomized trials give it the nod. The second strongest case exists for pure cognitive therapy. There are three controlled trials, including one for which it was superior to a credible, active psychological placebo. However, all three trials are from the same center but did use different therapists.

Combinations of cognitive and behavioral therapeutic techniques have good cross-site replication and good follow-up data, but the results are inconsistent. Brief psychodynamic psychotherapy has shown strong results in two separate trials with good follow-up; however, the therapy appears to be different at different sites, leaving us awaiting replication.

In any event, the literature seems to clearly show the viability of psychological treatments for IBS. The time may be ripe for large-scale direct comparisons of psychological and drug treatments for this widespread, chronic condition.

—*Edward B. Blanchard*

See also CHRONIC DISEASE MANAGEMENT; IRRITABLE BOWEL SYNDROME: PSYCHOSOCIAL ASPECTS

Further Reading

Blanchard, E. B. (2001). *Irritable bowel syndrome: Psychosocial assessment and treatment.* Washington, DC: American Psychological Association.

Blanchard, E. B., Schwarz, S. P., Suls, J. M., Gerardi, M. A., Scharff, L., Greene, B., et al. (1992). Two controlled evaluations of multicomponent psychological treatment of irritable bowel syndrome. *Behaviour Research and Therapy, 30,* 175-189.

Guthrie, E., Creed, F., Dawson, D., & Tomenson, B. (1991). A controlled trial of psychological treatment for the irritable bowel syndrome. *Gastroenterology, 100,* 450-457.

Payne, A., & Blanchard, E. B. (1995). A controlled comparison of cognitive therapy and self-help support groups in the treatment of irritable bowel syndrome. *Journal of Consulting and Clinical Psychology, 63,* 779-786.

Whorwell, P. J., Prior, A., & Faragher, E. B. (1984). Controlled trial of hypnotherapy in the treatment of severe refractory irritable-bowel syndrome. *Lancet*, 1232-1234.

IRRITABLE BOWEL SYNDROME: PSYCHOSOCIAL ASPECTS

Irritable bowel syndrome (IBS) is a functional gastrointestinal disorder that consists of abdominal pain or discomfort combined with altered stool frequency or consistency. The behaviors, illness experiences, and clinical outcomes of people with IBS are closely related to psychosocial factors such as life stress, psychological state, abuse, social support, and coping strategies.

IBS is currently viewed within a biopsychosocial context, which incorporates both the physical and psychosocial factors accountable for the illness. Psychosocial factors can affect physical factors, such as gut physiology (i.e., stress can increase the rate of colonic contraction). Gut function can also negatively affect a person's psychosocial state (i.e., frequent exacerbations of abdominal pain can lead to further anxiety and depression and increased vigilance to symptoms). A potentially vicious cycle can then be created between the two, which can worsen IBS symptoms and psychological disturbances.

LIFE STRESS

Patients with IBS appear to have an exaggerated gastrointestinal response to stress. While anxiety and stress can cause gastrointestinal urgency, cramps, or diarrhea in all people, the effect of stress on people with IBS is even greater. Stressful life events (such as a death in the family, a surgical procedure, employment or financial problems, or marital difficulties) are associated with the onset of symptoms in more than half of people with IBS. One study found that stress causes altered stool patterns and abdominal pain in a larger number of people with IBS than controls (73% and 84% of IBS patients respectively, as compared with 54% and 68% of controls). The result of these gastrointestinal changes can be increased bowel symptoms, physician visits, and disability days for people with IBS.

Psychological State

Psychological states can affect people's illness perception, which can result in greater health care seeking behavior. Their symptom intensity, illness behavior (defined as how symptoms are evaluated, perceived, and acted upon), and perceptions of symptom status can also be affected. It is therefore not surprising that psychological disturbances are more common in people with IBS that seek medical attention than in people with IBS who do not solicit medical assistance (IBS nonpatients). In contrast, the prevalence of psychosocial disturbances and the personality profiles of IBS nonpatients are similar to those found in the general population. IBS patients seeking medical attention suffer from a high prevalence of psychiatric and psychological disturbances such as anxiety, depression, phobias, and somatization. Somatization is defined as the expression of psychological stress through physical symptoms, and it tends to occur more often during times of stress. IBS patients also tend to have higher levels of hypochondriasis and hysteria than both nonpatients and controls. Other personality factors common to IBS patients are the minimization of emotional concerns, excessive concerns about health or bodily functions, and the continual need for reassurance about their health.

A life-events score is an individual's measure of the desirability of life events and of their impact and effect on the person's life (a measure of "good or bad"). If the summation of the life events is positive, then the individual is given a positive life-events score. IBS patients tend to have lower positive life-event scores than IBS nonpatients, signifying that IBS patients may perceive life events more negatively than people without IBS.

Coping Strategies

While coping strategies are generally helpful, some can be maladaptive and influence the clinical outcome of IBS. In a recent study, women with IBS who perceived an inability to decrease symptoms and exhibited catastrophizing behaviors—defined as pessimism and maladaptive coping related to pain (e.g., "I feel it's never going to get any better")—had a poorer clinical outcome during the 1-year follow-up. The negative effect of coping strategies on IBS is independent of the effects of abuse or psychological factors.

Therefore, the clinical outcome of IBS is strongly affected by coping skills or strategies.

The social learning of coping strategies and illness behaviors is also an influential factor in IBS. IBS symptoms are often found throughout families: the children of IBS patients exhibit similar patterns of illness behavior and seek medical attention for similar gastrointestinal symptoms as their parents. These behaviors were probably learned through childhood reinforcement and modeling of gastrointestinal symptoms.

Abuse

Many IBS patients have a history of abuse (physical, sexual, and emotional), especially during childhood. In a tertiary referral center, it was found that, of women with functional gastrointestinal disorders, 53% reported sexual abuse and 13% physical abuse. The connection between abuse and IBS most likely stems from abused patients' catastrophizing coping strategies and difficulty judging harmful stimuli. In fact, a history of abuse is the strongest predictor of poor treatment outcome for IBS patients. As compared to nonabused IBS patients, IBS patients with a history of abuse tend to experience an increase in severity of IBS, psychological disturbances, frequency of physician visits, and surgery throughout their lifetime. In addition, they have decreased daily function and a poorer clinical outcome than nonabused IBS patients.

—Anthony Lembo
and Rebecca Fink

See also CHILD ABUSE, CHILD NEGLECT, AND HEALTH; COMORBID MENTAL AND OTHER PHYSICAL DISORDERS; IRRITABLE BOWEL SYNDROME: PSYCHOLOGICAL TREATMENT

Further Reading

Creed, F. (1999). The relationship between psychosocial parameters and outcome in irritable bowel syndrome. *American Journal of Medicine, 107,* 74S-80S.

Drossman, D. A. (1999). Do psychosocial factors define symptom severity and patient status in irritable bowel syndrome? *American Journal of Medicine, 107,* 41S-50S.

Drossman, D. A., Creed, F. H., Olden, K. W., Svedund, J., Toner, B. B., & Whitehead, W. E. (1999). Psychosocial aspects of the functional gastrointestinal disorders. *Gut, 45*(Suppl. 2), II25-II30.

Koloski, N. A., Talley, N. J., & Boyce, P. M. (2001). Predictors of health care seeking for irritable bowel syndrome and nonulcer dyspepsia: A critical review of the literature on symptom and psychosocial factors. *American Journal of Gastroenterology, 96,* 1340-1349.

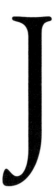

JOB STRAIN AND HEALTH

Job strain results when work is organized in a way that allows workers little job decision latitude and requires high levels of psychological job demands. The interaction of job decision latitude and psychological job demands to create job strain is figuratively depicted as a cross-tabulation.

EXPLANATION

Job strain results from how work is organized. Work systems are often organized to maximize how much a worker does and to ensure that the quality of the work done is at a consistently high level. To maximize how much a worker does, companies will increase production requirements to the point where quality is not sacrificed. To ensure consistently high levels of quality, the job is often simplified by reducing task variety or the skills required to get the job done. The manufacturing assembly line represents one type of work system where production requirements are high, quality is consistent, and the tasks to be done are simple and repetitive. In today's computerized workplaces, information systems monitor the worker and keep the worker moving at a fast pace, such as in customer service centers or catalog order centers. The worker must also meet customer demands. Once one call is completed, the next one is queued up for the worker by the information system. These work systems give rise to job strain because the worker has little latitude in what is being done or how to do it, yet high psychological demands are created by production

requirements and customer demands. In many job strain studies, these types of jobs are classified as high strain, as shown in Figure 1. Hereafter, high strain will be referred to as the hazardous work condition created by combining psychological job demands and job decision latitude.

Job strain occurs in all occupations within all industries. Thus, there are certain common work system indicators of both psychological job demands and job decision latitude. Psychological job demands are the result of the amount of work a person has to do, the job's mental requirements, the need to coordinate multiple tasks and requests from multiple people in order to get the job done, and time constraints regarding how quickly the work must be completed. Job decision latitude is the combination of task authority and skill discretion. Task authority is the degree to which the worker controls how to do the job. In high-strain work, this authority can reside with the information system or other machine. For example, in the U.S. Postal Service, people who sort the mail typically work at large multiple-position letter sorting machines. The worker sits in front of a machine that automatically grabs a letter and puts it into a window for the worker to visually scan. This is done every second for 45 minutes. Based on the address, the worker keys in a code using a special keyboard that sends the letter through the machine into a bin on the other side of the machine. People in this job have no authority to determine how they do the work. It can also reside with a supervisor or even the customer. Skill discretion relates to the ability of the worker to be creative in the use of skills and the development of new skills. A worker whose primary job is data entry has the potential opportunity to develop additional skills using other software if courses are available and work is organized to allow the person to take the classes and practice the new skills. Combining task authority and skill discretion to form job decision latitude captures to what degree workers have control over what they do and how they do it. This is also referred to as job control giving rise to the phrase demand-control model (DCM), a phrase often used instead of job strain.

The DCM predicts that high-strain work affects illness and disease in three possible ways (Karasek & Theorell, 1990): (1) a worker exposed to high-strain work on a daily basis will respond by releasing stress hormones that circulate in the blood. This physiological stress can increase the person's chances of developing high blood pressure and cardiovascular disease; (2) working in these conditions will cause psychological strains such as job-related tension, mental strain, and alienation that can lead to depression. Mental health problems like depression can also affect stress hormone levels, and (3) the psychological strain and physiological stress can lead a person to smoke, drink, abuse illegal substances, or have sleep problems. The emotional exhaustion can encourage sedentary behavior that can eventually result in obesity and the chronic health problems associated with obesity such as Type 2 diabetes.

The DCM shown in Figure 1 also predicts that work high in psychological demands and job decision latitude produces active learning and greater self-efficacy at work (Schnall, Belkic, Landsbergis, & Baker, 2000). The opposite of active work is passive work, where there are both few psychological demands and little job decision latitude. While less researched, this type of work may affect morbidity and mortality through the alienation and boredom it creates (Amick et al., 2002). In today's more dynamic economy, it

may also be a marker for job insecurity, since people in this type of work develop few skills on the job.

The public health implications of the DCM are threefold. First, high-strain work is a hazardous work condition. Second, passive work is a potentially hazardous work condition. Third, these hazardous work conditions can be improved through changes in work systems design that increase job control or psychological demands. Most important, work system redesign has been shown to be effective and to improve both satisfaction and productivity (see Capelli et al., 1997, for a discussion of work redesign).

DEVELOPMENT AND DETAILS

The DCM was originally developed by Robert Karasek (1979). He identified the three factors (task authority, skill discretion, and psychological job demands) that combine to create the four work environments depicted in Figure 1, when analyzing the 1969, 1972, and 1977 U.S. Quality of Employment Surveys. The measures are part of a broader survey, the Job Content Questionnaire (JCQ), which has been translated into multiple languages (see Karasek et al., 1998, where information on permission to use the JCQ is available, or go to www.uml.edu/Dept/WE/jcq.htm). The original JCQ (version 1.1) was developed in 1985 and updated in 1995 (version 1.5). In the United States, a common approach is to use a reduced question set including nine questions on task authority and skill discretion and five psychological work demands questions. Workers respond by endorsing how much they agree or disagree with statements about their work (the response scale varies from *strongly agree* to *strongly disagree).*

Researchers from many countries have used the instrument. The measures demonstrate strong reliability across country and gender. Cronbach's alphas, a measure of how consistently all the questions used to measure the job demands and decision latitude scales relate to each other and to the scales, range from an average of 0.73 for women and 0.74 for men. (A successful scale has a Cronbach alpha of 0.7 or greater.) In the Cornell Heart Study, the test-retest reliability (i.e., the ability of people to answer the same questions at two points in time the same way) of both decision latitude and psychological demands were 0.64 (reported in Schnall et al., 2000).

Some researchers interested in job strain have been unable to ask workers to answer questions. For these

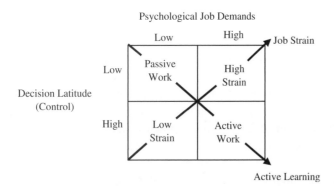

Figure 1   Job Strain or Demand-Control Model

researchers, a job exposure matrix has been constructed in both the United States and in Sweden (Johnson & Stewart, 1993; Schwartz, Pieper, & Karasek, 1988). To create a job exposure matrix, individual answers to JCQ questions are aggregated up to the occupational level (e.g., carpenter, nurse, teacher). For example, the information from the 1969, 1972, and 1977 Quality of Employment Surveys was pooled to create a sample of 3,000 men and 1,500 women. This information can then be used in other studies where only a standard occupation measure, for example, the three-digit international classification of occupations, is known. Job decision latitude and psychological job demands exposures can be linked to individuals by using their occupational information. One advantage is that job strain can be studied in data sets that do not contain any self-reported information. A second advantage arises from the fact that the workers reporting health problems are not the ones reporting work conditions. Thus, there is no likelihood of exposure misclassification due to health, because those with health problems underreport job decision latitude or overreport psychological job demands. One disadvantage occurs because the variability in psychological job demands and job decision latitude is between occupations, even though there is a lot of within-occupation variability. For example, not all nurses do the same work, but they are in the same occupation. A nurse working in the operating room has higher levels of psychological job demands than a nurse working in a private practice. Similarly, a nurse in a private practice has higher levels of job decision latitude compared to an operating room nurse. When individual self-reported data exists, the operating room nurse will be classified as high strain, while the private practice nurse will be classified as low strain (see Amick et al., 1998, for an example of how nurses are classified with self-reported measures). This level of specificity is missed when only the occupation, nursing, is used where all nurses will be assigned the same score. It is commonly recognized that job decision latitude varies between occupations, but psychological job demands vary as much within as between occupations. Until methods are developed for objective job strain exposure assessment, self-report and job exposure matrix measures will both continue to be widely used.

In statistical analysis, three methods have been commonly used to estimate the risk of illness, injury, psychological state, or mortality. First, researchers will create scales and then split the scales on the median to create the rows and columns in Figure 1. What results from this cross-classification are four groups: (1) high strain (jobs like bus driver, nurse's aide, or assembly line worker), (2) low strain (jobs like natural scientist, repairman), (3) active (jobs like physician, farmer, and bank officer), and (4) passive (jobs like janitor and night watchman). Scores above the job demands median and below the job decision latitude median are combined to create high strain. The high-strain group is compared to the low-strain group to estimate an effect as suggested by the arrow in Figure 1, yet often high strain is compared to all other groups. More recently, the active group is considered to have the "healthiest" work conditions and the other three groups are compared to it. This also allows estimating the passive work effect. Second, the job demands scale is multiplied by the reciprocal of the job decision latitude scale, and then those with the 20% highest scores are classified as high strain. This group is often termed "hazardous psychosocial work" and is compared to all other work. Hallqvist, Diderichsen, Theorell, Reuterwall, and Ahlbom (1998) have suggested that the best cutoff may be 10% to improve sensitivity of detecting biologically relevant exposure. Third, the psychological job demands measure is divided by job control to create a ratio. The ratio reflects a true measure of the ability of the person to use job resources to manage demands. The higher the score, the more likely the person is to be in a high-strain job. Researchers argue that this is more appropriate, since splitting measures on the median can lead to problems in hypothesis testing (Type II error).

Debate about measurement and analysis issues remain. Because of the implicit interaction of job decision latitude and psychological job demands, some researchers argue that the only appropriate way to estimate a combined effect is through including both main effects and interaction effects in the statistical model (Kasl, 1998). However, other approaches, such as estimating a synergy index (an approach to calculating a multiplicative interaction effect in epidemiology), have been used and may be as appropriate. Suffice it to say that at this moment, there is no single agreed upon method for job strain risk estimation.

A more recent concern is how to cumulate exposure over a person's working life. In most studies, job strain is measured at one point in time. Without multiple points of measurement of job decisions latitude and psychological job demands, the duration of exposure cannot be estimated. Duration has been examined in 5-year periods by Johnson and Stewart (1993), while Amick and colleagues (2002) examined the complete working life course. To date, no evidence indicates how long a worker can do high-strain work and remain risk free.

EXAMPLES

To illustrate the main high-strain hypothesis and the secondary active work hypothesis, two studies are briefly presented. As part of the Stockholm Heart Epidemiology Program (SHEEP), a case-control study of job strain and first hospitalization or fatal myocardial infarction, Hallqvist and colleagues (1998) used a synergy index to represent the multiplicative effects of decision latitude and job demands. These effects are hypothesized in Figure 1. When the synergy index is greater than 1.0, it indicates that there is greater than an additive effect of job decision latitude and job demands. A simple additive effect would not indicate a job strain effect. They found that the synergy index was 4.0, indicating a strong multiplicative effect.

Amick and colleagues (2002) prospectively examined the mortality risk for workers who spent their lives in high strain work or passive work. Figure 2 shows the study results. Using the median split methodology, a nonsignificant elevated risk for high-strain work

and a significant elevated risk for passive work were found. The results suggest that if workers spend their working lives in passive jobs, their chances of dying within 10 years following their last job are 35% greater than workers who spend their working lives in active jobs.

Both sets of findings indicate the importance of the broader conceptualization offered by the job strain model as opposed to the simple characterization of psychological job demands and job decision latitude.

—Benjamin C. Amick III

See also EFFORT-REWARD IMBALANCE; OCCUPATIONAL HEALTH AND SAFETY; WORK-RELATED STRESS AND HEALTH

Further Reading

Amick, B. C., III, Kawachi, I., Coakley, E. H., Lerner, D. J., Levine, S., & Colditz, G. A. (1998). Relationship of job strain and iso-strain to health status in a cohort of women in the U.S. *Scandinavian Journal of Work, Environment & Health, 24,* 54-61.

Amick, B. C., III, McDonough, P., Chang, H., Rogers, W. H., Duncan, G., & Pieper, C. (2002). The relationship between all-cause mortality and cumulative working life course psychosocial and physical exposures in the United States labor market from 1968-1992. *Psychosomatic Medicine, 64,* 370-381.

Cappelli, P., Bassi, L., Katz, H., Knoke, D., Osterman, P., & Useem, M. (1997). *Change at work.* New York: Oxford University Press.

Hallqvist, J., Diderichsen, F., Theorell, T., Reuterwall, C., & Ahlbom, A. (1998). Is the effect of job strain due to interaction between high psychological demand and low decision latitude? *Social Science and Medicine, 46,* 1405-1411.

Johnson, J. V., & Stewart, W. F. (1993). Measuring work organization exposure over the life course with a job-exposure matrix. *Scandinavian Journal of Work, Environment, and Health, 19,* 21.

Karasek, R. A. (1979). Job demands, job decision latitude, and mental strain: Implications for job redesign. *American Society for Quality, 24,* 285-308.

Karasek, R. A., Brisson, C., Kawakami, N., Bongers, P., Houtman, I., & Amick, B. (1998). The job content questionnaire (JCQ): An instrument for internationally comparative assessments of psychosocial job characteristics. *Journal of Occupational Health and Psychology, 3,* 322-355.

Karasek, R. A., & Theorell, T. (1990). *Healthy work: Stress, productivity, and the reconstruction of working life.* New York: Basic Books.

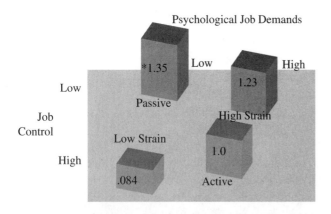

Figure 2   Working Life Course Job Strain Exposure in a Nationally Representative Sample of U.S. Workers From 1968 to 1992[a]

a. Risk estimates adjusted for age, race, gender, year, family income, family size, retirement, unemployment, baseline disability.
*p < 0.001.

Kasl, S. V. (1998). Measuring job stressors and studying the health impact of the work environment: An epidemiologic commentary. *Journal of Occupational Health and Psychology, 3,* 390-401.

Schnall, P., Belkic, K., Landsbergis, P., & Baker, D. (2000). The workplace and cardiovascular disease. *Occupational Medicine State of the Art Reviews, 15,* 1-189.

Schwartz, J. E., Pieper, C. F., & Karasek, R. A. (1988). A procedure for linking psychosocial job characteristics data to health surveys. *American Journal of Public Health, 78,* 904-909.

JOHN HENRYISM AND HEALTH

As defined by James, Hartnett, and Kalsbeek (1983), John Henryism (JH) is a "strong behavioral predisposition to cope actively with psychosocial environmental stressors." The construct is characterized by three major themes: (1) efficacious mental and physical vigor, (2) a strong commitment to hard work, and (3) a single-minded determination to succeed. The JH model takes its name and is inspired in part by the story of John Henry, the "steel-driving man." According to the legend, John Henry was a widely admired African American railroad worker in the late 19th century who, in an epic steel-driving competition, defeated a steam-powered drill. However, soon after rallying his strength to win the contest, John Henry died suddenly from mental and physical fatigue.

For James, the fabled actions of John Henry served to illuminate the empirical literature describing the relation between psychosocial stress and hypertension among those of low socioeconomic status (SES). It is well known that lower SES populations are routinely exposed to chronic, unremitting psychosocial and environmental stressors (i.e., low job control, financial difficulties, familial instability, discrimination, exposure to violence, lack of health care resources). In order to manage these persistent psychosocial stressors, some may adopt a high-effort or "active" style of coping, which may constitute an adaptive coping response among those with access to adequate educational or occupational resources. However, utilization of an active coping disposition may entail deleterious health outcomes among those without sufficient material resources (that may serve to buffer active coping efforts). Syme's (1979) seminal review posited that prolonged high-effort coping with adverse psychosocial

stressors might largely account for the inverse relation between SES and hypertension.

The JH hypothesis extends this literature by arguing that high JH may heighten the blood pressure of those in lower socioeconomic strata via the increased sympathetic nervous system arousal promoted by frequent high-effort coping. Or more formally, "the inverse association between socioeconomic status and blood pressure will be much more pronounced (i.e., more striking) for individuals who score high on JH than for those who score low" (James, 1994).

This entry reviews the theoretical underpinnings of the JH model, discusses empirical findings investigating the concept, and presents future directions for JH research.

EMPIRICAL INVESTIGATIONS OF THE JH CONSTRUCT

James's group initially conducted three cross-sectional studies of the JH hypothesis in rural, eastern North Carolina. Their 1983 pilot study examined a sample of 132 Black men, aged 17 to 60, who were members of the poor, predominately African American community. Findings revealed that at high JH, low levels of educational attainment (< 12 years) were marginally associated with higher resting blood pressure. Though these results were not statistically significant, the findings suggested a need for additional investigation.

The initial study was also designed to validate an early version of the JH Scale of Active Coping (JHAC12). The 12-item, 5-point Likert-type scale measures the three primary JH themes. Five response options for each item extend from *completely true* to *completely false.* Each item is reverse-coded and summed to derive a total JH score that ranges from 12 to 60 (with higher scores representing higher levels of JH). The JHAC12 has demonstrated acceptable internal consistency in samples of Black and White men and women. Adult samples tend to score near the high end of the JHAC12 range.

The second of James and colleagues (1992) studies extended the pilot findings to a sample including Black and White men and women. Lower SES was marginally associated with increased blood pressure for Black but not for White participants. Similarly, JH was found not to be predictive among Whites. However, among low SES African Americans, high levels of JH were associated with higher resting diastolic blood pressure and a threefold increase in hypertension prevalence. Surprisingly, the level of hypertension seen among high JH, high SES subjects was quite low, suggesting that among this rural population, high JH might protect against elevated blood pressure.

These early studies also demonstrated that JH was positively associated with a host of other lifestyle factors including life satisfaction, perceptions of good health, being married, having children, being employed, having a high-status, better-paying job, and church attendance. JH was inversely associated with education and age after adjustment for other demographic and psychosocial variables.

James's group focused their 1992 study on a much larger sample of African Americans from eastern North Carolina. The sample was drawn from a county that was more urbanized and socioeconomically diverse than in their previous studies. The traditional JH hypothesis was not supported. James reasoned, however, that the inverse association between SES and hypertension would be pronounced among low SES individuals who also reported higher levels of perceived stress. He suggested, though, that elevated perceived stress alone would be insufficient to spur elevated blood pressure. Rather, he argued (consistent with the JH model), that high effort coping with the elevated levels of perceived stress among low SES individuals would be associated with higher blood pressure levels. Indeed, post hoc analyses revealed significantly elevated blood pressure levels among low SES, high JH subjects, but only among those who reported high levels of perceived stress.

A host of other investigations have examined the influence of JH on measures of cardiovascular functioning. Wright and colleagues showed that high JH predicted higher blood pressure, higher total peripheral resistance, and lower resting cardiac index among Black and White adolescents. The highest levels of resting cardiovascular dysregulation were found among low SES adolescents who were high in JH. More recently, Merritt, Bennett, Sollers, Edwards, and Williams (in press) found that high JH and low education were associated with elevated diastolic and mean arterial pressure (MAP) responses and inhibited recovery responses to laboratory stressors.

Contrary to the traditional JH hypothesis, Light and colleagues (1995) found that high JH and high job status predicted elevated work blood pressure among women and Black adults. This was consistent with findings by McKetney and Ragland (1996), who found that high JH young adults with high levels of educational attainment showed marginally higher resting blood pressure. In a sample of Nigerian civil servants, Markovic, Bunker, Ukoli, and Kuller (1998) found a nonsignificant trend toward higher blood pressure levels among higher SES workers with high JH.

Despite these compelling findings, a host of other studies have failed to support the JH hypothesis. As with any construct, null findings may be influenced by myriad potential confounding factors. With respect to JH, however, some themes have emerged. First, a number of investigators have examined the effect on health outcomes of JH in isolation. JH certainly has value as one of few empirically supported, culturally patterned coping models, and this empirical approach has proven fruitful in some studies. However, examining JH solely opposes the traditional JH hypothesis, which is posited as an interaction with SES.

Next, there has been significant reliance on objective indicators of SES (most often education and/or income) in JH studies. While low SES is a critical component of the JH hypothesis, objective measures do a poor job in differentiating the more proximate social, environmental, and psychological characteristics that may drive the utilization of the JH style (e.g., James's finding that the low SES × high JH interaction predicted elevated blood pressure only among those reporting high levels of perceived stress). Thus, assessment of stressors in the home, occupational, and residential environment may prove efficacious in improving the predictive utility of the model.

Of some concern has been JH's external validity, a subject that has received little empirical attention. A major question is whether the JH construct can be applied outside of rural southern communities characterized by economic deprivation (where it has often been studied). With some exceptions, those studies utilizing more economically and geographically diverse samples have failed to confirm James's original JH hypothesis.

Finally, there does appear to be support for JH as a mode that is particularly relevant to the experience of African Americans. Many of the JH findings suggest that JH is more predictive of adverse outcomes among African Americans compared to Whites. The JH hypothesis has been confirmed almost exclusively in Black American populations, with the exception of a study conducted in a Dutch sample. Research conducted among European Americans shows no consistent pattern.

OTHER CONSIDERATIONS

Gender

There is some evidence to suggest that the traditional JH hypothesis may better capture the experience of African American males. Although a number of studies have found no difference in JH scores between men and women, at least one investigation has explicitly examined whether gender differences in JH predict hypertension prevalence.

In a sample of 600 African American men and women, high JH men were approximately 50% more likely to be hypertensive than were high JH women. High JH women were actually at decreased risk for hypertension. Interestingly, there was no support for the traditional JH × SES interaction, nor a three-way interaction with gender. This finding is consistent with those suggesting that women's coping behaviors are distinct from those of their male counterparts. Clearly, this issue deserves additional empirical attention.

Job Status and Workplace Factors

Conceptually, occupational factors constitute a major component of the JH pattern. Few JH studies, however, have addressed workplace concerns specifically. James and colleagues studied the interaction between JH and a variety of workplace factors in the prediction of resting blood pressure. Among Black males they found that high job success was associated with lower diastolic blood pressure, but only among those with low levels of JH. High JH men who felt that being Black had hindered their job success were found to display elevated diastolic blood pressure and lower levels of perceived job success. James posited that low JH men may have been "less ambitious" in their perceptions of job success.

Light and colleagues' (1995) study examining the association between job status and JH extended these findings. Her sample was better educated (65% of whom were college graduates) and had significantly higher job status (roughly 72% held white-collar positions). Light's findings are notable because they challenge the traditional JH hypothesis—that high JH and low SES interact to affect blood pressure. In the study, Blacks with high status jobs (in comparison to White

men and women) displayed higher levels of both systolic and diastolic blood pressure at work (using ambulatory measurement) and at home (resting casual blood pressure). That the majority of Blacks with high status jobs were also high in JH (71%, compared to 36% for White participants) supports James's assertion that individuals high in JH may have higher occupational goals and aspirations than those low in JH. James, however, argued that the psychosocial stressors encountered with attempts to achieve and maintain these goals would be associated with deleterious outcomes among those of low SES. Light's extension to this argument suggests that such psychosocial stress may not be uniformly associated with SES, but also with ethnicity. Interestingly, however, and as Light notes, though individuals may place themselves at risk for elevated blood pressure, the JH behavior pattern may be a quite adaptive means of achieving higher perceived job success (while risking blood pressure elevations) when one is of high SES.

Investigation of Biological Mechanisms and Clinical Outcomes

The JH model has been rigorously investigated in association with cardiovascular parameters, primarily blood pressure. These efforts, however, are far from comprehensive, given the model's potential association with other health outcomes not directly related to cardiovascular dysfunction. The increasing number of findings detailing the importance of the HPA-axis in mediating exposure to chronic stress and negative affect make it a useful domain for future investigation. A recent pilot study by Bennett, Merritt, Edwards, Sollers, and Williams (n.d.) demonstrated an association between high JH, high job demands, and dysregulated cortisol secretion. Other ongoing investigations are actively examining the relations between JH and other neuroendocrine parameters. Additional research is increasingly evaluating the utility of the JH model among clinical samples, including those with cancer and pain-related disorders.

Refinement of the JH Assessment Instrument

The assessment of JH can, at times, present analytic and interpretive difficulties. Scores on the 12-item JH Scale Active Coping Scale (JHAC) are often quite high for both Blacks and Whites. These high-scale scores (normally averaging 50-54 out of 60) have been found in many JH investigations and can make meaningful differences between high and low JH groups that are difficult to discern. James, Strogatz, Wing, and Ramsey (1987) attributed the high scores to the possibility of social desirability biases in the scale. High JH levels may be found because the construct taps factors such as hard work and determination, which are core American values (i.e., the Protestant work ethic). Some work has investigated the development of a JH-structured interview that would more systematically access the three key components of JH. Such an instrument, however, would not be useful in epidemiological investigations. Upcoming research is more vigorously examining the psychometric properties of the JHAC12.

CONCLUSION

This entry has reviewed evidence linking the JH model and SES with health outcomes. Because African Americans have historically suffered a lack of directed research attention, many argue the importance of identifying and elucidating the unique characteristics accompanying ethnic minority status. Compelling both conceptually and in its empirical application, the primary strength of the JH model may lie in its transdisciplinary approach to the identification of factors responsible for the promotion of ethnic disparities in health outcomes. Despite the model's appeal, significant empirical questions remain that should spur a new generation of JH research.

—*Gary G. Bennett*

See also AFRICAN AMERICAN HEALTH AND BEHAVIOR; CULTURE AND HEALTH; HEALTH DISPARITIES; STRESS, APPRAISAL, AND COPING

Further Reading

Bennett, G. G., Merritt, M. M., Edwards, C. L., Sollers, J., & Williams, R. B. (n.d.). *High effort coping, job demands, and the cortisol response to awakening.* Unpublished manuscript.

Harburg, E., Erfurt, J. C., Hauenstein, L. S., et al. (1973). Socio-ecological stressor areas and Black-White blood pressure: Detroit. *Psychosomatic Medicine, 35,* 276-296.

Jackson, L. A., & Adams-Campbell, L. L. (1994). John Henryism and blood pressure in Black college students. *Journal of Behavioral Medicine, 17,* 69-79.

James, S. A., Hartnett, S. A., & Kalsbeek, W. D. (1983). John Henryism and blood pressure among Black men. *Journal of Behavioral Medicine, 6,* 259-278.

James, S. A., Keenan, N. L., Strogatz, D. S., Browning, S. R., & Garrett, J. M. (1992). Socioeconomic status, John Henryism, and blood pressure in Black adults: The Pitt County Study. *American Journal of Epidemiology, 135,* 59-67.

James, S. A. (1994). John Henryism and the health of African-Americans. *Culture, Medicine, and Psychiatry, 18,* 163-182.

James, S. A., Strogatz, D. S., Wing, S. B., & Ramsey, D. L. (1987). Socioeconomic status, John Henryism, and hypertension in Blacks and Whites. *American Journal of Epidemiology, 128,* 664-673.

Light, K. C., Brownley, K. A., Turner, J. R., Hinderliter, A. L., Girdler, S. S., Sherwood, A., et al. (1995). Job status and high-effort coping influence work blood pressure in women and Blacks. *Hypertension, 25,* 554-559.

Markovic, N., Bunker, C. H., Ukoli, F. A., & Kuller, L. H. (1998). John Henryism and blood pressure among Nigerian civil servants. *Journal of Epidemiology and Community Health, 52,* 186-190.

McKetney, E. C., & Ragland, D. R. (1996). John Henryism, education, and blood pressure in young adults: The CARDIA study. *American Journal of Epidemiology, 143,* 787-791.

Merritt, M. M., Bennett, G. G., Sollers, J., Edwards, C. L., & Williams, R. B. (in press). Low educational attainment, John Henryism and cardiovascular reactivity and recovery to personally-relevant stress. *Psychosomatic Medicine.*

Syme, S. L. (1979). Psychosocial determinants of hypertension. In E. Oresti & C. Klint (Eds.), *Hypertension determinants, complications, and intervention* (pp. 95-98). New York: Grune & Stratton.

K

KEY INFORMANTS

The term *key informant* is best understood in the context of ethnographic or qualitative research in naturalistic settings (LeCompte & Schensul, 1999). These settings are often termed "the field" (DeWalt & DeWalt, 2002; Pelto & Pelto, 1978). The field is a sociophysical setting whose boundaries are defined in terms of institutions and people of interest and their associated activities in geographic space. For ethnographers, the field is any naturalistic geographic/social setting or location where a selected research problem is to be studied—a neighborhood, a network of clinics or emergency rooms, a group of buildings, or a school system. When ethnographic or qualitative researchers go to the field, they leave their own communities, institutional settings, and familiar behavioral and cognitive patterns to "enter" another social world—the world where the research will be conducted (Bernard, 2000; Miller & Crabtree, 1994; Werner & Schoepfle, 1987).

Ethnographic research is never "autobiographical." It requires that the researcher separate stereotypes, opinions, and judgments from accurate or "objective" observation and effective recording of the words, meanings, and opinions of research participants. Researchers thus must recognize and suspend their biases (LeCompte & Schensul, 1999). "Entry" is more than *going into* a medical clinic, a crack house, or a school; it requires that researchers transform themselves into instruments of data collection. Ethnographic research calls for engagement in direct learning through physical and social involvement in the field setting. Knowing, for ethnographers, is first and foremost experiencing by observing, participating in conversations and daily activities of members of the community under study, and recording these observations (Bernard, 2000; DeWalt & DeWalt, 2002). In the process, ethnographers learn what residents of the field already know—the language of the setting, the rules guiding social relationships, and the cultural patterns, expectations, and meanings that people share. Learning these rules, norms, boundaries, and behaviors is the task of ethnography. The first step in learning is establishing the relationships through which socialization can take place (Schensul, Schensul, & LeCompte, 1999).

The process of establishing personal relationships in the field is referred to as "building rapport" (Mischler, 1986; Schensul et al., 1999). Good ethnographers build trusting relationships easily. While sensitive to their surroundings and to appropriate timing especially with respect to sensitive questions (e.g., questions about sexual behavior or drug use), they quickly make efforts to ask questions that enable them to learn new things. One of the first steps in ethnographic field research in the field is the identification of those individuals who can help researchers to learn about the community and about the topic being discussed. These individuals, recognized as having special knowledge or expertise in a topic of interest to the researcher, are referred to as "key informants" (Bernard, 2000). Key informants are those knowledgeable individuals who are willing to share their knowledge with researchers once or repeatedly. According to Gilchrist (1992), "Key informants differ from other informants by the nature of their position in a culture and by their relationship to the researcher which is generally one of longer duration, occurs in varied settings and is more intimate" (p. 71).

Some qualitative researchers are critical of the term *key informant*, suggesting that it is symbolic of the power that researchers have traditionally held over the communities or other settings in which research is conducted. They suggest that "outside" researchers partner with local experts in the generation of knowledge (Clifford, 1988; Marcus & Fischer, 1986; Reason & Rowan, 1990). Others feel that the term *informant* refers to someone who is informing outsiders about behaviors or beliefs that communities wish to keep private. These views reflect different opinions about the appropriate relationship of the researcher to the community of study and the potential power imbalance between researchers and those researched. However, the term *key informant* can apply to anyone with specialized information or expertise, regardless of the mode of relationship, balance of power, or approach to qualitative research the researcher prefers.

Key informants provide depth and breadth of information. Key informants may have broad knowledge of a community or service system (e.g., superintendents or elected officials). They may introduce researchers to networks of people involved in specific roles and activities (physicians, drug dealers, alternative healers). Features of social geography (locations of commercial sex workers, romantic beach sites or hotels, which pharmacies older adults use) can be readily explored with the appropriate key informants. They may have expertise in specific topics ("over-the-counter remedies for arthritis," new drug trends in the community). Interviews with key informants reveal the domains and some of the subdomains of culture (i.e., the broad "coding categories" to be explored in further interviews and observations) (Fontana & Frey, 1994; Miller & Crabtree; 1994).

Researchers seeking for key informants will find that administrators, friends of friends, public figures, and other gatekeepers or people who provide entry to the research site constitute the best sources of information. People researchers know and trust can tell which individuals might make good candidates for key informant interviews. For each key informant, the researcher should have information about their possible area(s) of expertise, how to locate them, whatever information is available about their lifestyle, associations, schedule, and contacts. Once contacted and

interviewed, each key informant may be able to suggest others with related expertise or connections to the community.

Spradley (1979), a well-known ethnographer, notes that "although almost anyone can become an informant, not everyone makes a good informant" (p. 45). What makes a good key informant? Good key informants are natural researchers, interested in the purpose of the research and in exploring the topic in their own settings, together with as well as in the absence of the ethnographer. They are able to relate to a variety of different settings, sectors, networks, and individuals, and are prepared to link the ethnographer with these informational resources. The best key informants are clear about the boundaries of their own expertise. They alert their research partners to their own knowledge gaps. Key informants are often risk takers, willing to associate with the ethnographer despite questions about the research and the identity and intentions of the researcher. Usually they are experienced, having lived for a number of years in the research setting.

Qualitative researchers often make the mistake of interviewing a key informant only once. A single interview can provide an orientation to a subject or community, but the information that can be obtained from the first 60- to 90-minute interview is limited. This interview provides ideas and clues that can be probed in repeat interviews over a much longer period of time. Key informants often play a central role in their communities or networks, and can be very helpful in deepening the researcher's knowledge, tracking trends, and introducing researchers to others. Developing trust takes time. The quality and depth and detail of information is generally directly related to the intimacy and trust that develops between a researcher and a key informant. There are numerous examples of key informants in the anthropological literature. A typical key informant is the young man who found it very interesting to discuss the evolution and structure of the drug trade in a northeastern city. He was proud of the development of his own drug-dealing networks, clear about his plans for the future, and able to provide much helpful information over time with respect to new drug trends, and problems presented by the introduction of new drugs into the urban setting (Schensul et al., 2000).

Researchers approach key informants for interviews with open-ended questions. In the case of a clinic administrator, for example, the first question might be "Tell me about the kinds of health problems you see here." Subsequent questions might address location, types of patients/clients, where they go for help and services, how they manage their problems, the cost of help, difficulties in delivering services, and so on. Interviews are recorded by hand or by tape recording and transcribed verbatim. They are then coded by categories (such as those that constitute the above-mentioned topics of discussion) and subcategories as they emerge from the data. Interviews across key informants may be triangulated to verify already identified patterns and codes or to identify new ones (cf. Schensul et al., 1999). These interviews lead to further questions and more structured interviews with a larger sample of respondents to explore variations in the expression of cultural patterns or domains.

Key informants offer valuable information and emotional and social support to researchers new to a setting, as well as those seeking to explore new ideas and hunches with local experts. There are, however, limitations to the data that key informants provide. Information obtained from key informants must be complemented by other data sources such as interviews, observations, elicitation techniques, and surveys. Key informants do not represent every perspective in the community. They may also represent perspectives that diverge significantly from the norm. Furthermore, key informants may bias their information especially in the early stages of a relationship, when trust is evolving. Researchers must be able to situate key informants to interpret their contributions. Finally, researchers must triangulate a variety of data sources and seek for "saturation" (the point at which no new information is offered), in order to improve the validity of information provided by a single key informant source.

—Jean J. Schensul

Further Reading

Bernard, H. R. (2000). *Social research methods: Qualitative and quantitative approaches*. Thousand Oaks, CA: Sage.

Clifford, J. (1988). *Predicament of culture: Twentieth-century ethnography, literature and art*. Cambridge, MA: Harvard University Press.

DeWalt, K., & DeWalt, B. (2002). *Participant observation: A guide for fieldworkers*. Walnut Creek, CA: AltaMira.

Fontana, A., & Frey, J. H. (1994). Interviewing: The art of science. In N. Denzin & Y. Lincoln (Eds.), *The handbook of qualitative research* (pp. 361-376). Thousand Oaks, CA: Sage.

Gilchrist, V. (1992). Key informant interviews. In B. F. Crabtree & W. Miller (Eds.), *Doing qualitative research* (pp. 70-92). Newbury Park, CA: Sage.

LeCompte, M., & Schensul, J. (1999). Introduction to research methods. In J. Schensul & M. LeCompte (Eds.), *Ethnographer's toolkit: Vol. 1*. Walnut Creek, CA: AltaMira.

Marcus, G., & Fischer, M. (1986). *Anthropology as cultural critique: An experimental moment in the human sciences*. Chicago: University of Chicago Press.

Miller, W., & Crabtree, B. (1994). Clinical research. In N. Denzin & Y. Lincoln (Eds.), *The handbook of qualitative research* (pp. 340-352). Thousand Oaks, CA: Sage.

Mischler, E. (1986). *Research interviewing: Context and narrative*. Cambridge, MA: Harvard University Press.

Pelto, P. J., & Pelto, G. H. (1978). *Anthropological research: The structure of inquiry* (2nd ed.). Cambridge, UK: Cambridge University Press.

Reason, P., & Rowan, J. (Eds.). (1990). *Human inquiry: A sourcebook of new paradigm research*. New York: John Wiley.

Schensul, J., Huebner, C., Singer, M., Snow, M., Feliciano, P., & Broomhall, L. (2000). The high, the money and the fame: Smoking bud among urban youth. *Medical Anthropology, 18*, 389-414.

Schensul, S., Schensul, J., & LeCompte, M. (1999). *Essential ethnographic methods. Ethnographer's toolkit: Vol. 2*. Walnut Creek, CA: AltaMira.

Spradley, J. (1979). *The ethnographic interview*. New York: Holt, Rinehart & Winston.

Werner, O., & Schoepfle, M. (1987). *Systematic fieldwork: Foundations of ethnography and interviewing*. Newbury Park, CA: Sage.

KUOPIO ISCHEMIC HEART DISEASE RISK FACTOR STUDY

The Kuopio Ischemic Heart Disease Risk Factor (KIHD) Study is an epidemiological study of risk factors for atherosclerosis (a buildup of plaque in the arteries that can lead to heart attack and/or stroke), ischemic heart disease, related disorders (e.g., hypertension), and death in middle-aged and older adults from Kuopio, Finland, and surrounding communities. More than two decades ago, this area in eastern Finland was found to have one of the highest rates of heart disease among men in the world. The KIHD Study was designed to examine both traditional risk factors (e.g., cholesterol and blood pressure levels) and unknown or suspected risk factors (e.g., psychological characteristics) for cardiovascular diseases (CVD), in part to attempt to understand the high rates of heart disease in eastern Finland. When the study began in the mid-1980s, only males were invited to participate, in part because the high rates of heart disease observed in eastern Finland were noted in men, but also because at that time it was not as well understood as it is today that heart disease also is the leading cause of death in women. The most recent wave of data collection, obtained between 1998 and 2001, includes females in the study. Published findings from the KIHD Study to date have demonstrated that several important social, psychological, behavioral, and biological characteristics influence the development and progression of heart disease in men and are associated with increased risk of dying.

BACKGROUND

Dr. Jukka T. Salonen of Finland and Dr. George A. Kaplan of the United States jointly initiated the KIHD Study in 1984. They designed the study to be one of the most comprehensive studies of risk factors for CVD ever conducted by including assessments of a large number of biological, behavioral, psychological, social, economic, and environmental characteristics thought to influence risk for atherosclerosis and heart disease. As such, the study is highly multidisciplinary, with investigators from many areas of medicine, public health, epidemiology, and psychology contributing to the study. The KIHD Study was one of the first epidemiological studies to utilize state-of-the-art, noninvasive techniques to measure the extent and severity of atherosclerosis. Atherosclerosis is measured in the carotid arteries in the neck and the femoral arteries in the thigh. These sites are relatively easy to image with ultrasound technology, and plaque buildup in these sites is generally a good indicator of the overall amount of atherosclerosis found throughout the body.

KIHD investigators use annual linkages with the Finnish National Death Registry, the Finnish Cancer Registry, the social security institute of Finland, and hospital discharge records to record the health status, work and retirement history, as well as the experience of heart attacks, strokes, cancers, and deaths of KIHD

Study respondents. This multidisciplinary and comprehensive study has enabled investigators to address many previously unanswered research questions to better understand the development and progression of CVD.

STUDY POPULATION AND PROTOCOL

The KIHD Study originally recruited 2,682 men, who entered the study at the ages of 42, 48, 54, or 60 years old in two separate groups, called cohorts, over a 5-year period (1984-1989). All participants completed a comprehensive baseline examination that included interviews, paper-and-pencil questionnaires, laboratory tests, and physical measures. Four years later, a follow-up examination was undertaken on surviving members of the second cohort, with 1,038 men participating. KIHD investigators completed a third examination on 854 surviving male respondents 7 years later, or 11 years after the baseline. At the same time, a cohort of 921 women, matched to the ages of the male participants (i.e., 53, 59, 65, or 71 years old), was enrolled in the study. The second and third examinations were comparable to the first and included comprehensive interviews, paper-and-pencil questionnaires, laboratory tests, and physical measures.

HEALTH OUTCOMES

A primary goal of the KIHD Study has been to assess the illness and mortality experience of the study population in relation to the broad array of risk factors that were measured. To track deaths among KIHD Study participants, researchers annually link with the National Death Registry, which is maintained for all Finnish citizens. They also track the illness experience of study participants by reviewing hospital discharge records and/or performing annual linkages with medical databases. For example, to obtain information on the occurrence of heart attacks or stroke among study participants prior to 1993, data were obtained through the World Health Organization's Monitoring of Trends and Determinants of Cardiovascular Disease (MONICA) registry for this region. However, because the MONICA project, which had tracked cardiovascular events in 26 countries, including Finland, was discontinued after 1992, investigators have obtained more recent information on heart attacks and strokes via computerized linkages to the national hospital discharge registry in Finland. Linkage with the Finnish

Cancer Registry provides information about the type and severity of any cancers experienced by study participants. Investigators also have studied health conditions experienced by participants by collecting data on various health measures at each examination. These include assessments of systolic and diastolic blood pressure, noninvasive measurement of atherosclerosis of the carotid and femoral arteries, self-report of acute and chronic health conditions (e.g., diabetes, respiratory diseases), fasting levels of insulin, total cholesterol and lipoproteins, triglycerides, and markers of inflammation. Together, the breadth of information on health status obtained from these various sources has enabled investigators to report on the health status of KIHD Study participants over time.

KEY FINDINGS

KIHD investigators have made important contributions to the understanding of the role that psychosocial factors play in CVD risk. For example, KIHD Study research has shown that socioeconomic factors (e.g., education, occupation, income, childhood socioeconomic status), emotional states (e.g., anger and hostility, hopelessness, alexithymia), stress, and behavioral factors (e.g., alcohol consumption, smoking, physical activity, diet) critically influence the development and progression of atherosclerosis, hypertension, heart attack, stroke, and mortality. KIHD investigators also have documented the important

effects that trace elements (e.g., serum ferritin, selenium, and mercury) and LDL oxidation have on these health outcomes, and have reported on the protective effects of antioxidants and on the influence of particular genetic polymorphisms and/or mutations on cardiovascular disease risk. Study results so far have been based on data from the male participants, but future reports from this study will examine how these risk factors affect the health of women.

—*Susan A. Everson-Rose*

See also ALAMEDA COUNTY STUDY; BOGALUSA HEART STUDY; FRAMINGHAM HEART STUDY; HARVARD ALUMNI HEALTH STUDY

Further Reading

Everson, S. A., Goldberg, D. E., Kaplan, G. A., et al. (1996). Hopelessness and risk of mortality and incidence of myocardial infarction and cancer. *Psychosomatic Medicine, 58,* 113-121.

Keys, A. (1980). *Seven countries: A multivariate analysis of death and coronary heart disease.* Cambridge, MA: Harvard University Press.

Ross, R. (1993). The pathogenesis of atherosclerosis: A perspective for the 1990s. *Nature, 362,* 801-809.

Salonen, J. T. (1988). Is there a continuing need for longitudinal epidemiologic research? The Kuopio Ischemic Heart Disease Risk Factor Study. *Annals of Clinical Research, 20,* 46-50.

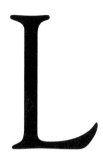

LATINO HEALTH AND BEHAVIOR

Health and behavioral data for Latinos have become increasingly available, and significant progress has been made in data collection methods. Although national data are available to provide an overview of health behaviors among Latino populations in comparison to Blacks and non-Latino Whites, less information is available by Latino subgroup. The examination of health behaviors is conducted within the broader definition of health as the social, physical, and mental well-being of an individual. It is also acknowledged that individual health behaviors are associated with socioeconomic status (SES) and the community health resources available to individuals to maintain their health status.

This entry has three objectives: to provide an overview of health status indicators for Latinos; to present empirical data on health behaviors of Latinos by age, gender, and subgroup when available; and to propose a framework for knowledge building to promote a new public health discourse on Latino health.

SOCIAL AND DEMOGRAPHIC PROFILE OF LATINOS

According to the 2000 census, 40 million Latinos live in the United States, representing 12.5% of the population. By the year 2050, Latinos are expected to constitute 25% of the U.S. population. Forty-five percent of Latinos live in the West, and 33% live in the South. Half of all Latinos live in just two states: California and Texas. Latinos are more likely to reside in metropolitan areas (46.4%) than non-Latino Whites (NLW) (21.2%), and more likely than NLW to live in households of five or more people (30.6% compared to 11.8%). Latino children currently constitute more than 15% of the total U.S. population of children, and 21% are under 14 years of age.

Nearly 60% of immigrants of color have resided in the United States for more than 10 years, most becoming U.S. citizens during that time. Close to 39% of Latinos are immigrants, compared to 61% of Asian Americans and 6% of non-Latino Blacks (NLB). Almost 25% of Spanish-speaking persons living in the United States speak little or no English. Differences in language proficiency by geographic location correspond to variations by region of the labor market experience of Latinos. Latinos have the lowest high school completion rate among all ethnic groups. With 6.8% of Latinos in the civilian labor force unemployed, compared to 3.4% of NLW, those who are employed are more likely to work in service occupations (19.4%) than are NLW (11.8%). Only 14% of Latinos are in managerial or professional occupations—with Mexicans as the least likely subgroup at 11.9%—compared to 33.2% of NLW.

In 1999, 22.8% of Latinos were living in poverty compared to 7.7% of NLW. Puerto Ricans are the most likely of all Latino subgroups to live below the poverty line (25.8%). Latino (36%) and NLB (37%) children are 3 times more likely to be poor than NLW (11%) children. Fifty-four percent of Latinas are either poor or near poor.

Latinas have the highest birth and fertility rates. Among subgroups, Mexican American women have the highest birth (26.4 per 1,000) and fertility (112.1

per 1,000) rates, and Cuban American women have the lowest birth (19.0 per 1,000) and fertility (75.5 per 1,000) rates. Although 87% of Latino children are U.S. citizens, either born or naturalized, they have limited access to primary and preventive health services. Even after adjusting for family income and parental education, Latino children are significantly more likely than NLW children to have suboptimal health status, spend more days in bed for illness, and make fewer physician visits.

FIVE LEADING CAUSES OF DEATH FOR LATINOS

Although the top two leading causes of death for Latinos, NLW, and NLB are the same—heart disease and cancer—age-adjusted mortality rates for these two diseases are lower than rates for the total population, NLW, and NLB. Latinos have higher age-adjusted mortality rates for diabetes, homicide, chronic liver disease, and HIV infection than the total population and NLW. Puerto Ricans (406.1 per 100,000) have higher age-adjusted all-cause mortality rates than Cubans (299.5 per 100,000) or Mexican Americans (348.4 per 100,000). Puerto Ricans, 25-54 years of age, are particularly at increased risk of death compared to NLW, Cubans, and Mexican Americans.

ACCESS TO HEALTH CARE SERVICES

Latinos are the least likely to have health insurance of all racial/ethnic groups: 67% of all Latinos compared to 86% of NLW and 80% of NLB. These rates are lower for Mexican Americans (61%) than for Puerto Ricans and Cubans (81% and 79%, respectively). The percentage with usual source of care, a good measure of access to health care, mirrors these health insurance coverage rates. Mexican Americans are the least likely to have a usual source of care (75%). Twelve percent of Latino children under age 18 lacked a usual source of care, compared to 5% for NLB and 4% for NLW. Persons who cannot identify a regular or usual source of care are much less likely to obtain preventive services or diagnosis, treatment, and management of acute and chronic health conditions.

HEALTH STATUS

Recent surveys provide useful insights regarding the burden of disability and disease among the Latino population. One measure, self-perceived health status, is a commonly used indicator of overall health status. Data from the National Health Interview Survey show that 16.2% of all Mexicans, 14.1% of all Cubans, and 17.5% of all Puerto Ricans report that they were in fair or poor health once differences in age distributions were taken into account—much higher than for the total population (10.8%) or NLW (9.3%).

CHRONIC HEALTH CONDITIONS

Less likely to use health services, Latinos with health conditions are also less likely to know that they have the disease. Although Latinos are more likely to develop diabetes than NLW (3.5 per 1,000 compared to 2.9 per 1,000), they are less likely to be aware that they have diabetes. The National Health and Nutrition Examination Survey (NHANES) found that 38% of Mexican Americans with diabetes were not previously aware that they had diabetes, compared to 33% of NLW.

NHANES data show that Mexican Americans are more likely to have high blood pressure (22% of Mexican American women compared to 19.3% of NLW women). Among diagnosed hypertensives, 12% of Mexican Americans had their blood pressure under control compared to 18% of NLW. The risks of the most common cancer sites—prostate, breast, and lung cancers—are lower for Latinos than they are for NLW. However, the incidence rate of cervical cancer was almost 1½ times higher for Latino women than for NLW women. The active asthma prevalence rate among Puerto Rican children (11%) is almost twice as high as that of NLB children (6%) and 3 times that of NLW children (3%).

Both Latino men and women have an AIDS case rate that is much higher than NLW men and women. Latinos' case rate is 58.2 per 100,000 compared to NLW case rate of 17.2 per 100,000, while Latinas' case rate is 16.6 per 100,000 compared to NLW women's case rate of 2.4 per 100,000. Given the higher risk of HIV/AIDS among Latinos, the lower rate of condom use by a partner among unmarried Latino women, 15-44 years of age, is of concern. Tuberculosis cases are also twice as high for Latinos (13.6 per 100,000) than the total population or NLW.

Latino adults are slightly more likely to report a major depression episode and Latino adolescents are slightly more likely to report a suicide attempt than

Table 1   Preventive Health Care Behaviors (in percentages)

	Hispanic	Mexican American	Non-Hispanic White	Non-Hispanic Black
Teeth cleaned during past year (> = 18 years)[a]	64.4	—	73	64.8
Dental sealants				
8 years[b]		10	29	11
14 years	—	7	18	5
Routine doctor visit in past year (> = 18 years)[c]	67.1	—	71.7	81.6
Pap smear in past 3 years (> = 18 years)[c]	86.2	—	87.1	88.5
Mammogram within past 2 years (> = 50 years)[c]	83.6	—	79.8	83.5
Blood pressure checked during past year (> = 18 years)[a]	82.9	—	88.7	91.7
Fully immunized 19- to 35-month-old children[d]	69	—	76	68
Flu shot in past year (age adjusted, > = 65 years)[e]	52.1	—	65.5	48.3
Pneumonia shot in past year (age adjusted, > = 65 years)[f]	33	—	57.9	34.6
Cholesterol checked (> = 18 years)[e]	64.4	—	76.4	69.9
Ever had blood stool test (> = 18 years)[e]	20	—	33.1	25.9
Aspirin therapy among persons with diabetes > = 15 times per month (age adjusted, > = 40 years)[f]	—	8	25	8
Prenatal care during first trimester[g]	74.4	72.9	88.5	74.3

Sources: a. 1999 Behavioral Risk Factor Surveillance Survey; b. 1988-1994 National Health and Nutrition Examination Survey; c. 2000 Behavioral Risk Factor Surveillance System; d. 2000 National Immunization Survey; e. 2001 National Health Interview Survey; f. 1988-1994 National Health and Nutrition Examination Survey; g. 2000 Natality, National Vital Statistics System.

NLW. Living in the United States is related to elevated risk for mental health problems—Mexican American adolescents and adults living in the United States have higher rates of depressive symptoms, illicit drug use, and suicidal ideation than Mexicans. Schizophrenia rates are slightly lower among Latinos than NLW. However, Latinos with mental illness (e.g., depression, schizophrenia) are less likely to receive treatment for their illness.

PREVENTIVE AND RISK HEALTH BEHAVIORS

Lack of access to health care also impedes usage and participation in preventive behaviors and services, among them, routine check-ups, Pap smears, mammograms, clinical breast exams, and prenatal care. Consistent evidence shows that individuals who practice one preventive behavior are more likely to practice other preventive behaviors. When exploring likelihood of screening mammography, women who engaged in such preventive health measures as Pap smears, cholesterol measurement, and seat belt use

were more likely to obtain screening mammography. Evidence shows that access to health care (insurance) and engaging in other healthy behaviors were more important predictors of preventive behaviors than ethnicity.

Rates of preventive health care behaviors for Latinos are consistently lower than for NLW and similar or lower than for NLB (see Table 1). Considerable effort has been made during the past few years to encourage women to have breast checks, mammograms, and Pap smears. This has resulted in an apparent elimination of disparities in use of these services for Latinas, yet these data may not reflect rates for Latinas who are migrant farm workers, seasonal workers, or distressed inner-city residents. In 2000, 86.2% of Latinas 18 years of age and older had received a Pap smear during the previous 3 years; 83.6% of Latinas over the age of 50 had received a mammogram.

Table 2 presents national data on risk and preventive health behaviors among Latinos. These data demonstrate that the pattern of higher rates of diabetes among Latinos is likely to continue given the

Table 2   Risk and Preventive Health Behaviors (in percentages)

	Hispanic	Mexican American	Non-Hispanic White	Non-Hispanic Black
Folic acid consumption by nonpregnant women > = 400 mcg daily (15-44 years)[a]	—	13	23	18
Fruits > = 2 daily servings[b] (age adjusted, > = 2 years)	32	29	27	24
Vegetables > = 3 daily servings[b] (age adjusted, > = 2 years)	2	2	(3% U.S.)	—
Saturated fat intake < 10% caloric intake (age adjusted, > = 2 years)[c]	—	39	35	31
Calcium intake > = mean intake (age adjusted, > = 2 years)[c]	—	44	49	30
Smokers (age adjusted, > = 18 years)[d]	16	—	24.5	22.2
Environmental tobacco smoke exposure among nonsmokers (age adjusted, > = 4 years)[c]	—	53	63	81
Overweight (6- to 19-year-olds)[c]	—	15	10	14
Obese adults (age adjusted, > = 20 years)[d]				
Men	22.1	—	22.5	27.5
Women	26.8	—	20.5	36.7
At least 1 drink during past month (> = 18 years)[e]	49.7	—	56.3	44.7
Driven with too much to drink (> = 18 years)[f]	5.6	—	4.3	3.7
Five or more drinks at one occasion > = 12 times per year (age adjusted, > = 18 years)[d]	8.3	—	10.7	5.3
No alcohol and illicit drugs during past month (12-17 years)[f]	79	—	77	82
No leisure time physical activity (age adjusted, > = 18 years)[d]	78.9	—	65	75.1
Vigorous physical activity (Grades 9-12)[g]	61	—	67	56
Responsible sexual behavior (Grades 9-12)[g]	84	—	85	84
Condom use by partner, unmarried females (18-44 years)[h]	17	—	24	22
Have functional smoke alarm on every floor in residence (age adjusted)[i]	81	—	89	86

Sources: a. 1991-1994 National Health and Nutrition Examination Survey; b. 1994-1996 Continuing Survey of Food Intake by Individuals, USDA; c. 1988-1994 National Health and Nutrition Examination Survey; d. 2001 National Health Interview Survey; e. 1999 Behavioral Risk Factor Surveillance Survey; f. 1998 National Household Survey on Drug Abuse; g. 1999 Youth Risk Behavior Surveillance System; h. 1995 National Survey on Family Growth; i. 1998 National Health Interview Survey.

higher risk of overweight among Latino children and adolescents, the high rates of obesity among Latino adults, and low rates of leisure-time physical activity. Latino rates of alcohol consumption are intermediate between those of NLW and NLB. Current smoking rates, and rates of exposure to environmental tobacco smoke among nonsmokers, are lower for Latinos than NLW and NLB. Although educational campaigns to increase folic acid consumption among women of reproductive age target all women and those living along the U.S.-Mexico border, nonpregnant Latinas

15-44 years of age (13%) are still less likely to consume the recommended level of folic acid (at least 400 mcg per day) than NLW and NLB women (see Table 2).

Linked to self-care practice and preventive behaviors is belief in susceptibility, self-efficacy, and health locus of control. Self-care education could increase individuals' internal health locus of control, thus leading them to choose self-care over medical care or no care in the face of certain common illness symptoms. For example, Mexican-born women were less likely to perform breast self-exam than U.S.-born women of Mexican descent not only because of lower SES, lack of health insurance, fewer health professional interventions, and less motivation to engage in other self-care practices, but also because they had a stronger belief in their perceived susceptibility to cancer and its seriousness and had a stronger belief in the role of fate and powerful others (physicians) in determining their health.

Disparities persist in rates of preventive health care behaviors, particularly for the use of flu and pneumonia shots among the elderly. Use of dental sealants for 8- and 14-year-old Latinos is half that of NLW. As documented in the Institute of Medicine's recent report *Unequal Treatment* (Smedley, Stith, & Nelson, 2002), Latinos have lower access to quality health care even within similarly insured populations. These disparities are more pronounced for newer diagnostic and treatment procedures. For example, only 8% of Latinos with diabetes who are at least 40 years of age take aspirin at least 15 times per month—one third of the rate for NLW.

SOCIOCULTURAL PROTECTIVE BEHAVIORS

Health disparities are buffered at times by protective factors, which include ethnic-specific values and behaviors that are culturally sanctioned. Protective behaviors such as reliance on family members for information and instrumental support, low-fat nutritious eating habits, attitudes and value on motherhood and children, and low use of alcohol, tobacco, and illicit substances have not been adequately measured, with few exceptions, in prior studies. These health behaviors and psychosocial resources represent important mediators in understanding health disparities.

Although Latinos currently have lower rates of heart disease and stroke, there are two trends that are of concern. The first trend is that while Latinos' rates of obesity, diabetes, and high blood pressure are higher than NLW groups, they are less likely to engage in leisure-time physical activity. The second trend is that U.S.-born Mexican Americans have higher rates of certain risk factors such as smoking and alcohol consumption than those born in Mexico. These trends may lead to higher rates of heart disease and stroke for Latinos, which has been observed in recent studies.

The San Antonio Heart Study used Framingham risk equations to predict cardiovascular disease (CVD) risk in Mexican Americans. The follow-up of the San Antonio Heart Study found a 38% higher all-cause mortality rate and a 30% higher CVD mortality rate for Mexican Americans as compared to NLW. While U.S.-born Mexican Americans showed greater mortality rates than NLW, Mexican immigrants did not. In explaining the excess risk for U.S.-born Mexican Americans, Stern and Wei (1999) concluded that immigrants from Mexico had very low mortality despite low SES due to a "healthy migrant effect," that is, the role of the protective factors that Mexicans bring with them. These findings point out the importance of conducting longitudinal studies for Latinos and analyzing results by birthplace/generation.

Noteworthy is that some studies show that as low-income Latino immigrants integrate into society, as measured by number of years in the United States and English-language proficiency, we observe a deterioration of protective factors, resulting in Mexican Americans and other Latinos becoming more likely to smoke, drink alcohol, be overweight, and have diabetes. Although these observations appear to be generalizable for all immigrants, for Latino immigrants—often living in greater degrees of poverty than other immigrants—the decrease in protective factors increases their burden of disease and disability.

Recent data show that U.S.-born Mexican Americans with higher education and English-language proficiency tend to have better health outcomes, while less educated U.S.-born Mexican Americans have worse health outcomes. These intragroup differences may be a function of their higher SES and greater access to health care services, while the less favorable outcomes of poor U.S.-born Mexicans may be explained by both their lower SES and the stressors associated with the continual process of acculturation. Perceived social acceptance—one measure of acculturation—should be explored as a possible predictor of service use, particularly preventive health services. Arcia, Skinner, Bailey, and Correa (2001) found that perceived social acceptance is a measure of perception, not of cultural behavior, and is therefore independent of language use, proficiency, and the cultural orientation of current or desired environments. Lack of social receptivity is a form of institutional discrimination and influences individuals' choice of their degree of active participation in society.

Protective behaviors may contribute to lower levels of perceived stress by the Latino community and may mitigate the detrimental effects of poverty on health status and outcome, particularly for Mexican immigrants. The relatively good health outcomes of Mexican-origin individuals may in part result from the protective effect of strong family and cultural ties, social behaviors, the healthy migrant effect, and underreporting of mortality and poor birth outcomes due to misclassification of Mexican-origin individuals on death certificates. The Latino or Mexican "epidemiologic paradox" (exemplified by high poverty but favorable infant mortality and low birth weight rates) has been coined in reference to the similar birth outcomes of Mexican-origin women with NLW women, and more recently for the entire Latino population. Latinas born on the island of Puerto Rico experienced fewer stressful life events and were less likely to engage in negative health behaviors during pregnancy than U.S.-born Puerto Rican women, despite such risk factors as low human capital, meager financial resources, and residence in disadvantaged neighborhoods. The healthier outcomes may be accounted for by such protective factors as strong family support and a Latino cultural orientation.

Health behaviors such as sleep, nutrition, exercise, and substance use can be highly associated with family cohesiveness, environment stressors, perceptions of health status, value of health, and definitions of taking care of one's health. Family cohesiveness has also been linked to disease management, with high levels of family cohesiveness resulting in good diet and exercise. More complete measures of culture-specific protective factors that promote favorable health behaviors and reduce risk behaviors require additional attention and inquiry.

The study of the role of culture-specific behaviors and female kin in differences in infant outcome between Mexican American and Mexican immigrant mothers shows that the extended family kin network and the women's perception of the infant as important to her role in life are positively associated with her self-care practices. Similar conclusions were drawn by Mendias, Clark, and Guevara (2001), who found that women of Mexican origin living in the United States perceive themselves primarily as mothers and wives—highly valued roles in Mexican culture—and, because they see the family and their role in the family as important, they believe their own health to be important. Other studies have found that life events and perceived stress can influence birth outcome and use of alcohol, tobacco, and illicit substances. The impact that psychosocial factors, such as stress and depression, have on specific health habits can be linked to a sense of powerlessness that is directly related to many poor health behaviors and negative attitudes toward the health care system.

Although stress is associated with community-level effects and depression, the role of social support shows highly variable results. For low-income Latinos, economic strain and worry, risk of violence and danger in the community, and institutional discriminatory practices are all highly stressful. These psychosocial antecedents as mediators in Latino health merit inquiry. Health behaviors, such as substance abuse, are highly related to stressors, and parental depression is highly associated with the aforementioned factors, less healthy behaviors, and less favorable health and well-being outcome for their children. Recent national data demonstrating Latino heterogeneity in health behaviors and outcomes provide an important opportunity to propose a framework for guiding the new generation of research.

LINKING THE FACTORS THAT CONTRIBUTE TO LATINO HEALTH BEHAVIORS AND OUTCOMES

The integration of multiple frameworks can provide a broader understanding of the dimensions of difference in health behaviors and outcomes among Latino subgroups and inform public health interventions to promote progress in reducing social class and racial and ethnic-specific disparities. Some consensus exists in the scientific public health community that multiple factors—economic, biological, environmental, psychosocial, access to health care and quality of services received, institutional racism, and political, legal, and structural factors (e.g., lack of outreach, immigrant and migrant status)—contribute to health outcomes. Evidence-based literature suggests that poverty is associated with a cluster of negative quality-of-life effects that are detrimental to health behaviors and outcomes. These include such health risks as undetected chronic or infectious diseases, nutritional deficiency, poor work conditions, unfavorable environmental and housing conditions, and racial and institutional discrimination, all of which contribute to chronic stressors in a support-limited environment. For example, 14.2% of Mexican American families reported food-insufficiency, compared to 6.7% of NLB and 2.1% of NLW.

In many ways, the acknowledgment of the multiple effects of poverty on quality of life and health

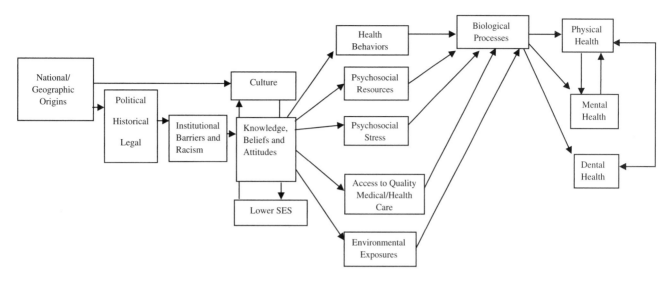

Figure 1   Framework for Understanding the Relationship Between Hispanic/Latino Ethnicity and Health

Source: Adapted from Williams, D. R. (1993). Race in the Health of America: Problems, Issues, and Directions. *MMWR*, 42, RR-10, 9.

outcome is not new to public health. The role of poverty has been, however, elevated as an important factor (under the rubric of social inequality, privilege and health, SES gradient) in understanding health outcomes of low-income groups.

Studies have failed, however, to examine the multi-system-level factors that are linked to individual, family, and community health and that contribute to health disparities in poor, Latino subgroups. There is ample evidence to suggest that limited economic and educational resources contribute to less nutritious eating habits, less access to appropriate health care resources, especially for low-income Latinos, higher rates of drug and alcohol use, and less access to quality education, sanitation, and safety services.

Factors associated with Latino health access and mortality and morbidity patterns suggest that preventive, risk, and protective health behaviors intersect to influence health outcome. However, the protective factors also seem to decrease with persistent intergenerational poverty and changes in family structure variables. When data are available by subgroup, Puerto Ricans and Mexicans have the worst rates among Latinos for many health indicators, including self-assessed health status, percentage of population below the federal poverty level, adolescent birth rate, and infant mortality rates. These subgroups are more multiracial than other Latino subgroups, and their poorer health outcomes illustrate the intersectional effects of

racial and ethnic status on health disparities in the United States. Differential effects of preventive, risk, and sociocultural protective behaviors are linked with subgroup membership.

Figure 1 proposes a set of direct and mediating variables that may contribute to elucidating the relationship between Latino ethnicity and health outcome (with the caveat that the strength of each variable will be dependent on age, race, gender, access to health care services, and subgroup membership). The framework accounts for the unique political, social, and structural factors that Latinos in general, and underserved Latino subgroups in particular, confront in U.S. society.

Latinos share different modes of historic incorporation, different forms of institutional responsiveness and treatment based on national/geographic origin, race, indigenous background, SES, and dominant language spoken. The political, historical, and legal context of the position of each Latino subgroup has directly shaped the nature and extent of the institutional barriers and racism that are strongly associated with the disproportionate number of Latinos in poverty. For example, Black Puerto Ricans and Dominicans have lower SES and worse health outcomes than other Puerto Ricans and Dominicans. Low SES or poverty is strongly linked with individual factors such as knowledge and beliefs about their symptoms, health care practices, attitudes toward the health care system, adherence to recommended treatments, and health behaviors toward seeking, accepting, and using health care services. These can be associated with individuals' perception of their social acceptance, which can be more a measure of institutional discrimination than of any of the individuals' characteristics.

These individual factors are strongly shaped by low educational levels and lack of access to relevant knowledge as a result of limited English-language and literacy proficiency and cultural-specific context. Although sociocultural factors may play a role in disease susceptibility, few studies have expended any effort in explaining how culture may be injurious or protective to health. Identified protective health factors include favorable health practices and psychosocial resources in the form of family, community, and societal support. In contrast, the rates of protective factors may decrease with time in the United States. Although risk factors are similar for all groups, risk factors are usually linked with ethnic-specific groups due to their context of poverty and health-delimiting correlates, limited access to health care, and the community context (such as exposure to violence, environmental pollutants). Jointly, these aforementioned factors contribute to psychosocial stressors. Accordingly, these risk factors for Latinos may contribute to changes in biological processes, such as higher rates of diabetes and cardiovascular diseases. The cumulative effects of these processes intergenerationally are likely to influence the overall well-being and health outcome of Latinos.

IMPLICATIONS FOR
PROMOTING HEALTH BEHAVIORS
AND ADVANCING LATINO HEALTH RESEARCH

A new theoretical discourse on the role of SES (poverty), not culture, may help to dispel the cultural attribution and deficit model that has dominated the public health literature on Latinos. The greater likelihood of living in poverty places Latinos at increased risk of disease and disability. Poverty is significantly associated with residence in resource-poor neighborhoods, greater likelihood of being exposed to environmental and occupational hazards, and greater likelihood of intentional and unintentional injury. Social environments can be linked to high levels of perceived stress, low levels of family cohesion and stability, and feelings of powerlessness, leading to low self-efficacy. These psychosocial variables may be

associated with poor health behaviors and health outcomes, as Phillips (1994) found when examining factors associated with healthy and unhealthy eating habits and intent to change eating habits among low-income, ethnic minority groups.

A major implication is that reduction in health disparities requires interventions to reduce poverty and increase access to health-promoting resources. For example, family economic security should be increased for low-income working poor by providing a living wage and a comprehensive form of family support for health, day care, and job development.

Future research on Latinos must be grounded in a more comprehensive "reality-based" conceptual context that accounts for resource-poor community contexts, racism, and discrimination in accessing health care so as to supplement the few studies identified by the recently released Institute of Medicine study, *Unequal Treatment*. Equally important are developing a health research agenda and funding priorities that are relevant and consistent with health data that show a disproportionate impact on Latinos, including ambulatory-sensitive conditions, diabetes, asthma, and obesity, and incorporate a more comprehensive view that includes the social, physical, and economic environment. A national strategic data collection plan requires implementation to monitor the health status and behaviors of Latinos by birthplace, subgroup, gender, and urban/rural residence and includes the residents of Puerto Rico. Community-based participatory research principles should be incorporated,in all human subject research conducted with state or federal funds. Community-based participatory research studies should be monitored to ensure that the researchers engage and sustain a solid partnership with the community to ensure appropriate interpretation of the data.

Significant progress has been made in mapping and profiling the overall health status of Latinos in the United States in the past decade. The national disease prevention and health promotion agenda for the year 2010, Healthy People 2010, now has "eliminating disparities" as one of its two overarching goals. For the first time, single targets are set for all racial and ethnic groups and baseline and monitoring data will be routinely published for Latinos and other racial/ethnic groups. This is an important first step toward achieving the goal of eliminating health disparities. Considerable effort is now needed to better understand the factors associated with health behaviors so as to improve our understanding of the reasons underlying ethnic specific disparities.

—*Ruth E. Zambrana and
Olivia Carter-Pokras*

See also ACCULTURATION AND HEALTH; AFRICAN AMERICAN HEALTH AND BEHAVIOR; ASIAN AMERICAN/PACIFIC ISLANDER HEALTH AND BEHAVIOR; HEALTH DISPARITIES

Further Reading

Aguirre-Molina, M., Molina, C., & Zambrana, R. E. (Eds.). (2001). *Health issues in the Latino community.* San Francisco: Jossey-Bass.

Arcia, E., Skinner, M., Bailey, D., & Correa, V. (2001). Models of acculturation and health behaviors among Latino immigrants to the U.S. *Social Science and Medicine, 53, 1,* 41-54.

Carter-Pokras, O., & Zambrana, R. E. (2001). Latino health status. In M. Aguirre-Molina, C. Molina, & R. E. Zambrana (Eds.), *Health issues in the Latino community* (pp. 23-54). San Francisco: Jossey-Bass.

Centers for Disease Control and Prevention. (1993). Use of race and ethnicity in public health surveillance. Summary of the CDC/ATSDR Workshop. *Morbidity and Mortality Weekly Report, 42,* 1-28.

Hajat, A., Lucas, J., & Kington, R. (2000). *Health outcomes among Hispanic subgroups: United States, 1992-95.* Advance data from Vital and Health Statistics, No. 310. Hyattsville, MD: National Center for Health Statistics.

Mendias, E. P., Clark, M. C., & Guevara, E. B. (2001, April). Women's self-perception and self-care practice: Implications for health care delivery. *Health Care for Women International, 22,* 3.

Perez, S. (Ed.). (2000). *Moving up the economic ladder: Latino workers and the nation's future prosperity: State of Hispanic America 1999.* Washington, DC: National Council of La Raza.

Phillips, K. (1994). Correlates of healthy eating habits in low-income Black women and Latinas. *Preventive Medicine, 23,* 781-787.

Smedley, B. D., Stith, A. Y., & Nelson, A. R. (Eds.). (2002). *Unequal treatment: Confronting racial and ethnic disparities in health care.* National Academies of Science. Washington, DC: Institute of Medicine.

Smedley, B. D., & Syme, S. L. (2000). *Promoting health: Intervention strategies from social and behavioral research.* Washington, DC: Institute of Medicine.

Stern, M. P., & Wei, M. (1999). Do Mexican Americans really have low rates of cardiovascular disease? *Preventive Medicine, 29,* 90-95.

Therrien, M., & Ramirez, R. R. (2001). *Current population reports: The Hispanic population in the United States, population characteristics March 2000.* Washington, DC: U.S. Census Bureau, Department of Commerce.

Williams, D. R. (1996). Racism and health: A research agenda. *Ethnicity & Disease, 6,* 1-6.

Zambrana, R. E., & Carter-Pokras, O. (2001). Health data issues for Hispanics: Implications for public health research. *Journal of Health Care for the Poor and Underserved, 12, 1,* 20-34.

LIPIDS: PSYCHOSOCIAL ASPECTS

Lipids are fats that circulate in the blood, and include cholesterol, triglycerides, and phospholipids. Lipids are usually transported in the blood from one tissue site to another in the form of lipoproteins, which are combinations of lipids and proteins. The most well-studied and clinically relevant of these lipoproteins are high-density lipoprotein (HDL) and low-density lipoprotein (LDL), but the major lipoproteins also include chylomicrons, very low density lipoprotein, intermediate-density lipoprotein, and Lp(a). Total cholesterol concentrations include cholesterol from all of the lipoproteins. Because about 70% of cholesterol in the blood is carried by LDL, there is a strong relationship between LDL-cholesterol and total cholesterol.

Lipids play a central etiological role in atherosclerotic cardiovascular disease (CVD). Evidence from epidemiological studies, clinical investigation, and basic science research has concluded that persistently elevated concentrations of total cholesterol, LDL-c, and probably triglycerides predispose individuals to higher risk of developing atherosclerotic heart disease and thrombosis, and high concentrations of HDL-c are cardioprotective.

DETERMINANTS OF LIPIDS

Both genetic and behavioral factors have influences on lipid and lipoprotein concentrations, and the influence is about equal in magnitude. Among the most important genetic influences are gender, inherited factors, ethnicity, and age. However, it is the behavioral factors that affect lipid levels that are of particular interest to behavioral scientists. For example, moderate alcohol consumption and exercise each modestly increase HDL-c with little or no effect on cholesterol or LDL-c. The use of exogenous estrogens in women also increases HDL-c in addition to lowering LDL-c levels. In contrast, cigarette smoking lowers HDL-c, and obesity and a diet rich in saturated fat increases LDL-c somewhat. However, even when considered together, these genetic and behavioral factors explain less than half the variability in lipid levels between individuals.

Anxiety and depression have been implicated in the development and progression of CVD, although the mechanisms linking these variables to disease end points are not known. Because much of the variability in lipid levels is also unexplained, investigations of how and whether mood states, such as anxiety and depression, are associated with lipid concentrations have been initiated.

MOOD AND LIPIDS

Several different mood states have been examined in relation to cholesterol and other lipids. These include depression, anxiety, hostility and aggression, and impulsivity, although the majority of the work in this area has focused on depression and anxiety. For example, depression has typically been found to be associated with low cholesterol levels, while anxiety is typically found to be associated with high cholesterol levels, as discussed below. While these general patterns in the literature have emerged, there is still no definitive consensus regarding the mechanism linking mood and cholesterol, and the nature of the causal relationship between mood states and lipid levels is not yet known.

The lifetime incidence of depression in the United States today is approximately 13% in men and 21% in women, and is increasing. Depression is a significant risk factor for death among cardiac patients, although the mechanism linking depression to risk of death is not yet adequately explained. Studies of depression and cholesterol levels generally have focused on a few, separate groups of individuals. Either clinical depression or dysphoria has been examined among healthy, hypercholesterolemic patients enrolled in lipid-lowering (primary prevention) trials; among cardiac patients enrolled in lipid-lowering (secondary prevention) trials; among large groups of healthy individuals enrolled in epidemiological studies; among postpartum women who experience a prominent and sudden drop in blood cholesterol after giving birth; and among one or a few hypercholesterolemic individuals (single-case study) undergoing pharmacological lipid lowering. Relatedly, cholesterol concentrations have been examined in psychiatric patients at elevated risk for suicide.

Most lipid-lowering trials have revealed the expected decrease in cardiovascular-related deaths but also a surprising increase in non-illness-related mortality primarily due to an increase in deaths from suicide, homicide, accidents, and violence. Although the findings are intriguing, these large trials have not been adequately designed for the examination of psychiatric outcome measures, and the link between non-illness-related mortality rates and mood simply cannot be adequately tested in these studies. However, they have provided a clear rationale for smaller-scale investigations to specifically test the putative relationship between cholesterol and negative mood.

The majority of these investigations have reported an inverse relationship between cholesterol and depressive states, and this holds for studies of those with spontaneously low cholesterol as well as for investigations of hypercholesterolemic individuals undergoing lipid lowering. However, there are some disparate results, with a few studies showing no relationship, and even a few showing a positive relationship. All of these investigations tend to vary with regard to the assessment of depression, the use of psychiatric versus healthy populations, and various, likely important characteristics of the population examined (gender, age, ethnicity).

The investigation of postpartum women, although small in number, has reported more consistent findings. Pregnancy increases cholesterol concentrations by about 40%, and blood levels of cholesterol drop rapidly following birth. Most, although not all, studies of healthy women have shown a moderate, inverse relationship between serum cholesterol levels and depressed mood in the postpartum period. Thus, these data support the notion that precipitous decreases in blood cholesterol have negative effects on mood, and thus suggest that the change in lipid concentrations is causing the mood effects.

The findings for anxiety patients are in contrast to those among depressed patients. Generally, elevated total cholesterol levels have been reported among subjects with anxiety disorders, particularly panic disorder. This is somewhat difficult to reconcile with the data on depression, because anxiety and depression frequently coexist. Thus, several investigators have examined blood cholesterol levels among patients with both anxiety and depression. Among those with major depressive disorder, the presence of current or past anxiety diagnosis is associated with increased blood cholesterol. However, those with a diagnosis of generalized anxiety disorder or panic without depression have higher blood cholesterol than those with a diagnosis of anxiety disorder or panic with comorbid major depression. In general, a relationship between trait anxiety and lipid levels in individuals without anxiety disorders has not emerged.

What might explain these sometimes contradictory findings? At least some of the discrepancies can be explained by examining the specific populations tested. For example, evidence for a relationship between transient depressed mood and lipid levels among nondepressed populations is stronger than is the evidence among clinically depressed patients. Evidence for a negative relationship between cholesterol and depressed mood among those treated for lipid lowering is more consistent among primary prevention trials than among secondary prevention trials. At least one study has determined that age is an important determinant of the relationship between cholesterol and depression; a negative association of lipid levels and depression was found only among older individuals. With regard to anxiety, the presence or absence of comorbid depression is an important factor to consider, as is the presence or absence of sleep panic. Finally, uncovering the causal relationship between cholesterol and mood states will clarify the mechanisms involved.

MECHANISMS

How do psychosocial factors influence lipid concentrations in the blood? Anxiety, depression, and hostility, as well as stress, may exert influences on lipids directly, indirectly, or both. For example, stimulation of the sympathetic nervous system, as occurs during anxiety, aggression, and with some other mood states, increases blood pressure, catecholamine concentrations, and cortisol release. Ultimately, lipolysis, or the release of stored lipids into the circulation, occurs, resulting in changes in circulating lipid levels. Arousal of the autonomic nervous system also alters lipid metabolism by influencing regulation of lipoprotein

lipase and hepatic lipase, the enzymes responsible for the metabolism of specific lipoproteins. Cholesterol influences neuronal membranes, and can influence the production and metabolism of several neurotransmitters. The best documented of these effects is the reduced serotonergic function that occurs with decreased cholesterol levels. Serotonin has prominent effects on mood, such as depression, aggression, and impulsivity, and thus provides a putative mechanism linking decreased cholesterol with negative mood states.

More indirectly, affect and mood changes alter behaviors, such as diet, exercise, interpersonal interaction, and sleep patterns. Many such behaviors have already been established as important influences on lipid concentrations in the circulation.

There is a strong public health focus on reducing blood cholesterol levels. Low cholesterol, either induced or naturally occurring, can have complex influences on psychosocial factors, and particularly mood.

—*Catherine M. Stoney*
and Diane Bonfiglio

See also Anxiety, Heart Disease, and Mortality; Heart Disease: Anger, Depression, and Anxiety; National Cholesterol Educational Program (NCEP)

Further Reading

Agargun, M. Y. (2002). Serum cholesterol concentration, depression, and anxiety. *Acta Psychiatrica Scandinavica, 105*, 81-83.

LONELINESS AND HEALTH

Loneliness has been defined as the unpleasant experience that occurs when a person's network of social relationships is deficient in some important way, either quantitatively or qualitatively. Loneliness can be mild and fleeting but it can also be a persisting, distressing experience. Robert Weiss has identified two main types of loneliness: social loneliness stemming from the absence of an adequate social network, and emotional loneliness stemming from the absence of emotional attachments provided by intimate relationships. The proportion of people who acknowledge loneliness varies as a function of various factors including the exact wording of the question posed (the nature of the loneliness described, the time span involved, etc.). Nonetheless, loneliness is clearly a widespread phenomenon. In one benchmark national survey of U.S. residents, 26% said they had felt "very lonely or remote from other people" in the past few weeks. Among adults in 18 countries, U.S. participants ranked high (fourth) in the extent of their loneliness, with the Japanese and Italians being highest in loneliness and the Danes being lowest.

Sociologists dating back to Durkheim have seen social ties as the mortar of society, arguing that when people feel alienated and lonely society is prone to breaking down. Consistent with this view, among adolescents loneliness has been associated with running away from home and delinquent acts such as gambling, theft, and vandalism. Similarly, sex offenders have been found to be high in loneliness and a correlation exists between suicidal ideation and loneliness. Loneliness can be a costly, serious problem for individuals and for society as a whole.

LONELINESS AND MENTAL HEALTH

Taking the American Psychiatric Association's widely known *Diagnostic and Statistical Manual of Mental Disorders (DSM-IV)* as a standard for mapping the terrain, there are numerous varieties of deficient mental health. These have been grouped into such categories of disorders as childhood, anxiety, mood, personality, psychosis, eating, substance abuse, and sleeping. A number of researchers have examined loneliness as a correlate of mental health (for earlier reviews, see Jones & Carver, 1991, and Ernst & Cacioppo, 1999). They have generated a reasonable-sized body of work on anxiety, mood, and personality but fewer investigations on other topics. In contrast to the extensive evidence developmental psychologists have gathered showing that children rejected by their peers are vulnerable to loneliness, researchers have done very few investigations on loneliness and childhood *DSM-IV* disorders per se. Some researchers have studied clinical populations, although undoubtedly a majority have administered paper-and-pencil measures to students or community residents. Thus, many of their findings apply more to mental health tendencies among members of the general public than to individuals with clinically diagnosed psychopathologies. In any case, numerous noteworthy correlations have been found.

Anxiety and Mood

Several studies have shown that the more loneliness people report, the more likely they are to report anxiety. Complementing self-reports, trait lonely individuals have high mean levels of cortisol, a physiological indicator of anxiety. Loneliness has also been implicated in various more specific forms of anxiety. For instance, Frieda Fromm-Reichmann saw loneliness as having much in common with panic states. Empirical studies find loneliness coupled with social anxiety in both children and adults. Not only has loneliness been included as a facet of posttraumatic stress disorder (PTSD), but also, among Israeli soldiers exposed to the stress of the 1982 Lebanon war, loneliness was an antecedent of combat-related psychopathology 2 years later.

During the 1970s, investigators observed a considerable concordance between loneliness and depression, so much so that they questioned if the two are separate phenomena. The answer is yes in the sense that statistical analyses have shown them to be distinguishable; logical analysis indicates that depression can result from any number of events whereas loneliness is a response to interpersonal deficits, and their correlates differ to some extent. More recent work shows that a self-critical form of depression is more closely associated with loneliness than a helpless, dependent variety. Complementing their greater depression, lonely individuals also report more negative and fewer positive feelings in response to mood scales. Lonely individuals are not a happy bunch.

Personality

In an early article published before World War II, Gregory Zilboorg portrayed the personalities of lonely individuals as manifesting narcissism, megalomania, and hostility. Clinical writing and some statistical evidence with clinical populations suggest that loneliness is common among adults with so-called borderline personalities. Such individuals have an unstable sense of self and unstable interpersonal relationships, are impulsive, have difficulty controlling their anger, and engage in "acting out behaviors." Correlational research shows loneliness is associated with several other personality characteristics such as low self-esteem, shyness, self-consciousness, neuroticism, pessimism, specific forms of perfectionism, and insecure attachment.

Psychoses

Loneliness is also a part of the experience of schizophrenics. In one study, older adult patients with residual-type schizophrenia mentioned that they felt their loneliness had increased over the course of their lives. In another study involving a small number of schizophrenics and control participants, schizophrenics were more lonely than controls. Interestingly, and seemingly at odds with discrepancy explanations of loneliness, the difference between actual and ideal social support was the same for both groups.

Eating Disorders

Loneliness appears to feed into eating disorders, although it is probably associated with both over- and undereating. Studies support the conclusion that obese as well as underweight individuals are lonely. With respect to loneliness, researchers have examined two specific eating disorders, bulimia and restraint. Bulimics are binge eaters who then purge themselves of their food. Two forms of complementary evidence show loneliness to be a characteristic of bulimics: (a) Among a sample of college students those matching the criteria for bulimia nervosa were higher in loneliness relative to participants not suffering from bulimia, and (b) older bulimics remember being lonely in their childhoods. Restrained eaters are individuals who think a great deal about food, have concern over their weight, and tend to diet to control it. Restrained eaters are lonely in their dispositions, yet when they are put in a lonely mood, their food intake is increased.

Substance Abuse

In half of the studies ($N = 4$) we could identify, loneliness was a risk factor associated with drug abuse. Apropos of alcohol abuse, a review of the relevant literature concluded alcoholics feel more lonely than most other groups. Loneliness is probably more closely associated with drinking during times of despair and unhappiness than social drinking. In young adults, loneliness predicts problem drinking (e.g., getting intoxicated). Those in treatment for alcoholism also show greater loneliness and, among advanced abusers, those high in loneliness show a poorer prognosis.

Sleep Disturbances

Loneliness and sleep disturbances are commonly mentioned features of bereavement. Do they also go together at other times in life? Yes, according to John Cacioppo and associates' recent research program in which people's sleep was monitored both in a laboratory and in their homes. Although lonely and nonlonely people spent about the same amount of time in bed, the lonely people slept a smaller proportion of that time. They took longer to get to sleep and woke up more often with the result being they were asleep less. Lonely people also complained of more sleepiness during the day. To the extent that sleep is a restorative behavior promoting longevity, sleep disturbances may be a pathway by which loneliness affects mortality independent of health behaviors such as not smoking.

LONELINESS AND PHYSICAL HEALTH

Beginning with Berkman and Syme's (1979) classic Alameda County Study, research has consistently indicated that measures of social contact and number of interpersonal relationships are related to physical health. After controlling for other risk factors, Berkman and Syme found that mortality rates among individuals with the lowest level of social contact were 2 to 3 times higher than among individuals with the highest level of social contact over a 9-year period. Subsequent reviews of research on the relationship between social relationships and health indicated that higher levels of social integration were consistently associated with reductions in the mortality rate (see Seeman, 2000).

Given that loneliness reflects a lack of interpersonal relationships or low levels of social contact, these data suggest that loneliness should also be related to measures of physical health. A number of longitudinal studies have found that loneliness predicts subsequent mortality. One recent study, for example, indicated that reports of loneliness predicted both 30-day and 5-year survival among heart bypass patients. Related to this finding, two studies that examined cause of death found loneliness to be associated with higher rates of death due to heart disease.

Loneliness is also associated with a variety of measures of physical health status. A number of studies have found loneliness scores to be significantly correlated with self-report ratings of health (e.g., how is your health, how does your health compare to others), with correlations ranging from $-.18$ to $-.55$. Loneliness correlates significantly with number of physical symptoms and number of illnesses. A recent study by Rook and her colleagues also found that loneliness was related to evidence of heart problems as detected in a physical examination of a community sample (Sorkin, Rook, & Lu, 2002).

One possible reason for this loneliness-health relationship involves preventive health behaviors. Loneliness has been found to be related to a variety of health-related behaviors, such as exercise, nutrition, relaxation, and substance use. Lonely individuals are less likely to engage in preventive behaviors. For instance, a study of older Canadian males and females found that users of psychotropic drugs (e.g., antidepressants) were more likely to be lonely (40%) than non-drug users (16%). Loneliness has also been found to predict health service use, with lonely individuals reporting more doctor visits and more frequent visits to the hospital emergency room.

The above suggests that there should be detectable physiological effects of high levels of loneliness on the body. Research by Jan Kiecolt-Glaser and Ron Glaser at Ohio State University has documented one such physiological effect of loneliness. They found that loneliness predicted several indices of immunocompetence. Studies they conducted using medical students and psychiatric patients showed that loneliness was related to immune system functioning of participants (see Kennedy, Kiecolt-Glaser, & Glaser, 1988). Supporting these results, a cross-sectional study by other researchers found that loneliness was related to lower numbers of CD4 cells in HIV-infected men. However, a longitudinal study found that higher levels of loneliness at baseline were associated with a *slower* rate of decline in CD4 cells over a subsequent 3-year period in HIV-infected men.

Causal Issues in Studying Loneliness and Health

A critical question in examining correlational relationships such as we have been reporting concerns the causal mechanisms involved: Does poor health lead to loneliness, or does loneliness produce poor health? Could they mutually influence one another? Perhaps there really is no direct causation, but rather one should think of third variables producing these correlations or mediating processes. For example, as discussed above, studies have consistently found that loneliness is related to depression, with correlations as high as .50 to .60. Studies have also found that measures of depression are related to subsequent mortality, suggesting that the loneliness-mortality relationship may be mediated by depression. Similarly, measures of loneliness are typically found to be strongly negatively related to measures of social support. Given that social support has been found to predict mortality, immune system functioning, cardiovascular disease, and other indicators of psychophysiology, relationships between loneliness and other measures of physical health may reflect the influence of social support on both loneliness and physical health.

To address these issues, Russell and his colleagues examined the relationship between loneliness and mortality while controlling for the influence of measures of interpersonal relationships (including social support) and depression among the elderly. A structural equation modeling analysis was conducted examining the ability of measures of social contact (i.e., social network size, social support, club involvement, and church attendance), loneliness, morale (i.e., depression, anxiety, and life satisfaction), and physical health (i.e., functional status, illnesses, doctor visits, and medications) to predict subsequent 12-year mortality. Results indicated that loneliness predicted subsequent mortality net of measures of social support and depression, through the mediating effects of physical health status. Loneliness was found to mediate the effects of social support on physical health and mortality, whereas the measures of morale were unrelated to subsequent mortality. These results therefore suggest that loneliness is related to physical health and mortality net of the influence of either depression or social support.

CONCLUSION

In sum, loneliness has been associated with a variety of manifestations of poor mental and physical health. Solitude may be a wellspring of creativity and personal growth. Yet the experience of loneliness is a gnawing, pathogenic discomfort.

Most lonely people would be happy to overcome their loneliness. Using their own strategies and natural processes of recovery, people by themselves often overcome loneliness that is precipitated by such life course events as going away to school or the death of a partner. A variety of approaches have been offered by professionals and even loneliness "businesses" (e.g., cruise companies) for helping people alleviate their loneliness. Professional strategies range from community-based interventions, such as helping people gain control over some aspect of their lives, to psychoeducational approaches to social skills training to group or individual therapy. In general, treatment outcome research testifies that such interventions have beneficial effects in comparison to waiting-list or placebo control conditions. Preventive lessons can also be learned from the growing body of knowledge of how factors beyond the individual (e.g., culture, environmental design, social policies) contribute to loneliness. Existentialists may be correct that loneliness is an inherent part of the human condition. But there does not need to be as much of it; less alienating lifestyles and societies can be fostered.

—*Daniel Perlman and
Daniel W. Russell*

See also SOCIAL INTEGRATION, SOCIAL NETWORKS, AND HEALTH; SUPPORT GROUPS AND HEALTH

Further Reading

Akerlind, I., & Hornquist, J. O. (1992). Loneliness and alcohol abuse: A review of evidences of an interplay. *Social Science and Medicine, 34*, 405-413.

Berkman, L. F., & Syme, S. L. (1979). Social networks, host resistance, and mortality: A nine-year follow-up study of Alameda County residents. *American Journal of Epidemiology, 109*, 186-204.

Cacioppo, J. T., Ernst, J. M., Burleson, M. H., McClintock, M. K., Malarkey, W. B., Hawkley, L. C., Kowalewski, R. B., Paulsen, A., Hobson, J. A., Hugdahl, K., Spiegel, D., & Berntson, G. G. (2000). Lonely traits and concomitant physiological processes: The MacArthur social neuroscience studies. *International Journal of Psychophysiology, 35*, 143-154.

Ernst, J. M., & Cacioppo, J. T. (1999). Lonely hearts: Psychological perspectives on loneliness. *Applied and Preventive Psychology, 8*, 1-22.

Jones, W. H., & Carver, M. D. (1991). Adjustment and coping implications of loneliness. In C. R. Snyder & D. R. Forsyth (Eds.), *Handbook of social and clinical psychology: The health perspective* (pp. 395-415). New York: Pergamon.

Kennedy, S., Kiecolt-Glaser, J.-K., & Glaser, R. (1988). Immunological consequences of acute and chronic stressors: Mediating role of interpersonal relationships. *British Journal of Medical Psychology, 61*, 77-85.

Seeman, T. E. (2000). Health promoting effects of friends and family on health outcomes in older adults. *American Journal of Health Promotion, 14*, 362-370.

Sorkin, D., Rook, K. S., & Lu, J. L. (2002). Loneliness, lack of emotional support, lack of companionship, and the likelihood of having a heart condition in an elderly sample. *Annals of Behavioral Medicine, 24*(4), 290-298.

LOW BIRTH WEIGHT: PSYCHOSOCIAL ASPECTS

The health of a society is often judged by the health and well-being of its mothers and infants. Social inequalities in health in the United States are reflected in a high incidence of low birth weight; a much higher rate than seen in other developed nations and not markedly affected by advances in medicine and technology. Low birth weight is a leading cause of infant mortality and morbidity. It also represents an enormous economic cost to society, both in short-term medical costs and long-term loss of human capital. Rates of low birth weight vary greatly among American populations of different race, economic status, and class; in particular, the disparity in low birth weight between African American and White populations is a striking and persistent public health problem.

Prevention of low birth weight requires an understanding of factors that cause both *fetal growth retardation* and *shortened gestation*. Well-known obstetrical risk factors for low birth weight include maternal cigarette use, alcohol use, low prepregnancy body weight, poor weight gain during pregnancy, vaginal tract infections, and multiple gestations. Unfortunately, randomized trials of smoking cessation programs, enhanced prenatal care, nutritional programs, and prophylactic treatment of women at high risk for infection have been disappointing.

It has long been recognized that maternal African American race, unmarried marital status, low education attainment, and impoverishment are major sociodemographic risk factors for infant low birth weight. The mechanisms underlying these associations are incompletely understood and appear independent of the medical risk factors listed above. The psychosocial context of pregnant women is associated with overall health and reproductive outcome. This context includes their individual vulnerabilities or resilience to psychosocial stressors, their family environments and social networks, and work and neighborhood contexts, as well as the broader context of contemporary American society.

MATERNAL CONTEXT

Psychosocial stress. Current thinking places maternal stress as the key link between the social, psychological, and biological environments that determine pregnancy outcome. Women living in socioeconomic deprivation or who are socially or psychologically vulnerable experience more stress than resilient women or women living in more advantaged contexts. Both direct/biological (e.g., via hormonal or immunologic pathway) and indirect/behavioral (via risky health behavior) mechanisms linking stress to low birth weight have been posited. These pathways are not mutually exclusive, and interactions between stress, maternal behavior, and maternal physiology are active areas of current research.

Stress is a complex construct. In epidemiological studies, different aspects of maternal stress that have been associated with an increased risk of low birth weight include the experience of stressful life events before and during pregnancy, anxiety (both general and pregnancy specific), depression, perceived stress, work-related stress, and unplanned pregnancy. Results are fairly consistent across studies, with increased stress associated with both shorter gestation and fetal growth restriction. Chronic stress appears to be more relevant than acute stressful events. The interaction between the presence of stressors, maternal perceptions of stress, coping resources, and vulnerability/resilience is an area of active research.

Social networks and social support. During pregnancy, the social support that a woman receives from family and friends, colleagues, and neighbors moderates the impact of stressors and may act as a buffer against the risk of low birth weight. Methodological difficulties in studying the subtleties of social support are highlighted by ethnographic studies, which suggest that women do not always perceive extensive and active social networks as supportive in relation to their pregnancies. Nevertheless, evidence from several decades' worth of observational studies is strongest for a protective role of support from an intimate partner, rather than from other sources, and for emotional, rather than instrumental, support. Unmarried women have consistently been shown to have a higher risk of both fetal growth restriction and preterm delivery, which may be due in part to a lack of intimate support. There is also accumulating evidence that exposure to intimate-partner violence, whether or not it results in physical harm, increases the risk of low birth weight.

Since the 1970s, several randomized trials of social support interventions have been conducted among high-risk women, variously defined as having a previous low birth weight infant, being in a high-stress situation, or having low social support. In most cases, nurses, midwives, or social workers delivered the social support interventions during repeated home visits throughout the pregnancy. As with studies of enhanced prenatal care and health behavior modifications, results have been consistently disappointing. It is likely that the quantity, frequency, and content of the interventions delivered in randomized trials are inadequate to overcome the long-term and pervasive lack of social support among women whose lack of support or isolation puts them at risk of low birth weight.

Socioeconomic status and social class. Low maternal socioeconomic status is a risk factor for infant low birth weight. However, the strength of the associations between socioeconomic status and low birth weight varies by the unit of analysis (i.e., maternal/paternal/family education, occupation, or income). Researchers often select the unit of analysis based on their hypothesized conceptual model. For example, if maternal health behaviors are considered to mediate the effects of social position on pregnancy outcomes, maternal education may be a more relevant factor than father's occupation. If resiliency to stressors is considered to be important, then family social class may modify this factor. Greater attention to the conceptualization of pathways leading to low birth weight is increasingly apparent in the epidemiological literature, but much remains to be learned about the role of social position in reproductive health.

Delineation of the etiologic role of psychosocial factors in reproductive health requires stratified analyses of race and socioeconomic status/social class. African American women with a college-level education have excess rates of very low birth weight and preterm delivery compared to college-educated White women. However, traditional socioeconomic variables, including maternal education level, do not fully capture the impact of race on socioeconomic status. On average, African Americans who attend college earn less than White high school dropouts, and female-headed African American and White households show differences in terms of income. Since discrimination and African American disadvantage is so pervasive in the United States, researchers have been unable to fully control for socioeconomic status.

SOCIAL CONTEXT

Multilevel statistical analyses of the effect of the social environment are the latest burgeoning of a long tradition of inquiry into the effects of the environment on maternal and child health. Important developments in multivariable statistical methods allow contemporary researchers to attempt to disentangle the effects of individual race and socioeconomic status from the effects of residential segregation, socioeconomic, and social class context.

Race/ethnicity. Although the incidence of low birth weight decreases for African Americans and Whites as the number of individual-level risk factors declines, the improvement is faster among Whites, resulting in a wider racial disparity in low birth weight rates in low-risk women. This has led some investigators to suggest that the smaller birth weights and shorter gestations are genetically determined in African Americans. However, the birth weight patterns of infants of African-born women are similar to those of infants of U.S.-born White women. Moreover, regardless of socioeconomic status, infants of African-born Black women have a reduced low birth weight rate compared to infants of comparable U.S.-born Black women. The increased risk of low birth weight among African American women is perpetuated across generations. As data inconsistent with a genetic hypothesis accumulate, social and psychophysiological hypotheses are advanced.

Mexican American infants of U.S.-born mothers have a greater risk of low birth weight rate than infants of Mexican born mothers. This differential persists independent of obstetrical and sociodemographic characteristics; this supports the hypothesis that psychosocial factors related to women's life-long minority status are detrimental to reproductive outcome.

Racial discrimination. Although racism is a deep-rooted and multilayered phenomenon in the United States, there is a paucity of published data on the relationship between women's exposure to racism and pregnancy outcome. Exposure to interpersonal racism is both an acute and chronic stressor for African Americans. An exploratory study found that among a sample of low-income African Americans maternal perception of exposure to racial discrimination during pregnancy was a risk factor for very low birth weight.

Residential segregation. In the United States, the geographic separation of the races is a long-standing reality. Interestingly, the racial composition of communities in which women reside affects their pregnancy outcomes. In 1950, Yankauer conducted a study of residential segregation by race and infant mortality in New York City. He found that areas with high proportions of births to non-White mothers had high population density, unsanitary conditions, lack of recreational areas, high rents for poor housing, and high rates of infant mortality. In a more recent study, residence in a predominantly African American community was associated with a decreased risk of low birth weight among African American women independent of individual socioeconomic status. The limited available data suggest that residence in neighborhoods with recent fluctuations in racial composition is associated with an increased risk of preterm delivery for African American women. A woman's experiences with stress and social support may explain this phenomenon.

Neighborhood context. The economic/class structure and unequal distribution of resources in society also contributes to population variation in low birth weight. A study found that the proportion of low birth weight infants in different Chicago neighborhoods rose for African Americans and Whites as the census tract median family income fell regardless of maternal age, education, or marital status.

Poor neighborhoods are characterized by (a) a higher prevalence of hazards to healthy pregnancy (e.g., reduced availability of healthful foods, increased levels of crime); (b) fewer protective resources (e.g., accessible prenatal care clinics); and (c) increased tolerance of health-compromising behaviors (e.g., more tolerance of smoking during pregnancy). Neighborhood deprivation, measured by such variables as unemployment and median income, has been consistently associated with increased risk of low birth weight and, in studies presenting race-specific analyses, it is clear that these relationships are more pronounced for African American women than for White women.

Absolute levels of affluence or poverty may be less important for health than relative inequalities. Positive income incongruity, defined as living in a more affluent neighborhood than expected, given a family's marital and educational status, was associated with a decreased risk of very low birth weight in a population-based study in Chicago.

Interactions between neighborhood-level and individual-level risk factors are likely to be important but have been addressed in few studies. One study reported numerous such interactions, including a greater increased risk of low birth weight among women with low education living in high-crime areas than among comparable women living in low-crime areas. More research is needed to clarify the relationships between the environments in which women live, their perceptions of these environments, and their resilience/vulnerability to environmental influences on reproductive health.

Societal context. The effect of changing politics, policies, and economic health at the state and national levels is likely to have profound effects on health, although these are generally difficult to document, due to long time lapses between triggering events and most health outcomes. An economic recession, with adverse effects on diet and physical activity at the population level, would not be mirrored by an increased incidence in cardiovascular disease until many years later. In contrast, pregnancy lasts a very short time. No studies in the United States have examined the impact of economic trends on pregnancy outcomes, but one interesting study, based on Scandinavian data, found an association between quarterly national unemployment levels and rates of very low birth weight over two decades.

Low birth weight is the major factor underlying the persistently poor international rating of the United States on infant mortality. An expanding literature highlights an important association between a woman's exposure to psychosocial stress during pregnancy and infant birth weight. Novel conceptual models that take into account pregnant women's neighborhood and social contexts are needed to help us better understand the psychophysiological mechanisms underlying racial and ethnic group differences in infant birth weight.

—*Kate E. Pickett and*
James W. Collins Jr.

See also Socioeconomic Status and Health

Further Reading

Collins, J., & David, R. (1990). The differential effect of traditional risk factors on infant birth weight among Blacks and Whites in Chicago. *American Journal of Public Health, 80,* 679-681.

Collins, J. W., Jr., David, R. J., Symons, R., Handler, A., Wall, S. N., & Dwyer, L. (2000). Low-income African-American mothers' perception of exposure to racial discrimination and infant birth weight. *Epidemiology, 11,* 337-339.

Dunkel-Schetter, C. (1998). Maternal stress and preterm delivery. *Prenatal and Neonatal Medicine, 3,* 39-42.

Hogue, C. J., Hoffman, S., & Hatch, M. C. (2001). Stress and preterm delivery: A conceptual framework. *Paediatric and Perinatal Epidemiology, 15*(Suppl. 2), 30-40.

Kramer, M. S., Goulet, L., Lydon, J., et al. (2001). Socioeconomic disparities in preterm birth: Causal pathways and mechanisms. *Paediatric and Perinatal Epidemiology, 15*(Suppl. 2), 104-123.

Lewit, E., Schuurmann, B. L., Corman, H., & Shiono, P. (1995). The direct cost of low birth weight. *Future of Children, 5,* 35-56.

Pearl, M., Braveman, P., & Abrams, B. (2001). The relationship of neighborhood socioeconomic characteristics to birthweight among 5 ethnic groups in California. *American Journal of Public Health, 91,* 1808-1814.

Pickett, K. E., Ahern, J., Selvin, S., & Abrams, B. (2002). Social context, maternal race and preterm birth: A case-control study. *Annals of Epidemiology, 12,* 410-418.

M

MEDICAL PSYCHOLOGY

Medical psychology "is the application of psychological concepts and methods to medical problems" (Rachman, 1977, p. vii). In a broader sense, medical psychology refers to the health care, research, and educational linkages of the discipline of psychology with medicine in the understanding, treatment, and prevention of illness and the promotion of health. Initially, the linkage was focused on child development and mental health and, as psychology developed as a life science, expanded to the broader purview of physical health. Psychology's unique contributions stemmed from the application of behavioral science modes of inquiry, methods of investigation and analysis, and reliance on empirical verification to matters of health and illness.

The expansion of medical psychology from a focus on mental health to physical health was facilitated by the recognition of the limitations of the biomedical model that incorporated assumptions of mind/body dualism. In contrast, the biopsychosocial model (Engel, 1977) recognized that biological, psychological, and social processes act together in health and illness and must be considered simultaneously in the etiology, diagnosis, treatment, and prevention of illness and the promotion and maintenance of health.

The emergence of the biopsychosocial model provided the foundation for the integration of behavioral science and biomedical science approaches to matters of health and illness and spawned the development of a new, interdisciplinary, field of behavioral medicine. Psychology's contributions to this new field are reflected in the emergence of two subareas within the discipline: health psychology and pediatric psychology. The emergence of new fields and subareas indicates that the interplay of psychology and medicine continues to be dynamic and synergistic.

Examples of major areas of research and health service include adaptation to illness such as coronary heart disease, sickle cell disease, and diabetes; adherence to medical regimens; stress management, pain management, and treatment of anxiety and depression, eating disorders, and sleep disorders; psychoneuroimmunology; promotion of health-enhancing lifestyle behaviors; and prevention of disease and injury.

—*Robert Joseph Thompson Jr.*

Further Reading

Engel, G. L. (1977). The need for a new medical model: A challenge for biomedicine. *Science, 196,* 129-136.

Rachman, S. (1977). *Contributions to medical psychology* (Vol. 1 [Vol. 2, 1980, Vol. 3, 1984]). Oxford, UK: Pergamon.

METABOLIC SYNDROME AND STRESS

The metabolic syndrome is a constellation of cardiovascular risk factors that is common among adults in industrialized societies. The key risk factors are glucose intolerance, insulin resistance, raised fasting serum triglycerides, and raised blood pressure.

Localization of body fat in the abdomen and low-level inflammation are often present within the cluster of risk factors. An individual with the metabolic syndrome may well be in good health but is more likely than others to develop Type 2, or maturity onset, diabetes and to experience a heart attack. Furthermore, there are indications of a causal connection between metabolic syndrome and accelerated decline of cognitive function. The metabolic syndrome is reversible. Effective treatment and prevention of the metabolic syndrome has the potential to reduce the burden of several key degenerative diseases.

Some ethnic groups, including those of South Asian origin, are particularly at risk of diabetes and coronary heart disease and are primary targets for intervention. Socially disadvantaged individuals are a further at-risk group. Prevalence of the metabolic syndrome, and each of its lipid and nonlipid components, is linked with low social status, and parallels the step-wise and inverse social gradients in risks for diabetes and cardiovascular disease. One approach is to treat individual risk factors as they are identified, for example, raised blood sugar (hyperglycemia) with an insulin-sensitizing drug, high blood pressure with a beta-blocker. This would entail medicalization of a large proportion of the adult population. Another approach is to prevent, or at least reduce, the probability that the metabolic syndrome will develop. To do so requires an understanding of its causes.

Accumulating evidence suggests the metabolic syndrome is a key component of the *social biology* of health inequalities. The characteristic and common pattern of the metabolic disturbances involved amount to a homeostatic alteration. There appear to be common causes, which are psychosocial, cultural, and behavioral in nature. Several causes of the metabolic syndrome are linked with low social status, including physical inactivity and, putatively, chronic stress.

The metabolic syndrome is also known as the insulin resistance syndrome and Reaven's syndrome X, after Gerald Reaven's description of the risk factor complex in 1988.

NATURE OF THE METABOLIC SYNDROME

The metabolic syndrome is not a disease, but it can be thought of as a disease precursor state. Presence of the syndrome increases the probability that diabetes and cardiovascular disease may develop (see below).

An individual is considered to have prevalent metabolic syndrome when a characteristic group of cardiovascular risk factors is detected. There is no universally accepted definition. The core features of the metabolic syndrome are disturbances of lipid and carbohydrate metabolism, and raised blood pressure. An abdominal distribution of fat, increased heart rate, and evidence of low-level inflammation are also signs of the syndrome.

Clinical and biochemical tests are needed to establish whether an individual has the metabolic syndrome. The clinical measurements are resting blood pressure and waist circumference (or the ratio of waist to hip circumference). A fasting venous blood sample serves to provide measures of serum triglycerides, HDL cholesterol, and glucose. A more sensitive measure of impaired glucose tolerance is obtained by carrying out a standard 75-g oral glucose tolerance test (OGTT). The plasma glucose level at 2 hours after drinking the glucose solution provides a measure of insulin-mediated glucose uptake. A high 2-hour glucose level (7.8-11.0 mmol/l [140-200 mg/dl] on the World Health Organization [WHO] definition) reflects a degree of glucose intolerance and insulin resistance that is intermediate to normal (< 7.8 mmol/l [140 mg/dl]) and diabetic levels (> 11.0 mmol/l [200 mg/dl]). Compared with a fasting glucose measurement, the OGTT requires more time and may not be practicable.

There are two approaches to defining the metabolic syndrome. Neither is rigid, but depends on risk scores: finding adverse levels among the group of risk factors, typically three or more of five. Cut points have been agreed on by the Third Adult Treatment Panel of the U.S. National Cholesterol Education Program to provide a low-cost diagnostic definition that does not include an OGTT (see Table 1). A similar definition was proposed by WHO in 1999.

Alternatively, population-based surveys and epidemiological studies use cut points based on the observed distribution of relevant risk factors. The metabolic syndrome has been defined, for example, on the basis that three or more of the following five variables are within the sex-specific adverse 20% (top quintile) group: serum triglycerides, HDL cholesterol (bottom quintile), 2-hour glucose, systolic blood pressure, and waist-hip ratio. Diabetics and those on hypotensive medication are assigned to the top glucose and blood pressure quintiles, respectively.

Table 1   ATPIII Definition of Metabolic Syndrome (defined by the presence of three or more of the five risk factors)

Waist circumference	*men*	> 102 cm (40 in)
	women	> 88 cm (35 in)
Serum HDL cholesterol	*men*	< 40 mg/dl (1.0 mmol/l)
	women	< 50 mg/dl (1.3 mmol/l)
Serum triglycerides		≥ 150 mg/dl (1.7 mmol/l)
Blood pressure		≥ 130/ ≥ 85 mmHg
Fasting glucose		≥ 110 mg/dl (6.1 mmol/l)

NOTE: ATPIII = Third Adult Treatment Panel of the U.S. National Cholesterol Education Program.

Using the "quintile" definition, prevalence of the syndrome was 12% among healthy male and female office workers about 50 years old (Whitehall II Study, 1991-1993; Brunner et al., 1997).

Different ATPIII (Third Adult Treatment Panel of the U.S. National Cholesterol Education Program) cut points for men and women for waist circumference and HDL cholesterol are a reflection of the distinct distributions of these variables in the two sexes. Distributions of the relevant risk factors may also differ by ethnic group. Inclusion of 2-hour glucose among the five variables is a strength of the quintile definition of the metabolic syndrome since the OGTT is a dynamic test of glucose handling that constitutes a metabolic challenge.

A representative survey of American adults found, using the ATPIII definition, that prevalence of the metabolic syndrome was 24%. The survey (3rd National Health and Nutrition Examination Survey, $N = 8,814$) was carried out in 1988-1994, and in the decade since the continuing rise in overweight and obesity in the United States suggests that prevalence of the syndrome is likely to have risen to an even higher level. Prevalence was 7% among 20- to 29-year-olds, rising to more than 40% among those over 60 years of age. Prevalence was similar in women and men. Mexican Americans had the highest prevalence (32%), compared with European and African American ethnic groups.

There is some debate about the clinical and epidemiological utility of the metabolic syndrome concept. The core risk factors are associated with one another (see Table 2) and cluster together in multivariate statistical analysis. The associations are moderately strong, with correlations of magnitude 0.2-0.5. Consequently, there may be considerable variation in the level of one risk factor given a particular level of another. Since each component of the metabolic syndrome is a risk factor for cardiovascular disease, it is to be expected that individuals with the syndrome are at higher risk of disease than those without it. Validity of the syndrome concept thus depends in some researchers' views on the extent to which the whole is greater than the sum of the parts. This question has not yet been resolved, in part because consensus has not been reached about definition. The value of a concept is that it provides a unifying framework within which to understand the metabolic disturbances that precede diabetes and cardiovascular disease.

METABOLIC SYNDROME AND DISEASE

The main component risk factors of the metabolic syndrome, namely, impaired glucose tolerance, insulin resistance, central obesity, and disturbances of lipoprotein metabolism characterized by raised serum triglycerides and low HDL cholesterol, are each associated with increased risk of coronary heart disease. These linkages have been demonstrated in a large number of epidemiological studies in Caucasian, South Asian, and Native North American populations.

The metabolic syndrome has been shown to predict coronary heart disease. The Botnia Study, for example, followed 3,606 Finnish and Swedish adults for 7 years and found that risk of the disease was considerably higher among those who had the metabolic syndrome at baseline, on the basis of the WHO definition, compared with those who did not. Cardiovascular mortality was 12.0% in participants with the syndrome, and 2.2% among those without it.

The metabolic syndrome is associated with increased probability of developing Type 2, or maturity

Table 2   Correlation Coefficients for Metabolic Syndrome Variables

	Body Mass Index	Waist-Hip Ratio	Triglycerides	HDL Cholesterol	LDL Cholesterol	2-Hour Insulin
Men						
Body mass index						
Waist-hip ratio	0.65					
Triglycerides	0.37	0.41				
HDL cholesterol	−0.30	−0.30	−0.47			
LDL cholesterol	0.13	0.18	0.24	−0.10		
2-hour insulin[a]	0.29	0.31	0.28	−0.21	0.08	
2-hour glucose[a]	0.11	0.14	0.16	−0.12	0.03	0.52
Women						
Body mass index						
Waist-hip ratio	0.57					
Triglycerides	0.38	0.45				
HDL cholesterol	−0.35	−0.36	−0.42			
LDL cholesterol	0.21	0.25	0.39	−0.20		
2-hour insulin[a]	0.26	0.33	0.28	−0.20	0.14	
2-hour glucose[a]	0.14	0.16	0.17	−0.08	0.10	0.46

SOURCE: Data from Whitehall II Study, Phase 3 examination (1991-1993).

a. 2-hour blood sample from 75-g oral glucose tolerance test.

onset, diabetes. Although progression is not inevitable, impaired glucose tolerance is a major risk factor for diabetes. Obesity and insulin resistance are further key aspects of the linkage between metabolic syndrome and diabetes. In the Whitehall II Study, obese men and women (body mass index > 30 kg/m²) were at high risk of having metabolic syndrome compared to those with normal body weight (odds ratios 15.8 in men, 18.9 in women). In the Atherosclerosis Risk in Communities Study (ARIC), approximately one quarter of obese participants were insulin resistant, and the obese were many times more likely to develop Type 2 diabetes than those of normal weight. In some populations, including South Asians, central obesity, reflecting accumulation of body fat in and around the abdomen, is a more important explanatory factor for glucose intolerance than the overall degree of obesity. One possible explanation is that abdominal fat is more resistant to the action of insulin than adipose tissue at other anatomical sites.

Evidence is accumulating that individuals with the metabolic syndrome may be at particular risk of decline in cognitive ability, particularly memory. Younger as well as older Type 2 diabetics show impaired performance on tests of immediate and delayed memory, and verbal fluency. Individuals with nondiabetic glucose intolerance, a characteristic of metabolic syndrome, display similar cognitive impairments. Insulin resistance in combination with raised blood pressure has also been linked with low scores on tests of mental arithmetic and verbal fluency.

Lipid disturbances are associated with Alzheimer's disease. The ε4 allele of the apolipoprotein E gene (APOE 4) is a risk factor for Alzheimer's dementia, as well as cardiovascular disease. APOE codes a protein involved in transport of lipids in the circulation and, by mechanisms not well understood, the apoE protein influences the rate of accumulation of amyloid plaques that are characteristic of Alzheimer's disease. Although trial data are lacking, retrospective studies show that the cholesterol-lowering statin drugs may offer some protection from the disease. This is further evidence for the role of lipids, and potentially metabolic syndrome, in the development of Alzheimer's disease, since the statins raise HDL cholesterol levels. In summary, the core features of the metabolic syndrome are each separately linked with risk of accelerated decline in cognitive ability, and if present simultaneously in the same individual they may exert synergistic effects.

METABOLIC SYNDROME
AND SOCIAL INEQUALITIES IN HEALTH

The metabolic syndrome is a social phenomenon. Characteristically, its prevalence is highest in the lowest social stratum, declines in steps across the middle classes, and is lowest in the highest stratum. This inverse and stepwise social gradient can be seen as a reflection of the differing patterns of environment and experience encountered at different levels of the social hierarchy. With this perspective, the metabolic syndrome appears to be the product of the interplay between biological endowment and social circumstances. These complex effects provide some insight to the mechanisms accounting for the social patterns of chronic disease in urban populations.

The Whitehall studies, among other epidemiological studies, have shown that socioeconomic position is a powerful predictor of premature coronary heart disease. In the Whitehall cohorts, occupational status (Civil Service employment grade) is a better predictor of disease than the combination of smoking, serum cholesterol, and blood pressure, the classic risk factors. These observations point to the fact that social and economic organization is an important determinant of population health. The Whitehall II Study further shows that social differences in mean serum cholesterol and blood pressure are small, and explain very little of the social gradient in coronary heart disease, while smoking can account at most for one third of it.

The metabolic syndrome appears to be the biological mechanism responsible for translating social position into cardiovascular risk. In the Whitehall II cohort, each of the components of the syndrome, with the exception of systolic blood pressure, exhibits an inverse gradient with occupational status. The probability of being in the lowest (adverse) 20% of the distribution of HDL cholesterol levels is two- to threefold greater in the office-support grade than in the senior administrative grade (odds ratio [95% confidence interval] 1.93 [1.5-2.5] in men, 3.00 [2.0-4.5] in women, test for trend $p < .001$ in both sexes). Similar gradients are observed for 2-hour glucose, serum triglycerides, plasma fibrinogen, and waist-hip ratio. Using the quintile definition (described above), the metabolic syndrome is strongly linked with lower occupational position (see Figure 1) (odds ratio for lowest vs. highest grade [95% confidence interval] 2.16 [1.6-2.9] in men, 2.75 [1.6-4.8] in women, test

for trend $p < .005$ in both sexes). These findings are replicated in other population-based surveys in Europe and North America, which show, for example, that central obesity is relatively common in lower social classes, and relatively rare in higher classes.

The metabolic syndrome is socially patterned. It also appears to be a powerful biological explanation for the inverse social gradient in coronary heart disease. This is evident in a prospective analysis of incident fatal and nonfatal coronary events in the Whitehall II Study. In multiple logistic regression analysis, metabolic syndrome variables measured at baseline account statistically for about half of social inequality in heart disease incidence. This is an important observation. The metabolic syndrome, in these men and women, is a better explanation for the inverse social gradient in coronary heart disease than is smoking.

METABOLIC SYNDROME AND STRESS

Stress can be physical, mental, or emotional in nature. It implies some external pressure that places demands on the capacity to respond. If the individual rises to the occasion without going beyond usual limits, then balance and equanimity will quickly return. This, at a basic level, is success: the ability to survive and if possible to flourish despite the impositions of the environment. Success and stress are, however, not opposites. Instead, we can see that stress leads to two types of outcome. One is a return to previous stability, the other a transition, temporary or permanent, to some alternative state.

The metabolic syndrome is a particularly common "alternative state" today, but this was not the case in the past. In pre-industrial societies, metabolic syndrome and Type 2 diabetes were rare if not unknown. But under current conditions in Westernized societies, prevalence of the metabolic syndrome among 50-year-olds is 10% to 30%, and diabetes approximately half of that, depending on the population in question and the syndrome definition used. Given this vast and growing global burden, it is appropriate to suspect that certain features of modern life are stressful. At the same time, we should bear in mind that never in history has life expectancy been so high within the populations in question, largely as a result of material living standards rather than the health care we may be fortunate enough to receive.

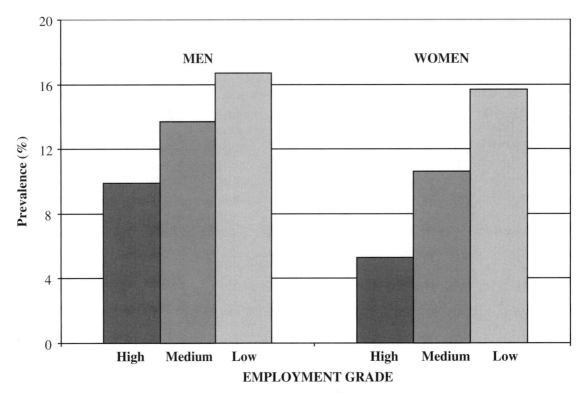

Figure 1   Prevalence of the Metabolic Syndrome by Civil Service Employment Grade (adjusted for age)

SOURCE: Whitehall II Study (Brunner et al., 1997).

Two biological pathways appear to be important to the emergence of the metabolic syndrome as a public health problem. Both can be seen as stress mechanisms arising from modern living conditions, though they are different in nature. The first is the consequence of our industrialized food supply together with the virtual elimination of need for physical activity. The second results from the mental and emotional distress of living in a hierarchical, complex, and competitive society, where the high status and economic success of the few bring fabulous rewards that will never be shared by the many.

An abundance of food and a low requirement for energy expenditure are defining characteristics of Westernized society. On the input side, it is possible to buy 70% of a woman's daily energy requirement (1900 calories) for $3.60, as a hamburger meal with a large serving of fries and Coke. On the output side, vigorous physical activity off the sports field is almost unheard of, and even moderate activity is unnecessary. These are prime conditions for generating a population that is overweight if not obese. However, biology and arithmetic are not so simple. Considering that 1 gram of fat is equivalent to only some 10 calories, a daily excess of energy intake over expenditure of as little as 1% (20 calories) would over a year convert to substantial weight gain. It is clear that there are homeostatic mechanisms to ensure this does not happen. Physiological control of appetite and diet-induced thermogenesis are able to regulate weight with exquisite sensitivity.

Yet the recent explosion of obesity indicates that weight regulation is not functioning well enough for 40% to 50% of the adult population. The explanation appears to lie partly in our food-saturated and sedentary environment, and partly in a widely inherited tendency to obesity. James Neel's thrifty genotype hypothesis proposes that Type 2 diabetes is the product of a genetic predisposition to store fat efficiently in times of plenty. Such a trait would have survival advantage during food scarcity and rarely lead to diabetes. In present conditions, when energy-dense food is abundant and prolonged physical activity unnecessary, this trait is often likely to lead, first, to obesity, second, to insulin resistance, and then to impaired glucose tolerance. Chronic physical inactivity adds to this process not only because energy expenditure and resting metabolic rate are low. Lower muscle mass and muscle blood flow are linked with insulin resistance, glucose intolerance, and low HDL cholesterol levels. A combination of aerobic endurance training and circuit-type resistance training appears to be an optimal program for reversing the disturbances characteristic of the metabolic syndrome, as well as for preventing its development.

The second mechanism is firmly located at the heart of modern life. Basic material needs are not the preoccupations they once were, but unemployment, low autonomy at work, excessive overtime, social isolation, and loss of a sense of control in the frenzy of aspiration appear to be bad for physical as well as psychological health. There is biological plausibility and growing evidence that chronic psychosocial stress may contribute to risk of metabolic syndrome, and later to Type 2 diabetes and coronary heart disease.

Robert Sapolsky and others have made a compelling case for the damaging effects of modern societies, particularly for those near the bottom of the socioeconomic scale. The key argument is an evolutionary one. Humans are adapted to respond to the challenge of external threats with an autonomic reaction, followed by a rise in cortisol secretion. This defense, or fight-or-flight, mechanism is useful in an emergency, but if repeatedly activated, may be maladaptive in the urban environment. The price of this maladaption is the metabolic syndrome.

The launch of the defense reaction is familiar to us. Rapid release of epinephrine from the adrenal medulla and norepinephrine from sympathetic nerve endings produces cognitive arousal, sensory vigilance, bronchodilation, increased heart rate, raised blood pressure, and energy mobilization. The effect of this neuroendocrine response is to prepare for physical exertion, not for a call to credit control. The second neuroendocrine pathway, the hypothalamic-pituitary-adrenal (HPA) axis, comes into action more slowly, and is more sustained. This component of the stress response involves release of cortisol from the adrenal cortex. Cortisol serves to protect the individual from the potentially malign effects of inflammation and infection, and the accompanying host response. But it also antagonizes the effects of insulin, acting to mobilize energy reserves by raising blood glucose and promoting fatty acid release from adipose tissue. In a physically inactive situation, these superfluous energy substrates increase hepatic lipoprotein output, and the circulating triglyceride level.

Repeated autonomic and HPA stimulation, particularly in combination with a sedentary lifestyle, is therefore a plausible cause of metabolic syndrome.

During the past 20 years, longitudinal epidemiological studies have been set up to test the psychosocial hypothesis of coronary heart disease causation. Evidence is accumulating that low control at work, lack of social support, and depressed mood predict incident disease. Whether chronic psychosocial stress is an important cause of atherosclerosis, exerting its effects independent of behavioral factors such as diet and smoking, remains at present uncertain.

A component question is whether there are psychosocial causes of the metabolic syndrome. If this were demonstrated, there would be a direct biological mechanism to link stress with heart disease. A recent addition to the evidence is a case control study comparing metabolic syndrome cases with healthy controls. The study tested the hypothesis that disturbances in neuroendocrine function and cardiac autonomic activity contribute to development of the metabolic syndrome. Urinary outputs of cortisol and norepinephrine metabolites were measured over 24 hours. Cardiac autonomic activity was obtained from analysis of digitized electrocardiogram recordings. Cortisol metabolite and normetanephrine (3-methoxynorepinephrine) outputs were higher among cases than controls (0.49, 0.45 standard deviations [SD], respectively, both $p < .05$). Heart rate was higher (72.3 vs. 64.5 beats/min, $p = .002$) and heart rate variability was lower (-0.72 SD, $p < .001$) among cases. Multiple regression models showed that psychosocial factors (employment grade, self-reports of household assets, and job strain) accounted for 37% of the link between metabolic syndrome and normetanephrine output, and about 15% for cardiac autonomic activity. Health-related behaviors (smoking, diet indicators, physical activity, and alcohol consumption) accounted for 5% to 18% of neuroendocrine differences.

This study simultaneously linked the two major neuroendocrine stress axes and cardiac autonomic activity with the metabolic syndrome. Output of cortisol and norepinephrine metabolites was higher among cases than controls. Heart rate variability was lower, indicating sympathetic predominance and reduced vagal tone. Psychosocial factors and health-related behaviors each explained a part of the neuroendocrine disturbances that accompany the syndrome. Follow-up of individuals who had metabolic syndrome at baseline but not 5 years later showed that the neuroendocrine changes are partially reversible. This is the first evidence that chronic psychosocial stress contributes to development of metabolic syndrome, although confirmatory prospective studies are required.

—*Eric Brunner*

See also ALLOSTATIS, ALLOSTATIC LOAD, AND STRESS; CARDIOVASCULAR REACTIVITY; STRESS: BIOLOGICAL ASPECTS

Further Reading

ANON. (2001). Executive summary of the Third Report of the National Cholesterol Education Program (NCEP) Expert Panel on Detection, Evaluation, and Treatment of High Blood Cholesterol in Adults (Adult Treatment Panel III). *Journal of the American Medical Association, 285*, 2486-2497.

Brunner, E. J. (1997). Stress and the biology of inequality. *British Medical Journal, 314*, 1472-1476.

Brunner, E. J. (2000). Toward a new social biology. In L. F. Berkman & I. Kawachi (Eds.), *Social epidemiology.* New York: Oxford University Press.

Brunner, E. J., Hemingway, H., Walker, B. R., Page, M., Clarke, P., Juneja, M., Shipley, M. J., Kumari, M., Andrew, R., Seckl, J. R., Papadopoulos, A., Checkley, S., Rumley, A., Lowe, G. D. O., Stansfeld, S. A., & Marmot, M. G. (2002). Adrenocortical, autonomic and inflammatory causes of the metabolic syndrome: Case-control study. *Circulation, 106*, 2659-2665.

Brunner, E. J., Marmot, M. G., Nanchahal, K., Shipley, M. J., Stansfeld, S. A., Juneja, M., & Alberti, K. G. M. M. (1997). Social inequality in coronary risk: Central obesity and the metabolic syndrome. Evidence from the WII Study. *Diabetologia, 40*, 1341-1349.

Eriksson, J., Taimela, S., & Koivisto, V. A. (1997). Exercise and the metabolic syndrome. *Diabetologia, 40*, 125-135.

Ford, E. S., Giles, W. H., & Dietz, W. H. (2002). Prevalence of the metabolic syndrome among U.S. adults: Findings from the Third National Health and Nutrition Examination Survey. *Journal of the American Medical Association, 287*, 356-359.

Kuper, H., & Marmot, M. G. (2003). Job strain, job demands, decision latitude, and risk of coronary heart disease within the Whitehall II Study. *Journal of Epidemiology and Community Health, 57*(2), 147-153.

Marmot, M. G., & Wilkinson, R. G. (1999). *Social determinants of health.* Oxford, UK: Oxford University Press.

McEwen, B. S. (1998). Protective and damaging effects of stress mediators. *New England Journal of Medicine, 338*, 171-179.

McKeigue, P. M., Ferrie, J. E., Pierpoint, T., & Marmot, M. G. (1993). Association of early-onset coronary heart disease in South Asian men with glucose intolerance and hyperinsulinemia. *Circulation, 87*, 153-161.

Neel, J. V. (1962). Diabetes mellitus: A "thrifty" genotype rendered detrimental by "progress"? *American Journal of Human Genetics, 14*, 353-362.

Sapolsky, R. M. (1998). *Why zebras don't get ulcers: An updated guide to stress, stress-related diseases, and coping.* New York: W. H. Freeman.

MINNESOTA MULTIPHASIC PERSONALITY INVENTORY (MMPI/MMPI-2)

The Minnesota Multiphasic Personality Inventory (MMPI/MMPI-2) is a 567-item true-false questionnaire that is currently the most widely used objective measure of psychopathology and personality in the world. Psychologist S. R. Hathaway and psychiatrist J. C. McKinley developed the original MMPI in the late 1930s at the University of Minnesota. The MMPI was constructed through a series of empirical studies that statistically identified items distinguishing groups of patients with various psychiatric conditions from a normative group (visitors to the University of Minnesota Hospital). This process yielded a set of 10 dimensional scales that measured facets of emotional disturbance such as somatic preoccupation, depression, antisocial attitudes and behaviors, persecutory ideation, anxiety, and thought disorder as well as personality traits such as introversion and gregariousness. Scores that fell 2 (1.5 for the MMPI-2) standard deviations above the mean of the normative group were designated clinically significant. Importantly, scales that identified general defensiveness and minimization or exaggeration of self-reported symptoms were also included in the instrument. The inclusion of validity scales was an innovation that remains a significant asset for the clinician when using the MMPI-2 because the accuracy of the patient's self-report can be reliably determined before inferences are made regarding the presence or absence of symptoms. Over the years, supplementary and focused content scales were derived from the MMPI item pool to assess clinically relevant phenomena such as posttraumatic stress disorder and substance abuse.

In 1989, a restandardization procedure that included the development of a diverse and nationally representative normative sample yielded the MMPI-2. The new normative sample consisted of 2,600 men and women from throughout the United States and encompassed individuals from a wide range of socio-economic, educational, and ethnic backgrounds. The MMPI-2 retained the original validity and clinical scales; however, outdated items were eliminated and items were revised to improve item comprehension. Furthermore, new item content was added to reflect contemporary clinical issues such as drug and alcohol abuse, suicidal ideation, and Type A behavior. Moreover, new validity and content scales were added to address contemporary clinical and interpretive concerns.

The MMPI-2 is used in a wide variety of settings to screen for psychopathology and aid in clinical decision making. The broad acceptance of the MMPI-2 is a result of the objective nature of the instrument and the extensive 60-year history of accumulated research supporting the validity of the MMPI/MMPI-2 in clinical judgment and decision making. Beyond the use of the MMPI-2 in employment screening, forensic evaluation, and outpatient and inpatient psychiatric settings, the MMPI-2 is widely used in medical settings. Scales associated with somatic preoccupation, Scale 1 (Hs), the potential to react to stress by developing physical symptoms, Scale 3 (Hy), and the report of a wide range of somatic symptoms and a preoccupation with bodily functions (Health Concerns) have been extensively studied in medical settings. These studies have established the predictive validity of the MMPI/MMPI-2 in medical and behavioral health settings. For example, individual attributes tapped by the items on the MMPI-2 Scale 3 (Hysteria) are associated with becoming disabled as a result of a work-related injury and remaining disabled after treatment. Importantly, the MMPI/MMPI-2 was administered prior to the injury, suggesting that the instrument was able to identify personal attributes and psychological factors that hindered recovery from injury and led to extended disability.

Within medical and behavioral health settings, the MMPI-2 is frequently used to screen for psychopathology and fitness to undergo medical treatments or procedures such as organ transplantation. The instrument is also used to determine the capacity to benefit from intensive treatment regimens or actively participate in physical rehabilitative programs.

As part of a comprehensive evaluation, the MMPI-2 can provide valuable information regarding the emotional response to an acute or chronic medical condition and provide information regarding substance abuse issues in patients being treated with potentially addictive analgesics.

The MMPI-2 can indicate how typical an individual's psychological response to a particular injury or medical condition is and also quantify this response relative to other patients. For example, chronic pain patients generally produce three MMPI-2 profile clusters. These three clusters include groups marked by elevations on both the 1 and 3 scales, a group marked by multiple clinical scale elevations associated with significant distress and maladjustment, as well as a group with all the MMPI-2 clinical scales falling within the normal range. Within the context of treatment for chronic pain, the MMPI-2 can identify how the person is presenting himself or herself for treatment, describe the emotional response to the pain, and determine how common such response is relative to others experiencing chronic pain. Chronic pain patients who produce profiles that fall within normal limits are coping with their pain with less distress and emotional sequelae than those who produce elevations on multiple MMPI-2 clinical scales. Given this information, interventions can be tailored to address the differences in emotional response to the chronic pain syndrome.

The use of the MMPI-2 in behavioral health settings provides the clinician with objective and clinically relevant information regarding the psychological response of patients to their medical condition. Originally, the MMPI was thought to be useful in identifying individuals whose physical complaints were "functional" or nonorganic in nature. On the contrary, rather than determining the nature of self-reported physical complaints, the MMPI-2 provides useful information regarding the psychological context within which the physical complaints occur and the emotional response to the medical condition. Specifically, the MMPI-2 serves as an objective measure of how well patients are emotionally coping with their condition, their psychological approach to medical interventions or procedures, and the relative degree of emotional turmoil and distress experienced within the context of their condition.

—Paul A. Arbisi and James N. Butcher

MOTIVATIONAL INTERVIEWING

Motivational interviewing (MI) is a client-oriented counseling method that was developed originally by William Miller and Stephen Rollnick for the treatment of people with addictive behavior such as alcohol use. It motivates people by helping them to recognize the difference between their current behavior and future personal goals and values (Miller & Rollnick, 2002). MI helps people explore the difficulties they have with their current behavior and make commitment to change.

PRINCIPLES AND ELEMENTS OF MOTIVATIONAL INTERVIEWING

Some of the principles of MI include expressing empathy or understanding of a client's behavior, avoiding argumentation with the client, and supporting a client's self-confidence toward changing the current behavior. Key elements used in MI are reflective listening and eliciting self-motivational statements. Through reflective listening, clients are allowed to express their views of the problem, even if the provider does not agree with the client. This way, the provider appreciates a true understanding of the client's perspective and experience. MI helps clients to develop and make statements that will encourage them to change their current problem behavior. Such self-motivational statements help clients understand and see how their problem behavior affects their future personal goals and values (Miller & Rollnick, 2002). Other elements employed in MI include giving clients feedback on their behavior, giving advice only when solicited, putting the responsibility for change on the client, and providing clients with a menu of options for behavior change.

APPLICATION OF MOTIVATIONAL INTERVIEWING IN HEALTH BEHAVIOR

The broadest application of MI is in the area of addictive behaviors. It is only recently that MI is beginning to be used in improving treatment adherence and outcomes in other areas of health behavior change such as obesity and diabetes, HIV risk factor modification, dietary adherence, fruit and vegetable intake, mammography screening, eating disorders, smoking cessation, and physical activity. There are currently several randomized controlled trials funded by the National Institutes of Health (NIH) testing the effectiveness of MI in improving medication adherence in hypertensive and HIV patients. As part of the Behavioral Change Consortium at the NIH, there are at least 15 current NIH-funded studies where MI is being tested as a primary or adjunct intervention for health behavior change, with different types of counselors and delivery modalities (see http://www1.od.nih.gov/behaviorchange/).

—*Gbenga Ogedegbe*

See also ALCOHOL ABUSE AND DEPENDENCE: TREATMENT; HEALTH PROMOTION AND DISEASE PREVENTION

Further Reading

Emmons, K. M., & Rollnick, S. (2001). Motivational interviewing in health care settings: Opportunities and limitations. *American Journal of Preventive Medicine, 20,* 68-74.
[Information on the practice of motivational interviewing]. http://www.motivationalinterview.org/
Miller, W. R., & Rollnick, S. (2002). *Motivational interviewing: Preparing people for change* (2nd ed.). New York: Guilford.
Resnicow, K., et al. (2001). A motivational interviewing intervention to increase fruit and vegetable intake through Black churches: Results of eat for life trial. *American Journal of Public Health, 91,* 1686-1693.

MULTILEVEL METHODS, THEORY, AND ANALYSIS

The term *multilevel* relates to the levels of analysis in public health research, which usually, but not always, consist of individuals (at lower level) who are nested within spatial units (at higher levels). Multilevel methods, meanwhile, consist of quantitative procedures that are pertinent when (a) the observations that are being analyzed are correlated; (b) the causal processes are thought to operate at more than one level; and/or (c) the research interest is especially in describing the variability and heterogeneity in the population, rather than average values.

Multilevel methods are specifically geared toward the statistical analysis of data that have a *nested* structure. The nesting, typically, but not always, is hierarchical.

For instance, a two-level structure would have many level-1 units nested within a smaller number of level-2 units. For instance, in educational research—the field that provided the impetus for multilevel methods—level-1 usually consists of pupils who are nested within schools at level-2. Such structures arise routinely in health and social sciences, such that level-1 and level-2 units could be workers in organizations, patients in hospitals, or individuals in neighborhoods, respectively.

MULTILEVEL DESIGNS

The existence of nested data structures is neither random nor ignorable; for instance, individuals differ but so do the neighborhoods. Differences among neighborhoods could either be directly due to the differences among individuals who live in them, or groupings based on neighborhoods may arise for reasons less strongly associated with the characteristics of the individuals who live in them. Regardless, once such groupings are established, even if their establishment is random, they will tend to become differentiated. This would imply that the group (e.g., neighborhoods) and its members (e.g., individual residents) can exert influence on each other suggesting different sources of variation (e.g., individual-induced and neighborhood-induced) in the outcome of interest and thus compelling analysts to consider covariates at the individual *and* at the neighborhood levels. Ignoring this multilevel structure of variations not simply risks overlooking the importance of neighborhood effects but has implications for statistical validity.

To put this in perspective, in an influential study of progress among primary school children, Bennett (1976), using single-level multiple regression analysis, claimed that children exposed to a "formal" style of teaching exhibited more progress than those who were not. The analysis while recognizing individual children as units of analysis ignored their grouping into teachers/classes. In what was the first important example of multilevel analysis using social science data, Aitkin, Anderson, and Hinde (1981) reanalyzed the data and demonstrated that when the analysis accounted properly for the grouping of children (at lower level) into teachers/classes (at higher levels), the progress of formally taught children could not be shown to significantly differ from the others.

What was occurring here was that children within any one class/with one teacher, because they were taught together, tended to be similar in their performance thereby providing much less information than would have been the case if the same number of children had been taught separately. More formally, the individual samples (e.g., children) were *correlated* or *clustered*. Such clustered samples do not contain as much information as simple random samples of similar size. As was shown by Aitkin et al. (1981), ignoring this autocorrelation and clustering results in increased risk of finding differences and relationships where none exist.

Clustered data also arise as a result of sampling strategies. For instance, while planning large-scale survey data collection, for reasons of cost and efficiency, it is usual to adopt a multistage sampling design. A national population survey, for example, might involve a three-stage design, with regions sampled first, then neighborhoods, and then individuals. A design of this kind generates a three-level hierarchically clustered structure of individuals at level-1 nested within neighborhoods at level-2, which in turn are nested in regions at level-3. Individuals living in the same neighborhood can be expected to be more alike than they would be if the sample were truly random. Similar correlation can be expected for neighborhoods within a region.

Much documentation exists on measuring this "design effect" and correcting for it. Indeed, clustered designs (e.g., individuals at level-1 nested in neighborhoods at level-2 nested in regions at level-3) are often a nuisance in traditional analysis. However, individuals, neighborhoods, and regions can be seen as distinct structures that exist in the population that should be measured and modeled.

A Typology of Multilevel Data Structures

The idea of multilevel structure can be recast, with great advantage, to address a range of circumstances where one may anticipate clustering. Health outcomes and behaviors as well as their causal mechanisms are rarely stable and invariant over time, producing data structures that involve repeated measures, which can be considered a special case of multilevel clustered data structures. Consider the *repeated cross-sectional design* that can be structured in multilevel terms with neighborhoods at level-3; year/time at level-2 and individuals at level-1. In this example, level-2 represents repeated measurements on the neighborhoods (level-3) over time. Such a structure can be used to investigate what sorts of individuals and what sorts of neighborhoods have changed with respect to health outcomes. Alternatively, there is the classic *repeated measure or panel design* in which the level-1 is the measurement occasion, level-2 is the individual, and level-3 is the neighborhood. This time, the individuals are repeatedly measured at different time intervals so that it becomes possible to model changing individual behaviors within a contextual setting of, say, neighborhoods.

When different responses/outcomes are correlated, this lends itself to a *multivariate multilevel data structure* in which level-1 are sets of response variables measured on individuals at level-2 nested in neighborhoods at level-3. The *multivariate responses* could be, for instance, different aspects of health behavior (e.g., smoking and drinking). In addition, such responses could be a mixture of "quality" (do you smoke/do you drink) and "quantity" (how many/how much) producing *mixed multivariate responses*. The substantive benefit of this approach is that it is possible to assess whether different types of behavior and whether the qualitative and quantitative aspects of each behavior are related to individual characteristics in the same or different ways. In addition, we can also ascertain whether neighborhoods that are high for one behavior are also high for another and whether neighborhoods with high prevalence of smoking, for instance, are also high in terms of the number of cigarettes smoked.

While the previous examples are strictly hierarchical, in that all level-1 units that form a level-2 grouping are always in the same group at any higher level, data structures could be nonhierarchical. For example, a model of health behavior (e.g., smoking) could be formulated with individuals at level-1 and both residential neighborhoods *and* workplaces at level-2 not nested but crossed, also called *cross-classified structures*. Individuals are then seen as occupying more than one set of contexts, each of which may have an important influence.

A related structure occurs where for a single level-2 classification (e.g., neighborhoods), level-1 units (e.g., individuals) may belong to more than one level-2 unit, also referred to as *multiple membership designs*. The individual can be considered to belong simultaneously to several neighborhoods with the contributions of each neighborhood being weighted in relation to its distance (if the interest is spatial) from the individual.

MULTILEVEL ANALYSIS

Three constitutive components of multilevel analysis are identified and discussed with examples from public health research.

Evaluating Sources of Variation: Compositional and/or Contextual

A fundamental application of multilevel methods is disentangling the different sources of variations in the outcome. Evidence for variations in poor health, for instance, between different contexts can be due to factors that are intrinsic to, and are measured at, the contextual level. In other words, the variation is due to what can be described as *contextual, area,* or *ecological effects.* Alternatively, variations between places may be *compositional*; that is, certain types of people who are more likely to be in poor health due to their individual characteristics happen to be clustered in certain places. The issue, therefore, is not whether variations between different places exist (they usually do), but what is the primary source of these variations. Put simply, are there significant contextual differences in health between settings (such as neighborhoods), after taking into account the individual compositional characteristic of the neighborhood?

The notions of contextual and compositional sources of variation have general relevance and they are applicable whether the context is administrative (e.g., political boundaries), temporal (e.g., different time periods), or institutional (e.g., schools or hospitals).

Describing Contextual Heterogeneity

Contextual differences may be complex such that it may not be the same for all types of people. Describing such *contextual heterogeneity* is another aspect of multilevel analysis and can have two interpretative dimensions. First, there may be a *different amount* of neighborhood variation, such that, for example, for high-social-class individuals it may not matter in which neighborhoods they live (thus a smaller between-neighborhood variation) but it matters a great deal for the low social class and as such shows a large between-neighborhood variation. Second, there may be a *differential ordering*: Neighborhoods that are high for one group are low for the other and vice versa. Stated simply, the multilevel analytical question is, are the contextual neighborhood differences in poor health, after taking into account the individual composition of the neighborhood, different for different types of population groups?

Characterizing and Explaining the Contextual Variations

Contextual differences, in addition to people's characteristics, may also be influenced by the different characteristics of neighborhoods. Stated differently, individual differences may interact with context and ascertaining the relative importance of individual and neighborhood covariates is another key aspect of a multilevel analysis. For example, over and above social class (individual characteristic), health may depend on the poverty levels of the neighborhoods (neighborhood characteristic). The contextual effect of poverty can either be the same for both the high and low social class suggesting that while neighborhood poverty explains the prevalence of poor health, it does not influence the social class inequalities in health. On the other hand, the contextual effects of poverty may be different for different groups, such that neighborhood poverty adversely affects the low social class but does the opposite for the high social class. Importantly, neighborhoods at the lowest level of poverty are also areas with the least health disparities as compared with areas at the highest level of poverty.

Thus, neighborhood-level poverty is not only related to average health achievements but also shapes social inequalities in health. The analytical question of interest is, are the effects of neighborhood-level socioeconomic characteristics on health different for different types of people?

MULTILEVEL STATISTICAL MODELS

Like all statistical regression equations, multilevel models have the same underlying function, which can be expressed as

> Response = Fixed/Average Parameters +
> (Random/Variance Parameters).

While in a conventional regression model the random part of the model is usually restricted to a single term (that are called error terms or residuals), in the *multilevel regression model* the additional focus is on

expanding the random part of a statistical model. A simple two-level model with a response, a normally distributed measure of poor health, and a single continuous individual (compositional) predictor, age, centered about its mean, for a random sample of individuals at level-1 who are nested within, and drawn from, a group of neighborhoods at level-2 is considered. Since a particular individual is assumed to belong to one and only one neighborhood, and assuming that two individuals from the same neighborhood are correlated, thereby producing a hierarchic nested structure, they are also referred to as *hierarchical models*.

Variance Components or Random Intercepts Model

Multilevel models operate by developing models at each level of analysis and combine them to form a full multilevel model. In the illustration considered here, models would have to be specified at two levels, level-1 and level-2. The model at level-1 can be formally expressed as

$$y_{ij} = \beta_{0j} + \beta_1 x_{1ij} + e_{0ij}, \qquad (1)$$

where y_{ij} is the measure of poor health for the ith individual in the jth neighborhood. The term β_{0j} (associated with a constant) is the average poor health for the jth neighborhood; β_1 is the fixed marginal effect of age (x_{1ij}) on poor health. The individual or the level-1 residual term, e_{0ij}, as in the ordinary regression case, typically, is assumed to have a normal distribution with a 0 mean and a variance, σ_{e0}^2.

Within the framework of multilevel models, the coefficients at level-1 become outcome variables at level-2. Thus, the model at level-2 can be expressed as

$$\beta_{0j} = \beta_0 + u_{0j} \qquad (2)$$

Stated verbally, the average poor health for the jth neighborhood is decomposed into β_0 (the "grand" average for poor health across all neighborhoods) and u_{0j}, which is the effect specific to the jth neighborhood, that is, the differential contribution (positive or negative) that this neighborhood makes to the prediction of the individual poor health.

The new neighborhood-specific term u_{0j} can be treated in one of the two ways. One procedure for incorporating the differential contribution of neighborhoods into a model is to fit a different regression line for each place. In some circumstances, for instance, when there are fewer higher-level units (e.g., neighborhoods) and a moderately large number of individuals in each, this may be efficient. It may also be appropriate if the interest is in making inferences about just those neighborhoods. However, if some of the neighborhoods have very few individuals, and if our interest is to make inferences about the neighborhood in general, fitting a separate model for each neighborhood may not be a viable strategy.

On the other hand, if neighborhoods are treated as a (random) sample from a population of neighborhoods and the interest is in making inferences about the variation between neighborhoods in general, that would constitute a *multilevel statistical approach*. Just as individuals are treated as a sample from a population of individuals and where a sample is used to make inferences about the population rather than about each individual, the neighborhoods are instruments for making inferences about the relevant population of neighborhoods. Adopting this approach provides a model with two random variables, one at each level of the data structure, and it is this feature that makes it a *multilevel statistical model*. Consequently, u_{0j} can be treated in a manner similar to individual-level residuals.

Substituting the level-2 model (Equation 2) into level-1 model (Equation 1) and grouping them into fixed and random part components (the latter shown in brackets) yields the combined model, also referred to as *random-intercepts* or *variance components* model:

$$y_{ij} = \beta_0 + \beta_1 x_{1ij} + (u_{0j} + e_{0ij}). \quad (3)$$

Assuming independence of the residual terms at level-1 and level-2, e_{0ij} and u_{0j}, respectively, the variance at level-2, σ_{u0}^2, measures the neighborhood differences after accounting for the compositional effect of age. It is in this way that the multilevel model disentangles the compositional effects (e.g., individual age) from the contextual differences between neighborhoods. Stated differently, multilevel models allow *variance partitioning* by different levels and the proportion of variance attributable to the level of neighborhood is achieved by dividing the level-2 variance by the total variance, which is given in Equation 4. Such statistics, also known as *intra-class correlation*, or *intra-unit correlation*, or *variance partitioning*

coefficient, are of great interest since they provide direct clues to the level at which an action lies or does not lie.

$$\sigma_{u0}^2 / \sigma_{u0}^2 + \sigma_{e0}^2. \quad (4)$$

Random Coefficients or Random Slopes Models

The level-1 model described in Equation 1 can be extended to describe the *contextual heterogeneity* in poor health/age relationship. This can be achieved by allowing the fixed effect of age to randomly vary across neighborhoods in the following manner:

$$y_{ij} = \beta_{0j} + (\beta_{1j} x_{1ij} + e_{0ij}). \quad (5)$$

At level-2, there will now be two models:

$$\beta_{0j} = \beta_0 + u_{0j} \quad (6)$$

$$\beta_{1j} = \beta_1 + u_{1j}. \quad (7)$$

Multilevel models specify the different intercepts and slopes for each context as coming from a distribution at a higher level. Substituting the macro models in Equations 6 and 7 into the micro model in Equation 5 gives the following:

$$y_{ij} = \beta_0 + \beta_1 x_{1ij} + (u_{0j} + u_{1j} x_{1ij} + e_{0ij}). \quad (8)$$

The key change is that the age effect in neighborhood j in Equation 8 consists of a fixed average age effect across all neighborhoods, β_1, and a differential age effect that is specific to each neighborhood, (u_{1j}). Such models are also referred to as *random-slopes* or *random coefficient models* or *mixed models* since the model in Equation 8 is achieved by allowing the fixed age effect to vary across neighborhoods.

While random-slopes models address the issue of contextual heterogeneity in multilevel analysis, random-intercepts models disentangle the compositional and contextual sources of variation.

Key Characteristics of a Multilevel Statistical Model

Multilevel models are essentially concerned with modeling both the average and the variation around the average. To accomplish this, they consist of two sets of parameters: those summarizing the average relationships(s) and those summarizing the variation around the average at both the level of individuals and neighborhoods. Thus, in Equation 8, the parameters β_0 and β_1 are fixed and give the average poor health/age relationship. The remaining subscripted parameters in the brackets are random (allowed to vary) and represent the differences in poor health between neighborhoods and between individuals within neighborhoods.

Representing the between-neighborhood differences in Equation 8 are two terms, (u_{0j}, u_{1j}), associated with the constant, and x_{1ij}, respectively. However, it is not the neighborhood-specific values that are estimated by multilevel models. Rather, they estimate the variances and the covariance. Making the usual IID (identical and independent distribution) assumptions, the neighborhood differences at level-2 can be summarized through a *variance-covariance parameter matrix* consisting of two variances (σ^2_{u0}), (σ^2_{u1}) and one covariance (σ_{u0u1}), respectively. The level-2 variance-covariance coefficients, meanwhile, can be used to derive neighborhood-specific predictions, usually referred to as *posterior residuals*, thereby allowing the researcher to make neighborhood-specific inferences. The level-1 residuals $(e_{0ij}$: remaining difference for individual i in neighborhood $j)$ can be summarized in a variance parameter, σ^2_{e0}. The model assumes that the variance at level-1 is *homoskedastic* (i.e., constant at all ages). This assumption can be relaxed and if the variance at level-1 is *heteroskedastic* (i.e., different at different ages), then that can be accordingly modeled within the multilevel statistical approach.

Main Contextual Effects and Cross-Level Interaction Models

An attractive feature of multilevel models—one that is commonly used in health research—is their ability to model neighborhood and individual characteristics, and any interaction between them, simultaneously. Consider a micro model with a categorical individual variable, social class:

$$y_{ij} = \beta_{01} + \beta_{1j} x_{1ij} + e_{0ij}. \qquad (9)$$

The parameter β_{0j} gives the average health for neighborhood j for a base category (e.g., low social class) and β_{1j} estimates the differential for high social class in neighborhood j (associated with an indicator variable, x_{1ij}). As before, this requires specifying two macro models at the neighborhood level. Since

neighborhood characteristics vary at level-2, they are consequently specified as predictor variables in the level-2 model and not in the micro model specified in Equation 9. Thus, the two elaborated macro models underlying Equation 9 are

$$\beta_{0j} = \beta_0 + \alpha_1 W_{1j} + u_{0j} \qquad (10)$$

$$\beta_{1j} = \beta_1 + \alpha_2 W_{1j} + u_{ij,} \qquad (11)$$

where W_{1j} is a neighborhood poverty covariate that is hypothesized to account for the complex variation in neighborhoods. The separate specification of micro and macro models correctly recognizes that the contextual variables are predictors of between-neighborhood differences, after allowing for individual compositional variables. Combining the macro equations in Equations 10 and 11 yields the following:

$$y_{ij} = \beta_0 + \beta_1 x_{1ij} + \alpha_1 W_{1j} + \alpha_2 W_{1j} x_{1ij} \\ + (u_{0j} + u_{1j} x_{1ij} + e_{0ij}). \qquad (12)$$

Specifically, the α parameters now account for the contextual variations for the two social class groups and represent the relationship between neighborhood differences (after controlling for individual variable, social class) and the contextual variable, W_j. Thus, α_2 assesses the relationship between low social class (at the individual level) and the poverty of the neighborhood, and represents the differential contextual effect of poverty for high social class. This formulation makes clear that it is only through multilevel models that *cross-level interactions* between individual $(x_{1ij}$: the indicator dummy for high social class) and contextual characteristics $(W_{1j}$: the neighborhood poverty covariate) can be robustly specified and estimated. If both the parameters are significant, then such models are called the *cross-level interaction models*. If, however, the parameter α_2 is not significant, then this would suggest that the neighborhood poverty effect is the same for the two social class groups. The precise nature of the relationship will obviously depend on the size and direction of the individual and contextual fixed parameters, β and α, respectively.

Nonlinear Multilevel Models

While the preceding discussion considered a single normally distributed response variable for illustration, multilevel models are capable of handling a wide range of responses. These include *binary outcomes*; *proportions* (as logit, log-log, and probit models); *multiple categories* (as multinomial and ordered multinomial models); and *counts* (as Poisson and negative binomial distribution models). In essence, these models work by assuming a specific, nonnormal distribution for the random part at level-1, while maintaining the normality assumptions for random parts at higher levels. Consequently, the discussion presented in this entry focusing at the neighborhood level (higher contextual level) would continue to hold regardless of the nature of the response variable, with few exceptions. For instance, partitioning variances across individual and neighborhood levels in complex *nonlinear multilevel logistic models* is not straightforward and is a subject of applied methodological research.

MULTILEVEL ANALYSIS: GENERAL ISSUES

While the advances in statistical research and computing have shown the potential of multilevel methods for health and social behavioral research, there are issues to be considered while developing and interpreting multilevel applications. First, it is important to clearly motivate and conceptualize the choice of higher levels (e.g., neighborhoods) in a multilevel analysis. Second, establishing the relative importance of context and composition is probably more apparent than real, that is, the procedure to distinguishing the relative importance of context and compositional factors is somewhat problematic, and necessary caution must be exercised while conceptualizing and interpreting the compositional and contextual sources of variation. Third, it is important that the sample of neighborhoods belongs to a well-defined population of neighborhoods such that the sample shares exchangeable properties that are essential for robust inferences. Fourth, it is important to ensure adequate sample size at all levels of analysis. In general, if the research focus is essentially on neighborhoods, then clearly the analysis requires more neighborhoods (as compared to more individuals within a neighborhood). Last, like all quantitative procedures, the ability of multilevel models to make causal inferences is limited and innovative strategies including randomized neighborhood-level research designs in combination with multilevel analytical strategy may be required to convincingly demonstrate causal effects of neighborhoods.

SUMMARY

The multilevel statistical approach—an approach that explicitly models the correlated nature of the data arising either due to sampling design or because populations are clustered—has a number of substantive and technical advantages.

From a substantive perspective, it circumvents the problems associated with *ecological fallacy* (the invalid transfer of results observed at the ecological level to the individual level); *individualistic fallacy* (occurs by failing to take into account the ecology or context within which individual relationships happen); and *atomistic fallacy* (arises when associations between individual variables are used to make inferences on the association between the analogous variables at the group/ecological level). The issue common to the above fallacies is the failure to recognize the existence of unique relationships being observable at multiple levels and each being important in its own right. Specifically, one can think of an *individual relationship* (e.g., individuals who are poor are more likely to have poor health); an *ecological/contextual relationship* (e.g., places with a high proportion of poor individuals are more likely to have higher rates of poor health); and an *individual-contextual relationship* (e.g., the greatest likelihood of being in poor health is found for poor individuals in places with a high proportion of poor people). Multilevel models explicitly recognize the level-contingent nature of relationships.

From a technical perspective, the multilevel approach enables researchers to obtain statistically efficient estimates of fixed regression coefficients. Specifically, using the clustering information, multilevel models provide correct standard errors, and thereby robust confidence intervals and significance tests. These generally will be more conservative than the traditional ones that are obtained simply by ignoring the presence of clustering. More broadly, multilevel models allow a more appropriate and realistic specification of complex variance structures at each level. Multilevel models are also precision weighted and capitalize on the advantages that accrue as a result of "pooling" information from all the neighborhoods to make inferences about specific neighborhoods.

The discussion of multilevel methods and analysis in this entry was essentially illustrated with a hierarchical two-level structure of individuals at level-1 nested within neighborhoods at level-2. Additional statistical and analytical considerations can be identified while dealing with three-level, repeated-measures, multivariate, or cross-classified data structures. Also of note are research developments whereby multilevel perspective has been extended to survival and event history models, meta-analysis, structural equation modeling, and factor analysis.

—*S. V. Subramanian*

See also Ecosocial Theory; Income Inequality and Health; Neighborhood Effects on Health and Behavior

Further Reading

Aitkin, M., Anderson, D., & Hinde, J. (1981). Statistical modelling of data on teaching styles (with discussion). *Journal of the Royal Statistical Society A, 144,* 148-161.

Bennett, N. (1976). *Teaching styles and pupil progress.* London: Open Books.

For fundamental ideas underlying multilevel models, see

Goldstein, H. (1995). *Multilevel statistical models* (2nd ed.). London: Arnold.

Longford, N. (1993). *Random coefficient models.* Oxford, UK: Clarendon.

Raudenbush, S. W., & Bryk, A. S. (2002). *Hierarchical linear models: Applications and data analysis methods.* Newbury Park, CA: Sage.

For an applied perspective on multilevel models, see

Hox, J. (2002). *Multilevel analysis: Techniques and applications.* Mahwah, NJ: Lawrence Erlbaum.

Leyland, A. H., & Goldstein, H. (Eds.). (2001). *Multilevel modelling of health statistics.* Wiley Series in Probability and Statistics. Chichester, UK: Wiley.

Snijders, T., & Bosker, R. (1999). *Multilevel analysis: An introduction to basic and advanced multilevel modeling.* London: Sage.

Subramanian, S. V., Jones, K., & Duncan, C. (2003). Multilevel methods for public health research. In I. Kawachi & L. F. Berkman (Eds.), *Neighborhoods and health* (pp. 65-111). New York: Oxford University Press.

For hands-on practical tutorial-based learning, see

http://multilevel.ioe.ac.uk.

http://tramss.data-archive.ac.uk/Software/MLwiN.asp.

Rasbash, J., et al. (2000). *A user's guide to MLwiN, Version 2.1.* London: Multilevel Models Project, Institute of Education, University of London.

MULTIPLE RISK FACTOR INTERVENTION TRIAL (MRFIT)

The Multiple Risk Factor Intervention Trial (MRFIT) was a randomized controlled trial designed to assess ability of multiple behavioral interventions to prevent the development of coronary heart disease (CHD) in individuals at high risk. From 1973 to 1975, an initial screening involved 361,662 men 35 to 57 years of age at 22 clinical centers in 18 U.S. cities; 12,866 men were selected who were without definite evidence of CHD but who had an elevated risk of CHD death based on their high blood pressure, elevated serum cholesterol, and/or cigarette smoking. In other words, these were men at risk who were not sick.

Half of these men were randomly assigned to either their usual source of medical treatment (i.e., the usual care, or UC, group) or to an intervention designed to reduce CHD risk factors (i.e., the special intervention, or SI, group). All men attended annual visits for assessment of (a) standard risk factors including cholesterol, smoking status, and blood pressure; (b) symptoms of CHD (i.e., morbidity) including self-reported angina as well as stroke or definite clinical myocardial infarction; and (c) behaviors and psychosocial variables including diet, illness, socioeconomic status (e.g., participant's education and income), physical activity, life events (e.g., demotion, marriage, divorce, vacation). In addition to these annual visits, SI men attended intervention visits at 4-month intervals.

Goals for the SI included smoking cessation for men who smoked cigarettes and weight reduction for men who weighed > 115% of their desirable weight. A nutritional goal for all SI men was a reduction in intake of saturated fats and cholesterol, moderate reductions in total fat, and modest increases in polyunsaturated fats. In addition to behavioral interventions, drug treatment was initiated for SI men with a diastolic blood pressure (DBP) of ≥ 90 mm Hg. Drug therapy was increased ("stepped-up") until DBP was consistently below 80 mm Hg. Interventions designed to achieve the goals included an initial 10-week intensive intervention, an extended intervention for those with risk factors that persisted after the initial 10 weeks, and a maintenance program following the reduction in risk factors.

The intervention program included four behavioral methods. First, intervention during the initial 10-week period involved group meetings. Group intervention was preferred based on evidence that group cohesiveness improves group attendance, self-esteem, and therapeutic outcome. Second, "behavioral diagnosis" occurred during case conferences scheduled with biomedical, nutritional, and behavioral scientists following the initial 10-week intervention. Behavioral diagnosis involved identification of problematic behaviors (e.g., smoking), people and situations that support the particular behavior, consequences of stopping the behavior, and the consequences of not stopping the behavior. Third, individual behavioral techniques were implemented to address these problematic behaviors. Behavioral techniques included self-monitoring (e.g., daily diaries), goal setting and contracting, frequent feedback, support and positive reinforcement for behavioral change, development of a self-reward system, modeling of correct health behaviors, and relaxation. Fourth, wives or partners of participants were encouraged to participate in the intervention and effort was made to have wives or partners attend intervention meetings, particularly those designed to modify eating patterns and smoking. When applicable, interventions were offered that would help wives or partners modify their own behaviors to facilitate achievement of desired changes in the MRFIT participants.

At baseline, men's elevated risk for CHD was reflected in their high blood pressure (135/91 mm Hg, on average), elevated serum cholesterol (254 mg/dL, on average), and relatively high rate of smoking (59 %). When MRFIT ended in 1982, all men had been followed for at least 6 years and the average length of time from randomization to the end of the trial was 7 years. At the 6-year examinations, BP dropped to 1221/80 mm Hg in SI men and 127/84 mm Hg in UC men. Cholesterol was reduced to 235 mg/dL in SI men and to 241 mg/dL in UC men. Finally, smoking rates decreased to 32.6 % in SI (a 50% quit rate) and 46.7% in UC men (a 29% quit rate). Despite an unexpected decline in risk factors among UC men, the greater reduction among SI men provided good evidence that multiple risk factors for CHD could be simultaneously modified.

Deaths and their causes were ascertained during the trial and thereafter. During the trial, death from CHD did not differ significantly between groups, with 17.9 deaths per 1,000 in the SI group and 19.3 deaths per 1,000 in the UC group. Total mortality in the trial also did not differ, with 41.2 deaths per 1,000 in the SI group and 40.4 deaths per 1,000 in the UC group. Therefore, despite greater reductions in risk factors among SI men relative to UC men, this did not translate into lower mortality among SI men relative to UC men. This nonsignificant result could have been a result of lower than expected mortality and the unexpected reductions in risk factors among UC men. Alternatively, the effects of risk factor modification may only emerge after 7 years. To address this question, long-term mortality was assessed for the period from randomization through December 1990, representing a 16-year follow-up. During this longer follow-up period, CHD death rates still did not differ between UC and SI men. However, SI was associated with a significantly lower rate of heart attacks (a major specific type of CHD death), with 29 deaths per 1,000 in the SI group and 36 deaths per 1,000 in the UC group.

Although the MRFIT was a randomized clinical trial designed to test the effect of an intervention on multiple risk factors, questionnaires and interviews were administered to test additional hypotheses within prospective cohort and case control designs. In other words, characteristics of the MRFIT men at baseline and during the trial (assessed during annual visits) have been considered in relation to subsequent death during follow-up. Two cohorts have been considered: men recruited during the initial screening ($N = 361{,}662$) and men recruited into the MRFIT ($N = 12{,}866$). Within these cohorts, associations with mortality and morbidity have been considered for various characteristics, including risk factors (e.g., cholesterol, abnormal electrocardiogram), Type A behavior pattern and/or hostility, exercise, and life events.

—*Brooks B. Gump*

See also ALAMEDA COUNTY STUDY; BOGALUSA HEART STUDY; FRAMINGHAM HEART STUDY; HARVARD ALUMNI HEALTH STUDY; KUOPIO ISCHEMIC HEART DISEASE RISK FACTOR STUDY

Further Reading

Benfari, R. C. (1981). The Multiple Risk Factor Intervention (MRFIT): The model for intervention. *Preventive Medicine, 10*, 426-442.

Multiple Risk Factor Intervention Trial Research Group. (1982). Multiple Risk Factor Intervention Trial: Risk factor changes and mortality results. *Journal of the American Medical Association, 248,* 1465-1477.

Multiple Risk Factor Intervention Trial Research Group. (1996). Mortality after 16 years for participants randomized to the Multiple Risk Factor Intervention Trial. *Circulation, 94,* 946-951.

MULTIPLE SCLEROSIS: PSYCHOSOCIAL ASPECTS

Multiple sclerosis (MS) is a chronic, often disabling disease of the central nervous system (CNS) affecting approximately 350,000 people in the United States. Prevalence among women is about twice of that found in men. It is believed that the immune system attacks the myelin sheath around the axons of the CNS, resulting in lesions. Potential symptoms include, but are not limited to, loss of function or feeling in limbs, loss of bowel or bladder control, sexual dysfunction, debilitating fatigue, blindness due to optic neuritis, loss of balance, pain, cognitive dysfunction, and emotional changes. MS remains one of the most disabling illnesses in the United States.

There are several possible courses. Between 65% and 70% begin with a relapsing-remitting course marked by periodic disease exacerbations, which remit partially or fully over the course of weeks or months. Most relapsing-remitting courses eventually give way to a secondary-progressive course in which there is also worsening between exacerbations. Approximately 10% to 15% have a primary-progressive course in which there is a steady worsening of symptoms with no exacerbations. Small percentages of patients have other courses, including a benign course with few symptoms, or in rare cases, a malignant course characterized by rapid deterioration resulting in death.

NEUROPSYCHOLOGICAL SYMPTOMS

Point prevalence for neuropsychological impairment ranges from 40% to 60% while lifetime prevalence is likely considerably higher. Problems with processing speed, attention, and concentration; verbal fluency; and verbal memory are among the most common problems. However, visual-spatial learning, construction, and organization, as well as executive functions, can also be affected. Memory deficits are commonly thought to be due to retrieval problems, yet some studies have also documented problems in encoding and storage of information. More cognitively impaired patients may also show euphoria or pathological laughing and crying, a state characterized by bouts of uncontrollable laughing, crying, or both in response to nonspecific stimuli in the absence of a matching mood state. The neuropsychological symptom profile in MS is heterogeneous. Severity of deficits can vary too. For some MS patients, neuropsychological symptoms may be the first symptoms to appear, while other patients may show preserved cognitive functioning decades after diagnosis.

Neuropsychological evaluation is recommended for patients reporting cognitive deficits. This can identify the source of problems, which can facilitate the development of adaptive strategies. For example, most patients refer to cognitive symptoms as "memory problems." However, deficits in other areas such as attention and concentration or executive functioning can often masquerade as memory problems. Nevertheless, development of compensatory strategies may improve adaptation. Neuropsychological evaluation may also assist employers and family members in adjusting the environment to optimize performance and developing realistic expectations about the patient's abilities.

To date, computer- or human-assisted cognitive rehabilitation has not been shown to be effective in reducing cognitive impairment; however, rigorous trials have not been performed. Learning compensatory skills is generally presumed to be helpful, but such strategies have also not received rigorous testing.

PSYCHOLOGICAL SYMPTOMS

Patients with MS frequently present with a variety of psychological difficulties. It is widely believed that depression is the most common and most debilitating psychological problem associated with MS. Cumulative lifetime prevalence of major depressive disorder following MS diagnosis is approximately 50%, which is higher than seen in other medical patients or the general population. MS-related depression and distress account for a larger decrement in quality of life than does physical disability and are associated with decreased adherence to medical regimens. Depression may also have fatal consequences: The rate of suicide is 7.5 times that in the general population.

MS-related depression may have some unique etiological characteristics. MS-related depression is associated with reduced social support, avoidant coping, depressive cognitive styles, and many other psychosocial risk factors common to other populations. Depression is not related to the level of physical or cognitive impairment. However, there is evidence that MS pathophysiology and pathogenesis are related to depression. Specific MS brain lesions in the temporal and frontal regions are associated with increased risk of depression. Depression is also associated with disease exacerbation and CNS inflammation. Many of the cytokines involved in MS inflammation, including interferon gamma (IFN-γ) and tumor necrosis factor alpha (TNF-α), are also known to produce depressive symptoms including depressed mood, changes in appetite and sleep, and social withdrawal. Thus, we have proposed that depression is a symptom of MS, and not a psychological response to loss of function. This would explain the greater prevalence of depression in MS populations relative to other medical populations.

Anxiety symptoms are also common but have received less attention. Injection anxiety and phobia have emerged as significant problems since the primary disease-modifying medications for MS must all be administered by injection. Between 30% and 50% of all patients are unable to self-inject due to anxiety or phobia, and inability to self-inject results in decreased adherence. Anxiety can also aggravate depression in MS and is associated with increased rates of suicidal ideation.

Treatment for Depression

While depression is common, many studies have shown that it is treatable. Cognitive-behavioral therapy (CBT) and antidepressant medications are equally effective in reducing depressive symptoms, while supportive or insight-oriented treatments appear to be somewhat less. It should be noted that studies have focused on main effects and not on patient predictors of differential response. Therefore, it cannot be said that supportive or insight-oriented treatments are necessarily ineffective for any individual patient, but only that depression in patients with MS, as a population, is more likely to respond to CBT or antidepressant medications. For specific symptoms of pathological laughing and crying, antidepressant medication has been shown to be helpful.

Many patients with MS have mobility impairments or experience fluctuations in symptoms that prevent them from attending a clinic on a regular basis. Others may live far from specialized treatment. Alternative treatment delivery methods via telephone or the Internet might increase access to mental health treatment for these patients. A recent small trial has shown that telephone-administered CBT is effective in reducing depressive symptoms compared with a treatment as usual control condition. Moreover, adherence to disease-modifying medications was better for the active treatment group than the control condition.

Effects of Treatment for Depression on Multiple Sclerosis

There are at least two potential pathways by which depression might affect MS disease: indirectly by affecting behaviors that affect MS exacerbation or progression, or directly via effects on the immune system. There is some support for the indirect hypothesis. A longitudinal study of patients initiating an interferon medication found that depression was associated with decreased adherence to medications used to treat MS. But if the depression was treated either with psychotherapy or antidepressant medications, the risk of discontinuation was no greater than for patients reporting no depression. However, it should be emphasized that neither depression nor adherence have been linked to exacerbation rate or sustained progression of the disease.

Distress and depression may directly affect MS pathogenesis. Distress has been shown to predict sustained progression of MS impairment over the course of 1 year. Depression has been associated both with observed inflammation in the brain by Gd+ MRI and with increases in interferon gamma (IFN-γ; a lynchpin in MS exacerbation that has been shown both to precede and to cause MS exacerbation). Furthermore, successful treatment for depression reduces T cell production of IFN-γ. However, to date no study has examined the effect of treatment for depression on MS exacerbation or sustained progression.

Injection Anxiety

Recent work has suggested that brief, six-session CBT focused on desensitization, exposure, and cognitive restructuring is effective in teaching phobic patients to self-inject.

THE EFFECTS OF STRESS ON MULTIPLE SCLEROSIS

Many patients report that stress results in disease exacerbation. Both case control and longitudinal studies have shown that stress increases the risk of experiencing exacerbation. However, different types of stress may have differential effects. While chronic marital and job-related stress may increase the risk of clinical exacerbation, major negative life events, such as a death in the family, do not appear to alter disease activity. Furthermore, trauma, such as being under missile attack in a war zone, may reduce the risk of clinical exacerbation. Thus, it may be important to differentiate between relatively severe stressors and moderate but more chronic stressors when examining the relationship between stress and disease activity.

These relationships were recently confirmed in a study following patients with monthly gadolinium enhanced (Gd+) MRI scans (gadolinium is a dye that permits visualization of the breakdown in the blood-brain barrier). Major stressors, such as a death in the family, had no significant effect on subsequent Gd+ MRI brain lesions. However, interpersonal family and work conflict was shown to increase the risk of developing a new brain lesion 8 weeks later. While there is strong evidence that stress may increase risk of MS inflammation and exacerbation, the effect sizes are at best modest, suggesting the presence of moderating factors. There are many potential moderating factors, including genetic, disease, environmental, and psychological factors. A recent study has suggested that adaptive coping may reduce the effect of interpersonal conflict on the subsequent development of new Gd+ brain lesions.

—*David C. Mohr*

See also AUTOIMMUNE DISEASES: PSYCHOSOCIAL ASPECTS; CHRONIC DISEASE MANAGEMENT; DEPRESSION: TREATMENT; PSYCHONEUROIMMUNOLOGY; STRESS, APPRAISAL, AND COPING

Further Reading

Brassington, J. C., & Marsh, N. V. (1998). Neuropsychological aspects of multiple sclerosis. *Neuropsychological Review, 8*, 43-77.

Mohr, D. C., Boudewyn, A. C., Goodkin, D. E., Siskin, L. P., Epstein, L., Cheuk, W., & Lee, L. (2001). Comparative outcomes for individual cognitive-behavioral therapy, supportive-expressive group therapy, and sertraline for the treatment of depression in multiple sclerosis. *Journal of Consulting and Clinical Psychology, 69*, 942-949.

Mohr, D. C., & Cox, D. (2001). Multiple sclerosis: Empirical literature for the clinical health psychologist. *Journal of Clinical Psychology, 57*, 479-499.

Mohr, D. C., Goodkin, D. E., Bacchetti, P., Boudewyn, A. C., Huang, L., Marrietta, P., Cheuk, W., & Dee, B. (2000). Psychological stress and the subsequent appearance of new brain MRI lesions in MS. *Neurology, 55*, 55-61.

Mohr, D. C., Likosky, W., Dick, L. P., Van Der Wende, J., Dwyer, P., Bertagnolli, A. C., & Goodkin, D. E. (2000). Telephone-administered cognitive-behavioral therapy for the treatment of depressive symptoms in multiple sclerosis. *Journal of Consulting and Clinical Psychology, 68*, 356-361.

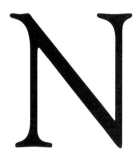

NATIONAL CHOLESTEROL EDUCATION PROGRAM (NCEP)

The greatest triumph of 20th-century cardiovascular medicine may not be recognized as the development of innovative surgical interventions, such as heart transplant, coronary artery bypass graft surgery, and various endovascular procedures, including percutaneous transluminal coronary angioplasty and stents, but rather as the movement toward prevention of coronary heart disease (CHD) through early detection and treatment of cardiovascular risk factors, including blood pressure and cholesterol. The National Cholesterol Education Program (NCEP) Adult Treatment Panel (ATP) of the National Heart, Lung, and Blood Institute (NHLBI) represents one such strategy that combines public health interventions at the social level (weight control, reduction of dietary saturated fat and cholesterol intake, increases in fiber consumption and physical activity) with aggressive medical management at the individual patient level through pharmacotherapy with therapeutic lifestyle changes and, if necessary, by adding drugs that lower cholesterol, such as HMG CoA reductase inhibitors or statins. Practice guidelines, such as NCEP-ATP, specify recommendations for behavioral changes for the general population, health care providers, and patients, which result in improved levels of cardiovascular risk and disease.

The current NCEP clinical practice guidelines (ATP-III) were released in May 2001, following the release of two previous guidelines (ATP-I, 1988, and ATP-II, 1993). NCEP recommends that all adults aged ≥ 20 years have their blood cholesterol measured every 5 years, with preference given to a complete lipoprotein panel, which measures fasting total cholesterol, low-density lipoproteins (LDL), high density lipoproteins (HDL), and triglycerides. (An alternative lab panel includes only a nonfasting total and HDL cholesterol with a complete lipoprotein panel for those with total cholesterol > 200 mg/dL or HDL < 40 mg/dL.)

LDL-lowering therapy results in reductions in total and coronary mortality, major coronary events, coronary procedures, and stroke. While the newest and most widely used pharmacologic agents are the HMG CoA reductase inhibitors (statins), other pharmacologic treatments include bile acid sequestrants, fibric acids, and nicotinic acid (niacin). Statins reduce LDL by 18% to 55% and triglycerides by 7% to 30%, and increase HDL by 5% to 15%. Statins have been demonstrated to reduce total and CHD mortality, as well as major coronary events and stroke. Patients treated with statins undergo fewer coronary procedures, including bypass and angioplasty.

NCEP ATP-III guidelines apply to both primary and secondary prevention, and identify a total cholesterol of < 200 mg/dL as desirable, 200 to 239 mg/dL as borderline high, and ≥ 240 mg/dL as high. LDL cholesterol levels are identified as optimal (< 100 mg/dL), near/above optimal (100-129 mg/dL), borderline high (130-159 mg/dL), high (160-189 mg/dL), and very high (≥ 190 mg/dL). HDL cholesterol levels of 40 to 59 mg/dL are ideal, whereas HDL levels < 40 mg/dL are considered low, and an independent cardiovascular risk factor. Triglyceride levels < 150 mg/dL are considered normal, 150 to 199 mg/dL are borderline high, 200 to 499 mg/dL are high, and ≥ 500 mg/dL are very high.

In NCEP ATP-III, the focus is on primary prevention, the goal of therapy being the lowering of low-density lipoprotein (LDL) cholesterol. NCEP ATP-III guidelines focus on cholesterol control by identifying those with elevated LDL, and targeting therapy (therapeutic lifestyle changes and medications) to meet LDL treatment goals, which vary according to overall cardiovascular risk (low, moderate, high). One of the major innovations of NCEP ATP-III is the emphasis on the clinical use of the Framingham risk score, which estimates the 10-year risk of CHD. This score can be easily calculated, and classifies individuals into low (< 10%), moderate (10-20%), or high (> 20%) risk of CHD in 10 years. Utilization of the Framingham risk score enables physicians to more accurately identify high-risk patients (it has greater predictive power than counting risk factors alone) and to intervene early and aggressively improving prevention of CHD events.

The major risk factors that modify LDL cholesterol treatment goals are cigarette smoking, hypertension, low HDL (< 40 mg/dL), family history of premature CHD, age (≥ 45 for men, ≥ 55 for women), and the presence of CHD (all clinical forms of atherosclerotic disease, including peripheral arterial disease, abdominal aortic aneurysm, symptomatic carotid artery disease, or diabetes, which is considered a "CHD risk equivalent," since its 10-year risk for CHD is about 20%). Another significant innovation in NCEP is the recognition of a growing public health problem, the "metabolic syndrome," which includes central abdominal obesity, hypertension, hyperlipidemia, and insulin resistance, as both a set of risk factors and a secondary target for therapeutic lifestyle changes and pharmacotherapy. (The age-adjusted prevalence of the metabolic syndrome is estimated by NHANES III to be nearly 25% for both men and women.)

Treatment goals for reducing LDL are as follows: For those with established CHD or CHD-risk equivalents, the LDL treatment goal is < 100 mg/dL; for those with multiple (2+) risk factors, the LDL treatment goal is < 130 mg/dL; and for those with zero or one risk factor the LDL treatment goal is < 160 mg/dL.

The awareness of one's own cardiovascular risk factors is a crucial first step in the prevention and management of cardiovascular disease. Reducing the burden of disease at the community level begins with a combination of public health interventions that reduce the average level of risk in the community with measurement and detection of risk factors at the individual level, and aggressive intervention in individuals identified at high risk.

Reducing the burden of disease at the community level begins with a combination of interventions that separately but simultaneously target both the general population and individuals at various levels of risk. Strategies to reduce the overall level of risk in the general population include public education and mass media campaigns (e.g., nutritional intervention programs such as Five a Day to promote increased consumption of fruits and vegetables), environmental changes (e.g., increased tobacco taxes, restrictions on smoking in public and workplaces, alterations in food composition), and mass medical screenings for risk factors (e.g., body mass index and waist-to-hip ratio for obesity, blood pressure for hypertension, blood sugar for diabetes, and blood cholesterol for hyperlipidemia). Targeting the individual involves increasing patient awareness of the importance of knowing his or her own risk factors and overall level of risk, knowing which risk factors can be modified and how to modify those risk factors, and working with his or her health care providers to reduce risk factors and overall level of risk. Recognizing the individual's readiness to change, and moving him or her from the precontemplator to the contemplator level is a crucial step in this process.

Healthy People 2000 represents a public health strategy aimed at bridging the population- and individual-focused approaches to improving the health status of Americans. One specific goal of Healthy People 2000 was to increase to 75% the percentage of adults aged ≥ 20 screened for high blood cholesterol within the preceding 5 years. Subsequently, Healthy People 2010 includes as a goal the reduction of the percentage of adults aged ≥ 20 with total blood cholesterol levels ≥ 240 mg/dL.

Recent prevalence data (1999) on cholesterol screening, based on the CDC's telephone-administered Behavioral Risk Factor Surveillance System (BRFSS), indicate that 74% of adults (age 20+) in the United States reported that they had had their blood cholesterol checked (this does not necessarily mean that the subtypes of cholesterol have been measured), and of those, 70% had this test within the past year, 24% had their test within the past 2 to 5 years, and 30% had been told that they have high blood cholesterol.

Men reported slightly higher percentages of elevated cholesterol (33.3%) as compared to women (28.4%). Self-reported rates of high blood cholesterol were slightly higher among Whites (29.7%) as compared to Blacks (26.0%), Hispanics (25.6%), and Asian/Pacific Islanders (27.3%). An additional trend observed was an increase in the percentage of individuals who were told that they have high blood cholesterol from 1991 to 1999. This trend most likely reflects better awareness and increased utilization of detection procedures, rather than a true increase in high blood cholesterol within the general population.

The Third National Health and Nutrition Examination Survey (NHANES III), conducted between 1988 and 1994, has shown declines in dietary intake of saturated fat and total fat, as well as reductions in blood cholesterol levels. From 1978 to the present, mean total cholesterol levels among U.S. adults have fallen from 213 mg/dL to 203 mg/dL, and the prevalence of high blood cholesterol (total cholesterol $\geq$ 240 mg/dL) has declined from 26% to 19%.

Taken together, these data indicate that significant behavioral changes in both patients and health care providers are taking place. Cholesterol levels are being measured more frequently, individuals with high blood cholesterol are being identified, and therapeutic lifestyle changes and pharmacotherapy are being utilized more frequently. At the same time, several studies have reported significant racial/ethnic disparities in the identification of high blood cholesterol and prescribing of cholesterol-lowering drugs for minorities.

ATP-III examined the necessity for special treatment considerations for different population groups varying by gender, age, and ethnicity. Several subgroups within the general population require specific modifications to cardiovascular risk factor management. These groups include patients with established CHD or at high risk for developing CHD and/or diabetes, younger adults (men aged 20-35, women aged 20-45), older adults (men $\geq$ 65, women $\geq$ 75), women aged 45 to 75, and those who are postmenopausal, and ethnic minorities. While the profiles of risk factors differ across these populations, the benefits of LDL reduction were recommended for all age, gender, and ethnic subgroups.

Several new developments that may give individuals greater choice and control over their risk factor monitoring and management deserve mention. These include the identification and testing of new cholesterol-lowering drugs with fewer side effects (such as myopathy and increased liver enzymes), and switching of drugs (such as statins) that require a physician's prescription to over-the-counter status (OTC switch), which, coupled with the availability of FDA-approved home cholesterol testing kits, have the capacity to make cholesterol self-management even more widely available and possibly at a lower cost.

New, emerging cardiovascular risk factors and pathophysiologic mechanisms, such as impaired glucose tolerance, lipoprotein (a), inflammation, thrombosis, and elevated serum homocysteine, as well as newer screening and/or diagnostic tests (such as C-reactive protein or CRP), are being examined in relationship to lipoproteins and LDL cholesterol reduction. Benefits of both risk factor reduction through diet and statin pharmacotherapy may extend beyond LDL management and cardiovascular disease. Statins may operate at multiple levels, including modification of the lipoprotein profile, reduction of vascular inflammation, and stabilization of vulnerable atherosclerotic plaque.

Individual clinical and public health interventions combined have the capacity to dramatically reduce levels of cardiovascular risk factors as well as cardiovascular morbidity and mortality. Readiness to change is required at all levels: the public, health care system, provider, and patient. Behavioral change must be promoted and supported at multiple levels. At the public level, changes in nutrition, physical activity, and smoking are needed. The physician and other health care providers need to routinely screen for lipids, calculate overall cardiovascular risk, and treat with both therapeutic lifestyle changes and appropriate medications. The individual patient needs to become aware of his or her lipid profile and overall cardiovascular risk, and needs to adhere to both lifestyle changes and medication regimens that reduce risk. Perhaps the greatest triumph of 21st century cardiovascular medicine will result from a better understanding of factors that inhibit or promote behavior change in individuals, and the effective incorporation of this knowledge into clinical practice.

—*Jonathan N. Tobin*
and Tania Zazula

See also ADHERENCE TO TREATMENT REGIMENS; ADOPTION OF HEALTH BEHAVIOR; BLOOD PRESSURE AND HYPERTENSION: PHYSICAL ACTIVITY; BLOOD PRESSURE, HYPERTENSION, AND STRESS; CARDIAC REHABILITATION; CHRONIC DISEASE

MANAGEMENT; HEALTH PROMOTION AND DISEASE PREVENTION; LIPIDS: PSYCHOSOCIAL ASPECTS; MULTIPLE RISK FACTOR INTERVENTION TRIAL (MRFIT); OBESITY: CAUSES AND CONSEQUENCES; OBESITY TREATMENT AND PREVENTION; PHYSICAL ACTIVITY AND HEALTH; TRANSTHEORETICAL MODEL OF BEHAVIOR CHANGE

Further Reading

LaRosa, J. C., He, J., & Vupputuri, S. (1999). Effect of statins on risk of coronary disease: A meta-analysis of randomized controlled trials. *Journal of the American Medical Association, 282,* 2340-2346.

National Cholesterol Education Program Expert Panel on Detection, Evaluation and Treatment of High Blood Cholesterol in Adults. (2001, May). *Third Report of the National Cholesterol Education Program (NCEP) Expert Panel on Detection, Evaluation and Treatment of High Blood Cholesterol in Adults (ATP-III).* Retrieved December 2002 from http://www.nhlbi.nih.gov and http://www.guidelines.gov

National Cholesterol Education Program Expert Panel on Detection, Evaluation and Treatment of High Blood Cholesterol in Adults. (2001). Executive summary of the Third Report of the National Cholesterol Education Program (NCEP) Expert Panel on Detection, Evaluation and Treatment of High Blood Cholesterol in Adults (ATP-III). *Journal of the American Medical Association, 285,* 2486-2497.

Nelson, K., Norris, K., & Mangione, C. M. (2002). Disparities in the diagnosis and pharmacologic treatment of high serum cholesterol by race and ethnicity: Data from the Third National Health and Nutrition Examination Survey. *Archives of Internal Medicine, 162,* 929-935.

Pasternak, R. C., Smith, S. C., Jr., Bairey-Merz, C. D. N., et al. (2002). ACC/AHA/NHLBI clinical advisory on the use and safety of statins. *Circulation, 106,* 1024-1028.

Reese, S., et al. (2001, September 7). State-specific trends in high blood cholesterol awareness among persons screened—United States, 1991-1999. *Morbidity and Mortality Weekly Report, 50,* 754-758.

Stamler, J., Daviglus, M. L., Garside, D. B., et al. (2000). Relationship of baseline serum cholesterol levels in three large cohorts of younger men to long-term coronary, cardiovascular, and all-cause mortality and to longevity. *Journal of the American Medical Association, 284,* 311-318.

The Third National Health and Nutrition Examination Survey (NHANES III) (1988-1994). (2002). Retrieved December 2002 from http://www.cdc.gov/nchs/about/major/nhanes/datatblelink.htm

Wilson, P. W., D'Agostino, R. B., Levy, D., et al. (1998). Prediction of coronary heart disease using risk factor categories. *Circulation, 97,* 1837-1847.

NATIONAL INSTITUTES OF HEALTH: HEALTH AND BEHAVIOR RESEARCH

The National Institutes of Health (NIH) is the primary federal agency responsible for basic research on the health and well-being of the population of the United States. With a 2002 budget of $23.5 billion, it pursues its mission to uncover fundamental knowledge about the nature and behavior of living systems and apply that knowledge to improve human health. Approximately 84% of the funds are distributed as grants and contracts to investigators in universities and other institutions. In addition, the NIH supports a smaller intramural program of research at the NIH campus in Bethesda, Maryland, and ancillary sites. As part of the quest to prevent and cure the full range of diseases and disorders, NIH has developed a long-term program of research on the behavioral and social aspects of health and illness. Health and behavior research, focusing on the behavioral and social sciences research linked to morbidity, mortality, and their causes and consequences, is a major component of the behavioral and social science research program of the NIH.

Historically, behavioral research has been supported since at least 1955 when the National Heart Institute (predecessor to the National Heart, Lung, and Blood Institute) funded its first behavioral research grant. Since those early beginnings, the behavioral and social sciences research program across the NIH has grown to an estimated $2.4 billion in fiscal year 2002.

While there has been a long and rich history of support for behavioral and social sciences research at NIH, in recognition of the key role that behavioral and social factors play in health, Congress saw a need to more fully integrate behavioral and social science into the programs of the NIH. In 1995, the congressionally mandated Office of Behavioral and Social Sciences Research (OBSSR) opened as a program office in the Office of the Director, NIH.

The mission of the OBSSR was to stimulate a broad integrated program of behavioral and social sciences research into the health research enterprise of the NIH. One of the first activities of the new office was to develop a definition of behavioral and social science research supported by the NIH. That definition is found below.

AREAS OF RESEARCH

The NIH supports both basic and clinical behavioral and social science research. Many studies have both basic and clinical components, and those investigations are often complementary.

Basic Research

Basic research in the behavioral and social sciences furthers understanding of behavioral and social functioning. As is the case for basic research in the biomedical sciences, basic behavioral and social sciences research does not address disease outcomes per se, but instead provides essential knowledge of fundamental processes and states.

Behavioral and Social Processes

Research on behavioral and social processes involves the study of human or animal functioning at the level of the individual, small group, institution, organization, or community. At the individual level, this research may involve the study of behavioral factors such as cognition, memory, language, perception, personality, emotion, motivation, and others. At higher levels of aggregation, it includes the study of social variables such as the structure and dynamics of small groups (e.g., couples, families, work groups), institutions and organizations (e.g., schools, religious organizations), communities (defined by geography or common interest), and larger demographic, political, economic, and cultural systems. Research on behavioral and social processes also includes the study of the interactions within and between these two levels of aggregation, such as the influence of sociocultural factors on cognitive processes or emotional responses. Finally, this research also includes the study of environmental factors such as climate, noise, environmental hazards, and residential environments and their effects on behavioral and social functioning.

Biopsychosocial Processes

Biopsychosocial research (also known as biobehavioral or biosocial research) involves the study of the interactions of biological factors with behavioral or social variables and how they affect each other (i.e., the study of bidirectional multilevel relationships).

Development of Procedures for Measurement, Analysis, and Classification

Research on the development of procedures for measurement, analysis, and classification involves the development and refinement of procedures for measuring and analyzing behavior, psychological functioning, or the social environment. This research is designed to develop research tools that could be used in other areas of behavioral and social sciences or in biomedical research.

Clinical Research

Clinical research in the behavioral and social sciences is designed to predict or influence health outcomes, risks, or protective factors. It is also concerned with the impact of illness or risk for illness on behavioral or social functioning. Clinical research may be divided into five categories.

Identification and Understanding of Behavioral and Social Risk and Protective Factors

Research on the identification and understanding of behavioral and social risk and protective factors associated with the onset and course of illness, and with health conditions, examines the association of specific behavioral and social factors with mental and physical health outcomes and the mechanisms that explain these associations. It is concerned with behavioral and social factors that may be health-damaging (risk factors) or health-promoting (protective factors).

Effects of Illness or Physical Condition on Behavioral and Social Functioning

Research in this category focuses on the consequences of illness for behavior. Included are such questions as the psychological and social consequences of genetic testing, behavioral correlates of head injury across developmental stages, emotional and social consequences of HIV infection or cancer, coping responses associated with chronic pain syndromes, effects of illness on economic status, and coping with loss of function due to disability.

Treatment Outcomes Research

Treatment outcomes research involves the design and evaluation of behavioral and social interventions to treat mental and physical illnesses, or interventions designed to ameliorate the effects of illness on behavioral or social functioning. This area also includes research on behavioral and social rehabilitation procedures.

In summary, behavioral and social science factors are key contributors to health outcomes. The research programs of the NIH are increasingly including behavioral and social sciences approaches aimed at understanding disease etiology and improving human health. Building on the important prior research on single diseases or processes, significant advances will likely come from work that takes an integrative approach to health by incorporating the methods and concepts of behavioral and social research with a more traditional biomedical approach.

—*Virginia S. Cain*

See also CENTER FOR THE ADVANCEMENT OF HEALTH; CENTERS FOR DISEASE CONTROL AND PREVENTION; HEALTH AND BEHAVIOR ORGANIZATIONS

Further Reading

Office of Behavioral and Social Sciences Research, National Institutes of Health, Department of Health and Human Services. (2003). Retrieved from http://obssr.od.nih.gov/

Singer, B. H., & Ryff, C. D. (Eds.). (2001). *New horizons in health: An integrative approach.* Committee on Future Directions for Behavioral and Social Research at the National Institutes of Health. Washington, DC: National Academy Press.

NEIGHBORHOOD EFFECTS ON HEALTH AND BEHAVIOR

Interest in geographical variations in health has a long history. However, the importance given to the examination of area differences in studying the causes of disease has varied over time. The focus on individual-level risk factors over the past few decades was generally associated with little interest in area characteristics as potential disease determinants. Recent years, however, have witnessed a resurgence of interest in how area or neighborhood characteristics may affect the health of their residents ("neighborhood health effects"). Several factors may have contributed to this trend. Chief among these has been a rekindling of interest in the social determinants of health and the recognition that social influences on health operate through many different processes, one of which may be the types of areas or neighborhoods in which people live. Simultaneously, there has been a growing discussion on the use of ecological variables in epidemiology. This discussion is related to a critique of the notion that all health determinants are best conceptualized as individual-level attributes. Research on neighborhood effects has fit into this emerging paradigm because it has conceptualized neighborhood context as potentially related to health, over and above individual-level attributes. In addition, recent discussions in sociology on the causes and consequences of residential segregation and urban poverty, together with neighborhood effects research in criminology and child development, have reinvigorated interest in the ways in which neighborhood context may affect individuals, including their health.

RESEARCH APPROACHES USED TO INVESTIGATE NEIGHBORHOOD HEALTH EFFECTS

Different research strategies have been used to investigate neighborhood or area health effects: ecological studies, contextual or multilevel studies, and comparisons of small numbers of well-defined neighborhoods. Ecological studies have examined variation in morbidity and mortality rates across areas in order to relate this variability to area characteristics. The sizes of areas examined have ranged from relatively large areas (such as counties), not really analogous to neighborhoods at all, to smaller areas (such as census tracts or block groups). The most common area characteristics investigated have been aggregate measures of the socioeconomic characteristics of residents or indices of deprivation constructed by combining several aggregate measures based on theoretical and/or empirical considerations. These studies have found that area deprivation is associated with increased mortality.

However, the use of these aggregate measures has often been accompanied by ambiguity regarding whether these variables are conceptualized as measures of area-level properties or simply as summaries of individual-level variables, and hence whether the objective is to examine how area constructs are related to health outcomes or document the area-level (or ecological) expression of a well-known individual-level relation. In addition, ecological studies cannot directly determine whether differences across areas are due to characteristics of the areas themselves or to differences between the types of individuals living in different areas.

The recognition of the need to separate out the effects of "context" (e.g., area or neighborhood properties) and "composition" (characteristics of individuals living in different areas) when examining area effects on health has led to a proliferation of reports involving contextual and multilevel analyses. Contextual and multilevel analyses require data sets including individuals nested within areas or neighborhoods. By simultaneously including both neighborhood and individual-level predictors in regression equations with individuals as the units of analysis, these strategies allow examination of neighborhood or area effects after controlling for individual-level confounders. They also permit the examination of individual-level characteristics as modifiers of the area effect. Multilevel analysis also allows the simultaneous examination of within and between neighborhood variability in the outcomes, and the extent to which between-neighborhood variability is "explained" by individual-level and neighborhood-level factors. Studies using these approaches have usually linked information on small area characteristics available in censuses to individual-level covariate and outcome data from surveys, epidemiological studies, or vital statistics data. For the most part, contextual and multilevel studies have been consistent in documenting "independent" associations of neighborhood socioeconomic characteristics with individual-level outcomes after controlling for individual-level socioeconomic position indicators. For example, living in a disadvantaged area appears to be associated with ill health, even after accounting for the personal income of persons living in different areas. However, the strength of the possible neighborhood or area effect is still under debate. Although contextual or multilevel studies are an attractive option in the investigation of neighborhood effects, their use raises a series of methodological challenges that are discussed in more detail below.

In contrast to the large-scale quantitative approaches summarized above, an alternative strategy has been to compare a small number of well-defined and purposely selected contrasting neighborhoods. These types of studies can incorporate knowledge on local history, sociology, and geography in defining neighborhoods. In addition, they may directly collect detailed information on neighborhood characteristics and health outcomes through combinations of quantitative and qualitative strategies. This approach has been used to document differences across neighborhoods in resources and services and relate these differences to differences in health behaviors. However, it is limited in the number and range of neighborhoods investigated and possibly in the generalizability of results. Its strength lies in the use of locally based definitions of neighborhoods (rather than administrative proxies) and in the feasibility of detailed assessment of a variety of neighborhood characteristics, which may help us understand the processes through which neighborhood environments could affect health.

CHALLENGES IN THE INVESTIGATION OF NEIGHBORHOOD HEALTH EFFECTS

A key challenge in the investigation of neighborhood health effects is specifying the specific processes through which neighborhood characteristics may affect health. This requires developing models of how features of residential areas may be related to specific health outcomes and empirically testing aspects of these models. In contrast to other fields, where the theory on the processes linking neighborhood characteristics to outcomes such as violence or child development have been well articulated, research on neighborhood health effects has only recently begun to articulate the processes that may explain the associations observed with health outcomes. The testing of aspects of these models also raises a series of important methodological challenges. Some of these challenges are specific to the investigation of neighborhood effects, and others pertain to the more general problem of the difficulties inherent in investigating complex causal processes using the quantitative methods usually used in public health and epidemiology. Analogous methodological challenges arise in research on "neighborhood effects" in fields other than health.

A first issue is the definition of *neighborhoods* or, perhaps more precisely, of the geographic area whose characteristics may be relevant to the specific health outcome being studied. In health research, the terms *neighborhood* and *community* have often been used loosely to refer to a person's immediate residential environment. The more generic term *area* has also been used. Clear distinctions between the terms *neighborhood*, *community*, and *area* are usually not made. Administratively defined areas have been used as rough proxies for neighborhoods or communities in many studies. There are multiple possible definitions of neighborhoods. The criteria used to define neighborhoods can be historical and geographical, based on people's characteristics or perceptions, or based on administrative boundaries. Boundaries based on these different criteria will not necessarily overlap, and alternative definitions may be relevant for different research questions. For example, neighborhoods defined based on people's perceptions may be relevant when the neighborhood characteristics of interest relate to social interactions or social cohesion, administratively defined neighborhoods may be relevant when the hypothesized processes involve policies, and geographically defined neighborhoods may be relevant when features of the chemical or physical environment (e.g., toxic exposures) are hypothesized to be important. More generally, the size and definition of the relevant geographic area may vary according to the processes through which the area effect is hypothesized to operate and the outcome being studied. Areas ranging from large to small with varying geographic definitions may be important for different health outcomes or for different mediating mechanisms. For some purposes, the relevant area may be the block on which a person resides, for others it may be the blocks around the residence, and for others it may be the geographic area in which services such as stores or other institutions are located. The size and definition of the area, the relevant processes, and the outcome being studied are linked. The development and testing of hypotheses regarding the precise geographic area that is relevant for a specific health outcome is a key challenge to neighborhood health effects research.

A second key issue is specifying (and measuring) the relevant area or neighborhood characteristics. To date, most existing research has examined how aggregate measures of neighborhood socioeconomic context are related to health outcomes. These associations are compatible with a wide range of processes relating neighborhood environments to

health. Establishing whether the associations observed reflect causal processes will require the direct empirical examination of the specific features of areas that may be related to different outcomes. The specification of these features is directly linked to theory on the processes hypothesized to be involved. The features of neighborhoods that are relevant are likely to differ from health outcome to health outcome but may include both material (physical or infrastructure) and social attributes. Material features may include, for example, availability of parks and recreational resources, density of fast-food stores, and toxic exposures. Social features may include social cohesion and social norms and values, which may, for example, influence the adoption of behaviors. In their proposed framework for conceptualizing, operationalizing, and measuring neighborhood effects on health, MacIntyre, Ellaway, and Cummins (2002) have referred to these two broad domains as features of material infrastructure and features of collective social functioning. To date, however, few studies have examined specific features of areas as predictors of health.

From a methodological point of view, examining the role of specific neighborhood or area characteristics is complex, because many of these dimensions may be interrelated (and thus difficult to tease apart) and may also influence each other. For example, features of the physical environments of neighborhoods may influence the types of social interactions, and vice versa. In addition, the processes involved, and the relevant neighborhood attributes, may differ from one outcome to another. For example, mechanisms involving resources and the physical environment may be more relevant for some outcomes (e.g., physical activity), whereas those involving social norms or contagion processes may be more important for others (e.g., smoking).

From the operational point of view, the measurement of specific characteristics of neighborhoods is complex. Options for the collection of this type of information include surveys of residents (which may be aggregated up to the desired area level) on objective and subjective characteristics of their neighborhoods, direct observation or videotaping and ranking of neighborhoods on prespecified criteria by raters (systematic social observation), and linking databases with geographically linked information (e.g., from public agencies) and estimating density and distance measures. The assessment of neighborhoods or areas presents a series of methodological challenges related to the measurement of ecological settings.

A crucial problem in the examination of neighborhood effects is how individual-level characteristics should be incorporated into the conceptual models and included in the analyses. The most common criticism of neighborhood effects is that they result from confounding by individual-level variables, that is, that differences across neighborhoods are not due to the effects of neighborhoods per se but rather to differences in the types of people living in different neighborhoods. The selection problem is a variant of this issue: People may be sorted into neighborhoods based on individual characteristics, and it may be these individual characteristics rather than neighborhood attributes that are related to health. The ideal solution to this problem is the use of experiments or randomized trials. Although some randomized trials of changes in neighborhood contexts have included health measures as outcomes, the vast majority of work remains observational. As a way to respond to the confounding and selection problem, observational studies have attempted to control for individual-level variables, most commonly indicators of social position, in order to determine whether associations are "independent" of individual-level attributes. Although this approach has served to revitalize interest in neighborhood health effects, it has several limitations in terms of estimating true causal effects of neighborhoods on health. To the extent that neighborhoods influence the life chances of individuals, neighborhood social and economic characteristics may be related to health through their effects on the achieved income, education, and occupation of their residents, making these individual-level characteristics mediators (at least in part) of neighborhood health effects rather than confounders. In addition, because socioeconomic position is one of the dimensions along which residential segregation occurs, living in disadvantaged neighborhoods may be one of the mechanisms leading to adverse health outcomes in persons of low socioeconomic position. For these reasons, although teasing apart the "independent" effects of both dimensions may be useful as part of the analytic process, it is also artificial.

Because disease is expressed in individuals, neighborhood factors necessarily exert their effect through individual-level processes, including behaviors and biological precursors of disease. For example, if neighborhood environments are related to cardiovascular

risk, they may exert their effects by influencing the behaviors of individuals. This raises questions regarding what individual-level variables should be controlled for in estimating neighborhood effects. Moreover, recent work has highlighted the limitations of multivariate adjustment strategies in estimating "independent" effects in situations (like the investigation of neighborhood effects) involving complex causal chains and numerous confounders and mediators. Further complexity results from the fact that in some cases, neighborhood and individual characteristics may mutually influence each other. For example, the availability of healthy foods in a neighborhood may influence the dietary behaviors of individuals, and individual behaviors may in turn affect food availability. In other words, individual properties may themselves shape neighborhood attributes. Understanding area or neighborhood effects may require the testing of hypotheses involving dynamic and reciprocal relations like these. The multivariate adjustment methods usually used in epidemiology (and used in the vast majority of neighborhood effects studies to date) are not well suited to the identification of causal neighborhood effects in these situations.

In addition to being mediators or confounders of neighborhood effects, it is likely that individual-level characteristics interact with neighborhood properties in shaping health outcomes. For example, gradients by individual-level income may be stronger in poor neighborhoods (where those with low income are unable to gain access to resources outside the neighborhood) than in rich neighborhoods (where the comparative advantage conferred by high income is not as great). Although a few studies have investigated interactions between neighborhood socioeconomic characteristics and individual-level social class indicators, results have not been fully consistent regarding the types of interactions present. The investigation of interactions requires large data sets and is precluded if correlations between neighborhood and individual-level variables are very high. Nevertheless, the development and testing of specific hypotheses regarding interactions may help enhance understanding of the processes though which neighborhood contexts may affect health.

Both cross-sectional and longitudinal study designs have been used to examine associations between neighborhood characteristics and health. Although several longitudinal studies have neighborhood differences in mortality or incidence of disease, most research has relied on the measurement of neighborhood environments at one point in time. Persons change neighborhoods over their life course, and neighborhoods themselves may also change over time. The cumulative or interacting effects of neighborhood environments measured at different times over the life course, the effects of duration of exposure to certain neighborhood conditions, the effects of changes over time in neighborhood characteristics, and the impact of moving from one neighborhood to another have not been systematically examined. The investigation of these longitudinal and life course dimensions will require study designs that follow both individuals and neighborhoods over time. More generally, there has been relatively little attention in existing research to the time scale over which any neighborhood effects are hypothesized to operate. Whereas for some health outcomes neighborhood characteristics measured simultaneously with the outcome may be relevant (e.g., availability of recreational spaces at a given point in time may be related to individuals' physical activity at the same point in time), for others longer time lags may be involved.

There has also been growing interest in increasing the use of experimental study designs in the investigation of neighborhood effects. One option is the inclusion of health outcome measures in randomized intervention studies, where, for example, families from disadvantaged neighborhoods are randomly assigned to move to low poverty areas. The randomization avoids the limitations (predominantly related to selection problems) inherent in observational studies. This approach, however, does not allow identification of the specific features of neighborhoods that are relevant, and also has limitations stemming from participation rates and dropouts.

Combinations of quantitative and qualitative research approaches may be especially useful in research on neighborhood health effects. There is a long history of ethnographic studies of how neighborhoods influence individuals within them. Qualitative studies may be helpful in understanding the processes involved as well as the dynamic interactions between area and individual characteristics, which may be difficult or impossible to examine using purely quantitative approaches. The combination of smaller-scale, in-depth approaches (qualitative and quantitative) focusing on a few contrasting neighborhoods with large-scale analyses of routinely available quantitative data on a large sample spanning a broader range of neighborhoods is a promising area.

An additional issue that has yet to be fully explored in research on neighborhood effects pertains to spatial dependencies across neighborhoods themselves. Aside from the need to account for these spatial dependencies in studies of neighborhood effects, investigation and quantification of these spatial dependencies may itself be of interest in terms of understanding the role of place in health. Just as individuals are interacting and interdependent parts of social groups, neighborhoods (as well as other geographically defined areas) are interdependent and interacting parts within larger wholes. For example, neighborhoods may play different roles within the social and economic structure of a city, and health-related differences across neighborhoods may be partly shaped by how neighborhoods relate to each other within the larger city structure. Only recently have these spatial processes begun to be directly investigated in neighborhood effects research, and applications to health outcomes remain rare. The presence of multiple levels as well as the roles of dynamic interactions within and between levels is a challenge in the investigation of neighborhood effects as it is for epidemiology generally.

The recent surge in neighborhood effects research in health has been fruitful in that it has stimulated thinking on the ways in which social processes (in this case the patterning of social and physical attributes across space) may influence health. Nevertheless, empirical research in this field remains plagued by complexities that make it difficult to definitively conclude from existing work whether neighborhood contexts are indeed causally related to health, and if so, what the mediating processes may be. Current research efforts focus on studies specially designed to test hypotheses regarding the specific processes through which neighborhood or area effects may affect specific health outcomes, and the time scale over which these effects may operate.

—*Ana V. Diez Roux*

See also ECOLOGICAL MODELS: APPLICATIONS TO PHYSICAL ACTIVITY; ECOSOCIAL THEORY; SOCIOECONOMIC STATUS AND HEALTH

Further Reading

Diez Roux, A. V. (2001). Investigating neighborhood and area effects on health. *American Journal of Public Health, 91*, 1783-1789.

Jones, K., & Duncan, C. (1995). Individuals and their ecologies: Analysing the geography of chronic illness within a multilevel modelling framework. *Health Place 1*, 27-40.

Kaplan, G. A. (1996). People and places: Contrasting perspectives on the association between social class and health. *International Journal of Health Services 26,* 507-519.

Katz, L. F., King, J., & Liebman, J. B. (2001). Moving to opportunity in Boston: Early results of a randomized mobility experiment. *Quarterly Journal of Economics, 116,* 607-654.

MacIntyre, S., Ellaway, A., & Cummins, S. (2002). Place effects on health: How can we conceptualise, operationalise and measure them? *Social Science and Medicine, 55,* 125-139.

MacIntyre, S., Maciver, S., & Sooman, A. (1993). Area, class, and health: Should we be focusing on places or people? *Journal of Social Policy, 22,* 213-234.

Pickett, K. E., & Pearl, M. (2001). Multilevel analyses of neighbourhood socioeconomic context and health outcomes: a critical review. *Journal of Epidemiology and Community Health, 55,* 111-122.

Raudenbush, S. W., & Sampson, R. J. (1999). Ecometrics: Toward a science of assessing ecological settings, with application to the systematic social observation of neighborhoods. *Sociological Methodology 29,* 1-41.

Robert, S. A. (1999). Socioeconomic position and health: The independent contribution of community socioeconomic context. *Annual Review of Sociology, 25,* 489-516.

Sampson, R. J., Morenoff, J. D., & Gannon-Rowley, T. (2002). Assessing "neighborhood effects": Social processes and new directions in research. *Annual Review of Sociology, 28,* 443-478.

Tienda, M. (1991). Poor people and poor places: Deciphering neighborhood effects on poverty outcomes. In J. Huber (Ed.), *Macro-micro linkages in sociology* (pp. 244-262). Newbury Park, CA: Sage.

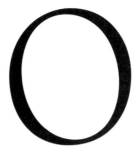

OBESITY: CAUSES AND CONSEQUENCES

The prevalence of obesity has increased dramatically in the past three decades and is a serious concern in the United States. According to the National Center for Health Statistics in 1999, 61% of American adults were classified as overweight or obese. The prevalence is even higher among African Americans and Hispanics; nearly two thirds of African Americans are overweight or obese. In addition, the number of overweight children has increased dramatically. Between 1963 and 1980, childhood obesity increased by 98% among 6- to 11-year-olds. Prevalence in children is estimated to be 14% to 22% (Strauss, 2002). Excessive weight is associated with a number of health problems and ultimately mortality. Being overweight also brings with it a number of psychological and social consequences.

DEFINING OVERWEIGHT AND OBESITY

When the energy a person consumes exceeds energy expenditure, weight gain results. One is considered to be obese when the body contains an excess of body fat (normally accounting for 25% of weight in women and 18% in men). Because body fat is difficult to measure, other indices have been developed to define obesity. Body mass index (BMI) is a commonly used metric in epidemiological studies for defining body weight and has a high correlation with direct measures of body fat. It is computed as weight in kilograms divided by height in meters squared. The World Health Organization and the National Heart, Lung, and Blood Institute have classified those with a BMI of < 18.5 kg/m^2 to be underweight, 18.5 to 24.9 kg/m^2 as healthy weight, 25 to 29.9 kg/m^2 as overweight, and $= 30$ kg/m^2 as obese. A BMI of 30 corresponds roughly to 40% above ideal weight.

BMI is frequently used as a guideline for establishing ideal weights because it has a strong relationship with mortality; at a BMI of 30, the risk of mortality increases approximately 30%. BMI does not take gender or frame size into account, is not a measurement of body fat, and does not assess for weight in specific areas of the body, but it is a useful heuristic in assessing body fat and calculating potential health risks.

DETERMINANTS

The determinants of body weight are not well understood, but there is increasing evidence that both genetics and environment play important roles.

Genetics

In families where one individual is obese, the likelihood that others will be obese as well doubles and is 7 to 8 times higher in families where there is extreme obesity (BMI > 45). In addition, obesity in children is more frequent in families where both parents are overweight. Genes are thought to explain 25% to 40% of the population variance in BMI. In studies of identical twins reared apart, genes account for 70% of the variance in BMI, whereas studies comparing adopted children and parents yield the lowest heritability levels (30% or less). Obesity-prone individuals may have increased appetite, diminished likelihood of being physically active, or metabolic differences in the way the body handles both calories consumed and expended.

Despite evidence of a strong genetic component in determining weight, the specific genes that influence body weight or predisposition to weight gain are not well known. One gene of interest, the *ob* gene, encodes a protein hormone called leptin. Higher concentrations of leptin are found in overweight individuals and increase proportionally with body fat. Leptin secretion leads to activation in brain areas involved in regulation of food intake and energy balance. Research on leptin as a body weight regulator is ongoing, but early studies have shown that some individuals injected with leptin serum lose weight, suggesting that some obese individuals may have developed leptin resistance, much like diabetics develop insulin resistance.

Environment

While genetics helps address obesity at an individual level, large population increases in obesity are explained by the environment. Many studies show that obesity rates in countries rise with modernization. This societal increase is a reflection of the "toxic food environment" in which Americans live.

In the United States, high-sugar, high-fat, and hence high-calorie junk food is affordable and convenient, and portion sizes are growing. The 8-ounce soft drinks of 50 years ago are now 16-ounce or 20-ounce bottles. Fast food chains promote larger-size "value meals" that can fulfill, in one meal, almost one entire day's recommended calorie intake. Children are often the targets of junk food promotion. More than 5,000 schools in the United States have contracts with fast food agencies to have outlets in the cafeterias. In addition, the average child watches 10,000 food advertisements on television each year, the majority of which are advertisements for sugared cereals, candy, fast foods, and soft drinks.

Compounding the problem of increasing energy expenditure is the increasing sedentary nature of modern societies. The Office of the Surgeon General's report on activity and health found that more than 60% of Americans do not obtain regular physical activity and 25% get no activity at all. The Centers for Disease Control and Prevention and the American College of Sports Medicine recommend 30 minutes of moderate activity three to five times per week. The population is far from this.

HEALTH RISK FACTORS

Approximately 280,000 deaths are attributable to obesity each year in the United States alone. Excess body weight is associated with a number of risk factors for coronary heart disease, such as hypertension, hyperglycemia, increases in low-density lipoprotein (LDL) and triglyceride levels, and decreases in high-density lipoprotein (HDL). These risk factors increase the likelihood of stroke, heart disease, and death. Distribution of fat also appears to affect health risks; excess upper-body fat is associated with hypertension, diabetes, and other medical problems.

Disease

Weight gains of more than 10 kg are associated with elevated incidence of hypertension and coronary heart disease. Risk of Type 2 diabetes increases even with weight gains of 5 kg between age 18 and midlife. Risk for developing endometrial and gallbladder cancer and gallstones are several times higher in obese individuals compared to average-weight individuals. Gallbladder disease among women in the highest BMI quartile is almost 3 times as high as women in the lowest, and twice as high among men. Osteoarthritis of the knees and hips are also strongly associated with body weight, but overweight women are less likely to become subject to hip fractures and breast cancer. Even modest weight loss of 5% to 15% is associated with improvements in blood pressure, lipids, and insulin sensitivity.

WELL-BEING

Psychological Effects and Consequences

Because of relentless social pressure to be thin, strong bias against overweight individuals exists, and hence many obese individuals suffer from guilt and shame. Research on whether obese individuals have more psychopathology overall is mixed. Most studies comparing obese and nonobese groups on psychological variables such as depression and anxiety have not found consistent differences; thus, it appears that not all obese individuals suffer psychological distress from their obesity. Body image dissatisfaction has been found to be consistently high in obese individuals, especially in adolescent girls and college-age women, which may increase the risks of habitual dieting or developing an eating disorder. It is probably the case that some obese individuals endure considerable distress and others do not, hence it is important to find what makes some more vulnerable than others.

Social Effects and Consequences

Obesity also has social and economic consequences. Direct health care costs attributable to obesity in 1995 were estimated at $51.6 billion, almost 6% of the total health care expenditure for that year. Physician visits attributable to obesity nearly doubled between 1988 and 1994, to 81.2 million visits per year. Using health care claims, obese employees had 21.4% more health care expenditures than lean employees, an increase comparable to risk factors such as smoking, high blood pressure, and high alcohol intake.

There are indirect costs attributable to obesity as well. In 1994, obese persons lost 39.2 million workdays; the lost productivity is estimated at around $3.93 billion. High-level absenteeism (seven or more absences due to illness during the previous 6 months) is twice as high among obese employees as average-weight employees, and moderate absenteeism (three to six absences) is 1.49 times as likely. In 1994, 5.9% of men and 4.7% of women with a healthy body weight were unable to work, compared to 5.6% and 7.9%, respectively, in the overweight population, and 9.6% and 12.6% in the obese population.

In addition to economic consequences of the condition, overweight individuals are less likely to get married and complete less schooling than average-weight individuals. In children, being overweight is associated with problems with peers, the consequences of which may extend far into the future.

One important factor in understanding the psychosocial consequences of obesity is the existence of bias and discrimination. Obese individuals are stereotyped as stupid and lazy, and they experience discrimination in many domains of life, including at school, with employment and promotions, and in medical settings. Negative attitudes about weight are conveyed through magazines, television, and everyday conversation; obesity is seen as a controllable condition and therefore overweight people deserve blame and scorn.

CONCLUSION

Obesity is an ever-increasing problem. Excess body weight brings greatly increased risk for medical and psychosocial problems. Body weight is partially determined by genetics, but the environment has a strong relationship with weight and might be improved by decreasing consumption of high-calorie foods and increasing physical activity. Research pertaining to the psychopathology of obese individuals is not uniform, but there is clearly psychological distress in a subset of the obese. Acceptance of overweight individuals may lead to less psychological distress and minimize some of the psychosocial effects of obesity.

—Shirley S. Wang and
Kelly D. Brownell

See also OBESITY IN CHILDREN: PHYSICAL ACTIVITY AND NUTRITIONAL APPROACHES; OBESITY IN CHILDREN: PREVENTION; OBESITY: PREVENTION AND TREATMENT

Further Reading

Ebbeling, C. B., Pawlak, D. B., & Ludwig, D. S. (2002). Childhood obesity: Public health crisis, common sense cure. *Lancet, 360,* 473-482.

Fairburn, C. G., & Brownell, K. D. (Eds.). (2002). *Eating disorders and obesity: A comprehensive handbook* (2nd ed.). New York: Guilford.

National Heart, Lung, and Blood Institute, National Institutes of Health. (1998). Clinical guidelines on the identification, evaluation, and treatment of overweight and obesity in adults: The evidence report. *Obesity Research, 6*(Suppl. 2), 51S-209S.

Strauss, R. S. (2002). Childhood obesity. *Pediatric Clinics of North America, 49,* 175-201.

Wadden, T., & Stunkard, A. J. (Eds.). (2002). *Handbook of obesity treatment.* New York: Guilford.

Wadden, T. A., Brownell, K. D., & Foster, G. D. (2002). Obesity: Responding to the global epidemic. *Journal of Consulting and Clinical Psychology, 70,* 510-525.

OBESITY IN CHILDREN: PHYSICAL ACTIVITY AND NUTRITIONAL APPROACHES

Obesity in youths has increased to epidemic proportions in the last two decades. This poses a serious health hazard. Obesity is often the precursor to other diseases, such as Type 2 diabetes and hypertension, that can lead to cardiovascular disease (CVD) in adulthood, and some of these complications emerge during the childhood and adolescent years. It is therefore imperative to intervene in childhood in order to retard or negate the appearance of obesity and CVD risk factors such as high levels of insulin, glucose, cholesterol, triacylglycerol, and blood pressure.

Decreased energy expenditure and increased energy intake are two of the major lifestyle behaviors thought to play a role in the development of obesity and consequent CVD. Decreases in moderate and vigorous physical activity (PA) and increases in sedentary activities such as television viewing, video game playing, and computer use have been associated with decreased energy expenditure. Other potential contributing factors are decreases in time spent in physical education at school, and the perception that neighborhoods may be unsafe for children to play in unsupervised. The increased availability and consumption of fast food, soft drinks, and other high-sugar or high-calorie foods and beverages are also thought to be contributors to the obesity epidemic. There are several possible settings for interventions targeting PA and nutrition in youths, including school, home, community, and medical offices. The focus here is on PA and nutrition interventions conducted in nonmedical settings.

Two of the important time periods that can be targeted with PA interventions in children and adolescents are during school and immediately after school. The small number of studies that have used interventions targeting health education and/or physical education classes have yielded mixed results. Some of the studies that measured adiposity using either body mass index or skin folds reported significant decreases in adiposity in youths who were exposed to an intervention compared to controls, while most reported no significant differences between the two groups. One study that had a comprehensive 2-year school-based intervention found a decrease in the prevalence of obesity and an increase in obesity remission in girls but not boys, and a decrease in television viewing in girls and boys. Another comprehensive 2-year study in middle schools found a decrease in adiposity in boys but not girls. Few studies have measured the effect of the intervention on CVD risk factors. Some studies found beneficial effects on blood pressure, total cholesterol (TC), high-density

lipoprotein cholesterol (HDLC), and TC/HDLC. In some cases, these changes were gender specific. Other studies found no significant effect of the intervention on lipids, cholesterol, or insulin and glucose. The disparities in the results may be due to several factors, including (a) whether the intervention occurred in the classroom, during physical education, or both, (b) the length of the intervention (i.e., 8 weeks to 3 years), (c) the age range of the subjects, and (d) the actual content of the intervention.

Fewer studies still have been conducted in the after-school time period, when youths are likely to engage in sedentary activities such as television viewing while consuming high-calorie, high-fat snacks. In one study, 79 obese 7- to 11-year-olds were randomized to either (a) a group that engaged in PA for the first 4-month period and then ceased PA for the next 4 months or (b) a group that served as a control for the first 4 months and then engaged in PA for the next 4 months. The goal of this study was to investigate the effect of PA on body composition (primarily adiposity), CV fitness, CV risk factors, and free-living diet and PA. Compared with the 4-month periods of no-PA, favorable changes were seen during the 4-month periods of PA in percentage of body fat, vigorous PA, insulin, and triacylglycerol. In another study, 81 obese 13- to 16-year-olds were randomized to one of three groups: (1) lifestyle education (LSE) sessions only, (2) LSE plus moderate-intensity PA, or (3) LSE plus vigorous PA; the energy expenditure for the two PA groups was controlled by having the moderate-intensity group exercise longer each session. The PA reduced percentage of body fat, although there was no clear effect of intensity. Favorable changes were seen in triacylglycerol, TC/HDLC, and diastolic blood pressure. In a study without a control group, 12 weeks of PA after school resulted in decreased adiposity in obese 11- to 14-year-old African American and Hispanic girls. The results of these studies indicate that controlled PA interventions held in the after-school hours can favorably impact adiposity and CVD risk factors in youths.

Nutrition interventions have targeted two school settings: providing nutrition information in the classroom and modifying the food items and choices offered by the school. Most studies that modified the foods offered by the school found decreases in fat intake during school lunch and decreased energy intake and increased fruit and vegetable intake as measured by 24-hour recalls. One 2-year study found no effect on fat intake. Studies that provided nutrition education found beneficial changes, including decreased intake of foods high in cholesterol and fat, decreased fat intake, increased fiber intake, increased fruit and vegetable intake, and choosing healthier snacks.

Studies whose goal it is to change both youths' PA and nutrition behaviors are hard to implement successfully, and even then can yield varying results. Outcome measures are often limited to the actual behaviors, that is, fat intake or time spent doing PA, and may sometimes include measures of adiposity. Few studies have measured actual CVD risk factors, which may incur beneficial changes even in the absence of changes in adiposity. Therefore, interventions need to be designed and tested that are comprehensive in nature. Furthermore, in order to measure the impact of these interventions on CVD risk, outcome measures also need to be comprehensive, including adiposity and several CVD risk factors.

—*Paule Barbeau*

See also OBESITY: CAUSES AND CONSEQUENCES; OBESITY IN CHILDREN: PREVENTION; OBESITY: PREVENTION AND TREATMENT; SCHOOL-BASED HEALTH PROMOTION

Further Reading

Crespo, C. J., Smit, E., Troiano, R. P., Bartlett, S. J., Macera, C. A., & Andersen, R. E. (2001). Television watching, energy intake, and obesity in U.S. children: Results from the third National Health and Nutrition Examination Survey, 1988-1994. *Archives of Pediatric and Adolescent Medicine, 155,* 360-365.

Fardy, P. S., White, R. E., Haltiwanger-Schmitz, K., Magel, J. R., McDermott, K. J., Clark, L. T., et al. (1996). Coronary disease risk factor reduction and behavior modification in minority adolescents: The PATH program. *Journal of Adolescent Health, 18,* 247-253.

Gortmaker, S. L., Peterson, K., Wiecha, J., Sobol, A. M., Dixit, S., Fox, M. K., et al. (1999). Reducing obesity via a school-based interdisciplinary intervention among youth: Planet Health. *Archives of Pediatric and Adolescent Medicine, 153,* 409-418.

Gutin, B., & Barbeau, P. (2000). Physical activity and body composition in children and adolescents. In C. Bouchard (Ed.), *Physical activity and obesity* (pp. 213-245). Champaign, IL: Human Kinetics.

Harrell, J. S., McMurray, R. G., Gansky, S. A., Bangdiwala, S. I., & Bradley, C. B. (1999). A public health vs. a risk-based intervention to improve cardiovascular health in elementary school children: The Cardiovascular Health in Children Study. *American Journal of Public Health, 89,* 1529-1535.

Hill, J. O., & Peters, J. C. (1998) Environmental contributions to the obesity epidemic. *Science, 280,* 1371-1377.

Troiano, R. P., & Flegal, K. M. (1999). Overweight prevalence among youth in the United States: Why so many different numbers? *International Journal of Obesity and Related Metabolic Disorders, 23*(Suppl. 2), S22-S27.

OBESITY IN CHILDREN: PREVENTION

Obesity among children and youth, sometimes called overweight, is typically defined as a body mass index (calculated by dividing weight by height squared, and expressed as kg/m^2) greater than or equal to the 95th percentile for children of the same age and gender. The prevalence of obesity among children and youth increased rapidly in the United States and other industrialized countries during the period 1970 to 2000. Obesity rates are also rising among children in less industrialized countries and among adults globally. Although the causes of obesity include both genetic and environmental determinants, obesity ultimately results from an excess of energy intake via diet relative to energy expenditure via physical activity. Both energy intake and expenditure can be influenced by individuals and their social and physical environment, and hence are the foci for action to prevent or treat obesity.

Obesity during adolescence is the best single predictor of adult obesity, although this relationship is not strong for early childhood obesity. Some studies also indicate prenatal risks. Efforts to prevent obesity and reduce obesity risk among children and youth are thus particularly important, and are focused on factors that affect food intake and physical activity in household, school, and community environments.

Coincident with the increase in obesity among children and youth in recent decades has been a tremendous increase in the availability of foods for consumption and in advertising directed at children to promote consumption. There is consistent evidence for increasing inactivity in children's and adolescents' lives during this time, particularly increasing television viewing. Television viewing has been related to this increasing prevalence in multiple longitudinal and cross-sectional observational studies. This effect is most likely due to both the displacement of more vigorous activities by television and effects on diet. Foods are the most heavily advertised product on children's television, and television viewing time is associated with between-meal snacking. Both clinical and school-based randomized trials have demonstrated that reduction in time spent watching television reduces obesity. Television viewing reduction is thus one realistic target for preventive efforts in households.

Another opportunity for prevention includes anticipatory guidance counseling for parents from primary health care providers focused on potential sources of excess caloric intake, such as sugar-sweetened beverages and super-sized foods, as well as reductions in time spent watching television.

School-based programs represent an important channel for behavioral change because of near universal enrollment and the potential to affect behaviors of children that track into adolescence and adulthood. Coordinated school health programming can potentially impact student diet and activity levels via altering school-based curricula, activities, and environments. Randomized trials indicate the success of school curricula in improving diet, reducing television viewing, and reducing obesity.

Because 15% of children and youth are now overweight or obese, prevention of adult obesity needs to include treatment of children and youth. However, the only interventions that have shown long-term effectiveness in reducing obesity have been intensive clinical programs for obese children. These are intensive programs that require parental participation, professional staff, and focus on modifications in both diet and physical activity levels.

—*Steven L. Gortmaker*

See also OBESITY: CAUSES AND CONSEQUENCES; OBESITY IN CHILDREN: PHYSICAL ACTIVITY AND NUTRITIONAL APPROACHES; OBESITY: PREVENTION AND TREATMENT

Further Reading

Dietz, W. H., & Gortmaker, S. L. (2001). Preventing obesity in children and adolescents. *Annual Review of Public Health, 22,* 237-253.

Ebbeling, C. B., Pawlak, D. B., & Ludwig, D. S. (2002). Childhood obesity: Public-health crisis, common sense cure. *Lancet, 360,* 473-482.

Epstein, L. H. , Myers, M. D., Raynor, H. A., & Saelens, B. E. (1998). Treatment of pediatric obesity. *Pediatrics, 101*(3, Pt. 2), 554-570.

World Health Organization. (2000). *Obesity: Preventing and managing the global epidemic: Report of a WHO consultation* (WHO Tech. Rep. Ser. 894), 1-253.

OBESITY: PREVENTION AND TREATMENT

Obesity is a condition characterized by elevated fat mass. It is typically estimated by the body mass index (BMI; kg/m^2), which is highly correlated with measures of body fat. The World Health Organization (WHO) defines the desirable range as a BMI between 18.5 and 24.9, *overweight* as a BMI of 25 to 29.9, *obese* as a BMI of 30 or greater, and *morbidly obese* as a BMI of 40 or greater. These categories have been established to reflect physical health risks associated with increasing BMI.

Obesity increases risk for cardiovascular disease, diabetes, hypertension, stroke, gallbladder disease, respiratory disease, some kinds of cancer, and more. Risk is determined in part by the distribution of fat on the body, with intraabdominal adiposity putting individuals at greatest risk. Risk for increased mental health difficulties does not appear to increase with BMI. As a group, the obese do not experience greater psychiatric symptoms than their nonobese counterparts, although the subgroup of individuals who seek professional weight reduction treatment are more likely to report depression, anxiety, and binge eating.

By 1999, rates of obesity in the United States reached 27%, with an additional 34% of individuals meeting criteria for overweight. These figures represent a dramatic increase over the previous decade, with a particularly steep increase in children and adolescents. Obesity has become the single most expensive health problem in the United States, surpassing smoking and alcohol in its medical and financial impact; in 1995, obesity-related complications were estimated to cost the United States $99 billion. Furthermore, the stigma associated with obesity affects the quality of life of obese persons. Obese women are less likely to complete high school, less likely to marry, and have lower household incomes. Overweight individuals are subjected to prejudice and discrimination when seeking college admissions, employment, and housing.

The etiology of obesity is simultaneously simple and complicated. Simply, one gains weight when taking in more calories than are expended. How this imbalance comes about, however, represents the confluence of biological, psychological, and environmental factors. Between 25% and 40% of an individual's weight is genetically determined through the mechanisms of fat cell number, basal metabolic rate, weight gain in response to overfeeding, and other factors. The remainder is accounted for by an individual's behavior and its interactions with biology and an environment increasingly supportive of weight gain. Longitudinal research has shown that individuals who move from less modernized to more modernized countries gain weight. The latter environment is one in which individuals are constantly exposed to energy-dense, heavily advertised, inexpensive foods, and in which a more sedentary lifestyle is supported—what Kelly Brownell and colleagues refer to as the "toxic environment."

Demographic risk factors for obesity include age, gender (being female), ethnic minority status, lower socioeconomic status, and having a family history of obesity.

TREATMENT

Goals of Treatment

Most weight loss approaches will produce some initial weight loss, and some will produce significant loss. However, the data consistently show that few individuals will achieve long-term maintenance of significant weight loss. Thus, treatment goals of reaching the "ideal weight" have been replaced with goals of a loss of 5% to 15% of body weight, a figure associated with significant improvements in a variety of health indices. Furthermore, increasing physical activity and improving diet improve health indices independent of weight loss. Goals of modest weight loss, healthier eating, and increased activity are recommended.

Treatment Matching

Treatment matching is a strategy for selecting an appropriate level of treatment based on a patient's risk profile. Less intensive and expensive approaches are recommended for individuals with lower BMIs, such that for lowest risk persons a program of prevention of weight gain through self-directed efforts and/or primary care support may suffice. The more aggressive and expensive treatments, such as pharmacological approaches or bariatric surgery, are recommended for individuals with BMIs of > 30 and > 40 respectively. The more aggressive approaches carry with them greater risk of more serious side effects, and only in very overweight individuals is the potential benefit of decreased risk of obesity-related health problems deemed to outweigh the risk of these side effects. For all patients, less aggressive approaches should be tried before more aggressive ones are resorted to.

Self-Help and Commercial Programs

There exist very little data on commercial weight loss programs. Weight Watchers has reported a recent average loss of 5 kg in 6 months among its group members, and substantial and maintained losses have been reported for the Trevose Weight Loss Program. While these particular programs are inexpensive (Trevose is free and Weight Watchers charges $12/meeting), most others are not so and provide no data on efficacy. There exist virtually no data on the efficacy of self-help programs promoted through popular diet books, which are purchased by millions each year. Data are sorely needed before recommendations can be made with respect to these treatments.

Behavioral Treatments

Most professionally directed behavioral weight loss programs operate in academic settings and are therefore well researched. They typically include dietary restriction (1200-1500 kcal/day), behavioral strategies to help limit intake (particularly of energy-dense foods) such as self-monitoring, portion control, and stimulus control. Many programs also include a focus on increased activity.

A 20-week program induces an average loss of 9 kg, approximately 9% of initial weight. Without further treatment, patients regain one third of lost weight in the year following treatment, with increasing regain over subsequent years. With further follow-up support, maintenance improves. Longer treatment does produce greater weight loss, although the rate of loss slows with time. Physical activity, whether through structured exercise periods or exercise incorporated into one's lifestyle, is associated with superior maintenance of weight loss. Very low-calorie diets

(400-800 kcal/day) produce a more dramatic initial weight loss, but these patients regain more rapidly than those on the more traditional regimen. It should be noted that most research on these programs has included predominantly Caucasian samples, a problematic state of affairs, given the high rates of obesity in ethnic minority populations in the United States.

It is notable that family-based behavioral weight loss treatments for obese children *do* produce significant and enduring results: One review revealed that, at 10-year follow-up, nearly 30% of children were no longer obese. These interventions include a diet and physical activity component, behavioral strategies such as self-monitoring, stimulus control, and positive reinforcement, and typically require active participation on the part of at least one parent through parental modeling of appropriate eating and activity behaviors. Behavioral interventions for adolescents are less successful, likely due to less parental control over the adolescent's behavior, suggesting the urgency of addressing obesity in its early stages.

Pharmacological Treatments

The realization that obesity is a chronic condition suggests the use of long-term pharmacological treatments. Currently, two medications are FDA approved for the long-term treatment of obesity. Sibutramine (Meridia) is a serotonin-norepinephrine reuptake inhibitor that appears to act on receptors in the hypothalamus that control satiety. Sibutramine is associated with increased heart rate and blood pressure and is contraindicated for individuals with hypertension and cardiovascular disease. Orlistat (Xenical) is a lipase inhibitor that produces weight loss by blocking the absorption of about one third of the fat a person consumes. The blocked fat is excreted from the body through stool, resulting in an overall reduction in calorie absorption. Consuming high-fat meals while taking this medication leads to unpleasant side effects that include oily stool and fecal incontinence; thus patients are reinforced for adhering to a low-fat diet. Both medications produce losses of 7% to 15% of initial weight, with greater losses achieved when the medications are combined with behavioral programs.

When obesity is accompanied by binge eating, selective serotonin reuptake inhibitor (SSRI) antidepressants (e.g., Prozac, Zoloft, Paxil) have produced decreases in binge eating and thereby some weight loss.

Surgical Treatments

Given the risks associated with surgery in general, and surgery in obese individuals in particular, surgical treatments are recommended only for individuals with a BMI of 40 or greater or those with a BMI of 35 *and* additional health risk factors. Two types of procedures are in current practice: gastric restrictive procedures and combined gastric restriction and malabsorption. The former includes vertical banded gastroplasty (VBG) and gastric banding. VBG involves the creation of a small gastric pouch at the base of the esophagus to limit possible intake. VBG produces initial average weight losses of 25% of initial body weight at 18 months. In gastric banding, the gastric reservoir is achieved through laparoscopic surgery by the application of a small belt below the esophagus; the size of the reservoir may be adjusted in an outpatient setting to suit patient needs. Reported weight losses associated with gastric banding reach up to 55% to 65% at 3-year follow-up.

Combined restriction and malabsorption procedures include the gastric bypass, the biliopancreatic diversion, and the duodenal switch. In the gastric bypass procedure, the pouch is created as in VBG, but the stomach and part of the intestine are bypassed by attaching the pouch to the jejunum. This procedure has produced average weight losses of 30% of initial weight during the first 18 months, with maintenance of a 25% loss up to 14 years later. The biliopancreatic and duodenal procedures are less common due to greater side effect profiles; they involve gastric resectioning and cholecystectomy and a lengthier bypass, and thus variations of malnutrition occur in a substantial minority of patients. Extensive evaluations generally precede surgery for the purpose of identifying contraindications and preparing the individual for the ensuing changes.

Over the years, significant advances have been made in surgical techniques and in the care of patients postsurgery; hence the risk of surgery has declined. The large weight losses are associated with dramatic improvements in health. Surgery for obesity can be life saving.

PREVENTION

Given the difficulty in treating obesity, prevention is the obvious alternative. Given the clear contribution of the environment to promoting weight gain, and the challenge in changing individual behavior within this environment, more macrolevels of intervention would seem an appropriate target. There exist little data on the prevention of obesity. However, a heart disease prevention program in Finland provides some evidence that macrolevel programs can be effective in producing clinically meaningful change. Some areas of the country saw a more than 75% reduction in premature deaths related to heart disease and stroke over a 20-year period following combined efforts of government and professionals at the policy level. Policy initiatives included setting and enforcing nutritional standards for food served in schools and at public catering outlets without a consequent increase in meal prices, as well as initiatives aimed at increasing physical activity.

Thus, prevention efforts must include not only encouragement of the individual to make personal change, but an environment that supports that change. Recent suggested targets of policy initiatives include controlling advertising, particularly to children; controlling sales conditions, for example, limited distribution of high-calorie/low-nutrient foods in schools; controlling pricing such that high-calorie/low-nutrient foods are more expensive and the sale of healthy foods is subsidized; and enhancing opportunities for physical activity, especially in demographically higher-risk populations.

CONCLUSION

The combination of prevalence, seriousness, and resistance to treatment make obesity one of the most significant public health problems of modern times. Advances have been made in treatment, but with the exception of surgery, weight losses tend to be modest and not well maintained. Prevention, therefore, must become top priority.

—Kathryn E. Henderson and
Kelly D. Brownell

See also OBESITY: CAUSES AND CONSEQUENCES; OBESITY IN
CHILDREN: PHYSICAL ACTIVITY AND NUTRITIONAL
APPROACHES; OBESITY IN CHILDREN: PREVENTION

Further Reading

Allison, D. B. (Ed.). (1995). *Handbook of assessment methods for eating behaviors and weight related problems: Measures, theory, and research.* Thousand Oaks, CA: Sage.

Brownell, K. D. (2000). *The LEARN program for weight management.* Dallas, TX: American Health.

Fairburn, C. G., & Brownell, K. D. (Eds.). (2002). *Eating disorders and obesity: A comprehensive handbook* (2nd ed.). New York: Guilford.

National Heart, Lung, and Blood Institute, National Institutes of Health. (1998). Clinical guidelines on the identification, evaluation, and treatment of overweight and obesity in adults-the Evidence Report. *Obesity Research, 6*(Suppl. 2), 51S-209S.

Puhl, R., & Brownell, K. D. (2001). Bias, discrimination, and obesity. *Obesity Research, 9,* 788-805.

Wadden, T. A., Brownell, K. D., & Foster, G. D. (2002). Obesity: Responding to the Global Epidemic. *Journal of Consulting and Clinical Psychology, 70,* 510-525.

Wadden, T., & Stunkard, A. J. (Eds.). (2002). *Handbook of obesity treatment.* New York: Guilford.

OCCUPATIONAL HEALTH AND SAFETY

Occupational health and safety is the field pertaining to the health and safety of the workforce. This field has been of societal concern since ancient times. The Edwin Smith Surgical Papyrus describes the treatment of injuries that were incurred by workers at the pyramid site in ancient Egypt (3000-2500 B.C.). Bernardino Ramazzini published the first Western textbook of occupational medicine in 1713. The pioneering work of Dr. Alice Hamilton in the 1920s served as a second of the initial steps toward the recognition of the field of Occupational Health and Safety in the United States.

Approximately 6,500 fatalities and 3,200,000 nonfatal injuries occur in the United States each year as a result of occupational injuries. In addition, there are about 862,200 occupational-related illnesses and 60,300 fatalities from occupational-related illnesses annually. Acute trauma is the leading cause of death and disability at work. Between 1980 and 1995, there were 16 deaths per day from trauma at work. Data from the National Institute for Occupational Safety and Health (NIOSH) reveal that $171 billion is spent each year in direct and indirect costs of occupational injuries and illnesses.

Each workplace has its own unique challenges. Selected occupational groups with hazards specific to their employment include workers in the hospital setting who are exposed to infectious agents such as hepatitis and HIV and to chemical hazards such as ethylene oxide. Firefighters face hazards such as smoke inhalation and medical sequelae thereof, and office workers face ergonomic hazards. According to the Bureau of Labor Statistics, the construction industry accounted for a greater proportion of fatalities than any other major industrial classification. In 1999, this industry accounted for 19.8% of the 6,023 occupational fatalities in the United States. Fatal falls accounted for 31.8% of the 119 fatalities. Selected occupational conditions of increased current concern are musculoskeletal disorders, exposure to poor indoor air quality, allergies, dermatitis, asthma, fertility and pregnancy abnormalities, hearing loss, infectious diseases, and violence and stress in the workplace. The modern workplace faces added stressors such as longer hours, shift work, compressed workweeks, and decreased job security.

Special populations such as the older worker, teen workers, and female workers may face hazards unique to their occupational group. According to the National Traumatic Occupational Fatalities data, workers aged 65 and older had a workplace fatality rate 2.6 times that of workers aged 16 to 64. Mining, agriculture, and construction saw the highest rates. Older men were at higher risk for fatalities caused by machines and older women for fatal falls and homicide. The number of older workers is projected to increase in the future. Young workers are also at risk; 70 teenagers die each year from work-related injuries in the United States, and 77,000 present to the emergency room with work-related injury. A study by NIOSH suggested that the three leading categories of work-related fatalities for 16- and 17-year-olds, namely, motor vehicle injuries, homicides, and machinery-related deaths, claim this age group at rates similar to or slightly higher than rates for adult workers.

It is projected that by the year 2008, women will represent 48% of the estimated 155 million workers. Compared to men, women appear to suffer disproportionately from some disorders. For example, musculoskeletal disorders account for 52% of injuries and illnesses suffered by female workers compared to 45% for men. In two thirds of the injuries resulting from workplace violence, the victims were women. Homicide, the leading cause of injury death in the workplace for women, accounts for 40% of these deaths. Hazards in the workplace may increase the risk of cancers unique to women, such as cervical and breast cancer. Women disproportionately comprise personnel in the health care industry, as 92% of the 4.3 million nurses and nurses' aides are women, thus exposing women to hazards unique to the health care setting.

The occupational medicine physician, the safety professional, and the management all work together to help provide a safe work environment. The occupational medicine physician provides care to workers who sustain work-related injuries and illnesses, and is responsible for establishing surveillance programs and instituting preventive measures in an effort to help provide a safe work environment. Safety professionals are concerned with the prevention and control of work-related injuries, illnesses, and other harmful events resulting from work. They are trained to recognize that occupational injuries and illnesses can be anticipated and prevented. They educate managers, supervisors, and employees regarding hazards that can cause injuries or illness, thus empowering them to help devise preventive measures. Ensuring a safe workplace cannot be accomplished without support from top management, however. In an effort to support occupational safety and health, management institutes preventive programs and provides occupational medicine services and proper personal protective equipment to employees. In addition, management helps to foster a climate at work where occupational health and safety is made a priority. The American College of Occupational and Environmental Medicine (ACOEM) is the nation's largest medical society dedicated to promoting the health of the worker. It was founded in 1916 and represents more than 6,000 physicians and other health care professionals specializing in the field of occupational medicine. ACOEM provides educational activities to physicians and nurses interested in this field. Occupational medicine became a distinct specialty within the American Board of Preventive Medicine in 1954. Occupational medicine training programs exist for physicians, nurses, and safety professionals who choose this field. In 2002, there were 37 sponsored graduate medical training programs in occupational medicine.

In 1971, the Occupational Safety and Health Administration (OSHA) was created with the goal of reducing occupational hazards, promoting a safe and healthy culture, and maximizing its effectiveness and efficiency by strengthening its capabilities and infrastructure. OSHA provides training, information, and free workplace consultations to small businesses in matters concerning occupational health and safety. NIOSH is the federal agency mandated to conduct research to prevent injuries and illnesses in the workplace. This agency has tracked occupational injuries, illnesses, hazards, and exposures since its creation by the Occupational Safety and Health Act in 1970. NIOSH complements important statistical or surveillance activities carried out by other federal agencies such as the Bureau of Labor Statistics and by the private sector. NIOSH also analyzes and interprets existing data, undertakes data collection efforts to fill gaps in surveillance, provides support to state agencies to conduct occupational surveillance and associated prevention efforts, funds and conducts research on surveillance methods, and works with federal, state, and private sector partners to improve occupational health surveillance. NIOSH helped to establish the National Occupational Research Agenda (NORA) in 1996. NORA provides a framework by which to guide occupational safety and health research for the occupational health and safety community.

The cost of occupational injury and illness is borne by every member of the society. It is estimated that the worker and family bear 30% in lost wages and lost overtime opportunities as well as medical expenses arising from undiagnosed work-related conditions, work-related conditions not compensated, and compensation not fully replacing wages. Other costs are associated with pain and suffering and loss of status and self-esteem to the worker and family. The employer is estimated to bear 40% of the cost in workers' compensation premiums, the impact on productivity, retraining, administrative expenses, loss of morale, and other intangible factors. The taxpayer, by way of the government, bears about 30% of the cost, inasmuch as the government provides support services and medical care for indigent, injured, or ill workers who were previously employed or who lack workers' compensation benefits.

In summary occupational health and safety affects every aspect of our society, every age group and every occupation. Occupational morbidity and mortality are important public health problems in the United States. There have been strides in this field, especially during the latter half of the 20th century. Since the establishment of OSHA in 1971, workplace deaths have decreased by 50% and occupational injury and illness rates decreased 40%, although U.S. employment doubled from 56 million workers at 3.5 million worksites to 111 million workers at 7 million sites. Occupational

health and safety needs to be an integral part of any organization's mission, values, and operational responsibilities and is a core need of every business. The field of occupational health and safety must continue to make strides in order to improve the quality of the lives of individuals and of society as a whole.

—*Judith Green-McKenzie and Edward Emmett*

See also CENTERS FOR DISEASE CONTROL AND PREVENTION; NATIONAL INSTITUTES OF HEALTH

Further Reading

American College of Occupational and Environmental Medicine. (2003). Retrieved from http://www.acoem.org.

Derr, J., Forst, L., Yun Chen, H., & Conroy, L. (2002). Fatal falls in the construction industry, 1990-1999. *Journal of Occupational and Environmental Medicine, 43* 853-860.

Kissner, S., & Pratt, S. (1997). Occupational fatalities among older workers in the United States. *Journal of Occupational and Environmental Medicine, 39,* 715-721.

LaDou, J. (Ed.). (1997). *Occupational and environmental medicine* (2nd ed.). Stamford, CT: Appleton & Lange.

McCunney, R. J. (Ed.). (2003). *A practical approach to occupational and environmental medicine* (3rd ed.). Philadelphia: Lippincott, Williams & Wilkins.

National Institute for Occupational Safety and Health. (2003). Retrieved from http://www.cdc.gov/niosh

Plog, B. (Ed.). (1996). *Fundamentals of industrial hygiene* (4th ed.). Itasca, IL: National Safety Council.

Zenz, C. (Ed.). (1994). *Occupational medicine* (3rd ed.). St. Louis, MO: C. V. Mosby.

OPTIMISM, PESSIMISM, AND HEALTH

The concepts of optimism and pessimism concern people's expectations for the future. These concepts have ties both to centuries of folk wisdom and to a class of psychological theories of motivation, which as a group are called expectancy-value theories. These theories suggest how optimism and pessimism come to be reflected in people's behavior and emotions. These reflections, in turn, represent pathways by which this personality disposition may influence people's health.

A little theoretical background: Expectancy-value models begin with the idea that behavior is aimed at attaining desired goals. Without a valued goal, no action occurs. The other core concept is expectancies: confidence or doubt about attaining the goal. If a person lacks confidence, again there is no action. Only with sufficient confidence do people engage (and remain engaged) in goal-directed efforts. These ideas apply to specific values and focused confidence; they also apply to optimism and pessimism, in which the "confidence" is simply broader in scope.

From these principles come many predictions about optimists and pessimists. When confronting a challenge, optimists should display confidence and persistence, even if progress is difficult and slow. Pessimists should be more doubtful and hesitant. Adversity should exaggerate this difference. Optimists believe adversity can be handled successfully, pessimists anticipate disaster. This can lead to differences in efforts to take precautions, differences in actions relating to health risks, and differences in persistence in trying to overcome health threats.

Behavioral responses are important, but overt behavior is not the only response when people confront adversity. People also experience emotions in such situations. Difficulties elicit many feelings, reflecting both distress and challenge. The balance among such feelings differs between optimists and pessimists. Because optimists expect good outcomes, they are likely to experience a more positive mix of feelings. Because pessimists expect bad outcomes, they should experience more negative feelings—anxiety, sadness, and despair. A good deal of research has found evidence of such emotional differences.

HEALTH-RELATED BEHAVIORS

There are several ways in which this personality dimension may relate to health. One pathway derives from the fact that some health problems arise directly as consequences of people's behavior. That is, some actions themselves are health risks. For example, smoking is a health risk. So is unsafe sex, driving without a seat belt, and eating a high-fat diet. Yet some people engage in all of these behaviors, whereas others take better care of themselves and avoid risk behaviors. Why this difference? Perhaps one reason some people fail to take precautions is lack of confidence. That is, they may lack confidence that taking proper steps will produce better outcomes for

themselves. If this were so, optimists should engage in more health-protective behaviors, and fewer risky behaviors, than pessimists.

On the other hand, it might be argued that optimists will expect the best, no matter what they do. This may make them feel impervious to any danger stemming from risky behaviors. If this were so, optimists would be less likely to take precautions than pessimists. The existence of these two lines of argument, making opposite predictions, makes it clear how important research is. Without collecting evidence, we would never know which line of argument is closer to the truth.

Studies bearing on this question have been done, however, and most of the evidence favors the position that optimists engage in health-promoting actions more than pessimists. Some of this evidence comes from studies of people with no salient health concerns, and relates to general health-promoting actions such as eating well, taking vitamin supplements, getting adequate sleep, using sunscreen, and so on. Some of the evidence comes from patient samples, who do have particular health concerns. It has been found, for example, that optimists exert greater efforts in a cardiac rehabilitation program, exercising more and reducing body fat more than pessimists. There is also evidence from other studies that optimists exert greater efforts toward recovery from surgery.

These findings suggest that the first line of reasoning is more correct than the second. This, in turn, appears to tell us something about the nature of optimism. Specifically, optimists do not seem to have naïve faith that everything will work out well for them, even if they do nothing to help. Rather, they seem to accept the fact that they have a role in many outcomes and that they must take active steps to ensure that positive outcomes emerge. Optimism thus appears to be a positive force for active self-care and self-protection, provided opportunities to take such steps present themselves.

GIVING UP AND HEALTH

There is a flip side to this picture of optimists as being more deeply involved than pessimists in the pursuit of desired goals. Specifically, the reduced efforts of pessimists confronting adversity sometimes slide all the way into giving up. This giving-up response itself can have adverse health consequences.

Several kinds of health-relevant behaviors seem to reflect a giving-up tendency. One of them is alcohol consumption, which at high levels is a health risk. Excessive alcohol consumption is often seen as reflecting the giving up of efforts to deal with one's problems. If so, pessimists should be more vulnerable than optimists to alcohol abuse. Results from two studies fit this picture. In one, among women with a family history of alcoholism, pessimists were more likely than optimists to report drinking problems. Another study examined people who had already been treated for alcoholism and were now entering an aftercare program. This study found that pessimists were more likely than optimists to drop out of the program and return to drinking. These two studies converge in showing that pessimists display a form of disengagement—alcohol consumption—more than optimists.

People can give up in many ways, of course. Alcohol dulls awareness of failures and problems. People can also turn their backs on their problems by distracting themselves. Even sleeping can help people escape from situations they prefer not to face. Sometimes, though, giving up is more complete. Sometimes people give up not just on specific goals, but on all the goals of their lives, by committing suicide. Several studies have found pessimism to be a key indicator of suicide risk. Although many people might not immediately think of suicide as a "health" outcome, it would be hard to argue against the idea that suicide interferes with good health.

POTENTIAL PHYSIOLOGICAL PATHWAYS

Another potential pathway by which optimism may relate to health is more complicated and less well mapped out than those described thus far. Experiences of intense distress, hopelessness, and giving up have physical concomitants; so do positive emotions and engagement in strenuous efforts. Many believe physiological responses such as these play roles in health outcomes. These responses might influence a person's likelihood of getting a disease in the first place, they might influence the progression of diseases, they might even influence mortality. Since the emotional and behavioral responses that induce the physical responses are themselves linked to optimism and pessimism, it seems likely that optimists and pessimists may differ in at least some of the physiological responses they experience when under stress.

There are two distinct issues here. The first is whether optimism relates to health events that are not plausibly accounted for by the sorts of behavioral pathways discussed earlier. The second is what kind of pathway would account for the association. With respect to the first issue, evidence is accumulating that differences in optimism-pessimism relate to differences in health-related events. With respect to the second issue, there is less to say. Research on pathways is at an early stage, and much less is known.

Studies of relations between optimism and health parameters have examined several different health indicators. One rather simple one is blood pressure regulation. This study involved 3 days of monitoring of blood pressure during normal activities. Results indicated that pessimists were more likely to have elevations in blood pressure than optimists. This study should not be taken as clear evidence that pessimism leads to hypertension, but it does suggest that further examination of the issue is warranted.

Several studies have examined differences in well-being following medical procedures. For example, one study of coronary bypass surgery included measures of patients' progress through the surgery. Two kinds of indirect evidence suggested that pessimists fared more poorly than optimists even on the operating table. Specifically, pessimists were more likely to display two markers during surgery that are widely taken as indicants of myocardial infarction. Thus, pessimists may have been at greater physical risk during the bypass surgery itself. Subsequent research with bypass patients focused on a problem that often arises after major surgery: the need for the patient to be readmitted to the hospital because of a deterioration in condition. This study found that optimistics were less likely to be rehospitalized, either for problems related to postsurgical infection or for problems related to the coronary artery disease.

The successful management of disease can be reflected in many ways. Another reflection is the process of disease progression and worsening, which can be either rapid or slow. Many chronic or incurable diseases produce a sequence of new symptoms over time. An example is HIV infection. HIV infection initially has no observable symptoms. Eventually, it produces a variety of symptoms that become increasingly debilitating.

Researchers have examined development of such symptoms in men who were HIV-positive but symptom-free, as a function of psychological variables related to pessimism. The men completed a measure of stoic or fatalistic preparation for the worst, an index that has been characterized by its developers as reflecting disease-specific pessimism. In this sample of men, all of whom initially were symptom-free, pessimistic responses to this measure predicted earlier symptom onset.

These researchers also studied survival time among patients whose disease had already progressed to AIDS. By the end of the study, 82% of the men had died from complications related to the disease. Disease-specific pessimism was related to shorter survival times. It was as though individuals with this attitude were preparing to die, and death then came to them more quickly.

Another project bearing on issues of disease progression and mortality examined a sample of cancer patients whose cancer had returned after earlier treatment. All the patients had completed a measure of pessimism about the future. They were followed for 8 months. By then, approximately one third of them had died. Greater pessimism predicted shorter survival time.

One more study, conducted in Finland, examined the relationship between a sense of hopelessness about the future and mortality in a sample of over 2,000 middle-aged Finnish men who had been treated for cancer or heart attacks. Hopelessness was assessed by two items: "I feel that it is impossible to reach the goals I would like to strive for" and "The future seems for me to be hopeless, and I can't believe things are changing for the better." These men were followed for 6 years. Those who had reported higher degrees of hopelessness had greater disease-specific mortality—and all-cause mortality—than men with less hopelessness.

Why were pessimistic people in these various studies more vulnerable than people who were more optimistic? Why were pessimists more likely to end up back in the hospital after heart surgery? Why were pessimistic cancer and HIV patients quicker to progress toward death? The answers—the mediating processes—are not clear. Perhaps pessimists give up the struggle, and this leads to physical changes that permit infection and disease to gain a greater foothold. Perhaps something about remaining engaged in the fight keeps the defenses of the body hard at work. Speculations about potential mechanisms currently revolve around neuroendocrine and immune responses. At present, however, there is little solid knowledge about the mechanisms underlying these effects. What is known is only that optimism works to people's physical benefit and pessimism to their detriment. Isolating the mechanisms underlying these effects is an important part of the agenda for the future.

—*Charles S. Carver*

See also EXPLANATORY STYLE AND PHYSICAL HEALTH; HAPPINESS AND HEALTH; HOPELESSNESS AND HEALTH; OPTIMISM AND PESSIMISM: MEASUREMENT

Further Reading

Carver, C. S. (2001). Depression, hopelessness, optimism, and health. In N. J. Smelser & P. T. Baltes (Eds.), *International encyclopedia of the social and behavioral sciences* (Vol. 5, pp. 3516-3522). Oxford, UK: Elsevier.

Carver, C. S., & Scheier, M. F. (2002). Optimism. In C. R. Snyder & S. J. Lopez (Eds.), *Handbook of positive psychology* (pp. 231-243). New York: Oxford University Press.

Chang, E. C. (Ed.). (2001). *Optimism and pessimism: Implications for theory, research, and practice.* Washington, DC: American Psychological Association.

Scheier, M. F., Matthews, K. A., Owens, J. F., Schulz, R., Bridges, M. W., Magovern, G. J., Sr., et al. (1999). Optimism and rehospitalization following coronary artery bypass graft surgery. *Archives of Internal Medicine, 159,* 829-835.

OPTIMISM AND PESSIMISM: MEASUREMENT

Research has shown that optimism and pessimism are important influences on emotional responses to health problems and health-related coping behavior. Optimism and pessimism have been defined differently—and therefore measured differently—by different researchers. Thus, there are a variety of measures available. By far the most commonly used measures are the Life Orientation Test (LOT) and the Attributional Style Questionnaire (ASQ), which measure two different kinds of optimism/pessimism. These measures are based on different theories, predict somewhat different kinds of behaviors and outcomes, and do not correlate strongly with each other—or with the many other types of optimism/ pessimism that researchers have identified.

THE LIFE ORIENTATION TEST

The LOT, developed by Michael F. Scheier and Charles S. Carver, is designed to measure "dispositional optimism." Dispositional optimism refers to a general tendency to expect positive outcomes, as opposed to dispositional pessimism, which refers to a general tendency to expect negative outcomes. These tendencies are sometimes referred to as "traits," or "generalized outcome expectancies." Reported alpha coefficients (a statistical measure of the internal consistency) range from about 0.75 to about 0.88, which indicates that the items intercorrelate with each other enough to support the assumption that they are all getting at the same psychological construct. Scheier and Carver have also shown that their measure has "discriminant validity," which means that it can be distinguished from measures of related constructs such as self-esteem and anxiety. As predicted, people who answer more optimistically on the LOT tend to use more active coping strategies and report fewer physical and psychological symptoms than people who answer less optimistically.

The original LOT included eight optimism/pessimism questions and four "fillers," which are questions included to disguise the purpose of the questionnaire. Answers to filler questions are not included when a measure is scored. The eight optimism/pessimism items include four items worded positively (i.e., where higher numbers indicate more optimism) and four items worded negatively (i.e., where higher numbers indicate more pessimism). The items are worded as descriptive statements: for example, "I'm always optimistic about my future," which is a positively worded item, or "I hardly ever expect things to go my way," which is a negatively worded item. For each item, respondents indicate the extent to which the statement is true of them, on a scale from 0 (strongly disagree) to 4 (strongly agree). Most researchers using the LOT reverse score the negatively worded items and then add together the scores for all eight items to create a total optimism score. This scoring follows both Scheier and Carver's original intentions, and the general assumption that optimism/pessimism is a *bipolar* dimension, with optimism at one end and pessimism at the other end. This implies that a lack of optimism is equivalent to the presence of pessimism, and the lack of pessimism is equivalent to the presence of optimism.

More recently, several researchers have argued that optimism/pessimism refers to two separate *unipolar* dimensions, instead of one bipolar dimension. They argue that the positively worded LOT items measure optimism (or a lack thereof), while the negatively worded items measure pessimism (or a lack thereof), *and* that these two dimensions are not highly correlated. People may score high (or medium or low) on optimism *and* high (or medium or low) on pessimism, so that one could be both highly optimistic *and* highly pessimistic, or neither optimistic *nor* pessimistic. Some studies have found that the presence of pessimism predicts different outcomes (e.g., higher ambulatory blood pressure) than the absence of optimism. The LOT (and its revised and extended forms, described below) can be scored to obtain either an overall optimism score, or separate optimism and pessimism scores, so researchers often use both scorings and compare the results. For separate optimism and pessimism scores, one sums the responses to the positive items to obtain an optimism score, and the responses to the negative items to obtain a pessimism score.

In 1994, Scheier and Carver revised the LOT by taking out two items that were too similar to questions used to assess coping. The revised scale (LOT-R) correlates very highly with the original LOT. In 1997, Edward C. Chang and his colleagues published an Extended Life Orientation Test (E-LOT), with six items assessing optimism and nine items assessing pessimism. The E-LOT correlates highly with the LOT, but the former has slightly better "psychometric properties," which means that it has greater internal consistency and more clearly distinguishable relations to other measures.

THE ATTRIBUTIONAL STYLE QUESTIONNAIRE

The Attributional Style Questionnaire (ASQ) has also been widely used by researchers. This measure follows from work by Martin E. P. Seligman, in which he and his colleagues explore how people understand the events that happen to them and how that understanding influences their coping and health. Most of their work has focused on vulnerability to depression in response to negative life events. They theorize that individuals who respond to negative events by attributing them to stable, global, and internal causes are more likely to become depressed. Attributions are the causal explanations we give for events. *Stable* attributions refer to causes that are relatively immune to change over time (e.g., ability as opposed to effort). *Global* attributions are to causes that should influence many domains (e.g., being generally unlucky), as contrasted with more *specific* attributions (e.g., having a bad day). *Internal* attributions are to causes within the individual (e.g., skill or absence thereof), as opposed to *external* causes (e.g., a vindictive boss). When something bad happens, people who believe that something within them, something that is unlikely to change, and something that influences most aspects of their life has caused the event are likely to be debilitated or depressed as a result. Seligman calls this way of explaining negative events a "pessimistic attributional style" in contrast to an "optimistic attributional style," where negative events are attributed to external, unstable, and specific causes. He and his colleagues use those terms interchangeably with pessimism and optimism respectively. Assessing attributional style is an indirect way of getting at an optimistic or pessimistic outlook.

The original ASQ presented respondents with six negative and six positive events and asked them to write down one major cause and provide ratings of stability, globality, and internality for each event. For stability, respondents are asked, "In the future, will this cause again be present?" For globality, they are asked, "Is this cause something that just affects this type of situation, or does it also influence other areas of your life?" For internality, they are asked, "Is the cause of this due to something about you or something about other people or circumstances?" All responses are on seven-point scales, and are generally summed to create a total pessimism score. Globality and stability tend to correlate with each other (and combined are sometimes referred to as hopelessness), while neither correlates very highly with internality.

The first ASQ was not very reliable. In 1988, Christopher Peterson and Paul Villanova introduced the Expanded Attributional Style Questionnaire (EASQ), which includes 24 negative events (e.g., "You go out on a date, and it goes badly") and has greater internal consistency than the original ASQ. The EASQ correlates modestly with the LOT and LOT-R, which suggests that they are getting at somewhat different constructs. The EASQ also correlates moderately with the other major measure of attributional style developed by Peterson and his colleagues:

the Content Analysis of Verbatim Explanations (CAVE). CAVE is a method of analyzing written or spoken content (e.g., speeches, interviews) for attributional style. Events and attributions are identified in a text, and trained judges rate each attribution on stability, globality, and internality. There is also a version of the ASQ for children, though the meaning of attributions by young children is a matter of contention.

OTHER OPTIMISM/PESSIMISM MEASURES

The Optimism-Pessimism Instrument (OP), developed by William N. Dember and his colleagues, is another self-report measure that generates separate optimism and pessimism scores. The OP contains 18 positive items, 18 negative items, and 20 filler items, to which respondents indicate their agreement (strongly agree, agree, disagree, strongly disagree). Both O and P scores from the OP correlate moderately to strongly with the LOT and moderately with the ASQ. The OP is designed to measure positive and negative outlooks in a very broad way and contains many items that tap into constructs other than optimism and pessimism specifically.

Neil D. Weinstein developed a measure of "unrealistic optimism." Respondents indicate the likelihood, relative to similar others, of negative and positive events happening to them in the future. Those who are unrealistically optimistic—that is, who think positive events are more likely and negative events less likely to happen to them than to others—may engage in risky health-related behavior. His measure is moderately related to other measures of optimism.

Julie K. Norem and her colleagues have developed the Defensive Pessimism Questionnaire (DPQ), which is designed to measure domain-specific optimistic and defensively pessimistic strategies. Seventeen items, which respondents rate according to how true they are for them, measure two components of defensive pessimism: negative expectations and reflectivity. Reflectivity refers to how much people mentally rehearse what might happen before an event. Those who score high in both pessimism and reflectivity tend to use defensive pessimism to cope with anxiety. Those who score low on both dimensions use strategic optimism, which involves setting high expectations and distracting oneself before an event. Both groups tend to perform better than other anxious people or dispositional pessimists. The DPQ correlates moderately with the LOT and E-LOT and weakly with the ASQ. It is designed to tap into strategies that are specific to particular domains; thus, academic, social, recreational, and health versions of the scale have been used in research.

The Optimism-Pessimism Test Instrument (OPTI), developed by Deborah J. Stipek, Michael E. Lamb, and Edward F. Zigler, consists of 20 short stories, each of which is read by the tester. The child being tested is then asked to choose between a positive outcome or a negative outcome to the story. The total number of positive outcomes chosen is the optimism score.

—Julie K. Norem

See also EXPLANATORY STYLE AND PHYSICAL HEALTH; HAPPINESS AND HEALTH; HOPELESSNESS AND HEALTH; OPTIMISM, PESSIMISM, AND HEALTH

Further Reading

Chang, E. C. (Ed.). (2001). *Optimism and pessimism: Implications for theory, research, and practice.* Washington, DC: American Psychological Association.

Chang, E. C., D'Zurilla, T. J., & Maydeu-Olivares, A. (1997). Optimism and pessimism as partially independent constructs: Relations to positive and negative affectivity and psychological well-being. *Personality and Individual Differences, 23,* 433-440.

Dember, W. N., Martin, S., Hummer, M. K., Howe, S., & Melton, R. (1989). The measurement of optimism and pessimism. *Current Psychology: Research and Reviews, 8,* 102-119.

Marshall, G. N., Wortman, C. B., Kusulas, J. W., Hervig, L. K., & Vickers, R. R., Jr. (1992). Distinguishing optimism from pessimism: Relations to fundamental dimensions of mood and personality. *Journal of Personality and Social Psychology, 62,* 1067-1074.

Norem, J. K. (2001). *The positive power of negative thinking: Using defensive pessimism to harness anxiety and perform at your peak.* New York: Basic Books.

Peterson, C., & Villanova, P. (1988). An Expanded Attributional Style Questionnaire. *Journal of Abnormal Psychology, 97,* 87-89.

Scheier, M. F., Carver, C. S., & Bridges, M. W. (1994). Distinguishing optimism from neuroticism (and trait anxiety, self-mastery, and self-esteem): A reevaluation of the Life Orientation Test. *Journal of Personality and Social Psychology, 67,* 1063-1078.

Stipek, D. J., Lamb, M. E., & Aigler, E. F. (1981). OPTI: A measure of children's optimism. *Educational and Psychological Measurement, 41,* 131-143.

Weinstein, N. D. (1980). Unrealistic optimism about future life events. *Journal of Personality and Social Psychology, 39,* 806-820.

P

PAIN: PSYCHOSOCIAL ASPECTS

Pain is a ubiquitous experience. Everyone experiences some kind of pain at some point in his or her life. Most common pain we experience is acute and transient in nature. It can be quite unpleasant, yet it does not cause any significant tissue damage or have long-term effects on our health. Such pain generally goes away on its own or with over-the-counter medical aids.

However, pain can also represent serious illnesses, or become disabling on its own as with a clinical pain disorder. Pain is one of the most common reasons for seeking medical care, accounting for more than 70 million office visits to physicians each year. Chronic and recurrent episodic pain are among the most common physical problems in the United States, with an estimated 90 million suffering from one or more pain syndromes.

Pain is a complex perceptual phenomenon. The International Association for the Study of Pain's (IASP) definition of pain reflects the complexity of pain as a phenomenological experience unique to each person. According to the IASP (1986) definition, pain is "an unpleasant sensory and emotional experience normally associated with tissue damage or described in terms of such damage." An important first step to understand pain is to clarify its difference from *nociception*. Nociception is a sensory process involving receptor activation (transduction), relay of information from the periphery to the central nervous system (transmission), and neural activity leading to control of the pain transmission pathway (modulation). Pain,

on the other hand, is an integrated perceptual process. Nociception may lead to pain perception, but it is not sufficient to account for pain as a clinical presentation. Thus, nociception is not synonymous with pain. The former is a physiological phenomenon, whereas the latter is a perceptual one, involving higher central nervous system mechanisms.

CONCEPTUALIZATIONS OF PAIN

In general, pain is considered as a warning sign implicating a disease or injury, and thus, many people consider it a "physical phenomenon." Scholars and clinicians have conventionally accepted this assumption for centuries. On the other hand, when pain could not be accounted for by physical findings only, as in many cases of clinical pain syndromes, pain was considered as "mental." Cartesian mind-body dualism dominated for centuries as a way of understanding pain, in which pain was somatic if there is an organic cause accounting for the experience or pain is "psychological" otherwise. It is only in the past quarter century that there has been a significant paradigm shift in thinking about pain as an integrated perceptual experience.

Sensory Model

Traditionally, there has been an implicit assumption that an isomorphic relationship exists between pain and nociception; pain was viewed as a sensory experience that should directly and linearly correspond to the degrees of noxious sensory stimuli impinging on the individual. Based on this model, the extent of organic pathology must account for the presence and extent of pain.

However, recent advancement in neural imaging helps us understand that the linear relationship between pathology and pain rarely exists. There are a large number of patients with severe pain syndrome whose exact pathology cannot be objectively identified, despite undergoing thorough diagnostic testing. It is also common to see patients who undergo an identical operation vary widely not only in their reports of postoperative pain severity but also in their responses to treatment. Conversely, imaging studies using computed tomography (CT) scans and magnetic resonance imaging (MRI) often reveal the presence of significant pathology in about a third of asymptomatic individuals.

Psychogenic Perspectives

When the presence of pain cannot be explained by physical pathology, conventional medical thinking was to consider those symptoms as psychological in origin. Similarly, if the pain is disproportionate to objectively determined physical pathology or if a patient does not respond to medical treatment targeted to modify nociceptive input, then pain is assumed to be also psychological. Psychological distress or specific ("pain prone") personality is believed to manifest itself as "physical" pain. The psychogenic model exists as an alternative model to the sensory model; thus pain is either somatic or psychological. If the report of pain occurs in the absence of or is "disproportionate" to objective physical pathology, ipso facto, the pain must be "all in their head." However, the model has not produced any empirical support, and the assumptions and logic of the model have been repeatedly questioned.

Toward an Integrated Model: Gate Control Model

Melzack and Wall (1965) were the first to integrate physical and psychological factors in pain perception with three dimensions incorporated: sensory-discriminative, motivational-affective, and cognitive-evaluative. This model, widely known as gate control theory, proposes that a mechanism in the dorsal horn of the spinal cord acts as a gate keeper that controls neural transmission of nociceptive events. The gating mechanisms are considered to be supported by the inhibitory activity in A-beta (large-diameter) and the facilitatory activity in the c (small-diameter) fiber in the dorsal horn. In addition, the model postulates that the cortical variables, such as anxiety, memory, and attention, interact with the spinal gating system to determine the final product: pain perception. The validity of the model has been challenged over the years; however, the model stimulated the development of comprehensive models that may explain how psychological factors modulate human pain experience.

BIOPSYCHOSOCIAL MODEL OF CHRONIC PAIN

The biopsychosocial view provides an integrated model for pain that incorporates purely mechanical and physiological processes as well as psychological and social contextual variables that may cause and perpetuate chronic pain. In contrast to the biomedical model's emphasis on the disease process, the biopsychosocial model views illness as a dynamic and reciprocal interaction between biological, psychological, and sociocultural variables that shape the person's response to pain.

The biopsychosocial model presumes at its core physical changes in the muscles, joints, or nerves that generate nociceptive input to the brain. At the periphery nociceptive fibers transmit sensations that may or may not be interpreted as pain. Such sensation is not yet considered pain until subjected to higher-order psychological and mental processing that involves perception, appraisal, and behavior. Perception involves the interpretation of nociceptive input and identifies the type of pain (i.e., sharp, burning, punishing, cruel). Appraisal involves the meaning that is attributed to the pain and influences subsequent behaviors. The individual may choose to ignore the pain and continue working, walking, socializing, and engaging in previous levels of activity or may choose to leave work, refrain from all activity, and assume the sick role. In turn, this interpersonal role is shaped by responses from significant others that may promote the healthy and active response or the sick role. The biopsychosocial model has been instrumental in the development of cognitive-behavioral treatment approaches for various clinical pain disorders.

PSYCHOLOGICAL CONTRIBUTORS TO PAIN

This section reviews specific psychological factors that have been shown to influence pain experience, based on the biopsychosocial model.

Learning Factors

Pain is an unavoidable part of human lives. No learning is required to activate nociceptive receptors. Pain is inherently aversive, prompting us to escape from it, and subsequently avoid, modify, or cope with pain or cues associated with potentially painful experience.

At the acute stage of pain, healing of tissue damage causing pain is essential. However, at some point, we all need to resume our normal life activities. Unfortunately, some people develop a conditioned fear to physical activities, because such activities may temporarily aggravate pain. Avoidance of pain is a powerful rationale for reduction of activity. Many pain patients express fear of aggravating their pain, and muscle soreness associated with exercise functions as a justification for further avoidance. Although it may be useful to reduce movement in the acute stage, limitation of activities can be chronically maintained not only by pain but also by anticipatory fear well after the healing period is over. Over time, fear of pain and avoidance of activities may become generalized to a wide range of life functioning including work, leisure, and sexual activities.

From the operant learning paradigm, overt behaviors indicative of pain can be reinforced and thus maintained via environmental contingency. When a person experiences pain, the immediate behavior is to escape from it. Or a person may limp or brace the affected area in order to protect the area. Such behaviors are adaptive and appropriate. However, these behaviors can be maladaptively maintained via reinforcement. For example, suppose that limping and groaning are always followed by sympathetic attention and solicitous help from a significant other; the positive consequence of the pain behavior reinforces the behavior and thus, the likelihood of the same behavior recurring increases. Although such behavior is likely appropriate and adaptive during the active healing of the tissue damage, once the learned behavioral pattern is established, the behavior may be governed under the control of external contingencies of reinforcement, not by the initial purpose of protecting the injured area. In a case of chronic pain, therefore, pain behavior may indicate the learned pattern of responding to the environment, rather than the adaptive pattern of protecting the body from injury.

It should be noted that the pain sufferer does not consciously emit pain behaviors to obtain reinforcers. It is more likely to be the result of a gradual process of shaping the behaviors. Thus, a person's response to life stressors as well as how others respond to the pain sufferer can influence the experience of pain in many ways, but are not the cause of the pain condition. In this regard, it is also important not to make the mistake of viewing pain behaviors as *malingering*. Malingering involves the patient *consciously and purposely* falsifying a symptom (e.g., pain) for specific secondary gain. In the case of pain behaviors, there is no suggestion of conscious deception but rather the unintended performance of pain behaviors resulting from environmental reinforcement contingencies. The person is typically not aware that these behaviors are being displayed, nor does he or she consciously intend to obtain a positive reinforcement by exhibiting the behaviors.

Social learning has received some attention in acute pain and in the development and maintenance of chronic pain states. From this perspective, the acquisition of pain behaviors may occur by means of "observational" learning and "modeling" processes. That is, people can acquire responses that were not previously in their behavioral repertoire by observing others exhibit behaviors. Children acquire attitudes about health and styles of symptom perception from their parents and others close to them. The culturally acquired perception and interpretation of symptoms determine how people deal with illness. The observation of others in pain is an event that captivates attention. This attention may have survival value, may help to avoid experiencing more pain, and may help to learn what to do about acute pain.

Cognitive Factors

Various cognitive factors influence the perception of pain as well as adaptation to pain. *Attentional* factors are important in pain experience since pain is a conscious experience. Such stories as an athlete continuing to play despite serious injury and starting to feel significant pain only after the game or an injured soldier's pain becoming unbearable only after retreating to a safe place have been told repeatedly among us. Our attentional resource is limited, and our sensory experience depends on the allocation of such resource. When the greater degree of attention is allocated toward bodily sensations, greater pain perception can be expected. Such process can be seen at the neural level; for example, distraction attenuates neural activities in the brain regions to which pain experience generally corresponds.

In addition, *beliefs* about pain interact with attention to and appraisal of sensory events. Thus, individuals expecting noxious experience may allocate greater attention and interpret sensory experience as more aversive than those who do not. Furthermore, if a person evaluates the sensory event to be pathological, the pain experience is likely to be potentiated. For example, consider a man waking up on Monday with chest pain. If he starts thinking of his friend who had a heart attack a few months ago and believes that chest pain signifies pathology in his cardiovascular system, his pain experience is likely to be substantially greater and aversive than if he considers his tendency to overdo extraneous activities over the weekend ("I must have strained my chest muscle"). Such experience is consistent with how the brain functions in terms of expectation about pain that likely contributes to the modulation of pain. Anticipation of pain alone (without actual pain experience) is known to evoke activities in the primary somatosensory cortex.

Plenty of experimental evidence exists on the effects of pain-specific thoughts on physiological reactions. Cues such as pain-related words may trigger physiological response in pain patients. Chronic regional pain patients tend to react strongly to pain-related stressors in a symptom-specific manner. For example, if a patient has back pain, she is likely to increase muscle tension in the paraspinal region in response to pain-related stressors but not in the other regions. Another patient with neck pain is likely to increase tension in the cervical area. Clearly, pain-related thought process, even in the absence of actual pain experience, can trigger the physiological responses that may contribute to an overall pain experience.

Maladaptive cognition, *cognitive error*, is known to significantly contribute to distress and disability associated with pain. Particularly, the extreme type of cognitive error, *catastrophizing*, is associated with greater pain experience as well as severe disability and poor outcome of pain treatment. Catastrophizing is an extremely negative style of thinking about one's plight no matter how unlikely such negative outcomes may be. Catastrophizing appears to be a particularly potent way of thinking that greatly influences pain and disability.

Moreover, if individuals believe that their pain is *uncontrollable*, pessimism and depreciation of their coping skills persist. On the other hand, if individuals believe that they are able to use coping skills effectively (*self-efficacy beliefs*), their tolerance to aversive situations increases. These cognitions seem to reciprocally influence physiological and behavioral aspects of pain. The positive effect of self-efficacy belief on pain experience seems to be mediated physiologically via the endogenous opioid system.

Successful self-regulation of pain depends on each person's specific ways of dealing with pain, adjusting to pain, and reducing or minimizing pain and distress caused by pain-coping strategies. Coping is a spontaneously employed action that has specific purpose and intention, and it can be assessed in terms of overt and covert behaviors. Overt, behavioral coping strategies include rest, medication, and relaxation. Covert coping strategies include various means of distracting oneself from pain, reassuring oneself that the pain will diminish, seeking information, and problem solving. Coping strategies are thought to alter both the perceived pain intensity and one's ability to manage or tolerate pain and to continue everyday activities.

The term coping may imply that it should always yield positive consequences; however, coping actually can be beneficial or detrimental in management of pain. Studies have found active coping strategies (e.g., efforts to function in spite of pain or to distract oneself from pain such as activity, ignoring pain) to be associated with adaptive functioning. Passive coping strategies (e.g., depending on others for help in pain control and restricted activities) were related to greater pain and depression. In a number of studies it has been demonstrated that if instructed in the use of adaptive coping strategies, the pain intensity decreases and tolerance of pain increases.

Affective Factors

As the IASP (1986) defines it, "Pain is unquestionably a sensation in a part or parts of the body but it is also always unpleasant and therefore also an emotional experience." The affective factors associated with pain include many different emotions, but they are primarily negative in quality.

The most studied negative affect in pain is depression. Depression as a clinical syndrome as well as depressed mood is quite prevalent in people suffering from pain. Approximately 50% of people who have chronic pain are depressed. Conversely, people with major depressive disorder exhibit diminished pain threshold and tolerance. The causal relationship between depression and pain has been debated for years. However, it is not likely to be a direct one but mediated by perceived functional interference and control over pain. Furthermore, the negative cognitions that are generally associated with depression no doubt contribute to the aversive nature of overall pain experience, as reviewed in the earlier section.

Fear and anxiety are a natural consequence of pain experience. How conditioned fear and anxiety may contribute to the maladaptation of people suffering from pain was reviewed in the earlier section. In addition, anxiety is known to potentiate pain severity during medical/dental procedures as well as postsurgically. Given these, it is not surprising that psychological treatment for pain patients generally includes the cognitive-behavioral strategies to better manage patients' anxiety and stress levels.

Another affective component particularly pertinent to chronic pain is anger. Anger has been widely observed in individuals with chronic pain. It is not just the experience of anger but how people manage their anger (i.e., expression of anger) that may influence the pain perception via the endogenous opioid system. Internalization of angry feelings is also strongly related to measures of pain intensity, depression, perceived interference, and reported frequency of pain behaviors.

Frustrations related to persistence of symptoms, limited information on etiology, and repeated treatment failures along with anger toward employers, the insurance and health care systems, family members, and themselves all contribute to the general dysphoric mood of these patients. The impact of anger and frustration on exacerbation of pain and treatment acceptance has not received adequate attention. It would be reasonable to expect that the presence of anger may serve as an aggravating factor, associated with increasing autonomic arousal and blocking motivation and acceptance of treatments oriented toward rehabilitation and disability management rather than cure, which are often the only treatments available for chronic pain.

CONCLUDING COMMENTS

Pain is a complex subjective phenomenon composed of not only a neural activity but also a range of psychosocial factors. The psychosocial factors clearly contribute to the interpretation of nociception as pain as well as the determination of how pain affects the person.

The assessment of pain is complicated by the fact that pain is a subjective experience. There is no "pain thermometer" that can accurately determine the amount of pain an individual feels. Then how do we know if and how much a person is hurting? We can only infer it from indications such as the severity of tissue damage, verbal pain complaints, or nonverbal pain behaviors. Even with tissue damage, it is impossible to specify how much pain *should* be experienced. For example, should a cut that is 1/2" long and 1/4" deep hurt twice as much as a cut that is 1/4" long and 1/8" deep? Nociception is a sensory process and pain is a perceptual process that requires attention and interpretation of the nociceptive input. Thus, nociception and pain are not synonymous.

The review of how the psychological factors are implicated as an integrated pain experience should clarify why the unidimensional sensory and psychogenic models are not adequate in understanding human pain experience.

Several multidimensional models have been developed with the two most widely discussed: the gate control theory and the biopsychosocial model. These are not competing models; indeed, they are actually complementary to one another.

As pain becomes chronic, the weight of psychological factors becomes greater, due to the increased complexity of the interaction among cognitive, behavioral, affective, and physiological aspects of pain. Various behavioral and cognitive techniques can be incorporated in the treatment of chronic pain, with the purposes of modifying maladaptive thinking, increasing self-efficacy, and acquiring skills to manage pain and stress. The comprehensive conceptualization of pain as the biopsychosocial phenomenon helps develop cost-effective treatment programs.

—*Akiko Okifuji*

See also CHRONIC PAIN MANAGEMENT; HEADACHES: PSYCHOLOGICAL MANAGEMENT

Further Reading

Chapman, C. R., & Okifuji, A. (in press). Pain: Basic mechanisms and conscious experience. In R. H. Dworkin & W. S. Breibart (Eds.), *Psychosocial and psychiatric aspects of pain: A handbook for health care providers.* Seattle, WA: IASP Press.

Fernandez, E., & Turk, D. C. (1989). The utility of cognitive coping strategies for altering pain perception: A meta-analysis. *Pain, 38*(2), 123-135.

Gatchel, R., & Turk, D. C. (Eds.). (1999). *Psychological factors in pain*. New York: Guilford.

International Association for the Study of Pain. (1986). Classification of chronic pain: Descriptions of chronic pain syndromes and definitions of pain terms. *Pain, 3,* S1-S226.

Melzack, R., & Wall, P. (1965). Pain mechanisms: A new theory. *Science, 150,* 971-979.

Turk, D. (1996). Biopsychosocial perspective on chronic pain. In R. Gatchel & D. Turk (Eds.), *Psychological approaches to pain management: A practitioner's handbook*. New York: Guilford.

PARTICIPATORY RESEARCH

A great deal of concern has been raised in recent years about the fact that many research results receive only limited use in actual practice. Part of the reason for the chasm between research and practice is that those who are to be the beneficiaries and users of research often wonder whether research done under highly controlled conditions, in far away communities, and with populations different from their own is applicable to their particular needs and constraints. Most efforts to improve the research-to-practice problem are "downstream" in the research process, in that they attempt to secure interest and adoption among potential users after the research is done. In contrast, participatory research represents an "upstream" approach that involves actively engaging practitioners, policymakers, and others in the research process itself—so they can help ensure that the research will be relevant to their needs and can assist in interpreting and applying the results in their community. Participatory research can therefore be defined according to a core set of three components: (1) systematic investigation (2) involving the intended beneficiaries and users of the research (3) for the purposes of education and taking action or effecting social change.

ORIGINS AND DEVELOPMENT OF PARTICIPATORY RESEARCH APPROACHES

Participatory research has had a rich and honored tradition in health and community development. It was widely applied and honed in various forms with varied names in developing countries, where it had a decidedly practical orientation aimed at enabling social change and community development projects to be conducted among populations suspicious of the motives of Western researchers. Among the variations of names for participatory research in health were the following:

- Participatory action research
- Participative research
- Conscientizing research
- Policy-oriented action research
- Empowerment evaluation
- Collaborative inquiry
- Dialectical research
- Emancipatory research
- Social reconnaissance
- Participatory learning research
- Participatory rural appraisal

While most investigators and participants paid at least some attention to all three of the components laid out in the definition of participatory research provided above, some laid greater emphasis on one component than the others. Those who emphasized the systematic investigation part tended to gravitate to models that put less importance on the product than on the research methodologies. Those who were concerned primarily with capacity building in the community emphasized the learning process at the possible expense of the research or the social change. Those for whom the primary concern was with social action might have sought it with some sacrifice or compromise of the scientific or the educational components.

The North American renaissance of participatory research has taken place in social, educational, and health services development and delivery, and more in urban settings, in contrast to the rural settings and agricultural focus of participatory research in developing countries. In health services, nursing has led the way with collaborative studies between academic nurses and hospital nursing administrators and staff. In this context, participatory research has been aimed at improving nursing roles and difficult working conditions that have resulted from changes in health care systems. In public health, the revival of participatory research has been most notable in minority health as a way of overcoming certain disparities in health.

As with the impetus in developing countries, the distrust of researchers has played an important part in this demand for greater participation. Native communities, for example, after decades of serving as subjects for behavioral surveys, health education program evaluations, and epidemiological and anthropological studies, have put the brakes on external researchers exploiting their circumstances with very little gain to themselves. Similarly, African Americans living in inner-city ghettos noticed that their lives have been described in research reports in unflattering, if sympathetic, ways, but they have seen little come of it besides embarrassment and shame cast on their communities.

These and other communities recognized that they still needed information about their circumstances that only original research could provide. Meanwhile, academic and public health researchers recognized that the data they needed could not be had without more active cooperation of communities. This convergence of needs led to a reworking of the power balance between researchers and the researched. Instead of being viewed simply as research objects and giving informed consent, those who were to be researched gave their knowledge and experience to help develop the research questions to be asked and the methods to be applied in their communities. Rather than being relegated to the role of victim, as described in studies of their health problems and conditions of living, they became active partners in identifying the key problems to be addressed and then in interpreting and using the research findings in program development, monitoring, and evaluation and in advocating for policy and program changes.

PARTICIPATORY RESEARCH IS AN APPROACH TO RESEARCH, NOT A METHOD

This description of the origins and development of participatory research might give the impression that it is a research method designed primarily for researcher-public interaction. Yet it is neither a research method nor is it limited to circumscribing the relationship between academic researchers and the public. Instead, participatory research is an approach that entails involving any and all potential users of the research as well as other stakeholders in formulating as well as applying the research. A broad and diverse range of research methods can be applied in the service of participatory research—epidemiological, experimental, survey, focus groups, qualitative

interviews, and observation. Which methods to apply within a participatory research approach depends on a determination of which methods will best address the research questions and which are feasible in the particular setting.

WHO SHOULD PARTICIPATE?

Whose participation needs to be solicited and engaged in participatory research depends on who would be affected most directly by the research results. Much of the discussion in participatory research has taken place within the context of community development and community programs, and therefore assumes that participatory research must of necessity engage the lay community. Community, in this context, is usually understood to be a local geopolitical entity, as in the term community-based participatory research. Both the need and opportunity for undertaking participatory research with groups other than community residents arise, however, if other groupings of people sharing common characteristics or interests or causes are considered, or if research is to be undertaken for other purposes besides community development. Participants can therefore also consist of those sharing a particular race, ethnicity, gender, sexual orientation, or health condition, as well as health and service agencies and organizations, practitioners, managers, policymakers, and legislators.

HOW MUCH PARTICIPATION IS NECESSARY?

What should be considered as the minimum and maximum degree of participation in order to label research as participatory? Maximum participation occurs when those whose participation is sought remain active partners throughout the study: from formulating the research questions, to selecting the methods, to collecting the data, to analyzing the data, to interpreting and applying the findings. At the other end of the spectrum, the minimal amount of participation that can still be considered as useful consists of involving stakeholders at least in the beginning of the study in identifying the research questions and in the concluding stages of interpreting and applying the findings. This demarcation of the range of participatory research clarifies its distinction from basic and applied research that typically involves only traditionally defined researchers in the research process while viewing all others as subjects of the research, and its distinction from action research where there is a commitment to action and analysis and where the research involves community development approaches but where those involved in the action situation (often practitioners in the practice setting) are still considered as subjects of the research.

How is it possible to determine the extent to which participation of nonresearchers should be incorporated into a given research project or a given phase of a research project? This depends in part on their wishes, in part on the participants' trust of the researchers, and in part on the complexity of the research methods and analysis. In general, there is little need (nor is there much justification) to drag volunteer participants through a labor-intensive and highly technical research process, so long as they have the opportunity to shape the research questions and to interpret and apply the findings.

USES OF PARTICIPATORY RESEARCH AND DEMANDS FOR ITS EXPANSION

At the same time as practitioners and communities are demanding to have a say in the research conducted in their patients or populations, legislators are calling for greater accountability of researchers to ensure that their research influences actual practice. There has also been a growing demand among funding agencies for participatory research, given its potential for education, action, and social change. The U.S. National Institute of Environmental Health Sciences (NIEHS), for example, sees participatory research as an opportunity to advance environmental science while addressing the environmental health concerns of community residents. The NIEHS and the Centers for Disease Control and Prevention (CDC) have announced research funding competitions that require all research projects to use participatory research approaches, while other federal and nonfederal agencies have also shown a growing tendency to support the use participatory research approaches in many of their grant programs.

The vast majority of research conducted today does not incorporate participatory research approaches. Should all research be participatory? A rule of thumb as to what research might benefit from participatory research approaches is that if the research findings are intended to be used by one or more particular groups, then the findings might be more likely to be used if

members of that group have been involved in the research—so that the research is conceptualized, constructed, interpreted, and applied to meet their needs as they perceive them, rather than only addressing what others perceive to be their needs.

Participatory research seeks to contribute to better use of science, better application of research results, and better dissemination of research findings. To ensure better use and application of research, it must be seen as relevant to the local and immediate circumstances of those who would use it. The research that is synthesized into "best practices" comes from carefully controlled trials in distant places under the direction and resources of equally foreign scientific groups. Local practitioners and policymakers have good reason to suspect that their circumstances are different from those represented in the studies that underpin the best practices. Participatory research offers them an opportunity to examine their own circumstances, to pilot test the best practices within their own context, and to adapt them to their own needs. This, in turn, provides valuable data to the research community as it seeks to extend the relevance of evidence-based guidelines and best practices into other areas of health and other populations. Health agencies can provide the bridge between university-based researchers and patient self-help groups and community-based projects, using participatory research at the clinical or agency level to adapt best practices, and at the community level to ensure relevance of the research to the community's needs and actions.

—Lawrence W. Green and
Shawna L. Mercer

See also CHURCH-BASED INTERVENTIONS; COMMUNITY-BASED PARTICIPATORY RESEARCH; COMMUNITY COALITIONS; CULTURAL FACTORS AND HEALTH; HEALTH DISPARITIES; IMMIGRANT POPULATIONS AND HEALTH; KEY INFORMANTS; SELF-EFFICACY; SOCIAL CAPITAL AND HEALTH

Further Reading

Green, L. W., & Mercer, S. L. (2001). Participatory research: Can public health researchers and agencies reconcile the push from funding bodies and the pull from communities? *American Journal of Public Health, 91*, 1926-1929.

Institute of Health Promotion Research, University of British Columbia. (1996). *Study of participatory research in health promotion: Review and recommendations for* the development of participatory research in health promotion in Canada. Ottawa: Royal Society of Canada. Available from http://www.rsc.ca/english/publications.html

Minkler, M., & Wallerstein, N. (Eds.). (2003). *Community-based participatory research for health*. San Francisco: Jossey-Bass.

PEPTIC ULCERS AND STRESS

EVIDENCE AND CONTROVERSY

- At 5:46 a.m. on January 17, 1995, a major earthquake devastated the Hanshin-Awaji area of Japan. More than 6,000 people were killed, and 300,000 had to be evacuated from their homes. During the next 2 months, there were 3 times as many bleeding ulcers detected at local hospitals as in the same period of the previous year.

- During 1971-1975, the National Health and Nutrition Examination Survey asked 2,511 Americans how much "strain, stress, or pressure" they were under. Ten years later, those who had felt under a great deal of stress were 3 times as likely to have an ulcer than those who felt no stress at all.

- Researchers found that 44% of English patients with new ulcers had been having serious, objective life difficulties during the past 6 months, as compared with only 9% of healthy people of similar age and background.

- Among Italian patients who had recently developed ulcers, those who scored in the highest third on an anxiety questionnaire were 4 times as likely to remain unhealed after a standard course of treatment.

- In a study of 2,109 Swiss ulcer patients, those classified by their physicians as under stress were twice as likely to relapse during the first year after cure.

There is a wealth of research demonstrating that people who are experiencing life stress are more likely to develop an ulcer of the stomach or the duodenum and that their ulcers are harder to cure. The stereotype of the frazzled executive reaching for his bottle of Maalox every time he slams down his telephone is misleading only in its suggestion that ulcers are more common in the rich than in the poor (in fact it is the other way around).

On the other hand, in recent years it has been widely stated that ulcers are caused not by stress but by an "ulcer germ," *Helicobacter pylori*. Since the early 1990s, the discrepancy between these two rival explanations has been confusing physicians as well as the lay public about the role of psychological factors in ulcer disease.

The hunch of an Australian scientist, Barry Marshall, who believed that bacteria might be involved in ulcers, was so revolutionary that it took 15 years to convince the medical community. We now know he was right: Helicobacter pylori lives in the stomach of most ulcer patients, and many people who suffered from ulcer pain for decades have been given permanent relief by a single brief course of antibiotics. The Helicobacter story has not only clarified the origins of one specific disease and improved the lives of many patients but has opened the door to a paradigm shift in medical science by suggesting that infectious agents may play a role in many chronic diseases, including heart attacks and cancer.

The relation between Helicobacter and ulcer is not so simple, however. It is true that most people with ulcers are infected, but so are a large percentage of healthy adults: Half of Americans over age 60, and 90% of all African adults, have Helicobacter pylori in their bodies, many of them without a twinge of indigestion. And, contrariwise, as many as one ulcer in four develop in people who have never had a Helicobacter infection, confirming that the ulcer story is larger than just Helicobacter pylori.

Helicobacter pylori usually settles into the body during childhood, but ulcers rarely develop before the age of 30, and only one in five people with Helicobacter pylori infections ever develops an ulcer. Clearly, additional factors, psychological or nonpsychological, must be involved if a person's relationship with his or her resident Helicobacter makes the leap from peaceful coexistence to ulcer. Similarly, only a small proportion of people who are coughed on by somebody with tuberculosis, or who have strep in their throats, become ill.

Barry Marshall himself has warned against overstating the implications of his discovery. To determine the toxic effects of Helicobacter pylori, Marshall once bravely downed a concoction of live bacteria. When he then looked inside his own stomach, he saw that the bacteria had caused inflammation—but not an actual ulcer. Based on this and other evidence, Marshall wrote that according to Koch's criteria, the standard method for proving that a given infectious agent causes a given disease, his germ had not been demonstrated to cause ulcer.

Important as it is to avoid overestimating the role of Helicobacter pylori in ulcer disease, it is equally vital to recognize a series of pitfalls that can lead to overestimating the role of stress.

For one thing, sick people like having explanations for their sickness, and stress is a popular one, especially when the disease is as notoriously "psychosomatic" as ulcer. Furthermore, being sick is in itself stressful. Ulcer patients have been consistently found to be more anxious, depressed, and hostile than control groups. But having constant stomach pain could itself lead to anxiety, depression, and irritability, so the psychological characteristics could result from the disease instead of the other way around.

Socioeconomic status constitutes a special pitfall in ulcer research. The poor are particularly likely to have ulcers, both because Helicobacter pylori infection is rampant in conditions of crowding and inferior hygiene and because heavy physical labor increases ulcer risk. Since the poor are also particularly likely to have stressful lives, a study that looks at the general population is likely to show an artifactually strong association between stress and ulcer.

HOW ULCERS DEVELOP

To understand the role of psychological factors, it is useful to review a few medical facts. An ulcer (sometimes called "peptic" after pepsin, an enzyme found in gastric juices) is an open sore where stomach acid has eaten its way into the lining of either the stomach itself or the duodenal bulb, located where the stomach ends and the intestine begins. Ulcers do not ordinarily occur lower down in the intestine, because bicarbonate pours into the mix just inches past the bulb and neutralizes the stomach acid.

In a way, it's a miracle we don't all have ulcers. Glands inside the stomach are constantly churning out hydrochloric acid, which gets the process of digestion going by reducing the food we have eaten to pulp. When a hungry person smells a juicy steak, the acidity of the stomach contents can be 10 times stronger than vinegar.

So why doesn't that same acid reduce the stomach itself to pulp?

One answer is that the entire gastrointestinal tube is coated with a thin layer of protective mucus. A second answer is buffering of acid by food: Stomach acidity hits its peak as we start eating, but the acid starts to be neutralized by the first chewed-up bite as soon as it emerges from the far end of the esophagus.

Under ordinary circumstances, there is a nice balance between acid production on the one side and protective forces like mucus and food on the other, so the lining of the stomach and the duodenum remains intact. Ulcer-promoting factors throw off that balance either by increasing gastric acid or by decreasing the protective forces.

Helicobacter pylori disturbs the balance chiefly by degrading the quality of the protective mucus. Cigarette smoking and having Type O blood help Helicobacter pylori to do its damage; they do not seem to cause ulcers in people who are not infected. Nonsteroidal anti-inflammatory drugs (NSAIDs) such as aspirin or ibuprofen, the chief causes of non-Helicobacter ulcers, also degrade the mucus defenses.

Other risk factors act by increasing the quantity of acid that ulcer-susceptible tissues are exposed to. A high level of pepsinogen in the blood, which runs in families, is associated with high rates of acid secretion, as is heavy physical labor. Abnormal gastric contractions can cause acid to stagnate at length in the stomach or to be dumped copiously into the duodenum. And skipping breakfast increases the contact between acid and the stomach and duodenal lining by prolonging the nighttime period when there is no buffering by food.

MECHANISMS OF STRESS

So how do psychological factors promote ulcers? The classic explanation is that stress puts the lining of the upper gastrointestinal tract at risk by stimulating the stomach to secrete high levels of acid. This is correct as far as it goes, since acid production is in fact stimulated by stress in human beings (though, curiously, not in monkeys, our close animal relatives).

But other physiological mechanisms seem at least as important in the pathway between stress and ulcer formation. Stress decreases blood circulation in the gastrointestinal tract, rendering it more susceptible to damage, and it can also affect gastrointestinal contractions. Life stress is known to interfere with the process of wound healing, which may contribute to the poor prognosis of ulcers in patients who are chronically anxious or experiencing a particularly difficult period. Psychological factors may directly disrupt a long-standing equilibrium between Helicobacter and its host, both because Helicobacter pylori flourishes in the presence of high acid levels and, conceivably, by affecting immune defenses against Helicobacter.

Stress can also promote ulcer formation indirectly, by influencing behavior. Many behavioral patterns associated with life stress and psychological distress—heavy alcohol consumption, cigarette smoking, irregular eating habits, sleeplessness—are also risk factors for ulcer. People also take more NSAIDs when they are under stress, whether because they are getting more headaches or in the hope an aspirin will calm them down or help them sleep. These behavioral concomitants of stress are extremely important, explaining about half of the causative effect of stress on ulcers. It is therefore vital for health care workers to discuss food and sleep rhythms and substance use with ulcer patients, emphasizing the chain of causality from stress to unhealthy behavior patterns to disease.

Beyond such counseling around health risk behaviors, there does not seem to be a major place for psychologically oriented interventions in the average patient with an ulcer. Modern medical therapy heals nearly all ulcers rapidly and easily, while chronic disease can almost always be avoided using Helicobacter pylori eradication therapy, early treatment of symptom recurrences, or in the worst case nontoxic maintenance regimens. The modest effect on ulcer symptoms from dynamically oriented individual psychotherapy or cognitive interventions hinted at in two clinical trials is dwarfed by the efficacy of modern medical therapy. In the one published head-to-head trial, a psychologically oriented intervention (group counseling) was significantly inferior to maintenance therapy with H_2-receptor blockers, and was in fact indistinguishable from placebo. In yet another trial, cognitive intervention was associated, disconcertingly, with significantly *increased* ulcer recurrence rates.

Midcentury medical lore held that hospitalization, by removing the ulcer patient from a stressful life situation, was in itself therapeutic. Recent confirmation that anxiety impedes ulcer healing lends credence to these older concepts, the weak results of published trials being due in large part to their enrolling unselected ulcer patients. Psychotherapy or cognitive-behavioral therapy may indeed have something to offer in the treatment of peptic ulcer, but only in a few highly motivated patients with high perceived stress levels and resistant disease.

PAST AND FUTURE

Ulcers were uncommon in 19th-century Europe and America but burgeoned after 1900, to the point that one out of eight people born around 1910 was destined for an ulcer. The ulcer epidemic happened to correspond with the rise of psychoanalysis and of psychosomatic medicine, whose proponents spotlighted the apparently overwhelming association of peptic ulcer with stress and the success of rest and relaxation in healing it. What was known at the time of ulcer physiology, which focused chiefly on excess secretion of gastric acid, jibed perfectly with a psychosomatic cause.

Ironically, as the origins of peptic ulcer were becoming clear in the 1980s, the epidemic was already receding—probably because hygienic improvements were preventing children from acquiring Helicobacter pylori from older friends and family members. So concepts of peptic ulcer have changed radically: In the middle of the 20th century it was a common and disabling disease, often required surgery, and was a model for the ability of psychological distress to cause disease. Fifty years later, ulcer is relatively uncommon, can usually be eliminated with a brief course of medication, and is a model for the ability of bacteria to cause unexpected damage.

It is tempting to take sides and consider the cause of ulcers either as stress or as Helicobacter pylori. The truth is more complex and more interesting: There is no single culprit. Peptic ulcer results from the massed effect of various risk factors, with different combinations active in any individual patient. In the same way, coronary artery disease has long been conceptualized in terms of risk factors, which include both high cholesterol and psychological stress. It is by now well accepted that stress can influence heart attacks, angina pectoris, and sudden death, but this discovery has not prompted fruitless debates over whether psychological factors are "the cause" of heart disease. As the novelty of Helicobacter pylori wears off, the medical community is likely to arrive at a willingness to embrace the complexity of mind-body interactions in understanding the causation of peptic ulcer as well.

—*Susan Levenstein*

See also ALLOSTATIS, ALLOSTATIC LOAD, AND STRESS; GASTRIC ULCERS AND STRESS; STRESS: BIOLOGICAL ASPECTS; STRESS, APPRAISAL, AND COPING

Further Reading

Anda, R. F., Williamson, D. F., Escobedo, L. G., Remington, P. L., Mast, E. E., & Madans, J. H. (1992).

Self-perceived stress and the risk of peptic ulcer disease: A longitudinal study of U.S. adults. *Archives of Internal Medicine, 152*, 829-833.

Gilligan, I., Fung, L., Piper, D. W., & Tennant, C. (1987). Life event stress and chronic difficulties in duodenal ulcer: A case control study. *Journal of Psychosomatic Research, 31*(1), 117-123.

Holtmann, G., Armstrong, D., Pöppel, E., Bauerfeind, A., Goebell, H., Arnold, R., Classen, M., Witzel, L., Fischer, M., Heinisch, M., Blum, A. L., & Members of the RUDER Study Group. (1992). Influence of stress on the healing and relapse of duodenal ulcers. *Scandinavian Journal of Gastroenterology, 27*, 917-923.

Jess, P., & Eldrup, J. (1994). The personality patterns in patients with duodenal ulcer and ulcer-like dyspepsia and their relationship to the course of the diseases. Hvidovre Ulcer Project Group. *Journal of Internal Medicine, 235*(6), 589-594.

Levenstein, S. (2002a). Commentary: Peptic ulcer and its discontents. *International Journal of Epidemiology, 31*(1), 29-33.

Levenstein, S. (2002b). Psychosocial factors in peptic ulcer and inflammatory bowel disease. *Journal of Consulting and Clinical Psychology, 70*, 739-750. Retrieved from http://www.apa.org/journals/ccp/press_releases/june_2002/special_issue/ccp703739.pdf

Levenstein, S., Prantera, C., Scribano, M. L., Varvo, V., Berto, E., & Spinella, S. (1996). Psychologic predictors of duodenal ulcer healing. *Journal of Clinical Gastroenterology, 22*(2), 84-89.

Loof, L., Adami, H., Fagerstrom, K., Gustavsson, S., Nyberg, A., Nyren, O., & Brodin, U. (1987). Psychological group counseling for the prevention of ulcer relapse. *Journal of Clinical Gastroenterology, 9*(4), 400-407.

Matsushima, Y., Aoyama, N., Fukuda, H., Kinoshita, Y., Todo, A., Himeno, S., Fujimoto, S., Kasuga, M., Nakase, H., & Chiba, T. (1999). Gastric ulcer formation after the Hanshin-Awaji earthquake: A case study of Helicobacter pylori infection and stress-induced gastric ulcers. *Helicobacter, 4*(2), 94-99.

Svedlund, J., & Sjodin, I. (1985). A psychosomatic approach to treatment in the irritable bowel syndrome and peptic ulcer disease with aspects of the design of clinical trials. *Scandinavian Journal of Gastroenterology* (Suppl. 109), pp. 147-151.

Wilhelmsen, I., Tangen, T., Ursin, H., & Berstad, A. (1994). Effect of short-term cognitive psychotherapy on recurrence of duodenal ulcer: A prospective randomized trial. *Psychosomatic Medicine, 56*, 440-448.

PHYSICAL ACTIVITY AND HEALTH

Physical activity is defined as any bodily movement produced by skeletal muscles that results in energy expenditure. Physical activity is a broad term that captures virtually every type of physically active behavior including competitive and recreational sports, active forms of transportation (e.g., cycling to work), leisure activities (e.g., hiking), occupational activities (e.g., firefighting), household chores (e.g., sweeping), and exercise. Exercise is a specific subtype of physical activity that is performed to improve health and/or physical fitness. It includes activities such as aerobic endurance training (e.g., swimming, jogging), strength training (e.g., lifting weights, doing push ups), and flexibility training (e.g., yoga, stretching).

A relationship between physical activity and health was first suggested by British researchers who found a greater incidence of heart disease among double-decker bus drivers than bus conductors (Morris, Kagan, Pattison, Gardner, & Raffle, 1966). The researchers surmised that conductors might have been less prone to heart disease than drivers because they were more physically active during their work day. The conductors climbed up and down the bus stairs all day collecting fares, while the drivers sat behind the wheel.

Since the bus driver study, considerable research has examined the association between physical activity and health. For example, a study of almost 17,000 Harvard alumni from 1962 to 1978 found that all-cause mortality (death by any cause) was 53% lower for men who participated in at least 3 hours of sports activity per week than for men who engaged in less than 1 hour of sports activity per week (Paffenbarger, Hyde, Wing, & Hsieh, 1986). These activity-related reductions in mortality are largely due to the health-promoting effects of being physically fit. Men and women who are very fit have approximately a 75% lower death rate than individuals who are very unfit. Fortunately, unfit, inactive people who start an exercise program and who become physically fit can decrease their risk of death by about 44% (Blair et al., 1995). Thus, it is never too late to start exercising—greater physical fitness is associated with lower mortality among adults of all ages.

If physically fit and active people are less likely to die, then it stands to reason that they are also less likely to get sick. Indeed, four decades' worth of research indicate that exercise reduces the risk of developing a variety of physical and mental health problems. Exercise is also an effective therapeutic modality for people with certain physical and mental health ailments.

EXERCISE AND PHYSICAL HEALTH

Most health researchers have focused on the relationship between physical health and *exercise* rather than on the relationship between health and other types of physical activity. Based on this research, it is now well established that a regular program of exercise reduces the risk or delays the onset of coronary heart disease, hypertension, colon cancer, and diabetes mellitus. The association between exercise and other diseases and disabling conditions such as stroke, arthritis, osteoporosis, and certain cancers (e.g., endometrial, breast, and prostate) is still under investigation, but it is believed that exercise may prevent or delay the progression of these conditions.

How Are Physical Health Benefits Achieved Through Exercise?

Long-term physiological adaptations underlie the health benefits associated with regular exercise. Regular endurance training leads to adaptations primarily in the cardiorespiratory system whereas strength training elicits adaptations primarily in the musculoskeletal system. Other types of exercise including flexibility, speed, and agility training also bring along positive physiological changes but are outside the scope of this summary.

Endurance exercise (aerobic exercise) is continuous activity that produces a short-term elevation in heart rate and breathing rate. It results in a slight increase in the cross-sectional area of trained muscle fibers, as well as improved fat-burning capacity and significant increases in the ability of muscle cells to deliver, uptake, and utilize oxygen (i.e., increased oxygen uptake or VO_{2max}). Regular participation in endurance exercise also results in a lower heart rate (number of beats per minute) at rest and during activity, and, just like any other muscle, the heart is strengthened as a result of exercise training. Consequently, each heart contraction becomes more forceful. This helps the heart to empty itself of blood more fully with each beat and results in an increased stroke volume (the volume of blood pumped per beat).

In people with hypertension (high blood pressure), exercise training can decrease resting blood pressure. Taken together, these exercise-related adaptations increase the efficiency of the heart and subsequently lead to improvements in cardiorespiratory fitness. Such improvements are equally achievable by both men and women regardless of their age and are associated with a dramatic reduction in morbidity and mortality from coronary artery disease, diabetes mellitus, colon cancer, and possibly stroke and other forms of cancer.

Strength training (resistance training/exercise) includes activities that challenge muscles by providing them with more than normal resistance to movement. Repeated bouts of exercise that involve lifting a moderate- to heavy-weight load with a smaller number of repetitions (6-8) will increase muscular strength. Increased strength is associated with increased muscle size (hypertrophy) and increased efficiency of communication between the nervous system (i.e., the brain) and the muscle. Repeated bouts of exercise that involve lifting a light- to moderate-weight load with a greater number of repetitions (10-12) will result in greater muscle endurance due to improved oxygen delivery and uptake in the trained muscle. There will also be some increase in strength due to an increase in muscle size. The *relative* amount of this increase is similar for men and women and remains fairly constant across the life span.

With increased strength, individuals are able to lift heavier loads, and with increased endurance, muscle fatigue is delayed. Resistance training can help to maintain posture and potentially delay the progression of osteoporosis (low bone density)—a common health concern for postmenopausal women. For older adults, exercise that promotes muscle strength and balance helps to prevent falls. Falls represent a major cause of morbidity and mortality among the older population.

Exercise Prescription to Improve Physical Health

There is a dose-response relationship between exercise and physical change, which means that the greater the dose of exercise, the greater the effects. There are different guidelines for prescribing endurance exercise versus resistance exercise. These guidelines indicate the amount of exercise needed to obtain physiological and, ultimately, health benefits.

To accrue the benefits of *endurance exercise*, the dose must take into account the frequency, intensity, and duration of the exercise regimen. The standard recommendation is that on most days of the week, individuals participate in 30 minutes of moderate-intensity exercise. Moderate-intensity exercise is activity that requires approximately 3 to 6 times as much energy as one expends while at rest. For most people, this is equivalent to brisk walking.

It is important to note that as long as these frequency, intensity, and duration aspects of the prescription are met, the training effects are similar regardless of the *type* of endurance exercise performed (e.g., jogging, swimming, brisk walking). Moreover, there is emerging evidence that people who engage in *traditional* endurance exercise programs (e.g., aerobics classes, swimming) accrue the same physiological and health benefits as people who opt for a program of *lifestyle* physical activity. Lifestyle physical activity programs encourage the incorporation of 30 minutes' worth of several short bouts of moderate-intensity exercise into daily routines (e.g., climbing stairs, walking to work, doing yard work), rather than trying to accumulate all 30 minutes of exercise in a single bout. The promotion of lifestyle physical activity as a form of exercise is a relatively new concept. Consequently, more research is needed to gain a better understanding of the long-term benefits of lifestyle physical activity on health.

To accrue the benefits of *resistance training*, the dose must take into account repetitions (number of times each exercise is repeated), weight of the load being lifted, and sets (number of times each series of repetitions is performed). Muscular *strength* is best developed by performing one-three sets of 6-8 repetitions of a resistance exercise (e.g., lifting and lowering a dumbbell) with a heavy weight, defined as 80% of the maximum amount of weight the individual can lift and lower once. Muscular *endurance* is best developed by performing a minimum of one set of 10-12 repetitions of a resistance exercise using lighter weights, defined as 40% to 50% of the maximum amount of weight that can be lifted and lowered once. The former training regime is more suitable for serious weight lifters and the latter regime is more suitable for average healthy adults. Resistance training should be performed 2-3 days/week with a day off between workouts to allow trained muscle groups time to recover. It is important to note that the health benefits of resistance training are manifested only in the area of the body that is being trained. Thus, exercisers should ensure that they are performing exercises that work the desired muscle group.

PHYSICAL ACTIVITY AND MENTAL HEALTH

Participation in various types of physical activity (e.g., sports, leisure, exercise) has been linked with a general sense of "feeling good." These positive, activity-induced feelings are associated with better mental health among the general population as well as individuals who are psychologically distressed.

In the general population, single, acute bouts of physical activity have proven effective for elevating mood (e.g., increasing feelings of energy and tranquility, decreasing feelings of anxiety and depression). Longer-term physical activity programs have proven effective for improving thoughts and feelings about oneself in general (i.e., self-esteem), and about specific aspects of oneself (e.g., body image, self-efficacy for performing physical tasks, perceptions of control over certain aspects of one's life). Interestingly, physical activity seems to have its greatest effects on the people who feel the worst about themselves. In other words, people in a bad mood or who have very low general and/or specific self-perceptions will show the greatest improvements along these dimensions as a result of physical activity participation. Moreover, exercise is important for preventing mental health disorders as fit individuals have a lower incidence of anxiety and depressive disorders than unfit individuals.

For individuals who are psychologically distressed, exercise may be an effective treatment strategy. Among individuals diagnosed with a mental illness such as an anxiety or depressive disorder, exercise has been found to be just as effective in reducing feelings of distress as many conventional therapies such as relaxation, occupational therapy, and drug therapy. Similarly, exercise can be an effective strategy for reducing pain and the psychological distress associated with a chronic pain condition (e.g., osteoarthritis).

How Are Mental Health Benefits Achieved Through Physical Activity?

To accrue the mental health benefits of physical activity participation, it is not essential to improve physical fitness. This suggests that unlike the *physical* health benefits of physical activity, the *mental* health benefits are not derived solely from physiological adaptations. Currently, it is unclear exactly how physical activity leads to improved mental health, but several psychologically and physiologically based explanations have been advanced. Psychologically based explanations include the propositions that exercise creates a sense of accomplishment, provides opportunities for social interaction, and distracts attention from daily stressors, thus contributing to improved mental health. Physiologically based explanation include the hypotheses that biochemicals that enhance feelings of well-being (e.g., endorphins, certain neurotransmitters) are released into the bloodstream as a consequence of physical activity and that activity elevates core body temperature, thus promoting decreased muscle tension and improving sleep quality. Individually, none of these explanations can fully account for the positive effects of physical activity on mental well-being. It is likely, however, that a combination of psychological and physiological mechanisms accounts for the effects.

Physical Activity
Prescription to Improve Mental Health

It is unclear exactly what dosage of activity produces the greatest mental health benefits. For instance, the frequency, intensity, and duration aspects of exercise seem to be of only modest importance in determining the extent to which exercisers experience improvements in depression and anxiety. This suggests that the exercise prescription can take many forms when the goal is to reduce depressive and anxiety symptoms. It does seem, however, that whereas most types of physical activity (e.g., exercise, sports) can enhance general and specific self-perceptions, only exercise reduces depression and anxiety. Thus, the type of physical activity may be an important consideration when prescribing exercise to improve certain aspects of mental health.

—*Amy E. Latimer and
Kathleen A. Martin*

See also CANCER AND PHYSICAL ACTIVITY; CARDIAC REHABILITATION; HEART DISEASE AND PHYSICAL ACTIVITY; PHYSICAL ACTIVITY INTERVENTIONS; PHYSICAL ACTIVITY AND MOOD

Further Reading

Blair, S. N., Kohl, H. W., III, Barlow, C. E., Paffenbarger, R. S., Jr., Gibbons, L. W., & Marera, C. A. (1995). Changes in physical fitness and all-cause mortality. *Journal of the American Medical Association, 273*, 1093-1098.

Lox, C. L., Martin, K. A., & Petruzello, S. J. (2003). *The psychology of exercise: Integrating theory and practice.* Scottsdale, AZ: Holcomb Hathaway.

Morris, J. N., Kagan, A., Pattison, D. C., Gardner, M. J., & Raffle, P. A. B. (1966). Incidence and prediction of ischaemic heart-disease in London busmen. *Lancet, 2*, 553-559.

Paffenbarger, R. S., Jr., Hyde, R. T., Wing, A. L., & Hsieh, C. (1986). Physical activity, all-cause mortality, and longevity of college alumni. *New England Journal of Medicine, 314*, 605-613.

Pollock, M. L., Gaesser, G. A., Butcher, J. D., et al. (1998). The recommended quantity and quality of exercise for developing and maintaining cardiorespiratory and muscular fitness, and flexibility in healthy adults. *Medicine and Science in Sports and Medicine, 30*, 975-991.

Sallis, J. F., & Owen, N. (1999). *Physical activity and behavioral medicine.* Thousand Oaks, CA: Sage.

U.S. Department of Health and Human Services. (1996). *Physical activity and health: A report of the surgeon general.* Atlanta, GA: Centers for Disease Control and Prevention.

PHYSICAL ACTIVITY INTERVENTIONS

The importance of physical activity has been well documented in the scientific literature. For example, in 1996, the Office of the Surgeon General's report stated that there is an expansive and strong body of scientific evidence that demonstrates that regular physical activity can prevent or control a number of chronic diseases and conditions, including cardiovascular disease, stroke, Type 2 diabetes, hypertension, obesity, osteoporosis, and certain types of cancer. When people engage in the recommended amount of physical activity, they can reduce their risk for many diseases and increase their overall level of health, functioning, and quality of life. Despite this knowledge, physical inactivity has been increasingly documented as a major public health issue in the United States as well as other industrialized nations. In light of the pervasiveness of physical inactivity, a growing amount of research has been aimed at developing effective interventions for promoting regular physical activity increases in a range of settings and populations.

Research on the behavioral epidemiology of physical activity has explored the prevalence of physical activity among different population segments, factors that may influence whether persons engage in physical activity or not, and what the characteristics of active versus inactive persons are. For example, in a study conducted by Caspersen and colleagues with adults in the United States, Canada, England, and Australia, it was found that, across these countries, approximately 30% of adults are sedentary. Sedentary was defined as engaging in no leisure-time physical activity. Additional research has found that there are differences in physical activity levels between different groups of people. The 1996 Office of the Surgeon General's report summarized the epidemiological findings of population-level studies of physical activity and reported that, among adults, women are less active than men, older people are less active than younger people, and that, as education and income decrease, inactivity increases. Additional research has shown that as children grow older, they become less physically active. Research with youth has also demonstrated that while boys tend to be more active than girls at most ages, by age 18, differences between boys and girls in physical activity levels are minimal.

In general, the epidemiological research demonstrates that the majority of the public needs to increase their physical activity levels to meet recommended guidelines. However, systematic attempts to promote regular physical activity participation have brought to light the many challenges of attempting to intervene on this complex health behavior. Such challenges include accurately assessing more moderate-intensity forms of physical activity, developing interventions that reach the large numbers of individuals who could benefit from physical activity increases, and identifying the most effective strategies for promoting sustained physical activity participation in the face of the many personal and environmental obstacles to being active that often occur across time.

The majority of the physical activity interventions that have been undertaken to date tend to target specific age groups, and typically have occurred at individual or interpersonal levels of impact. Therefore, this entry focuses on the current state of physical activity interventions within each age group. In addition, discussion focuses on the settings of the interventions (i.e., home, school, work, health care), and the channels through which the interventions take place (i.e., individual, group, environmental, policy).

PHYSICAL ACTIVITY INTERVENTIONS WITH YOUTH

Many intervention studies with youth ages 5 to 13 years (i.e., elementary and middle school-age populations) have been school based. These interventions have often focused on curriculum changes in physical education (PE) classes. One example of this is the SPARK study (Sports, Play and Active Recreation for Kids) conducted by Sallis and colleagues with 955 fourth- and fifth-grade children. The investigators compared an intervention delivered by trained classroom teachers or trained PE specialists with a control group. Students in these groups were compared on a variety of factors, including total minutes of PE per week, minutes of physical activity during PE, and use of quality teaching methods by the teachers. The researchers found that, compared to the control group, trained classroom teachers were able to almost double the number of minutes per week in physical activity during the PE classes. PE specialists were able to increase the number of minutes even more. However, Sallis and colleagues did not find that children increased their levels of physical activity outside of school, despite efforts to train the children in self-management techniques for increasing overall physical activity.

Other studies that have been conducted within school PE curricula have been successful as well. For example, the CATCH study (Child and Adolescent Trial for Cardiovascular Health), conducted by Luepker and colleagues, employed an intervention in PE classes for third- through fifth-grade students in 96 schools. Similar to the SPARK study, this intervention involved training PE specialists and PE teachers on ways to increase the time of enjoyable moderate and vigorous physical activity during PE class. Children in classes that received the CATCH intervention (vs. control classes) were able to increase their moderate and vigorous physical activity to 50% of class time, whereas controls were at 42% at the end of the 3-year study. The CATCH trial was also able to increase physical activity levels outside of school through a home/family component of the intervention.

Stone and colleagues conducted a recent review of physical activity intervention studies with youth and found that since 1980, 22 of the studies were school based and only 7 were community based. This is in contrast to the observation that children engage in much of their physical activity outside of school. At the time of that review, little attention had been given to middle school children. Since then, there have been an increasing number of studies that have focused primarily on middle school children. One study currently being conducted by Dzewaltowski and colleagues is the Healthy Youth Places Project. This study uses a school-based intervention, but takes a more ecological approach as well. The intervention being evaluated takes into account the places where middle school children spend most of their time, including the classroom, the lunchroom, and in afterschool programs, as well as evaluating the influence adults involved in these programs (i.e., school staff with an interest in health promotion) have on the children.

A second intervention trial conducted in middle schools by Sallis and colleagues also focused more on environmental and policy factors outside of the classroom. Unlike previous studies, this study did not use classroom education. Instead, the focus of the intervention was on changing school policies and environments to allow for more opportunities to engage in physical activity at school. This approach proved to be effective. Researchers found that, after 2 years, children in the intervention schools increased their physical activity levels over that of children in control schools. Interestingly, however, this effect was found only for boys and not for girls. Such ecological approaches deserve further attention in future intervention studies. In addition, gender-specific interventions may need to be designed to allow for improvement in both boys and girls.

PHYSICAL ACTIVITY INTERVENTIONS WITH ADOLESCENTS AND YOUNG ADULTS

There have also been studies employing interventions targeted at adolescents (approximately high school to college age). Stone and colleagues' review of youth intervention studies identified seven intervention studies conducted with adolescents as the target population. All but one of these studies involved interventions that were conducted through schools in PE classes. One school-based study, conducted by Killen and colleagues, was the Stanford Adolescent Heart Health Program. The focus of this study was on reducing risks for cardiovascular disease; thus, the intervention contained several components of risk reduction, including increasing physical activity, decreasing smoking, and adopting a "heart-healthy" diet. Participants in this study included 1,447 students ages 14 to 16 years in four different high schools. Two schools received the intervention and two schools served as controls.

As with the youth studies previously described, the intervention for this study was delivered within the context of students' regular PE classes. Students were exposed to 20 class sessions of intervention material in which they were given information about the topic under discussion, were taught skills to help them change negative health behaviors, and developed skills to resist outside factors that could influence whether they engaged in unhealthy behaviors. The control schools did not receive any instruction. It was found that students in the treatment schools gained more knowledge than those in the control schools. It was also found that more sedentary students in the treatment schools engaged in regular exercise at follow-up than those in the control schools.

A recent study called PACE+ (Patient-Centered Assessment and Counseling for Exercise Plus Nutrition), conducted by Patrick and colleagues, targeted adolescents in a primary care setting. This study is one of the first to employ a more ecological or community approach with adolescents, rather than using the school environment. The intervention for this study focused on increasing moderate and vigorous physical activity, as well as decreasing fat intake and increasing fruit and vegetable consumption. Participants were randomly assigned to either a mail-only, infrequent telephone and mail contact, or frequent telephone and mail contact intervention. Researchers found increases in moderate but not vigorous physical activity in all three groups across the 4-month study period.

A focus on school-based interventions can also be found in the college environment. The Project GRAD (Graduate Ready for Activity Daily) study, conducted by Calfas and colleagues, examined physical activity levels among college seniors, with a particular focus on the transition between college and subsequent employment settings. Participants included 338 college seniors who were randomly assigned to one of two conditions: a physical education course based on empirically supported behavior change concepts or a general health course, each lasting one semester. At the end of the semester, it was found that women in the intervention condition increased their total energy expenditure (total amount of activity), their amount of weight training, and their flexibility relative to controls. However, there were no observed effects for the men. A 2-year follow-up found no differences in physical activity between the two intervention groups; however, cognitive processes related to motivational readiness for physical activity were significantly improved for women even after 2 years. Although this study did not find any effects for men or any long-term effects on physical activity levels, it did demonstrate long-term success in improving the processes of change for women that have been found to be important predictors of physical activity in other studies.

As previously mentioned in the youth research area, studies on adolescents' and young adults' physical activity levels need further extension into community and ecological settings. Other data have demonstrated that children and adolescents obtain most of their physical activities from afterschool and community programs, such as local youth sports and extramural classes. However, few studies have attempted to employ physical activity interventions in these types of community settings.

PHYSICAL ACTIVITY INTERVENTIONS WITH MIDDLE-AGED ADULTS

Interventions targeting middle-aged adults tend to occur in more diverse settings, such as work and health care environments. Sallis and Owen point out that work settings have many advantages that individually based settings (such as home-based studies) may not have for this age group. For example, studies in worksites can reach a large population of adults with a variety of backgrounds, worksites already have usable communication systems and other resources that can be taken advantage of, and worksites usually have a group of staff interested in the health and safety of the workers. In addition, since at least some segments of the population generally work in one place for a while, researchers can often keep in contact with participants for a reasonably long period of time.

Despite these advantages, recent reviews have questioned the success of physical activity intervention studies in worksites. A review by Dishman and colleagues identified 73 studies of various types of worksite fitness or physical activity interventions conducted in a variety of work environments, including corporations, universities, and public agencies. Characteristics of the interventions in these studies were also varied and included health education/risk appraisal, exercise prescription, behavior modification, or a combination of these approaches. Some

studies involved a supervised intervention team where participants met with a member of the research team on a regular basis (either individually or in groups), whereas others used a nonsupervised intervention. Dishman and colleagues conducted a quantitative analysis (meta-analysis) of 26 of these studies. The average age of participants in these studies was generally mid- to late 30s. Their analysis revealed a small positive effect overall for the worksite studies examined. They also found that studies using randomized and controlled experimental designs demonstrated smaller increases in physical activity than studies using less rigorous scientific designs.

Based on their review, Dishman and his colleagues concluded that physical activity interventions at worksites do not appear to be effective in increasing physical activity. One of the reasons cited for this is that people do not tend to use work as a place for exercising. The authors state that future research in worksites should make better use of the resources in the organization. That is, rather than focusing on changing behavior at an individual level, future studies should incorporate a more ecological approach by making use of multilevel designs that incorporate personal, environmental, and organizational factors.

Health care settings also have the advantage of being able to reach a large portion of the population, especially for middle-aged and older adults. In fact, physical activity counseling from physicians has been recommended as part of routine medical care. A few studies have examined the influence of physician advice interventions. Sallis and Owen explained that these studies involve training physicians on how to give brief advice during typical office visits to help people overcome barriers. These studies have demonstrated that even very brief counseling from a physician can have a positive influence on amount of physical activity. Simons-Morton and colleagues conducted a formal review of research in health care settings and identified several factors that influence success in increasing physical activity. These factors included multiple contacts with patients, a behavioral approach, exercise supervision, providing equipment to patients, and long-term follow-ups.

PHYSICAL ACTIVITY INTERVENTIONS WITH OLDER ADULTS

In recent years, physical activity interventions with older adults have moved to the forefront of physical activity research. King and colleagues pointed out that the research in this area has grown because older adults (over 50 years old) are a fast-growing segment of the population, in addition to being among the most sedentary segments of the population. Furthermore, many of the negative health conditions that affect older adults are preventable or controllable with regular physical activity of even a moderate level.

King and colleagues conducted a recent review of studies of physical activity interventions aimed at older adults, which identified 29 studies since 1984 that were community based and employed an experimental or quasi-experimental design. Approximately half of the studies reviewed used a theoretical framework for designing the intervention. This review found that the interventions that were most effective in increasing physical activity were those that used behavioral or cognitive-behavioral interventions rather than those based only on education or instructional-type interventions. These researchers also found that regularly supervised, home-based approaches were generally as or more effective than classroom or group-based formats. In addition, continuing telephone contact with participants was found to be just as effective as in-person contact in maintaining physical activity levels for up to 2 years in this age group.

King conducted a second review of intervention studies with older adults and identified a number of factors that serve as correlates or predictors of physical activity for older adults. These include current level of physical health, age, gender, smoking status, education level, income, and body weight. In addition, one should consider participants' desires to increase physical activity, beliefs about the importance of physical activity, and self-efficacy (i.e., one's perception that one can successfully engage in physical activity if desired). This review also identified several program-related factors that need to be considered. These include physical activity structure (e.g., requiring participants to take classes, encouraging increases in daily walking around one's neighborhood) format (home based, facility based), complexity, intensity, convenience, financial costs, and psychological costs (e.g., embarrassment or self-consciousness in attending an exercise class). In addition, women in particular might benefit more from a social component to the program. Environmental factors that were identified as correlates of physical activity included social support, in which the desired

source of support may depend on the phase of the study (i.e., beginning an exercise routine vs. maintaining). Physician support and ease of access to exercise facilities appear to be important factors to consider as well.

The review by King and colleagues presented four main recommendations for future research in this area. One recommendation is that specific guidelines be developed for older adults regarding how much and what types of physical activity are needed. These guidelines should include strength, flexibility, and balance training. In addition, clearer definitions are needed regarding what exactly moderate and vigorous physical activities are when the target group consists of older adults. A second recommendation is that interventions that have been supported in prior research should be tested in a wider variety of subgroups, including those who are frail or who have chronic conditions or disabilities, ethnic minorities, low-income subgroups, rural elderly, those over age 85, and those who are socially isolated or depressed. A third recommendation is that protocols be developed that health care providers can use to efficiently assess the health status of older adults and recommend physical activity regimens that are more individually tailored to a person's specific needs. Last, these researchers recommend that environmental and policy-level approaches be rigorously studied. Specifically, more information is needed on what types of interventions that include environmental and policy changes would be effective in allowing physical activity to be incorporated more easily into people's daily lives.

FUTURE DIRECTIONS

As mentioned in the previous sections, there are several directions for further research in the physical activity intervention arena. For example, previous research has identified risks for physical inactivity that are associated with certain demographics, including persons with lower incomes, racial and ethnic minorities, and those with disabilities. People in these groups are less likely to be physically active compared to the general population, and therefore, interventions should be tailored to meet their specific needs. A review by Taylor and colleagues was able to identify 10 studies aimed specifically at various ethnic minority groups, some of which were also low income. The majority of these studies did not employ rigorous experimental designs, and only two reported reliable, positive changes in physical activity. In general, the 10 studies identified used poor-quality measures of physical activity. Future research with ethnic minority groups should use more rigorous scientific methods and validated measures of physical activity.

The same review identified only four studies conducted with people with disabilities. Each of these studies was conducted with a group that had a specific disability, and each reported increases in physical activity as a result of the intervention. Despite these positive findings, many disabilities have not been studied and will need to be examined in further research.

Another area of research requiring more attention is research on gender differences. As previously discussed, interventions have had mixed results for women and men. For example, a recent nationwide randomized clinical trial called the Activity Counseling Trial (ACT) reported gender differences in response to three physical activity interventions being evaluated. In this study, eligible primary care patients were randomly assigned to either an advice group (physician advice plus written materials), assistance group (physician advice, written materials, plus interactive mail and behavioral counseling), or counseling group (all of the above components plus regular telephone counseling and classes). At the 24-month follow-up, women in the assistance and counseling groups had higher scores on fitness measures than in the advice group. However, there were no differences found for men on either fitness measures or levels of physical activity. It can be concluded from such investigations that men and women likely have different needs regarding the best methods for increasing their physical activity levels.

Most of the interventions discussed in this entry were at the individual or group level. More work is needed in the area of environmental and policy interventions designed to increase physical activity. These types of interventions involve changing the social and physical environments in which people can be active. An example of an environmental intervention is a recent study conducted by Brownson and colleagues that involved examining the influence that walking trails in neighborhoods have on levels of physical activity. However, there have been very few studies at the environmental level.

Within the studies of individuals, there is a need for more intergenerational work. There has been at least one recent study, conducted by Ransdell and colleagues, that demonstrated some success in getting mothers and daughters to exercise together. Although not all studies involving children and their parents together have been successful, the success demonstrated by this small study should encourage other researchers to engage in larger-scale studies with an intergenerational design. The needs of both the parents and children (as well as, potentially, grandparents) need to be taken into consideration when designing these types of studies.

An additional issue that affects all types of intervention studies is the measurement of physical activity. Guidelines for amounts of physical activity have recently been applied to moderate physical activity. For many individuals, what constitutes "moderate activity" is not as clear and not as easily remembered as bouts of more vigorous physical activity. More work is needed in developing reliable and valid measures of moderate physical activity for all age groups.

Last, new technologies are having an influence on physical activity interventions. Recent research has begun to employ new technologies such as telephone-linked computer systems and Web-based formats for physical activity interventions. Controlled studies are needed comparing these different formats. A major issue for this type of research is ensuring that groups that may not have current ready access to such technologies, but likely will in the future, are included in these studies. It is possible that personality and demographic characteristics may influence receptiveness to these types of intervention formats.

In summary, research with physical activity interventions is making steady progress toward increasing physical activity levels among people of all ages. Many studies discussed above have demonstrated promising results. This entry highlights the need to take into account the optimal setting and channel for the intervention, which may be different for different age groups. Challenges to this area of research for all age groups include accurate measurement of moderate intensity physical activity, use of more environmental and policy-level approaches, further exploration of gender differences, and reaching subgroups of the population at particular risk for inactivity.

—Shannon Q. Hurtz and
Abby C. King

See also CANCER AND PHYSICAL ACTIVITY; HEART DISEASE AND PHYSICAL ACTIVITY; PHYSICAL ACTIVITY AND HEALTH; PHYSICAL ACTIVITY AND MOOD

Further Reading

Blair, S. N., & Morrow, J. R. (Eds.). (1998). Theme issue: Physical activity interventions [Special issue]. *American Journal of Preventive Medicine, 15*(4).

Brownson, R. C., Housemann, R. A., Brown, D. R., Jackson-Thompson, J., King, A. C., Malone, B. R., & Sallis, J. F. (2000). Promoting physical activity in rural communities: Walking trail access, use, and effects. *American Journal of Preventive Medicine, 18,* 235-241.

Calfas, K. J., Sallis, J. F., Nichols, J. F., Sarkin, J. A., Johnson, M. F., & Caparosa, S. (1999). Project GRAD: Two-year outcomes of a randomized controlled physical activity intervention among young adults. *American Journal of Preventive Medicine, 18,* 28-37.

Caspersen, C. J., Merritt, R. K., & Stephens, T. (1994). International activity patterns: A methodological perspective. In R. K. Dishman (Ed.), *Advances in exercise adherence* (pp. 73-110). Champaign, IL: Human Kinetics.

Dzewaltowski, D. A., Estabrooks, P. A., & Johnston, J. A. (2002). Healthy Youth Places promoting nutrition and physical activity. *Health Education Research: Theory and Practice, 17,* 541-551.

Killen, J. D., Telch, M. J., Robinson, T. N., Maccoby, N., Taylor, C. B., & Farquhar, J. W. (1988). Cardiovascular disease risk reduction for tenth graders. *Journal of the American Medical Association, 260,* 1728-1733.

King, A. C. (2001). Interventions to promote physical activity by older adults. *Journal of Gerontology, 56A,* 36-46.

Luepker, R. V., Perry, C. L., McKinlay, S. M., Nader, P. R., Parcel, G. S., Stone, E. J., et al. (1996). Outcomes of a field trial to improve children's dietary patterns and physical activity: The Child and Adolescent Trial for Cardiovascular Health (CATCH). *Journal of the American Medical Association, 275,* 768-776.

Patrick, K., Sallis, J. F., Prochaska, J. J., Lydston, D. D., Calfas, K. J., Zabinski, M. F., et al. (2001). A multicomponent program for nutrition and physical activity change in primary care: PACE+ for adolescents. *Archives of Pediatrics and Adolescent Medicine, 155,* 940-951.

Sallis, J. F., McKenzie, T. L., Alcaraz, J. E., Kolody, B., Faucette, N., & Hovell, M. F. (1997). The effect of a 2-year physical education program (SPARK) on physical activity and fitness in elementary school students. *American Journal of Public Health, 87,* 1328-1334.

Sallis, J. F., & Owen, N. (1999). *Physical activity and behavioral medicine.* Thousand Oaks, CA: Sage.

U.S. Department of Health and Human Services. (1996). *Physical activity and health: A report of the surgeon general.* Atlanta, GA: U.S. Department of Health and Human Services, Centers for Disease Control and Prevention, National Center for Chronic Disease Prevention and Health Promotion.

Writing Group for the Activity Counseling Trial Research Group. (2001). Effects of physical activity counseling in primary care. *Journal of the American Medical Association, 286,* 677-687.

PHYSICAL ACTIVITY AND MOOD

Physical activity is thought to have positive effects on mood and psychological well-being. Many people report feeling better after exercising, although this is by no means universal. It has also been proposed that regular physical activity relieves depression and helps people cope with stress. This entry examines the evidence underlying these claims, summarizing the information that has been obtained from several very different research paradigms. The implications of a favorable effect of physical activity on mood are far reaching, since they are relevant to the well-being of the population at large, the mental health of vulnerable individuals, and the maintenance of long-term adherence to physical activity programs.

POPULATION STUDIES

A number of cross-sectional population or epidemiological studies have assessed associations between levels of physical activity and mental health. Physical activity has been positively related to general well-being, and negatively associated with anxiety and depression, in representative population samples in several countries. Such associations might be due to the influence of a third factor. For instance, physical illness could lead to reduced physical activity and to poor psychological well-being, and low socioeconomic status is associated both with physical inactivity and with increased levels of mental ill health. However, in a nationally representative sample of 16-year-olds in the United Kingdom, participation in physically active sports and pastimes was found to be negatively associated with distress after adjustment for sex, socioeconomic status, and health. Interestingly, participation in nonactive social pastimes (such as pool and pinball games) was positively related to distress. In old age, maintenance of greater physical activity is associated with less depression and disability, and greater active engagement with social roles.

Epidemiological methods have also been used to examine relationships between changes in mood and physical activity over time. Much of the evidence indicates that physical activity reduces risk of subsequent depression. Thus, an analysis of the Alameda County, California, population cohort assessed the incidence of new cases of clinical depression over a 5-year period in 1,947 adults varying in physical activity. Greater physical activity at baseline was protective against future depression, after adjusting statistically for age, socioeconomic status, ethnicity, financial strain, chronic health problems, disability, body mass, alcohol, smoking, and social support. The evidence from both cross-sectional and longitudinal population studies therefore indicates that physical activity has a favorable effect on mood and psychological well-being.

ACUTE PHYSICAL ACTIVITY

A second source of evidence comes from studies assessing mood before and after individual bouts of physical activity. Do people feel better after they exercise, and if so, for how long? Studies of this issue have used a variety of psychological measures, and physical activity interventions that vary in type (e.g., running, bicycling, swimming), duration, and intensity. While the majority of research has shown positive mood effects after exercise, some investigators have argued that the reductions in anxiety that occur are no greater than those reported after a comparable period of quiet rest. Others have demonstrated transient increases in mental vigor and exhilaration lasting 15 to 20 minutes. There is some evidence that positive mood changes only occur after moderate but not intense exercise, which may lead to extreme fatigue and depressed mood. Investigating this issue is complicated by the fact that measures of mood may be confounded with the physical effects of activity. For example, assessments of states of anxiety typically include ratings of tension and shortness of breath, both of which might be elevated because of recent exertion. Clearly, the impact of physical activity also varies between populations. In trained athletes, the mood effects of activity may be dependent on how they feel they have performed on that occasion, while in a sedentary individual even moderate activity could lead to feelings of exhaustion.

One acute effect of physical activity that has been recorded in several studies is a reduction in physiological stress responsivity. The magnitude of blood pressure and heart rate responses to standardized mental stress tests are attenuated if stress testing is preceded by physical activity. This phenomenon is thought to last for at least 2 hours, but is not well understood. It may be due to neuroendocrine and autonomic nervous system activation during exercise, which blunts subsequent reactivity to stress. People who exercise regularly also report more positive moods at the end of the days on which they are active compared with rest days, and may perceive the minor hassles in their lives as less stressful. These acute effects could contribute to the impact of physical activity on mood and well-being over the longer term.

PHYSICAL ACTIVITY INTERVENTION STUDIES

The strongest evidence for the effects of physical activity on mood probably emerges from experimental intervention studies in which sedentary people are randomized to exercise and control conditions, and changes in mood are assessed. Work of this type has been carried out with healthy populations, in samples from the general community with symptoms of depression and anxiety, and in psychiatric populations. The impact of aerobic activity has generally been positive, with increases in positive mood and perceived coping ability together with reductions in anxiety and depression in people randomized to regular physical activity conditions. Depression has been a major focus of this research because of the clinical implications for the management of depressive illness, but the evidence for reductions in anxiety is just as strong. There is less convincing evidence for the influence of anaerobic (resistance) training than for aerobic activity.

However, problems with the design of studies prevent definite conclusions from being drawn. Many studies have been carried out with small samples of 20 to 50 participants. The fact that these individuals choose to take part in research on physical activity may mean that they are not representative of the larger population.

Few studies have used the gold-standard clinical trial intention-to-treat approach to analysis, in which all entrants to studies are analyzed irrespective of whether they completed the trial or dropped out. Since there is often a large drop-out in activity studies, a further selection bias is introduced; people who complete a trial may benefit psychologically, but those who drop out have probably not felt positive changes and are excluded from the analysis. It could therefore be that positive psychological changes with physical activity only occur in individuals who are predisposed to experience such effects. The duration of physical activity programs has generally been short, with few studies continuing for more than 12 weeks, and follow-ups have been limited.

Another important issue concerns the comparison conditions selected for the study. Unless these are matched with physical activity in terms of level of attention and contact with investigators, the amount of social involvement, and the sense of achievement that arises from successfully completing exercise assignments, then any positive mood changes might be due to these nonspecific factors, rather than more direct mechanisms.

There have been some convincing studies. For example, a comparison of a 4-month course of aerobic exercise, antidepressant treatment, or their combination, was carried out at Duke University with 156 older patients with depressive disorder. All groups showed similar reductions in depression over the treatment period, suggesting that physical activity stimulated similar changes to those produced by pharmacotherapy. Moreover, relapse during the 12 months following treatment was less frequent in the exercise than medication groups. Nonetheless, conclusions about the mood benefits of regular physical activity must remain tentative, not so much because of the accumulation of negative findings, but because of design limitations in much of the research to date.

MECHANISMS RELATING PHYSICAL ACTIVITY AND MOOD

The mechanisms underlying the effects of physical activity on mood are not well understood. Most studies of changes in mood following activity programs have found little correlation between cardiorespiratory fitness and psychological responses. This suggests that mood changes are unlikely to be simple effects of improved fitness. An early suggestion was that mood changes were due to increased levels of opioid peptides such as beta-endorphin, but trials using endorphin antagonists such as naltrexone have been inconsistent. Since these antagonists block endorphin responses, they should reduce any positive

mood change with exercise. But when they are administered in a double-blind fashion, so that neither the participant nor the investigator knows whether the active drug or placebo has been given, differences between conditions have been inconsistent. Monoamine neurotransmitters such as dopamine and serotonin may be involved, but convincing evidence from humans is lacking.

As noted earlier, episodes of reduced stress responsivity and enhanced mood follow individual bouts of exercise, so that the person exercising regularly may experience repeated periods of tranquility that could lead over time to generalized positive mood change. Another attractive theory is that the achievement of intermediate physical activity targets (e.g., running half a mile, swimming for 10 minutes) induces changes in self-concept and a sense of mastery that may generalize to heightened self-esteem and enhanced well-being. There are exciting possibilities for future research in teasing out the mechanisms underlying mood changes.

CONCLUSIONS

Evidence for a beneficial effect of physical activity on mood has emerged from several complementary types of research. Both cross-sectional and longitudinal epidemiological studies have rather consistently demonstrated that physically active people are less likely to be depressed and have more positive moods than are sedentary individuals. Acutely, exercise leads to enhanced positive mood in some individuals and to reduced postexercise stress responsivity. Intervention trials with sedentary individuals have generally endorsed the favorable effects of activity, but research design limitations prevent definitive conclusions from being drawn. The positive psychological effect of physical activity may be important from the public health perspective. Most of the health benefits of regular activity are long term, and so remain intangible for many years. The effects of activity on mood are more immediate, so they could provide greater short-term reinforcement of exercise habits. Greater attention to mood change may therefore help to sustain active lifestyles.

—*Andrew Steptoe*

See also DEPRESSION: TREATMENT; PHYSICAL ACTIVITY AND HEALTH; PHYSICAL ACTIVITY INTERVENTIONS

Further Reading

Babyak, M., Blumenthal, J. A., Herman, S., Khatri, P., Doraiswamy, M., Moore, K., Craighead, W. E., Baldewicz, T. T., & Krishnan, K. R. (2000). Exercise treatment for major depression: maintenance of therapeutic benefit at 10 months. *Psychosomatic Medicine, 62*, 633-638.

Biddle, S. J. H., & Mutrie, N. (2001). *Psychology of physical activity*. London: Routledge.

Morgan, W. P. (Ed.). (1997). *Physical activity and mental health*. New York: Taylor & Francis.

Sallis, J. F., & Owen, N. (1999). *Physical activity and behavioral medicine*. Thousand Oaks, CA: Sage.

Stephens, T. (1988). Physical activity and mental health in the United States and Canada: Evidence from four population surveys. *Preventive Medicine, 17*, 35-47.

Steptoe, A., & Butler, N. (1996). Sports participation and emotional wellbeing in adolescents. *Lancet, 347*, 1789-1792.

Strawbridge, W. J., Deleger, S., Roberts, R. E., & Kaplan, G. A. (2002). Physical activity reduces the risk of subsequent depression for older adults. *American Journal of Epidemiology, 156*, 328-334.

PLACEBOS AND HEALTH

Placebos are physically inert substances or procedures that are presented to patients in the guise of physically active treatments. Most placebos are capsules or pills that look exactly like the active drug to which they are being compared. However, sham surgery has also been used as a placebo. Placebo surgery involves making an incision and sewing the patient back up, without performing the surgical procedure.

The term *placebo* is Latin and means "I shall please." This reflects the historical use of placebos to placate patients whose complaints could not otherwise be treated. It also indicates a belief that while the placebos might please patients, they are not likely to produce real benefits. The misperception that placebos do not produce real benefits began to change during the 1950s and 1960s, as research revealed genuine changes in patients' conditions following placebo administration. Among the conditions that have been shown to be affected by placebos are asthma (including changes in bronchial constriction and dilation),

pain, anxiety, depression, gastric function (nausea and vomiting), general arousal (including blood pressure and heart rate, as well as subjective reports of arousal), sexual arousal, and skin conditions (contact dermatitis and warts). Besides producing therapeutic benefits, placebos sometimes mimic the side effects of active medications, although to a much lesser degree. The eventual result of the recognition of the placebo effect was the routine use of placebos as control treatments in the evaluation of new medications.

The magnitude of placebo effects varies from condition to condition. For example, placebos duplicate about 80% of the therapeutic benefit of antidepressants and about 50% of the pain-reducing effects of analgesics. The size of the placebo effect can also vary as a function of a number of other factors. For example, placebo capsules are more effective than placebo pills, and placebo injections are more effective than placebo capsules. The strength of the medication to which the placebo is being compared also affects the effectiveness of the placebo. Thus, placebo morphine is more effective than placebo aspirin. Two placebos are more effective than one placebo, and placebos with a recognized brand name are more effective than placebos administered as generic drugs. In general, the effectiveness of a placebo depends on amount of effect that the person expects to experience.

How is it that an inert substance can produce psychological and physical changes? Currently, the two most popular explanations of the placebo effect are classical conditioning and response expectancy. Classical conditioning is a phenomenon discovered by the Russian physiologist Ivan Pavlov, at the beginning of the 20th century. In classical conditioning, a stimulus (called an *unconditional stimulus*) that automatically elicits a response (called an *unconditional response*) is paired repeatedly with a neutral stimulus (called a *conditional stimulus*). After a number of such pairings, the conditional stimulus acquires the capacity to evoke a response (called a *conditioned response*). Generally, the conditional response is the same as the unconditional response, only weaker. In some cases, however, it appears to be the opposite of the unconditional response, in which case it may be referred to as a *compensatory response*.

As applied to placebo effects, conditioning theory posits the following sequence of events. Active medications are unconditional stimuli, and the therapeutic responses they elicit are unconditional responses. The pills, capsules, and injections by means of which the medications are delivered are conditional stimuli. Because these conditional stimuli are repeated paired with the active medications that produce the therapeutic benefits, they acquire the capacity to elicit these benefits as conditional responses.

Conditioning theory appears capable of explaining many placebo effects, but there are also some problems with this explanation. For one thing, the conditional response to morphine is an increase in sensitivity to pain (i.e., it is a compensatory response). However, the effect of placebo morphine is a reduction in pain sensitivity. Therefore, it cannot be due to classical conditioning. In fact, it seems to override the conditioning effect. Another problem with the conditioning model of placebo effects is that it does not account well for the existence of placebo effect throughout the history of medicine. Most of the substances that were used as medications before the 20th century (e.g., turpentine, crushed glass, worms, spiders, furs, feathers, crocodile dung, lizard's blood, frog's sperm, pig's teeth, rotten meat, fly specs, powdered stone, iron filings, and human sweat) are now recognized to have been placebos. Because they do not automatically produce therapeutic benefits, they cannot have functioned as unconditional stimuli for placebo effects.

Response expectancy theory rests on the discovery that the belief that an automatic subjective response will occur tends to elicit that response. Thus, the anticipation of anxiety makes people anxious, the belief than one will stay depressed forever is very depressing, and the anticipation of changes in pain alters the perception of pain. More generally, subjective experience appears to be due to a mix of external and internal factors. It is shaped partially by external stimuli and partially by the person's beliefs, expectations, and interpretations of those stimuli. As applied to the placebo effect, expectancy theory asserts that placebos produce their effects by changing people's expectations. A placebo antidepressant, for example, leads people to expect a change in their depression, and that expectation makes them feel less depressed. A shortcoming of expectancy theory is that it does not easily account for the physical effects of placebos.

It is important to note that conditioning theory and expectancy theory are not mutually exclusive. Specifically, classical conditioning may be one of the means by which expectancies are altered. Thus, if an active drug (the unconditional stimulus) repeatedly elicits a particular therapeutic benefit (the unconditional

response), it will also lead people to expect that benefit when they think they are taking the drug, and that expectation might produce the placebo effect (the conditional response).

—*Irving Kirsch*

Further Reading

Kirsch, I. (1997). Specifying nonspecifics: Psychological mechanisms of placebo effects. In A. Harrington (Ed.), *The placebo effect: An interdisciplinary exploration* (pp. 166-186). Cambridge, MA: Harvard University Press.

PREGNANCY OUTCOMES: PSYCHOSOCIAL ASPECTS

The outcomes of pregnancy include many different medical and psychosocial effects for mother and infant. Among the most significant are preterm delivery (PTD; birth at less than 37 weeks gestation) and low birth weight (LBW; less than or equal to 2500 grams). Infants born early are more likely to be LBW. The United States has surprisingly high rates of LBW and PTD compared to other nations. In 2001, of births in the United States, 11.9% were PTD and 7.7% were LBW. Both rates show increases in the past decade. LBW and its effects occur disproportionately among African American women. In 2001, of African American births in the United States, 13.1% were LBW compared to 6.7% of non-Hispanic Whites and 6.4% of Hispanics. For PTD, 17.6% of African Americans deliver early, 11.4% of Hispanics, and 10.6% of non-Hispanic Whites. These adverse outcomes occur among African Americans of all socioeconomic levels, not only among those who are poor, although poor women of all ethnicities are at greater risk of poor pregnancy outcomes as well.

The consequences of LBW and PTD include higher rates of infant death and a host of developmental and pediatric health complications. For example, prematurity is the leading cause of death in the first month of life. In addition, prematurity is a major contributor to developmental delays, chronic respiratory problems, and vision and hearing impairment. In addition to these significant developmental and health implications of adverse pregnancy outcomes, medical costs associated with PTD and LBW births are enormous. The average cost of a birth after 37 weeks gestation in the United States is less than $5,000 compared to more than $50,000 on average for infants born preterm, amounting to health care costs of close to $12 billion per year presently.

Because of the many adverse consequences of LBW and PTD, these outcomes are a high priority in public health and medicine. National health agendas have set goals for reductions in rates of PTD (to 7.6%) and LBW (to 5%) by the year 2010. A greater understanding of the etiology of early birth and of poor fetal growth is sought, as are strategies for prevention. In recent years, we have begun to develop stronger integrative models of the causes of adverse pregnancy outcomes, taking into account psychological, social, cultural, and biological factors, as well as demographic analyses of their etiology.

Medical risk factors such as hypertension, gestational diabetes, a prior PT or LBW delivery, and gynecological infections predict adverse outcomes such as PTD and LBW, but not terribly well. Availability and use of prenatal care throughout pregnancy predict better outcomes; lack of prenatal care contributes to the adverse outcomes of poor women. In addition, behavioral factors such as tobacco use (smoking), alcohol use, and drug use are known risk factors for adverse outcome. However, relatively high rates of LBW and PTD still occur in women who do not use substances. Therefore, attention has turned in recent years to a wide range of further behavioral and psychosocial factors possibly involved. Among these, stress has probably received the greatest attention.

Stress is broadly defined as demands that tax or exceed resources. Stressors are demands such as life events, chronic strain, and trauma. Stress responses include emotional, behavioral, and biological reactions to demands. In pregnancy, the stress variables studied most often are major life events, such as death of a close relative or a family member's job loss, and the emotional state of anxiety. Nearly three dozen studies have been done on stress and PTD alone. The subset of these that are prospective studies with larger samples, standardized measures of stress, and appropriate controls indicate that stress is a significant risk factor for PTD. In a series of studies, Christine Dunkel Schetter and colleagues have found that multidimensional stress measures predict PTD. The component of stress that seems to be most responsible is anxiety. Women who are more anxious *in general* during pregnancy and who are more anxious *about their pregnancies* deliver their babies earlier. These findings

appear to hold true for all ethnic groups, although emerging findings suggest that additional factors such as racism may figure importantly in the etiology of PT birth in African Americans.

Emerging research in several laboratories with human and animal models points to dysregulation of the maternal stress systems in the mediation of the relationship between stressful experience and early onset of labor. Acute stress elicits a cascade of biological responses involving many systems including the cardiovascular system, the endocrine system, the immune system, and the nervous system including the brain. Complex responses to stress that occur in humans in response to stress are well understood and provide a basis for our growing knowledge of stress in pregnancy. One feature that differs is that the fetus and the placenta both release stress hormones such as corticotropin-releasing hormone (CRH) in response to specific maternal stress hormones. High levels of maternal stress hormones such as cortisol and CRH have been implicated in PTD via their effects on the placenta and the fetus. Although the pathways and precise mechanisms are not fully worked out as yet, it appears that psychosocial stress and emotions in the mother can lead to physiological effects that influence the timing of delivery and in some cases, trigger early delivery. In addition, emerging research suggests effects of maternal stress on fetal development and on the offspring's health over the life span.

In addition to the fast-growing body of work on maternal stress and pregnancy outcomes, other findings point to personal resources such as a woman's degree of mastery, optimism, self-esteem, and social support in predicting fetal growth. Women who lack these resources are at higher risk of delivering an LBW infant, independent of the timing of delivery. In addition, recent results suggest that perceived racism and rumination over severely stressful life events among African American pregnant women predict LBW independent of their level of education, income, and medical risk. There is some evidence that these links are mediated by behavioral health factors such as substance use, lack of prenatal care, inactivity, and poor diet. However, this topic requires much further investigation before we will fully understand the risk factors and pathways.

It remains to be known whether there are vulnerable times in pregnancy such as the first trimester when stress may have its most potent effects. Some evidence points to critical times in early pregnancy. Further evidence points to prepregnancy states of the mother such as emotional stability and her family history of stress and birth as potent risk factors. Both prenatal risk factors and prepregnancy risk factors hold promise for future interventions that reduce rates of LBW and PTD.

There have been very few randomized, controlled trials testing psychosocial interventions in pregnancy in order to prevent LBW or PTD. A number of social support interventions have been tested but only one or two have been found effective. For example, Jane Norbeck and her colleagues in San Francisco targeted a group of low-income African American women who had inadequate social support and intervened to reduce LBW in this group by use of individual counseling sessions in which problems and successes in life were identified and meaning, self-esteem, and social support were bolstered. This intervention successfully reduced LBW by 13% from 22% in the control group to 9% in the intervention group. This study is promising although methodological limitations hinder our ability to draw strong conclusions about most interventions as yet.

Future directions include (1) the further development and refinement of theories of the etiology of PTD and LBW that combine biological, psychological, sociocultural, and medical knowledge, and (2) the development of intervention trials that are based in theory and, importantly, that test process variables allowing researchers to infer what the mechanism of effective interventions are.

—Christine Dunkel Schetter
and Christine M. Rini

See also PREGNANCY PREVENTION IN ADOLESCENTS

Further Reading

Barker, D. J. P. (1998). *Mothers, babies and health in later life.* Edinburgh: Churchill Livingstone.

Births: Final data for 2000. (2002). *National Vital Statistics Reports, 50*(5). Public Health Service Report No. 2002-1120. Retrieved from http://www.cdc.gov/nchs/data/nvsr/nvsr50/nvsr50_05.pdf

Dunkel Schetter, C., Gurung, R. A., Lobel, M., & Wadhwa, P. (2000). Stress processes in pregnancy and birth: Psychological, biological, and sociocultural influences. In A. Baum, T. Revenson, & J. Singer (Eds.), *Handbook of health psychology.* Hillsdale, NJ: Lawrence Erlbaum.

Hobel, C. J., Dunkel-Schetter, C., & Roesch, S. (1999). Maternal stress as a signal to the fetus. *Prenatal and Neonatal Medicine, 3,* 116-120.

March of Dimes. (2003). Retrieved from www.marchofdimes.com/peristats

Norbeck, J., DeJoseph, J. F., & Smith, R. T. (1996). A randomized trial of an empirically derived social support intervention to prevent low birth weight among African American women. *Social Science and Medicine, 43,* 947-954.

Rini, C., Dunkel-Schetter, C., Wadhwa, P. D., & Sandman, C. A. (1999). Psychological adaptation and birth outcomes: The role of personal resources, stress, and sociocultural context in pregnancy. *Health Psychology, 18*(4), 333-345.

Sapolsky, R. M. (1998). *Why zebras don't get ulcers: An updated guide to stress, stress-related diseases, and coping.* New York: W. H. Freeman.

PREGNANCY PREVENTION IN ADOLESCENTS

CURRENT STATISTICS ON ADOLESCENT PREGNANCY

Adolescent pregnancy includes women between the ages of 10 and 19 who conceive and give birth to children. Statistical data, based on recorded birth certificates from state vital statistics offices, are used to calculate the teen pregnancy rate. Adolescent pregnancy rates are compiled and distributed through the Center for Health Statistics and the Centers for Disease Control and Prevention (CDC, 2003). These data are often looked at by categories of ages: 10-14, 15-19, and 18-19. Age categories have been shown to reflect certain risk factors that can be anticipated due to a young woman's age and point of development, and predict deleterious health, social, and economic effects. Younger adolescents ages 10-14 show the greatest risk factors. Pregnant adolescents, under the age of 15, for example, have higher rates of complications and more premature and low-birth-weight babies than older mothers.

Vital statistics also offer information on adolescents who are married and not married at the time of the birth of their children. Marital status is important in relation to the incidence of adolescent births as well as the sociopolitical and moral debates about adolescent pregnancies.

Adolescent Birth Rates

The overall adolescent birth rate has fallen since the 1950s. There was a sharp increase in the birth rate in the 1980s, followed by a continuous decrease in the 1990s. Statistical data from the Center for Health Statistics indicate that birth rates for adolescents were at a historic low in 2001 (CDC, 2003). There were 45.3 births per 1,000 women ages 15-19, down 5% from 2000 and 24% lower than in 1990. For young adolescents ages 10-14, the rate per 1,000 women was 0.8; that figure was 8% lower than in 2000 and 34% lower than in 1990. For older adolescents ages 18-19, pregnancy rates were 76.1 per 1,000; that figure was down 3% from 2000 and 14% from 1990.

The U.S. teen birth rate remains the highest among developed countries. According to the latest data available, the rate is lowest in Japan at about 4 births per 1,000 women and is below 10 per 1,000 in a number of countries, including Denmark, Finland, France, Germany, Italy, the Netherlands, Spain, Sweden, and Switzerland.

Births to adolescents also vary a great amount based on race and ethnicity. Non-Hispanic Whites had a birth rate of 30.3 per 1,000 in 2001, non-Hispanic Blacks had a birth rate of 73.5 per 1,000, Native Americans had a birth rate of 56.3 per 1,000, Asian/Pacific Islanders had a birth rate of 19.8 per 1,000, and Hispanics had a birth rate of 86.4 per 1,000. Hispanics clearly have the highest birth rates of any group.

Increase in Births to Unmarried Adolescents

Despite the fact that the overall birth rates of adolescent women have decreased for 50 years, the proportion of unmarried adolescents who have children has continued to rise, from 14% in 1940 to 67% in 1990 and 79% in 2000 (CDC, 2001). These data are keeping alive an ongoing public debate about the unacceptability and the social problem of adolescent childbearing. Recent data from Child Trends (2001) indicate that 22% of births to unmarried adolescents are repeat (second or subsequent) childbirths. As the vital statistics indicate, however, an increase in unmarried teen pregnancy is not due to an overall increase in births to adolescents; rather, it is because fewer and fewer adolescents who give birth are married. This occurrence of unmarried adolescent pregnancies follows a broader social trend for women of all ages. Adolescent pregnancy, for example, accounts for only 28% of all unmarried pregnancies to women. This shows that the trend of giving birth outside of marriage is much larger for adult women than for adolescent women.

WHY IS ADOLESCENT PREGNANCY CONSIDERED A PROBLEM?

Pregnancy is not a disease to be prevented but a normal condition for females of childbearing ages who are sexually active and do not use contraceptives (Franklin, Corcoran, & Harris, in press). Adolescent pregnancy would not be a problem except that the pregnancy occurs in a certain social and developmental context that produces harmful or unwanted outcomes for herself and others. The social and developmental context of adolescent pregnancy, for example, is usually believed to be accompanied by negative and adverse health, social, and economic consequences for the young woman and her child. Many of these consequences, however, are intricately intertwined with the social and economic circumstances of adolescent women who are poor and who are also single parents or bear children outside of marriage. Poverty causes some researchers to question the social and economic validity of the core issues that are discussed as problems produced by adolescent pregnancy. It could be, for example, that the health, social, and economic problems associated with adolescent pregnancy would exist for these young women, even if they were not pregnant, because they are poor and lack education, resources, and skills.

PUBLIC FOCUS ON ADOLESCENT PREGNANCY PREVENTION

Public policies and concerns for adolescent pregnancy have focused mainly on pregnancy prevention. Most public debates center on moral and economic positions against childbirth to unwed, economically dependent, adolescent women. Public concerns against unwed pregnancy focus attention on the specific risk factors associated with adolescent pregnancies and the need for pregnancy prevention because of known health and social risks to the adolescent mother and her child. Public policies and pregnancy prevention programs focus on reducing risk factors associated with adolescent pregnancies, and on specific interventions for improving protective factors for vulnerable adolescent populations.

Health Factors

Obstetric health risks to adolescent mothers include such conditions as toxemia, anemia, cephalopelvic disproportion, and hypertension. Adverse health risks to the child include low birth weight, prematurity, and infant mortality. These conditions are probably overattributed to the physiologic immaturity of the adolescent. Sociodemographic factors, such as low socioeconomic status (SES), single status, and poor prenatal care, have confounded earlier studies in this area. When adolescents receive good medical care their risk for negative health outcomes substantially decreases. Ongoing relationships with health professionals, such as visiting nurses, have also been shown to reduce the repeat pregnancies of adolescents and to produce overall favorable impacts on the adolescent mother's health outcomes. The greatest health risks appears to be among adolescents who are 15 years of age or younger, because young pregnant adolescents may deny or conceal their condition, thus delaying health care.

Family Factors

Family composition and relationship functioning act as both determinants and protective factors against adolescent pregnancy. Adolescents from single-parent homes are sexually active at earlier ages than are those from two-parent families (see Corcoran, Franklin, & Bennett, 2000, for a review). Parental supervision and monitoring show positive results as a protective function as does explicit disapproval of sexual activity from parents, especially when it occurs in the context of a close mother-daughter relationship.

Socioeconomic Factors

Low SES has long been established as a significant contributing factor to premature pregnancy (Corcoran et al., 2000). Conversely, high SES is associated with low childbearing rates. Societal attitudes and the differences between education, income, and other opportunities are often used to explain differences in early childbearing among socioeconomic levels. Academic achievement and positive school experiences act as protective factors to prevent pregnancy. Research has shown that career and academic development are linked to the prevention of pregnancy.

Peer Group Factors

Peer group attitudes and behaviors influence an adolescent's decision to take on parenting at a young age. A large majority of girls say they received pressure from boys and other girls to be sexually active. Many girls reported being afraid of losing their boyfriends if they refused sex (Franklin et al., in press).

Religious Factors

Most of the research indicates that commitment to a religion acts as a protective factor against early sexual activity. Placing a high importance on religion and prayer, as well as attendance at parochial schools, appears to serve as a protective factor to the early onset of sexual intercourse (Franklin et al., in press).

Social Support Factors

Several risk factors for adolescent pregnancy have been shown in studies to be positively affected by providing adequate social support to adolescents: (1) birth weight, (2) maternal adjustment, (3) parenting behavior, (4) child development knowledge, (5) infant health outcomes, (6) family relationships, and (7) maternal satisfaction with pregnancy and prenatal and postpartum health care seeking (Franklin et al., in press).

Individual Psychological Factors

Substance use, sexual abuse, repeat pregnancies, and lack of academic achievement are the individual attributes most associated with risk for adolescent pregnancy (Franklin & Corcoran, 1999). Personal distress, social role conflicts (i.e., being a student and a mother), developmental crisis (i.e., still being a child and not being prepared for the demands of raising a child), and depression are also evident in pregnant and parenting adolescents. Adolescent pregnancy causes an emotional and situational crisis for young girls but does not appear to be associated with any particular psychological profile or disorder. Behavioral disorders can increase the risk for early sexual behavior in adolescents, but overall individual psychological attributes, such as self-esteem, do not predict pregnancy.

EFFECTIVE INTERVENTIONS FOR PREGNANCY PREVENTION

In 1997, Franklin, Grant, Corcoran, O'Dell, and Bultman performed a meta-analysis of 32 primary pregnancy prevention outcome studies. Three outcome variables—sexual activity, contraceptive use, and pregnancy rates—were included and analyzed as three separate and independent meta-analyses. Eleven moderator variables (e.g., age, gender, ethnicity) also were examined in relationship to the findings. These authors compared community-based versus school-based interventions and included in their study both clinic and no-clinic programs. The majority (approximately 80%) of the participants in the 32 adolescent pregnancy prevention programs evaluated in the meta-analysis were female youths from African American and Hispanic cultures.

Results indicated that the pregnancy prevention programs examined in the studies had no effect on the sexual activity of adolescents. Sufficient evidence was found, however, to support the efficacy of pregnancy prevention programs for increasing contraceptive use. A smaller but significant amount of evidence also supported program effectiveness in reducing pregnancy rates. Contraceptive knowledge building and distribution was found to be the most effective intervention for increasing contraceptive use and reducing pregnancy rates among adolescents. Moderator analysis showed that younger teenagers (under age 14) have higher pregnancy rates and do not perform as well on contraceptive use measures as older teenagers (age 15 and older).

A more recent narrative review of effective programs conducted by Kirby (2001) recommends several multicomponent programs targeting both sexuality and youth development activities. The Children's Aid Society program known as the Carrera program has been shown to reduce pregnancies for as long as 3 years, for example. Carrera is an expensive, comprehensive program that includes several types of interventions that are offered in combination with one another over time: (1) family life and sex education, (2) individual academic assessment and preparation for standardized tests and college prep exams, (3) tutoring, (4) self-expression activities through the use of the arts, and (5) comprehensive health and mental health care.

Several evidenced-based curricula for preventing adolescent pregnancy are also available for practitioners to use with adolescent groups. These curricula have clearly written manuals and materials and have been found to be effective in one or more experimental and quasi-experimental studies on pregnancy prevention. Some of the curricula have been widely tested in numerous studies and found to be effective.

Finally, experimental studies indicate that brief pre- and postnatal interventions and prolonged contacts and education with mothers after childbirth had substantive impacts on rapid, repeat childbearing. Interventions, such as nurse visitation in the home and ongoing educational classes, were found effective for decreasing rapid, repeat childbearing (Seitz & Apfel, 1999). Harris and Franklin (in press) also found that a brief, strengths-based, cognitive-behavioral group, "The Taking Charge" curriculum, delivered in a school setting was effective in helping pregnant and parenting adolescents improve school performance, increase problem-solving skills, and remain in school.

—*Cynthia Franklin, Jacqueline Corcoran,*
and Mary Beth Harris

See also PREGNANCY OUTCOMES: PSYCHOSOCIAL ASPECTS

Further Reading

Centers for Disease Control and Prevention. (2001). Births to teenagers in the United States, 1940-2000. *National Vital Statistics Reports, 49*(10), 1-24.

Centers for Disease Control and Prevention. (2003). Revised birth and fertility rates for the United States in 2000-2001. *National Vital Statistics Reports, 51*(4), 1-24.

Child Trends, Inc. (2001). *Facts at a glance, 12/99 overview.* Retrieved from http://www.childtrends.org/.8

Corcoran, J., Franklin, C., & Bennett, P. (2000). Ecological factors associated with adolescent pregnancy and parenting. *Social Work Research, 24,* 29-39.

Franklin, C., & Corcoran, J. (1999). Preventing adolescent pregnancy: A review of programs and practices. *Social Work, 45*(1), 40-52.

Franklin, C., Corcoran, J., & Harris, M. B. (in press). Risk, protective factors, and effective interventions for adolescent pregnancy. In M. W. Fraser (Ed.), *Risk and resilience in childhood and adolescents* (2nd ed.). Washington, DC: NASW Press.

Franklin, C., Grant, D., Corcoran, J., O'Dell, P., & Bultman, L. (1997). Effectiveness of prevention programs for adolescent pregnancy: A meta-analysis. *Journal of Marriage and the Family, 59*(3), 551-567.

Harris, M. B., & Franklin, C. (in press). Effects of a cognitive-behavioral, school-based, group intervention with Mexican-American pregnant and parenting mothers. *Social Work Research.*

Kirby, D. (2001). *Emerging answers: Research findings on programs to reduce teenage pregnancies.* Washington, DC: National Campaign to Prevent Teenage Pregnancy.

Seitz, V., & Apfel, N. H. (1999). Effective interventions for adolescent mothers. *Clinical Psychology: Science and Practice, 6,* 50-66.

PSYCHONEUROIMMUNOLOGY

Psychoneuroimmunology is the study of the interactions between brain, behavior, and the immune system. This field has developed from scientific information that the immune system does not operate autonomously. Rather, there are bidirectional communication pathways between the immune system and central nervous system with each having regulatory influences over the other. The presence of these neural-immune interactions provides the basis for the impact of behavioral and psychological factors on immunity and immune-mediated diseases. Conversely, given the ability of immune cell products to alter neural function, immune processes can affect behavior and emotion.

IMMUNE SYSTEM

The immune system is the body's defense against invading external pathogens such as viruses and bacteria and from abnormal internal cells such as tumors. Innate immunity refers to the body's resistance to pathogens that operates in a nonspecific way without recognition of the different nature of various pathogens, whereas specific immunity is acquired in response to the identification of non-self molecules called antigens. Macrophages and granulocytes are examples of nonspecific immune cells that react to tissue damage by consuming debris and invading organisms. Natural killer (NK) cells are another example of nonspecific immunity that acts to kill virally infected cells in a nonspecific way without need for prior exposure or recognition. In contrast, each T cell or B cell is genetically programmed to attack a specific target by secreting antibodies (B cell) or by killing cells of the body that harbor a virus (T cell).

Both innate and specific immunity are orchestrated by the release of interleukins or cytokines from immune cells; cytokines are protein "messengers" that regulate the immune cells. This cytokine network aids in the differentiation of the immune response and in the coordination of its magnitude and duration. For example, there are two main classes of cytokines secreted by the T cells. One class of cytokines, T helper type 1 (Th1) cytokines, supports T cell responses (e.g., the ability of T cells to kill virally infected cells), whereas another class of cytokines, T helper type 2 (Th2), supports an antibody-mediated humoral immune response. However, the immunoregulatory processes cannot be fully understood without taking into account the organism and the internal and external milieu in which innate and specific immune responses occur.

BIOLOGICAL CONNECTIONS BETWEEN THE CENTRAL NERVOUS SYSTEM AND IMMUNE SYSTEM

Autonomic Nervous System

The central nervous system and the immune system are linked by two major physiological systems, the hypothalamic-pituitary-adrenal (HPA) axis and the autonomic nervous system composed of sympathetic and parasympathetic branches. The sympathetic nervous system (SNS) is a network of nerve cells running from the brain stem (i.e., the phylogenetically "older" part of the brain that runs the body's physiological systems) down the spinal cord and out into the body to contact a wide variety of organs including the eyes, heart, lungs, stomach and intestines, joints, and skin. In organs where the immune system cells develop and respond to pathogens (e.g., bone marrow, thymus, spleen, and lymph nodes), sympathetic nerve terminals make contact with immune cells. Thus, sympathetic release of norepinephrine and neuropeptide Y, together with receptor binding of these neurotransmitters by immune cells, serve as the signal in this "hard-wire" connection between the brain and the immune system. In addition, sympathetic nerves penetrate into the adrenal gland and cause the release of epinephrine into the bloodstream, which circulates to immune cells as another sympathetic regulatory signal.

Many immune system cells change their behavior in the presence of neurotransmitters. Under both laboratory and naturalistic conditions, sympathetic activation has been shown to suppress the activity of diverse populations of immune cells including NK cells and T lymphocytes. In contrast, other aspects of the immune response can be enhanced. For example, catecholamines can increase the production of antibodies by B cells and the ability of macrophages to release cytokines and thereby signal the presence of a pathogen. Additional studies indicate that sympathetic activation can also shunt some immune system cells out of circulating blood and into the lymphoid organs (e.g. spleen, lymph nodes, thymus) while recruiting other types of immune cell into circulation (e.g., NK cells). In general, SNS activation can reduce the immune system's ability to destroy pathogens that live inside cells (e.g., viruses) via decreases of the cellular immune response, while sparing or enhancing the humoral immune response to pathogens that live outside cells (e.g., bacteria). Together, these observations are a cornerstone for understanding fundamental, neuroanatomic signaling between the autonomic nervous and immune systems.

Neuroendocrine Axis

The other way in which the brain can communicate with the immune system is via the HPA system. This process begins in the hypothalamus, an area of the brain that governs basic bodily processes such as temperature, thirst, and hunger. Following the release of neuroendocrine factors from the brain, the endocrine glands secrete hormones into the circulation, which reach various organs and bind to hormone receptors on the organs. Under conditions of psychological or physical stress, for example, the hypothalamus increases its release of corticotropin-releasing hormone (CRH) into a small network of blood vessels that descends into the pituitary gland. In response to CRH, the pituitary gland synthesizes adrenocorticotropic hormone (ACTH), which travels through the bloodstream down to the adrenal glands and triggers the release of a steroid hormone called cortisol from the outer portion of the adrenal glands. Cortisol exerts diverse effects on a wide variety of physiological systems, and also coordinates the actions of various cells involved in an immune response by altering the production of cytokines or immune messengers. Similar to sympathetic catecholamines and neuropeptide Y, cortisol can suppress the cellular immune response critical to defending the body against viral infections. Indeed, a synthetic analog of cortisol is often used to suppress excessive immune system responses (e.g., in autoimmune diseases such as arthritis, or allergic reactions such as the rash produced by poison oak). Cortisol can also prompt some immune cells to move out from circulating blood into lymphoid organs or peripheral tissues such as the skin. Even more remarkable about the interactions between the neuroendocrine and immune systems is that immune cells can also produce neuroendocrine peptides (e.g., endorphin, ACTH), which suggests that the brain, neuroendocrine axis, and immune system use the same molecular signals to communicate with each other.

Central Modulation of Immunity

Together, this converging evidence of brain-immune system interactions legitimizes the possibility that the brain has a physiological role in the regulation of immunity. Indeed, one key peptide involved in integrating neural and neuroendocrine control of visceral processes is CRH, and release of this peptide in the brain alters a variety of immune processes including aspects of innate immunity, cellular immunity, and in vivo measures of antibody production. Peripheral immune measures also change following lesioning of the brain (e.g., hypothalamus) or in response to the stimulation of certain brain regions. The brain controls immune cells in lymphoid tissue in the same manner it controls other visceral organs, namely, by coordinating autonomic and neuroendocrine pathways; when these pathways are blocked by specific factors that bind to sympathetic or hormone receptors, the effects of CRH or brain stimulation on immune function is also blocked.

BEHAVIORAL AND PSYCHOLOGICAL INFLUENCES ON IMMUNITY

Given that psychological responses are expressed in neural activity with accompanying changes in neuroendocrine and autonomic function, it is not surprising that behaviors and emotions are capable of altering immunity. One seminal example is classical conditioning of immune responses. Conditioned immune responses have also been found to retard disease progression in an animal model of autoimmune disease. In the clinical setting, immunosuppressive conditioning occurs in cancer patients who receive chemotherapeutic drugs, and conditioning processes are thought to contribute to biological effects of placebo.

Stress and immunity, animals. Considerable evidence has shown that stress can influence health outcomes, and this general concept has led to evaluation of the impact of experimental stressors on immunity. In animals, acute administration of stressors produces alterations of immunity that cannot be accounted for by the physical effects of the stress. Psychological components such as conditioned fear and uncontrollability induce altered immunity, and these effects are related in a dose-dependent manner to the severity of the stressor. Almost every component of the immune system has been found to respond to stress. Stressors (e.g., electric shock, social defeat, restraint, handling, maternal separation) decrease specific and nonspecific cellular immune responses and produce a shift in the expression of regulatory cytokines from those that drive cellular responses (e.g., Th1 cytokines) to those that enhance humoral immunity (e.g., Th2 cytokines). Stress can also alter the migration and distribution of immune cells between compartments in which decreases of immune function in one compartment (e.g., peripheral blood) may lead to increases in another area of the body (e.g., skin), through SNS-induced changes in expression of adhesion molecules on lymphocyte and vascular endothelium; adhesion molecules allow the immune cells to stick to the vessel wall and begin to move from the peripheral blood into the bodily tissues. Thus, conclusions that stress suppresses or enhances immune function with effects on immune competence must be interpreted in light of the high level of redundancy of the immune system and the ability of the immune system to compensate for changes in any one aspect.

Acute stress and immunity, humans. Acute laboratory stressors (e.g., mental arithmetic, public speaking, physical exercise) produce profound and rapid changes in the immune system due to the redistribution of immunoregulatory cells from lymphoid organs such as the spleen into the vascular space. Increases of NK cell activity, for example, follow increases in the number of NK cells in the circulation, whereas stress-induced decreases of lymphocyte proliferation are related to shifts in the relative number of T helper to T suppressor lymphocytes. Blockade of the adrenergic receptor attenuates the acute immunologic effects of stress, suggesting that sympathetic activation underlies these processes possibly through effects on adhesion molecule expression. Individuals who are aged or are undergoing chronic stress show exaggerated

responses to acute stress and are likely to take longer to recover from the administration of stress consistent with the notion that the effects of chronic stress accumulate with age and this "wear and tear" or "allostatic load" produces a dysregulation of the body's ability to respond to stress.

Chronic stress, depression, and immunity. In contrast to the effects of laboratory stress, chronic or naturalistic stressors such as bereavement, examination stress, or caregiving are associated with reliable decreases of cellular and innate immunity. A similar pattern of immune alterations is reported in patients with major depression, which is not surprising as individuals undergoing stress often report negative emotions and depressive symptoms and the presence of such affective symptoms is associated with greater immune alterations. When depressive symptoms resolve, a normalization of natural and cellular immune function occurs. Extension of these nonspecific immune findings to disease-specific immune measures has received recent attention, and both depressed and stressed persons show declines of cellular response to varicella zoster virus (i.e., shingles) and impairments in responses to vaccines including influenza, pneumococcal, and hepatitis B. Conversely, writing about a traumatic experience ameliorates emotional stress and increases antibody responses to hepatitis immunization.

Role of moderating variables. Heterogeneity in the effects of stress and depression on immunity can be accounted for by a number of factors such as age, gender, ethnicity, health behaviors (e.g., smoking, alcohol consumption), and coping or personality. Older adults show declines in cellular immunity, and the presence of comorbid depression, and possibly stress, further magnifies age-related immune alterations. Gender of the subject exerts differential effects on pituitary-adrenal and immune systems by modulating the sensitivity of target tissues, and women show exaggerated expression of cytokines that lead to inflammation. Such inflammatory responses to stress may place women at increased risk for autoimmune disorders. In contrast, declines of T cell and NK cell response appear to be more prominent in depressed men than depressed women. In regard to ethnicity, African American ethnicity interacts with a history of alcohol consumption to exacerbate immune abnormalities; alcohol dependence is associated with decreases of NK and cellular immune responses with a shift toward

Th2 cytokine response. Moreover, depressed patients who are comorbid for alcohol abuse or tobacco smoking show exaggerated declines of NK activity.

Other personal characteristics, such as coping and personality, that moderate neuroendocrine and sympathetic activity contribute to individual differences of immune responses to psychological stress. For example, coping and personality characteristics influence people's perceptions of external events, and it is the perception of stress (rather than the event itself) that triggers physiological stress responses by the sympathetic nervous system or HPA axis. To some extent, these effects are moderated by social factors in which social support is associated with immune enhancement, whereas disruption of social relationships (e.g., bereavement, divorce, feelings of loneliness) leads to down-regulation of certain immune parameters. Furthermore, psychosocial interventions designed to reduce distress, increase adaptive coping, and provide social support can improve NK and cellular immune responses.

SLEEP, CYTOKINES, AND IMMUNITY

Disordered sleep and loss of sleep are thought to adversely affect resistance to infectious disease, increase cancer risk, and alter inflammatory disease progression. Animal studies show that sleep deprivation impairs influenza viral clearance and increases rates of bacteremia. In humans, normal sleep is associated with a redistribution of circulating lymphocyte subsets, increases of NK activity, increases of certain cytokines (e.g., IL-2, IL-6), and a relative shift toward Th1 cytokine expression that is independent of circadian processes. Conversely, sleep deprivation suppresses NK activity and IL-2 production, although prolonged sleep loss has been found to enhance measures of innate immunity and proinflammatory cytokine expression. In clinical populations who show disordered sleep (e.g., depression, bereavement, alcoholism), alterations of natural and cellular immune function coincide with sleep loss and disturbances of sleep architecture. Decreases of sleep time and/or increases of rapid eye movement (REM) or "dream" sleep are associated with increases in the nocturnal and daytime expression of IL-6, possibly with consequences for daytime fatigue.

Bidirectional actions of cytokines on sleep have also been identified. In animals, cytokines have both somnogenic and inhibitory effects on sleep depending on the cytokine, plasma level, and circadian phase. In humans, much less is known about the sleep regulatory effects of cytokines. Expression of the Th2 or anti-inflammatory cytokine IL-10 prior to sleep predicts amounts of delta sleep during the nocturnal period. In contrast, peripheral administration of the proinflammatory cytokine IL-6 reduces delta sleep, and nocturnal levels of both IL-6 and TNF temporally correlate with increases of REM sleep, particularly during the late part of the night.

CYTOKINES' INFLUENCES ON THE CENTRAL NERVOUS SYSTEM AND BEHAVIOR

Not only does the brain participate in the regulation of immune responses, but the central nervous system receives information from the periphery that an immune response is occurring with consequent changes in both electrical and neurochemical activity of the brain. During immunization to a novel protein antigen, the firing rate of neurons within the brain (e.g., ventromedial hypothalamus) increases at the time of peak production of antibody; this part of the brain controls autonomic activity. Cytokines released by immune cells are increasingly implicated as messengers in this bidirectional interaction, and the release of IL-1 following activation of macrophages with virus or other stimuli induces alterations of brain activity and changes in the metabolism of central brain chemicals and neurotransmitters such as norepinephrine, serotonin, and dopamine in discrete brain areas. Much recent data have focused on how these cytokines signal the brain given their large molecular size and inability to cross readily the blood-brain barrier. It is now known that IL-1 and possibly other inflammatory cytokines communicate with the brain by stimulating peripheral nerves, such as the vagus, that provide information to the brain. In sum, the immune system acts in many ways like a sensory organ, conveying information to the brain that ultimately regulates neuroendocrine and autonomic outflow and the course of the immune response.

Immune activation leads to changes of peripheral physiology and behaviors that are similar to a stress response. With peripheral immune activation, proinflammatory cytokines are expressed in the central nervous system, CRH is released by the hypothalamus, and there is an induction of a pituitary-adrenal response and autonomic activity. Coincident with these physiological changes, animals show reductions in activity, exploration of novel objects, social interactions, food and water intake, and a willingness to engage in sexual behaviors. Taken together, this pattern of behavioral changes (i.e., sickness behaviors) is similar to that found in animals exposed to fear or anxiety-arousing stimuli, and can be reproduced by the central or peripheral administration of IL-1. In contrast, central administration of a factor that blocks IL-1 antagonizes these effects. These cytokine-brain processes are also implicated in increased sensitivity to pain stimuli that is found following nerve or tissue injury.

Human studies have begun to reveal links between peripheral cytokines and behavioral changes. Associations between cytokines and sleep have recently been extended to measures of daytime fatigue. In cancer survivors, the occurrence of fatigue is associated with increases of proinflammatory cytokines. Large doses of cytokines, given as immunotherapy for cancer or hepatitis C, frequently induce depression-like symptoms such as depressed mood, inability to experience pleasure, fatigue, poor concentration, and disordered sleep, which can be effectively treated by giving antidepressant medications. Finally, physiological activation of the immune system by bacterial products with the release of proinflammatory cytokines leads to increases of depressed mood and anxiety and decreases of verbal and nonverbal memory functions.

CLINICAL IMPLICATIONS OF PSYCHONEUROIMMUNOLOGY

The factors that account for individual differences in the rate and severity of disease progression are not fully understood, although increasing evidence suggest that behavior and multisystem physiological changes that occur during depression or stress come together to exacerbate the course of many chronic diseases. In the following sections, several pertinent disease examples are presented in relation to relevant psychoneuroimmunology processes.

Cardiovascular Disease

Atherosclerosis is now thought to be an inflammatory process that involves a series of steps, each of which appears to be affected by stress and/or depression (Coe & Lubach, 2003; Dantzer, 2001; Sanders & Straub, 2002). Activated macrophages within the vascular secrete proinflammatory cytokines, which, in turn, leads to expression of adhesion molecules. With recruitment of immune cells to the vascular cell wall or endothelium and the release of inflammatory cytokines, the vascular endothelium expresses adhesion molecules that facilitate further binding of immune cells. Importantly, psychological and physical stressors increase both release of proinflammatory cytokines and expression of adhesion molecules that tether ("slow down") and bind immune cells to the vascular endothelium. Moreover, it appears that depression is associated with activation of the endothelium. Acute coronary patients who are depressed show an increased expression of an adhesion molecule that is released following activation of the vascular endothelium (i.e., soluble intracellular adhesion molecule). Importantly, this molecular marker of endothelial activation, as well as IL-6, predict risk of future myocardial infarction.

Infectious Disease Risk

Compelling evidence has shown that inescapable stress, a putative animal model of depression, increases susceptibility to viral diseases such as herpes simplex, influenza, and Coxsackie virus infections via alterations in immune function. In humans, prospective epidemiological studies and experimental viral challenge studies show that persons reporting more psychological stress have both a higher incidence and a greater severity of certain infectious illnesses such as Epstein-Barr virus infections and the common cold. In most studies, immune correlates were not obtained although stress-related increases of IL-6 temporally predict greater symptom severity in persons inoculated with influenza A. Moreover, experimental vaccinations have been used as a probe to examine the disease-specific and integrated in vivo action of the immune system in relation to psychological stress.

Substance and alcohol dependence also increases the risk of infectious disease, possibly through effects on neuroimmune pathways. Chronic alcohol use is associated with decreases of NK cell responses and cytokine-stimulated NK activity, decreased cellular immunity, and a relative shift toward a Th2 cytokine response. The incidence and severity of tuberculosis, hepatitis C, and possibly HIV infection is increased in alcoholics, and further data show that exaggerated expression of the Th2 cytokine IL-10 prospectively predicts infectious disease complications in alcoholics recovering from surgery. Likewise, cocaine dependence is associated with an increase in the incidence and severity of HIV disease progression and hepatitis C seroconversion, which is thought to be driven by the pharmacological effects of cocaine on proinflammatory and Th1/Th2 cytokine expression and HIV replication.

HIV

HIV infection shows a highly variable course, and psychoneuroimmunology (PNI) relationships appear to play a significant role in influencing the rate of HIV disease progression across patients. Depression, bereavement, and maladaptive coping responses to stress (including the stress of HIV infection itself) have all been shown to predict the rate of immune system decay in HIV patients. Immune system decline and HIV replication are particularly rapid in patients living under chronic stress (e.g., gay men who conceal their homosexuality) and in patients with high levels of SNS activity (e.g., socially inhibited introverts). Tissue culture studies have shown that SNS neurotransmitters and glucocorticoids can accelerate HIV replication by rendering T lymphocytes more vulnerable to infection and by suppressing production of the antiviral cytokines that help cells limit viral replication. Current research is focusing on pharmacological strategies to block the effects of stress neuroendocrine hormones on chronic viral infections such as HIV.

Stress, Depression, and Rheumatoid Arthritis: Neuroimmune Mechanisms

In a negative feedback loop, proinflammatory cytokines stimulate the HPA axis that results in the secretion of glucocorticoids, which, in turn, suppresses the immune response. However, in autoimmune disorders such as rheumatoid arthritis, it is thought that the counterregulatory glucocorticoid response is not fully achieved. In animals that are susceptible to arthritis, there is a central hypothalamic defect in the biosynthesis of CRH, blunted induction of ACTH and adrenal steroids, and decreased adrenal steroid receptor activation in immune target tissues, which together contribute to weak HPA response, one that is not sufficient to suppress the progression of an autoimmune response. Rheumatoid arthritis patients also show a relative hypofunctioning of the HPA axis despite the degree of inflammation. Stress and

depression can lead to HPA axis activation and to increases of proinflammatory cytokines, and recent data suggest that stressful events, particularly those of an interpersonal nature, provoke symptoms of disease such as greater pain and functional limitations. Moreover, the presence of depression in rheumatoid arthritis patients undergoing stress is associated with exaggerated increases of IL-6, a biomarker predictive of disease progression. Conversely, administration of a psychological intervention that decreases emotional distress produced improvements in clinician-rated disease activity in rheumatoid arthritis patients, although immunologic mediators were not measured. Likewise, in the case of another autoimmune disorder, psoriasis, a stress reduction intervention, mindfulness meditation, was found to induce a more rapid clearing of the psoriatic lesions.

Cancer and PNI

Experimental studies conducted in animal models have shown that exposure to acute stress leads to decreases in NK cell function and facilitates the metastatic spread of NK-sensitive tumors. However, establishing the links between psychological factors, changes in the immune system, and the development and progression of cancer in humans has been more challenging. Stress, distress, and lack of social support are associated with changes in the immune system and related physiological systems in cancer patients. In addition, there is some evidence that these and other psychological factors are linked to disease outcomes, such as recurrence and survival. In metastatic breast cancer patients, group psychotherapy led to improvements in mood and increased survival time, controlling for initial staging and medical care during the follow-up period. Among patients with malignant melanoma, group psychotherapy was associated with decreases in distress, increases in active coping, and increases in NK cytotoxicity, as well as a higher rate of survival. Both baseline NK cytotoxicity and improvements in coping behavior were associated with disease outcomes in this study.

Although these results are compelling, research linking psychological variables to cancer onset and progression are inconsistent, and the role of the immune system in mediating any psychological effects on disease course is not established. Interactions between tumors and the immune system are complex and vary depending on the type of cancer as well as the stage of disease. The importance of the immune system in regulating the most common human tumors, such as breast and prostate cancer, is not fully defined. In addition, immunogenic tumors have rarely been investigated in PNI studies. Other physiological systems, such as the endocrine, may also play a role; for example, dysregulated cortisol rhythm is associated with both reduced NK activity and increased mortality in metastatic breast cancer patients.

—Michael Irwin, Julienne Bower, and Steve Cole

NOTE: This work was supported in part by Grants AA10215, AA13239, MH55253, T32 MH 18399, AG18367, AT00255, AR/AG41867.

See also ALLOSTATIS, ALLOSTATIC LOAD, AND STRESS; AUTOIMMUNE DISEASES: PSYCHOSOCIAL ASPECTS; CARDIOVASCULAR REACTIVITY; CAREGIVING AND STRESS; ENDOGENOUS OPIOIDS, STRESS, AND HEALTH; IMMUNE RESPONSES TO STRESS; METABOLIC SYNDROME AND STRESS; STRESS: BIOLOGICAL ASPECTS; WOUND HEALING AND STRESS

Further Reading

Ader, R. (2000). On the development of psychoneuroimmunology. *European Journal of Pharmacology, 405*(1-3), 167-176.

Coe, C. L., & Lubach, G. R. (2003). Critical periods of special health relevance for psychoneuroimmunology. *Brain, Behavior, and Immunity, 17*(1), 3-12.

Cohen, S., & Herbert, T. B. (1996). Health psychology: Psychological factors and physical disease from the perspective of human psychoneuroimmunology. *Annual Review of Psychology, 47*, 113-142.

Dantzer, R. (2001). Cytokine-induced sickness behavior: Mechanisms and implications. *Annals of the New York Academy of Sciences, 933*, 222-234.

Irwin, M. (2002). Psychoneuroimmunology of depression: Clinical implications. *Brain, Behavior, and Immunity, 16*(1), 1-16.

Kiecolt-Glaser, J. K., McGuire, L., et al. (2002). Psychoneuroimmunology and psychosomatic medicine: Back to the future. *Psychosomatic Medicine, 64*(1), 15-28.

Kronfol, Z., & Remick, D. G. (2000). Cytokines and the brain: Implications for clinical psychiatry. *American Journal of Psychiatry, 157*(5), 683-694.

Maier, S. F., & Watkins, L. R. (1998). Cytokines for psychologists: Implications of bidirectional immune-to-brain communication for understanding behavior, mood, and cognition. *Psychological Review, 105*(1), 83-107.

Sanders, V. M., & Straub, R. H. (2002). Norepinephrine, the beta-adrenergic receptor, and immunity. *Brain, Behavior, and Immunity, 16*(4), 290-332.

PSYCHOPHYSIOLOGY: THEORY AND METHODS

Psychophysiology studies the behavior of the individual in a biological context. It is an attempt to chart the mutual interactions between psychological processes and the workings of the body, giving equal emphasis to both. It is fundamental to psychophysiology that behavior and mental life cannot exist apart from the body. It follows that a full understanding of psychological processes depends on understanding the biological context from which they proceed. Because of its emphasis on integrating our understanding of mental and physiological processes, psychophysiology has contributed to research methods and theory building in behavioral medicine. It does this by helping to disentangle the relationships between psychology and biology in relation to good and poor health. From this perspective, psychophysiologists bring a physiological emphasis to the study of behavior and mental processes as they affect good and poor health.

The emphasis of psychophysiology, like that of behavioral medicine itself, is primarily on the whole person. However, it is necessary to measure the functions of specific systems, such as the cardiovascular system, endocrine system, or immune system, in the course of psychophysiological investigations. This calls for a methodology that allows emotional experience to be studied along with physiological functioning in ways that are unobtrusive and minimally invasive. This ensures that the person being studied is behaving in a normal manner, as in everyday life, and is not reacting unduly to the apparatus or laboratory setting. Psychophysiological principles have been used to study responses to stress in the laboratory, responses to stressors in daily life, and individual differences in such responses.

Behavioral medicine is both a science and an approach to clinical practice. Both parts are concerned with the influence of behavioral factors on health and disease. Behavioral medicine holds that states of health can be influenced by overt behaviors, such as dietary habits, and by covert behaviors, such as emotional states and stress responses. This perspective leads behavioral medicine researchers to ask questions about the ways that emotional states and stress responses can affect health through their influence on physiology.

The goal is to bring to light how our behaviors and our ways of perceiving and reacting to the world may affect our well-being for better or worse. Such research addresses questions in several major areas, including (1) how the body responds during positive and negative emotion states; (2) how a given person may differ from one time to the next in stress reactivity; (3) the ways in which persons differ from one another in their stress responses; and (4) on the positive side, establishing the effects of behavior on good health and longevity. To carry out such research, behavioral medicine draws in part on the theory and methods developed in the field of psychophysiology.

In laboratory studies, persons are often exposed to stressors to determine how they react to such challenges both emotionally and physiologically. The results are thought to indicate how emotionally relevant events and behavioral stressors can affect physiology in daily life and therefore whether they may contribute to disease. For example, a commonly used stressor is public speaking. This calls on the subject to make up a short speech and deliver it without notes. Public speaking is stressful because most persons wish to avoid the embarrassment of doing poorly and want to be seen as competent by observers in the laboratory. In this sense, the social world can be modeled in a small way in the laboratory. During public speaking, this process of social evaluation, along with the resulting fear and anxiety, produces substantial increases in heart rate and blood pressure and stress hormones, including catecholamines and cortisol. The person's mood states are assessed while he or she is at rest before the task begins and again at the end, using paper-and-pencil measures or brief interviews. Similarly, automated blood pressure monitors and other recording devices are used to measure cardiovascular functions at rest, during the preparation and delivery of the speech, and afterward during a recovery period. In this manner, the combined cardiovascular and psychological reactions of the person may be measured. Using public speaking as a stressor therefore provides information on how a person's physiological reactions are set off by psychological causes.

This research strategy can then be extended to compare different kinds of people in their physiological reactivity to stress. One common example is for the researcher to identify young, healthy individuals who have a family history of high blood pressure and also to find those with no such history. These family history groups can then be compared in the laboratory for differences their stress responses, perhaps using the public speaking stressor or some other method. This allows potential differences in stress reactivity to be assessed in relation to a family history of this prevalent cardiovascular disease. It is then possible to follow such persons for a period of years to establish which persons become hypertensive and which retain a normal blood pressure. Do persons from the family history group have a greater likelihood of becoming hypertensive in middle age? Are persons with greater reactions to stress more likely to become hypertensive, regardless of family history? Such studies therefore allow potential interactions between family history and stress reactivity to be studied. If persons with a family history of hypertension who are also highly reactive to social stress are much more likely to become hypertensive, then we would conclude that the family history created a biologically based risk factor that was enhanced by an elevated level of stress responsivity. In contrast, should risk of hypertension be increased equally by high reactivity in persons with and without a family history of hypertension, we would conclude that family history and reactivity tendencies contribute to hypertension risk in an additive manner.

Although the laboratory provides a well-controlled environment with an extensive range of measurement techniques, ambulatory methods have been used with increasing frequency outside the laboratory to document how challenges in persons' daily lives can affect cardiovascular, endocrine, or immune systems. Such methods measure the person's responses to naturalistic stressors, such as work stress, or challenges in the home, such as family conflict or the stress of caring for a chronically ill spouse. Such studies rely on small, lightweight monitors that can be worn comfortably as persons go about their daily routines. These monitors can make reliable measurements in a wide range of circumstances. Such systems are able to track heart rate, blood pressure, and physical activity. In addition, people usually report on their subjective state using brief paper diaries or personal digital assistants. As in laboratory studies, this ambulatory method may be used to estimate the interaction of stress responses and disease risk. Persons with and without a family history of hypertension may be compared as they go about their daily lives. As in the laboratory, persons with the largest or most prolonged reactions to stress at home or at work are suspected of having greater risk of future disease, and again they may be followed up for actual occurrence of hypertension in future years.

Although some research focuses on family history, other work seeks to connect psychological dispositions, such as hopelessness, depression, or hostile style, to disease risk. Studies using this strategy may compare highly hostile persons with nonhostile individuals with a specific hostility-provoking interaction, such as harassing comments during work on a difficult task. By measuring physiological reactions to such specific challenges in persons with different psychological characteristics, a clearer picture may be developed of the psychological and physiological interplay that is suspected of contributing to disease.

While much of this research focuses on negative emotion states, stress responses, and risk of disease, there is a growing interest in positive emotional states and in studying persons who tend frequently to experience the positive emotions of joy and happiness. As in the above examples, such persons can be selected for their emotion traits using a combination of self-report techniques and in laboratory tests of brain function. Persons high in typical positive affect can then be compared to those with less positive affective states in their resistance to the effects of stress and in their long-term states of health.

The research examples listed above all depend on testing persons while they are relaxed and resting, as well as when they are under stress or perhaps in a pleasurable mood. For these reasons, it is desirable to use measurement methods that do not cause discomfort or distress. Behavioral medicine research has therefore relied on methods of psychophysiological measurement that are noninvasive or minimally invasive and cause the volunteer no discomfort.

The examples above focused on the cardiovascular system, which can be studied using methods such as the electrocardiogram, blood pressure monitoring, impedance cardiography to measure pumping action of the heart and constriction of the blood vessels, and occasionally, fluid output to assess kidney function.

Stress research often uses additional methods to track responses of the endocrine system, involving collection of urine, blood, or saliva for measurement of stress hormones and other substances associated with stress and pain responses. Still other studies examine the immune system, here using minimally invasive techniques in the collection of blood for later measurement of the numbers of immune system cells and their biological activity. Closely related to these physiological measurements is the need to classify persons as to personality and temperament characteristics to establish relationships between acute stress responses or chronic allostatic responses in the lab or in daily life. These considerations call for use of interviews or paper-and-pencil measures of personality and mood states. Finally, the application of such psychophysiological techniques calls for appropriate selection of tasks and ways to analyze the data.

—*William R. Lovallo*

See also ALLOSTATIS, ALLOSTATIC LOAD, AND STRESS; BLOOD PRESSURE, HYPERTENSION, AND STRESS; CARDIOVASCULAR PSYCHOPHYSIOLOGY: MEASURES; CARDIOVASCULAR REACTIVITY; EMOTIONS: NEGATIVE EMOTIONS AND HEALTH; EMOTIONS: POSITIVE EMOTIONS AND HEALTH; GENERAL ADAPTATION SYNDROME; HEART DISEASE AND REACTIVITY; HOPELESSNESS AND HEALTH; HOSTILITY AND HEALTH; HOSTILITY: PSYCHOPHYSIOLOGY; IMMUNE RESPONSES TO STRESS; PSYCHONEUROIMMUNOLOGY

Further Reading

al'Absi, M., Bongard, S., Buchanan, T., Pincomb, G. A., Licinio, J., & Lovallo, W. R. (1997). Cardiovascular and neuroendocrine adjustment to public-speaking and mental arithmetic stressors. *Psychophysiology, 34,* 266-275.

al'Absi, M., Everson, S. A., & Lovallo, W. R. (1995). Hypertension risk factors and cardiovascular reactivity to mental stress in young men. *International Journal of Psychophysiology, 20,* 155-160.

Cacioppo, J. T., Tassinary, L. G., & Berntson, G. G. (Eds.). (2000). *Handbook of psychophysiology.* New York: Cambridge University Press.

Davidson, R. J. (2000). Affective style, psychopathology, and resilience: Brain mechanisms and plasticity. *American Psychologist, 55,* 1196-1214.

Everson, S. A., Kaplan, G. A., Goldberg, D. E., & Salonen, J. T. (1996). Anticipatory blood pressure response to exercise predicts future high blood pressure in middle-aged men. *Hypertension, 27,* 1059-1064.

Everson, S. A., McKey, B. S., & Lovallo, W. R. (1995). Effect of trait hostility on cardiovascular responses to harassment in young men. *International Journal of Behavioral Medicine, 2,* 172-191.

Glaser, R., & Kiecolt-Glaser, J. K. (Eds.). (1994). *Handbook of human stress and immunity.* San Diego, CA: Academic Press.

Kamarck, T. W., & Lovallo, W. R. (2003). Progress and prospects in the conceptualization and measurement of cardiovascular reactivity. *Psychosomatic Medicine, 65,* 9-21.

Lovallo, W. R. (1997). *Stress and health: Biological and psychological interactions.* Thousand Oaks, CA: Sage.

Powell, L. H., Lovallo, W. R., Matthews, K. A., Meyer, P., Midgley, A. R., Baum, A., Stone, A. A., Underwood, L.,

McCann, J. J., Janikula Herro, K., & Ory, M. G. (2002). Physiologic markers of chronic stress in premenopausal, middle-aged women. *Psychosomatic Medicine, 64,* 502-509.

Sausen, K. P., Lovallo, W. R., Pincomb, G. A., & Wilson, M. F. (1992). Cardiovascular responses to occupational stress in medical students: A paradigm for ambulatory monitoring studies. *Health Psychology, 11,* 55-60.

Schneiderman, N., Kaufmann, P., & Weiss, S. (Eds.). (1989). *Handbook of research methods in cardiovascular behavioral medicine.* New York: Plenum.

Turner, J. R., Sherwood, A., & Light, K. C. (Eds.). (1992). *Individual differences in cardiovascular response to stress.* New York: Plenum.

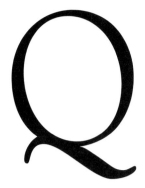

QUALITY OF LIFE: MEASUREMENT

There are two very different types of indicator in terms of which the performance of health care may be assessed. The first type, which may be termed the quantity of life, is concerned with the impact of health care on mortality. The second type of indicator is concerned with the quality rather than duration or survival of lives. An evaluation of contemporary health care that only assessed death rates would provide only a very skewed and limited assessment. However, while the measurement of death and survival may be considered a relatively clear and precise task, quality of life is concerned with experiences that are inherently personal and subjective. Nevertheless, confidence has grown in the last 30 years that quality of life can be measured with sufficient accuracy.

Recognition of the importance of quality of life in health care is often traced to the World Health Organization's declaration that health should be considered a state of complete physical, mental, and social well-being rather than merely the absence of disease. Health and illness often have wide-ranging impact on individuals, and the goal of health care is to address these broader impacts. Since the 1970s, an array of instruments in the form of questionnaires and interview schedules, together with models and principles of measurement, have been developed to assess these broader impacts of health and illness. Strictly speaking, in the context of health care, we are concerned with instruments to assess health-related quality of life, rather than quality of life determined by, for example, individuals' education or political environment

outside the realm of health care. However, terminology is not consistent, and instruments are often also referred to as "health status," "subjective health status," and "outcome" measures. An essential feature of such instruments is that, whenever possible, judgments of quality of life are made by the patient or layperson rather than the health professional because of the substantial evidence that patients and health professionals significantly differ from each other in their judgments about quality of life, and it is patients' views that are of ultimate concern.

USES OF QUALITY OF LIFE MEASURES

Health-related quality of life measures have been developed to fulfill a number of different purposes. First and most important is their use as measures of outcome in the evaluation of health care interventions. Whether the intervention is relatively simple, such as a drug, or is more complex, such as a new type of behavioral intervention or innovative form of clinic, health-related quality of life measures provide unique evidence of the impact of the intervention, in both positive and negative consequences, as viewed by patients. Thus, trials of new drugs intended to have positive effects on survival for patients with cancer, high blood pressure, or neurodegenerative disease will commonly now include measures to assess effects on aspects of quality of life such as mood, symptoms such as pain and nausea, family life, and social functioning. Such trials require that health-related quality of life be assessed before and after the study intervention as well as in control or comparison groups receiving either placebo or best available alternative treatment in order to specify the impact of the study intervention.

One particular type of quality of life instrument, discussed below, the utility or preference measure, is intended to provide a single global or net measure of the value of a health state to an individual, taking account of all gains and losses in specific areas of quality of life. It has been argued by health economists that these utility measures provide a unique form of outcome measure in evaluations that can be used to produce overall summaries of the net costs and benefits of health care interventions for purposes of planning and prioritizing services.

A second application is the use of health-related quality of life measures to assess the nature and level of health-related problems in a community or group of patients. Particularly as evidence accumulates that quality of life measures are strongly predictive of future health problems and also of future demands upon health care, such measures provide indicators that assist in the planning of services and identification of current or future need. A related but distinct third application is the use of quality of life measures in individual patient care, assessing the patient's needs, and progress in response to treatment. Evaluations of this application suggest that while health professionals find this novel form of information about their patients interesting and helpful, it does not improve the quality of their care and health outcomes.

Finally, quality of life measures can be used to understand problems in health care such as illness behavior and professional-patient relationships. Correlations between conventional laboratory or clinical measures of disease severity and patient-assessed health-related quality of life measures are usually modest rather than high. Health-related quality of life measures often provide better predictors of patients' illness behavior, satisfaction with care, adherence to regimens, and ability to cope with health problems.

TYPES OF MEASURE

Several different types of health-related quality of life measure have been developed. They have distinct properties and purposes. The first type to be developed was the "generic" measure, so called because they were intended to be applicable in content to the widest range of health problems and patient groups. One of the earliest of such generic instruments to be

widely used was the Sickness Impact Profile (SIP) (Bergner et al., 1976). The SIP comprises 136 statements about the individual for each of which the respondent selects the answer yes or no. Each item contributes to one of 12 scales or dimensions: ambulation, household management, emotions, eating, body care and movement, recreation, alertness, communication, mobility, social interaction, sleep and rest, work. Items are differentially weighted, based on panels' judgments of relative severity. Items can also be summed to produce physical, psychosocial dimension, and overall total scores. A similar instrument, the Nottingham Health Profile (NHP), comprises 38 questionnaire items with binary yes/no responses and six scales: energy, sleep, pain, social isolation, emotional reactions, and physical mobility (Hunt, McEwen, & McKenna, 1986).

By far the most commonly used generic instrument is the Short-Form 36-Item Health Survey (SF-36; Ware & Sherbourne, 1992). Its 36 items contribute to eight scales: physical functioning, social functioning, pain, energy, mental health, health perceptions, role limitations due to physical problems, and role limitations due to emotional problems. Two summary scores, physical and mental component, can be derived from the instrument. An advantage of SF-36 over SIP and NHP is that more than two response categories ("yes" or "no") are provided for each item. Respondents generally prefer questions with possible answers that permit expression of the extent or degree to which a problem is experienced (e.g., "all of the time," "some of the time").

More recently, numerous instruments have been developed intended to provide assessments of specific health problems, hence the term *disease-specific*. Evaluations such as randomized controlled trials to evaluate interventions to improve health-related quality of life increasingly have to detect ever more modest and subtle benefits and side effects. For this reason, it is argued that instruments have to be targeted at the very specific features of particular health problems rather than relying on questionnaire content that is intentionally general. As a result, for most common health problems, there now exist several specifically developed health-related quality of life instruments.

A typical example of a disease-specific instrument is the Western Ontario and McMaster Universities Arthritis Index (WOMAC; Bellamy, Buchanan, Goldsmith, Campbell, & Stitt, 1988). This instrument comprises 24 items assessing pain, stiffness, and physical function in osteoarthritis of the hip and knee. As an alternative instrument for arthritis, assessing a wide set of consequences of the disease than WOMAC, the Arthritis Impact Measurement Scale (AIMS) comprises 45 items assessing nine dimensions of arthritis impact: mobility, physical activity, activities of daily living, dexterity, household activities, pain, social activities, depression, and anxiety (Meenan, 1982). However, there are several other instruments purporting to assess health-related quality of life in relation to arthritis, differing in range and detail of item content, time-frame addressed by question length and complexity of instrument and extent of available evidence evaluating performance.

Generic and disease-specific instruments have contrasting advantages. Disease-specific measures are intended to provide highly relevant evidence of patients' experiences of a particular disease that may simply be missed by the more general and nonspecific information captured by generic instruments. By contrast, generic instruments may provide evidence of unexpected experiences not normally associated with a specific disease. They also permit comparisons of evidence across diseases and interventions for different diseases that cannot be achieved with disease-specific measures.

Both generic and disease-specific instruments normally have one feature in common, that the content comprises standard questionnaire items. It has been argued that it runs counter to the purpose of quality of life assessment to have invariant content to address issues that inevitably vary between individuals. To meet this criticism, a number of instruments have been developed that contain items that can be individualized by means of the respondent identifying his or her own personal health-related quality of life concerns for assessment. A simple example, also taken from the field of arthritis, is the McMaster-Toronto Arthritis Patient Function Preference Questionnaire (MACTAR; Tugwell et al., 1987). To complete this assessment, patients with arthritis identify their own activities limited by arthritis rather than respond to a standard list of questions; they rank activities chosen in order of preference to have them improved by treatment and subsequently rate extent of improvement in chosen activities. The principle of individualized instruments has been extended from the disease-specific context, and there now exist instruments such as the Schedule for the Evaluation of Individual Quality of Life that attempt to provide individualized questionnaire content that can be applied across all health care problems (O'Boyle, McGee, Hickey, O'Malley, & Joyce, 1992). Although efforts have been made to turn such instruments into self-completed questionnaires, the added complexity of tasks usually results in such instruments requiring an interviewer.

One final type of instrument is the utility-based or preference-based measure. As already mentioned, it differs from other measures largely in terms of its purpose. The purpose of such instruments is to derive an estimate of the net value to patients or society of health states, usually health states that can be attributed to health care interventions. The values or, in the language of this approach, the utilities associated with an intervention are combined with evidence of the costs of an intervention to provide an overall cost-utility analysis. Decision makers in health care are expected to favor those interventions that have a favorable ratio of costs and utilities.

The utilities associated with given health states are obtained from respondents by one of several experimental techniques employed in interviews. One approach (standard gamble) is to invite respondents to judge what level of risk of death they would be prepared (hypothetically) to face from a treatment that would restore them to normal health. The greater the risk, the lower the level of utility associated with a given health state. Another approach (time trade-off) invites respondents hypothetically to choose between a life spent in a state of ill health that is the object of the study and another life that is healthy but for a shorter duration. Again the assumption is made that the greater the time that respondents forgo, the worse the health state, that is, the lower its utility.

There are some inherent difficulties of comprehension and compliance by respondents in interviews to elicit utilities. For this reason, health-related quality of life instruments in the form of self-completed questionnaires have been developed that have the advantage of standard easy to answer response categories but with utility values assigned to response categories from prior experimental research. The most commonly used of such instruments is the EQ-5D, the core of which requires that respondents, in order to describe their health, choose from three different levels of severity of five simply presented dimensions of health (mobility, self-care, usual activity, pain, mood) (EuroQol Group, 1990). The health state selected has a numerical score determined by previous lay panels' judgments of the utilities associated with different health states. Attempts have also been made to derive utility values for the SF-36 questionnaire described above. Supporters of this approach argue that, by separating out descriptions of health states from how such states are valued, there is a clearer and more transparent approach to measurement than is usual in quality of life measures.

REQUIRED PROPERTIES OF MEASURES

For a quality of life measure to work well in the applications outlined earlier, it is essential that it have a number of measurement properties that can only be achieved by careful research in developing the instrument. The four key measurement properties required of an instrument are reliability, validity, responsiveness, and feasibility. These are considered in turn.

Reliability is concerned with the reproducibility and internal consistency of a measure. Reproducibility focuses upon whether an instrument produces the same results on repeated applications when respondents have not changed on the subject being assessed. Correlation coefficients provide evidence of the strength of association between repeated tests but are also essential to check for systematic shifts in mean score from an instrument. Retesting of an instrument is normally performed between 2 and 14 days after the first administration on respondents for whom there is other independent evidence that no important change has occurred in relevant aspects of health.

Internal reliability is a distinct requirement because, normally, constructs in health-related quality of life are measured by several questionnaire items that are combined to form a scale. The use of scales reflects a very basic principle of measurement: that several related observations will produce more reliable estimates of the intended construct than one single questionnaire item. However, for this to be true, the extent to which items are addressing a single construct has to be examined by calculating the extent of agreement between items of a scale. As the level of agreement falls between items intended to be a scale, it becomes more likely that the items are not internally consistent measures of a single construct.

The *validity* of a measure is determined by assessment of the extent to which it measures what it purports to measure. A fundamental issue, therefore, is determining the purpose of an instrument. An instrument validated for use in specific purposes requires further evidence of validity when applied for a new purpose or context. Two approaches to the assessment of validity are essential. First, face and content validity require judgments as to whether an instrument appears to measure its intended target and whether questionnaire items address the full range or scope of the intended construct. It is increasingly accepted that face and content validity are enhanced by the care and extent to which relevant patient groups have participated in the initial development of an instrument.

The second and more formal quantitative assessment of instruments examines construct validity. Here the pattern of associations of an instrument with other data is inspected; for example, a health-related quality of life scale may be expected to have associations with measures of disease severity, health care utilization, and emotional well-being. Crucially, construct validity is not established by one study but by an accumulating pattern of evidence.

Responsiveness assesses the extent to which an instrument can detect important changes over time within individuals, an essential feature of any instrument to be used in trials or other forms of evaluation of interventions. As with validity, there are several approaches to assessing responsiveness with no single method dominant. A range of statistical approaches essentially examine the amount of intraindividual change in an instrument in samples expected on other grounds to have experienced change. An alternative set of approaches use external criteria against which to judge change over time in an instrument. For example, patients may be asked (by means of a so-called transition question) to rate the extent to which their health-related quality of life has changed compared to a specific previous occasion. The responsiveness of a health-related quality of life instrument completed at the same time as the transition question and at the specific previous occasion would be judged by level of agreement of change score on the instrument with patients' transition questions.

One of the commonest problems that limits the responsiveness of instruments stems from so-called ceiling and floor effects. Because of the choice and wording of questionnaire items, it may be impossible for respondents to register further improvements or deterioration in health-related quality of life. It is common to consider instruments in which answers are highly skewed to one or the other end of the distribution of possible scores as more prone to such effects.

One last criterion needs to be applied to the evaluation of instruments in this field, *feasibility*. Especially as health-related quality of life instruments are usually completed by respondents when unwell, there is an imperative that they impose as little burden as possible in terms of length, complexity, or distressing content. It is standard practice to ask patients directly about the acceptability of an instrument as part of its development and evaluation. Other indicators of acceptability include the time taken to complete an instrument and its response rate. Feasibility also focuses upon the overall burden to investigators and others in administering and processing an instrument. Some instruments, especially those requiring administration by interview, may require more time to complete and process responses and training on the part of the interviewer. The extent of disruption to normal clinical activity is an important consideration.

There has been increasing interest in reducing the length of instruments to improve overall feasibility. It is quite often possible to produce shorter forms of health-related quality of life instruments with little or no loss of validity and responsiveness.

At present, only a minority of clinical trials use health-related quality of life instruments as measures of outcome, even when it is clear that they would be relevant to the questions addressed by the trial. This partly reflects lack of familiarity with their potential contribution. When they are used, inappropriate measures are often selected. As illustrated earlier with the example of arthritis, there are often several competing instruments from which to choose for any given health problem. More sensible use of appropriate measures of quality of life are more likely to emerge if studies are performed in which two or more instruments are completed at every assessment point over time by all patients. Only with such data can the comparative performance of different instruments against the criteria earlier described be more accurately assessed and understanding of instruments increase. Comparative longitudinal data from trials and similar studies are particularly needed to identify instruments most sensitive to changes in quality of life that matter to patients. In some fields such as cancer and rheumatology, professional consensus groups have also assessed available comparative evidence to determine which instruments are generally most useful. A view emerging from many reviews is that it is optimal practice in trials and evaluative studies to use both a disease-specific and generic health-related quality of life measure to cover a full spectrum of possible outcomes of interventions.

As applications of health-related quality of life measures increase, it becomes more important to focus on the interpretability of scores from such instruments. Whereas numerical values for familiar clinical measures such as blood pressure and hemoglobin are readily interpreted, this is not the case for measures of quality of life. Different approaches to increase interpretability have been adopted. One approach is to relate particular changes in score on an instrument to more familiar human experiences. Thus, it is possible to estimate the likely change in quality of life score of someone made redundant from work or bereaved; such change scores can then be related to changes in scores observed in clinical trials. Another approach is to calculate scores typical of healthy members of the community, and of patients attending ambulatory or inpatient care, and to use these scores as benchmarks of different levels of life, with poorest scores typically observed in inpatients and most favorable scores observed in healthy members of the community.

Alternatively, more use can be made of transition questions described earlier. Patients who complete health-related quality of life measures at two time points, for example, in a clinical trial before and after an intervention, can also at the second time point make judgments about whether they have noticed a change in dimensions assessed by the instrument. A comparison of health-related quality of life scores of patients noticing that they are a little worse (or better) can be made with the scores of those rating themselves as unchanged in order to estimate average change scores associated with perception of change. Such estimates can be treated as the smallest scores that will be treated as real change rather than noise or random error in an instrument; often referred to as "minimal clinically important change."

The principle that personal experiences of health and illness can be measured is now well established. Effort is now focused on improving the use and interpretation of measures of health-related quality of life to inform decisions about health care.

—*Ray Fitzpatrick*

See also Chronic Illness: Psychological Aspects; Cost-Effectiveness

Further Reading

Bellamy, N., Buchanan, W. W., Goldsmith, C. H., Campbell, J., & Stitt L. W. (1988). Validation study of WOMAC. *Journal of Rheumatology 15,* 1833-1840.

Bergner, M., Bobbitt, R. A., Kressel, S., Pollard, W., Gilson, B., & Morris, J. (1976). The Sickness Impact Profile: Conceptual formulation and methodology for the development of health status measure. *International Journal of Health Services 6,* 393-415.

Bowling, A. (1995). *Measuring disease.* Buckingham, UK: Open University Press.

EuroQol Group. (1990). EuroQol: A new facility for the measurement of health-related quality of life. *Health Policy 16,* 199-208.

Fitzpatrick, R., Davey, C., Buxton, M., & Jones, D. (1998). Evaluating patient-based outcome measures for use in clinical trials. *Health Technology Assessment 2,* 1-74.

Hunt, S., McEwen, J., & McKenna, S. (1986). *Measuring health status.* London: Croom Helm.

Meenan, R. F. (1982). The AIMS approach to health status measurement. *Journal of Rheumatology 9,* 785-788.

O'Boyle, C., McGee, H., Hickey, A., O'Malley, K., & Joyce, C. (1992). Individual quality of life in patients undergoing hip replacement. *Lancet 339,* 1088-1091.

Tugwell, P., Bombardier, C., Buchanan, W. W., Goldsmith, C. H., Grace, E., & Hanna, B. (1987). The MACTAR Patient Preference Disability Questionnaire. *Journal of Rheumatology, 14,* 446-451.

Ware, J., & Sherbourne, C. (1992). The MOS 36-item Short Form health survey (SF-36) 1: Conceptual framework and item selection. *Medical Care 30,* 473-483.

R

RACE AND HEALTH.
See HEALTH DISPARITIES

RAYNAUD'S DISEASE: BEHAVIORAL TREATMENT

Raynaud's disease is a disorder of peripheral blood vessels in which blood flow in the fingers and toes stops when they are exposed to cold. The attacks typically last about 5 to 15 minutes, may occur several times a day, and can be quite painful. Because the symptoms are localized, and because healthy individuals can be trained to increase their peripheral blood flow with behavioral methods such as biofeedback, these techniques have been used to treat persons suffering from Raynaud's disease.

The disease was first described by a French physician, Maurice Raynaud, in his doctoral thesis published in 1862. When exposed to cold, the digits first turn white, due to the cessation of blood flow. This is followed by a blue or cyanotic phase caused by depletion of oxygen in the remaining blood. During these periods, the digits feel numb or extremely cold. The attacks often end with a red or reactive hyperemic phase, in which burning and/or pain are experienced due to a sudden inrush of returning blood.

Blood flow in the fingers and toes is controlled by nerves that constrict small blood vessels to reduce blood flow and by chemicals that circulate in the blood. Raynaud thought that the attacks were caused by overactivity of these nerves. However, Thomas Lewis showed, in a few patients, that the attacks could occur even when these nerves were anesthetized, and our laboratory later verified this in a larger controlled study.

Lewis thought that the attacks were caused by an abnormality in the blood vessels themselves. Several laboratories have shown that the peripheral blood vessels of Raynaud's disease patients were oversensitive to chemicals that circulate in the blood, such as serotonin and norepinephrine, particularly during cooling. However, the amounts of these chemicals in the blood are not abnormally high. The most recent research suggests that the abnormality may lie in the signaling pathways that connect the biochemical receptors for norepinephrine and serotonin with the muscle fibers in the blood vessels that make them constrict.

Raynaud's disease runs in families, suggesting that genetic factors may be involved. However, specific genes that cause Raynaud's disease have not yet been identified. The disease is about four times more common in women than in men and affects about 4% of the population in the United States. Raynaud's symptoms can also occur in conjunction with other diseases, such as scleroderma, where it is referred to as secondary Raynaud's phenomenon. This entry focuses on primary Raynaud's disease.

BEHAVIORAL CONTROL OF PERIPHERAL BLOOD FLOW

Biofeedback comprises a set of techniques whereby a physiological function is measured and information immediately presented to the subject, who then learns to control it using mental methods. Finger temperature is generally used as an indicator of blood flow because it can be easily and inexpensively measured. Feedback can be given using meters, tones, lights, or digital displays.

Edward Taub first showed that normal volunteers could learn to raise and lower their finger temperature, using a variable intensity light as feedback. He also noted that success was dependent, to some extent, on the personality of the trainer. Francis J. Keefe then conducted several controlled studies showing that several combinations of brief temperature biofeedback and suggestions to increase finger temperature produced significant temperature elevations. He also showed that these effects were maintained 1 to 2 weeks after training. Our laboratory then replicated these findings and showed that the training effects were maintained outside the laboratory, in a different environment.

BEHAVIORAL TREATMENT OF RAYNAUD'S DISEASE

Behavioral treatments for Raynaud's disease have generally employed finger temperature biofeedback and/or autogenic training, a relaxation-based method using self-suggestions of warm imagery such as, "My hands are warm and heavy." Richard S. Surwit treated 30 patients who were randomly assigned to receive twelve 45-minute laboratory sessions in autogenic training, either alone or in combination with temperature biofeedback. Also, for 1 month, half the patients served as a waiting list control group for the other half and then received treatment. Subjects as a whole showed significant improvement in response to a cold stress test, but there were no significant differences in attack frequency reduction between treated subjects (32%) and waiting list controls (10%). Similar results were found in a subsequent study the following year.

Because the above studies combined biofeedback with autogenic training, our laboratory separated the methods. We compared finger temperature biofeedback, autogenic training, forehead muscle biofeedback (an irrelevant form of feedback used as a placebo control), and temperature feedback given during mild cold stress to the finger. We reasoned that this last procedure would better enable the patients to produce the feedback response in the natural environment, where it must be produced under cold conditions. There were eight patients in each group. The following winter, the patients who received temperature feedback alone, or in combination with cold stress, reported 66.8% and 92.5% fewer attacks respectively. These results were maintained at 2- and 3-year follow-up periods. The patients who received autogenic training or muscle biofeedback did not report significant symptom reductions. Interestingly, these patients did show signs of relaxation, such as decreased muscle tension and heart rate, whereas the biofeedback patients did not.

These last findings suggested that relaxation was not beneficial in alleviating Raynaud's attacks, and led us to study the mechanisms of temperature biofeedback. Another Raynaud's researcher, Jay D. Coffman, discovered that activation of a class of biochemical receptors in blood vessels (β-adrenergic receptors) could increase finger blood flow without relaxation. We blocked these receptors with a drug (β-blocker) injected into the artery that carries blood to the hand (brachial artery). When we did this during temperature biofeedback, the blood flow elevations stopped. This showed that β-adrenergic receptors are involved. We then anesthetized the nerves to the fingers during temperature feedback, but the temperature elevations still occurred. This showed that the nerve pathways are not needed for temperature biofeedback, just as they are not needed to produce a Raynaud's attack. Finally, we drew blood samples from the hand during temperature biofeedback and analyzed the blood for levels of two main chemicals that cause changes in blood flow: norepinephrine and epinephrine. We found that these levels did not change. Thus, the temperature and blood flow elevations occurring during biofeedback are probably caused by changes in a circulating chemical acting at β-receptors, without the involvement of the finger nerves. This mechanism appears to be independent of physiological relaxation.

Finally, the effects of temperature biofeedback with cold stress and a drug that increases blood flow (nifedipine) were tested in a large multisite, clinical study. Three hundred and thirteen patients were randomly assigned to receive ten 1-hour training sessions in temperature biofeedback or forehead muscle biofeedback (behavioral placebo), or to receive nifedipine or a pill placebo. Standard treatment protocols were followed by all five sites. Nifedipine-treated patients showed a significant reduction in attack frequency (66%) compared to placebo, but the temperature biofeedback patients did not. Examination of the data showed that the temperature biofeedback patients failed to learn to increase their finger temperature. The reasons for this are not known, but may have been due to the use of a standard protocol, without personalized interactions between the therapists and the patients.

—*Robert R. Freedman*

See also BIOFEEDBACK

Further Reading

Freedman, R. R. (1991). Physiological mechanisms of temperature biofeedback. *Biofeedback and Self-Regulation, 16,* 95-115.

Stetter, F., and Kupper, S. (2002). Autogenic training: A meta-analysis of clinical outcome studies. *Applied Psychophysiology and Biofeedback, 27,* 45-98.

REPRESSIVE COPING AND HEALTH

The origins of the term *repression* can be traced back to Sigmund Freud, who considered repression as a mechanism of stopping anxiety-reaching consciousness. The modern usage of repression also refers to repression as a way of not attending to negative, emotional information.

However, the use of the term has been considerably developed since the time of Freud. Nowadays, the most popular usage of repression recognizes it as an individual difference variable (or trait), and is thought of as a specific type of coping or defense mechanism that some people exhibit. Consequently, in this conceptualization of repression, individuals are said to have a repressive coping style or exhibit repressive defensiveness. The major defining characteristic of these individuals (who are usually termed *repressors*) is that they do not recognize their own emotional responses and they use a variety of strategies to avoid their negative emotions. They seem to be self-deceivers rather than impression managers, in that they expend a lot of resources in maintaining the belief that they are not prone to negative emotion (self-deception), rather than convincing other people that they are not prone to negative emotion (impression management). Repressors like to see themselves as rational, even-tempered, and calm individuals who are not prone to strong negative emotion.

What are the ramifications of possessing a repressive coping style? Although repressors appear to be psychologically healthy, and there is a lack of evidence that repressors suffer from psychological symptoms, this is not the same for physical health. There is considerable evidence that suggests that the repressive coping style may be associated with adverse physical health.

DEVELOPMENT OF RESEARCH ON THE REPRESSIVE COPING STYLE

Until the late 1970s, there was a lack of systematic research into repression, partly due to the difficulty in identifying repression for research purposes. One solution to this problem was to treat repression as an individual difference variable or trait and to measure it using questionnaires. One of the most successful early attempts to identify repressors involved using a questionnaire, the Byrne Repression-Sensitization Scale, and individuals who scored low on this scale were called repressors. However, the repression-sensitization scale is really a measure of trait anxiety and does not differentiate between people who are truly low on anxiety and repressors. This led to inconsistent results of laboratory experiments on repression using this measure, as the participants in the "repressor" group would be a mixture of truly low-anxious people and repressors, and the composition would vary with each sample in each experiment. Because of inconsistent findings, research into repression declined.

THE SEMINAL STUDY

Interest in repressive coping was rekindled by Dan Weinberger and colleagues in 1979 at Harvard University. Weinberger redefined repression based on the pattern of scores obtained from self-report questionnaires of defensiveness as well as trait anxiety. Weinberger added a measure of defensiveness because it had previously been shown to be a measure of repression, independent of anxiety. Individuals with a repressive coping style were defined as people who scored low on a measure of trait anxiety, but to differentiate them from truly low-anxious individuals who also scored high on a measure of defensiveness. In Weinberger and his coworkers' experiment, male students were asked to complete a task that included phrases with sexual content (e.g., "the prostitute slept with the student") or aggressive content (e.g., "his roommate kicked him in the stomach"). Physiological recordings were taken of heart rate, skin resistance, and forehead muscle tension. Repressors compared to nonrepressors (including truly low-anxious individuals) reported the lowest level of subjective distress, although physiological measures indicated that repressors were more stressed than nonrepressors. This pattern of response is a well-replicated finding. When repressors are put in potentially stressful situations, they report low levels of distress but high physiological arousal. This has been demonstrated in both males and females and in student, general population, and patient samples. Repressors are a substantial group, accounting for 10% to 20% of the population.

REPRESSORS AND AVOIDANCE OF NEGATIVE EMOTIONS

How do repressors manage to experience such low levels of negative emotion? There is considerable evidence from various studies that repressors use an avoidant style of processing negative information. For example, in a variety of laboratory tasks where participants are asked to attend to positive or negative information, repressors tend to avoid negative socially threatening information. Similarly, in laboratory tasks where individuals are asked to forget or remember negative words that can be related to themselves, repressors are better than nonrepressors at forgetting negative (but not positive) information.

Avoiding processing negative emotional material may result in poor recall of unpleasant memories, and a number of studies have demonstrated links between repressive coping and the accessibility of negative memories, as repressors also recall fewer negative (but not positive) autobiographical memories from both childhood and adulthood than nonrepressors.

REPRESSORS AND CHILDHOOD MEMORIES

It is important to establish that repressors do have something unpleasant to repress, as it is possible that repressors' poor recall of negative childhood memories may just mean they had a happy childhood, with no unpleasant memories to suppress. To explore this, an interview study was conducted by Lynn Myers and Chris Brewin investigating female repressors' childhood experiences. To address the issue of repressors avoiding negative emotion, repressors did not rate the emotionality of their experiences; this was undertaken by independent raters. This bypassed the possibility of repressors interpreting their experiences in a positive fashion. So, for example, in the interview there are a number of specific questions such as, "Did you feel you could go to your parents if you were upset or unhappy?" Independently of whether participants answer yes or no to this question, specific examples of occasions when they could/could not go to their parents are elicited and form the basis of the interviewer ratings. The results were that repressors' accounts of their childhood were more likely to be characterized by paternal antipathy, indifference, and lack of closeness than nonrepressors. The results of this study provide evidence that repressors do indeed have unpleasant memories to suppress.

DO REPRESSORS HAVE SIGNIFICANTLY WORSE HEALTH OUTCOMES?

It has been thought that not attending to bodily signs of distress, such as anxiety, can be detrimental to health. In fact, it has been suggested that attending to bodily signs is necessary for good health. Consistent with this thinking, there is a body of research linking repressive coping to poor physical health.

Cancer

There are a number of studies that suggest a link between repressive coping and cancer. Studies have found a higher incidence of repressors than nonrepressors among cancer sufferers in a variety of different age groups: children, adolescents, and adults. Also, in studies of breast cancer, where women have been followed up over time, repressors were more likely to display more rapid progression of the disease than nonrepressors. This link with cancer may be associated with problems of the immune system, as it has been demonstrated in adult and elderly samples that repressors have poor immune functioning.

However, these results should be interpreted with caution, since the majority of these studies have been cross-sectional—in other words they have taken place *after* patients have had a diagnosis of cancer. So, we do not know if these patients had a repressive coping style before or after diagnosis. If they developed a repressive coping style after diagnosis, this would be considered to be a reaction to having cancer and would not be seen as a risk factor for developing cancer. In longitudinal studies (those following a group of cancer patients over time), there are also limitations in that behavioral reasons why repressors may have a poorer outcome have not been investigated in the studies mentioned in this section. For example, repressors may not comply/adhere to treatment or follow recommended health behaviors, but we do not know that, as these behaviors have not been measured.

Heart Disease

There is evidence to suggest that at least male repressors may be at increased risk of cardiovascular disease through a number of different mechanisms: increased lipid levels, high physiological reactivity to stress, and reacting badly to potentially useful but upsetting information about heart disease.

Male repressors, but not female repressors, have been found to have raised blood lipid levels. In addition, studies suggest that repressors may be at risk due to high physiological arousal in stressful conditions. Certainly, one of the defining characteristics of the repressive coping style in both sexes is their high physiological reactivity to stress. It has also been shown that repressors have higher blood pressure levels than nonrepressors in response to psychological but not physical stressors.

Studies of predominantly male patients with heart disease examined the effect of repressive coping in terms of the efficacy of a cardiovascular education program. The main findings were that repressors tended not to acknowledge the type of lifestyle changes necessary for a successful recovery. Those repressors who did acknowledge these necessary changes were more likely to suffer from more complications (e.g., hospitalization for chest pain, heart attack). Therefore, repressors who did learn about risk factors related to their disease made a poor recovery.

Why is it harmful to teach repressors about cardiac risks? It may be that if repressors gain cardiac risk information, they are more highly aroused by this knowledge than nonrepressors. If this is the case, it may be important to deal with lifestyle changes in repressors via psychotherapeutic interventions.

Pain

Repressive coping has been linked to impaired pain perception. Typically, repressors require almost twice the amount of electrical stimulation than nonrepressors to elicit judgments of pain and discomfort. This may be seen in terms of repressors' failure to pay attention to distress. Similarly, chronic pain patients who exhibit a repressive coping style self-report low levels of psychological distress associated with pain, but they report higher levels of pain severity and perceived disability. They also tend to fare less well in pain programs.

Asthma

It has been shown that there is a higher incidence of repressors in asthma patients than would be expected. Repressors account for between 30% to 50% of asthma patients, whereas in the general population this figure is 10% to 20%. Studies have shown that although repressors reported high levels of adherence to their asthma medication, an objective measure of lung function was worse than nonrepressors. Again, this may be seen as a function of repressors self-reporting low levels of distress while experiencing bodily symptoms, in this case, poor lung functioning. However, similar issues apply to those mentioned in the section on cancer above. These results must be interpreted with some caution, as studies are cross-sectional, so that we do not know if these patients were repressors before or after diagnosis. If they developed this coping style after diagnosis, this would be considered to be a reaction to having asthma and would not be seen as a risk factor.

High Arousal

As well as high physiological arousal already mentioned, repressors appear not to pay attention to distress during minor surgical procedures, such as dental surgery and colonoscopy.

—*Lynn B. Myers*

See also EXPRESSIVE WRITING AND HEALTH

Further Reading

Byrne, D. (1964). Repression-sensitization as a dimension of personality. In B. A. Maher (Ed.), *Progress in experimental personality research* (Vol. 1, pp. 169-220). New York: Academic Press.

Myers, L. B. (2000). Identifying repressors: A methodological issue for health psychology. *Psychology and Health, 15*, 205-214.

Myers, L. B., & Brewin, C. R. (1994). Recall of early experience and the repressive coping style. *Journal of Abnormal Psychology, 103*, 288-292.

Singer, J. L. (Ed.). (1990). *Repression and dissociation*. Chicago: University of Chicago Press.

Weinberger, D. A., Schwartz, G. E., & Davidson, R. J. (1979). Low-anxious, high-anxious and repressive coping styles: Psychometric patterns and behavioral responses to stress. *Journal of Abnormal Psychology, 88*, 369-380.

RESEARCH TO PRACTICE IN HEALTH AND BEHAVIOR

Most health professionals would agree that practical decisions about how to treat individual patients should be based on the best available scientific evidence. The 1990s, however, brought a growing realization that scientific knowledge was exerting too little influence on usual clinical practice. A 1990 Institute of Medicine report concluded that less than 5% of medical treatment decisions were based on strong research evidence, about half were based on shared practitioner beliefs that had minimal scientific support, and half were based on personal opinion. Recognition of the dramatic gap between research and medical practice generated an impetus to develop "evidence-based medicine" that could help clinicians to choose treatments, insurers to manage risk, and regulators to set policy based on the "conscientious, explicit use of current best evidence " (Sackett et al., 1996). Implementation was challenging, requiring the assemblage of large, accessible electronic research databases and expert review groups to systematically compile, update, and evaluate the research evidence. The Cochrane Collaborative Group pioneered and continues to undertake expert reviews of evidence for the efficacy of different treatments catalogued by disease. Increasingly, the federal government invests resources to commission reviews of clinical research, create practice guidelines, specify standards of care and quality assurance procedures, and train health practitioners to use them.

The evidence-based movement that began in medicine is now being embraced by other disciplines (psychology, nursing, public health) that practice interventions to promote health. To improve the evaluation of evidence from clinical trials, many major medical journals (e.g., *Journal of the American Medical Association, British Journal of Medicine, Lancet*) and review groups have adopted the Consolidated Standards of Reporting Trials (CONSORT guidelines) (Moher et al., 2001). CONSORT specifies the full range of information that needs to be provided when reporting clinical trials. Behavioral medicine journals like *Health Psychology* and *Annals of Behavioral Medicine* are now beginning to adopt CONSORT criteria. The Clinical Psychology Division of the American Psychological Association has set out guidelines for considering a psychotherapy empirically supported, and maintains a list of treatments that qualify. Finally, a subcommittee of the Society of Behavioral Medicine has been mandated to develop guidelines that help clinicians make scientifically informed decisions about behavioral interventions to promote health.

HOW CLINICIANS MAKE TREATMENT DECISIONS

The evidence-based movement has made great strides toward systematizing scientific knowledge about which treatments improve health most cost effectively. Often, however, the best scientifically supported treatments are not the ones most widely practiced. The gap that now needs to be bridged, therefore, is the one that prevents current research knowledge from being applied as usual clinical practice. To understand what barriers impede translation from research to practice, it is helpful to consider how clinicians make treatment decisions.

When deciding how to treat a particular patient, practitioners respond to several classes of information: evidence, constraints, and patient/clinician factors (Mulrow & Cook, 1998). "Evidence" designates clinical and laboratory data describing the particular patient, as well as generalized research findings characterizing many patients affected by the same problem (i.e., basic research findings concerning the causes and distribution of the disorder, randomized clinical trials of treatments for the condition, and systematized reviews consolidating the findings regarding efficacious treatments).

"Constraints" are contextual, systems-level influences that limit or direct a clinician's decisional options. These include limitations on practitioners' time as well as on the range of treatments that third party payers will reimburse. Other constraints involve explicit policies or laws that designate specific treatments as best practice or as minimal standard of care. Explicit policy constraints often have an implicit parallel in shared professional beliefs about what constitutes optimal treatment and in public demand (often driven by media advertising) for treatments perceived as desirable. "Patient factors" that rightfully influence the choice of treatment include an individual's prior history of treatment successes and failures, as well as personal and cultural beliefs about which treatments are acceptable. For example, even though physician practice guidelines designate antidepressant medication as the first line treatment for depression, many patients refuse drug treatment or prefer treatment via psychotherapy; others begin and discontinue medications because of side effects; some proportion fail to adhere consistently; and another subset is unable to initiate medication because of concurrent medications or comorbid conditions, including pregnancy. Finally, an influential "clinician factor" is whether the practitioner has training, experience, and comfort in delivering an evidence-based treatment.

BRIDGING THE GAP BETWEEN RESEARCH AND PRACTICE

Science has increasingly penetrated the clinical decision-making process, and yet further progress remains needed. The evidence base is now accessible for clinicians to consult electronically for help in making treatment decisions. Simplest to use are synthesized, secondary reviews of treatment efficacy, like those provided by the Cochrane Collaborative (2003), National Guidelines Clearinghouse (2003), and Agency for Healthcare Research and Quality (AHRQ; 2003) practice guideline databases. Because these resources were developed for physicians, they often emphasize pharmacological over behavioral treatments. Psychosocial treatments are sometimes covered extensively (e.g., smoking cessation), but more often referenced as minimalist behavioral counseling that can be incorporated into a visit to a general medical practitioner. At the opposite extreme are fully manualized, multisession behavioral treatments delivered by trained therapists. These have generally been studied by psychologists, and their evidence base can be accessed by more laboriously searching psychINFO or Medline using the search filters "randomized controlled trial," "double-blind," "clinical trial," and "meta-analyses." Treatment manuals, usually unpublished, can often be obtained by contacting the researchers.

Efforts are under way to address system constraints that insulate practice from research knowledge. Examples include Robert Wood Johnson initiatives to heighten managed care's coverage of tobacco control interventions, tying insurance reimbursement to the extent of a treatment's basis in research support. Technological advances are easing the burdens that treatment places on practitioner and patient time. Increasingly, computerized "expert" systems are becoming available to perform assessments and tailor-make interventions accordingly. Telephone and Internet delivery channels are being implemented to make treatment accessible outside the logistical constraints of geography, scheduling, traffic, childcare demands, and time of day.

Still badly in need of systematization into the evidence base are client and practitioner factors that should meaningfully influence treatment. Research is only now beginning to characterize demographic and cultural disparities that moderate treatment outcome. Yet, on a daily basis, practitioners and clients actively negotiate treatment choices that balance real-world constraints, personal idiosyncrasies, and scientific knowledge. Only rarely does a client's condition match a clear prototype, with a well-founded treatment acceptable to both practitioner and patient. Often, no treatment has an adequate evidence base, or the presenting problem is ill defined or co-occurs with comorbidities whose relative urgencies are hard to prioritize. One treatment, a pharmacotherapy, may empirically be superior to alternatives, but it may have failed previously or provoked an allergy for the particular patient or be culturally unacceptable to him or her. There may be a validated manualized behavioral treatment for the condition, but not one that the clinician has practiced. Trying to follow an unfamiliar manual may detract from forming the kind of therapeutic alliance that is empirically validated to help clients initiate healthful behavior change. Such are the messy realities that practitioners confront daily and that frighten researchers striving for scientific clarity. Eventually, such complexities need to be addressed. Doing so will make the clinical research base more relevant to practitioners, who will in turn be empowered greatly by having their decisions more securely grounded in science.

—Bonnie Spring and
Sherry Pagoto

Further Reading

Agency for Healthcare Research and Quality. (2003). *Practice guideline databases*. Retrieved from www.ahrq.gov

Beutler, L. E. (2000). David and Goliath: When empirical and clinical standards of practice meet. *American Psychologist, 55,* 997-1007.

Chambless, D. L., & Ollendick, T. H. (2001). Empirically supported psychological interventions: Controversies and evidence. *Annual Review of Psychology, 52,* 685-716.

Cochrane Collaborative. (2003). Retrieved from www.cochrane.org/cochrane/revabstr/mainindex.htm

Davison, G. C. (1998). Being bolder with the Boulder model: The challenge of education and training in empirically supported treatments. *Journal of Consulting and Clinical Psychology, 66*(1), 163-167.

Donald, A. (2002). Evidence-based medicine: Key concepts. *Medscape Psychiatry & Mental Health eJournal, 7*(2), 1-6.

Moher, D., Schulz, K. F., & Altman, D. G. (2001). The CONSORT statement: Revised recommendations for improving the quality of reports of parallel-group randomised trials [Comment]. *Lancet, 357,* 1191-1194.

Mulrow, C., & Cook, D. (1998). *Systematic reviews: Synthesis of best evidence for health care decisions.* Philadelphia: American College of Physicians.

Nathan, P. E. (1998). Practice guidelines: Not yet ideal. *American Psychologist, 53,* 290-299.

National Guidelines Clearinghouse. (2003). Retrieved from www.guideline.gov/index.asp

Sackett, D. L., Rosenberg, W. M., Gray, J. A., Haynes, R. B., & Richardson, W. S. (1996). Evidenced-based medicine: What it is and what it isn't. *British Medical Journal 312,* 71-72.

Schulkin, J. (2000). Decision sciences and evidence-based medicine: Two intellectual movements to support clinical decision making. *Academic Medicine, 75,* 816-817.

Williams, J. K. (2001). Understanding evidence-based medicine: A primer. *American Journal of Obstetrics and Gynecology, 185,* 275-278.

RHEUMATOID ARTHRITIS: PSYCHOSOCIAL ASPECTS

Rheumatoid arthritis (RA) is an autoimmune disease characterized by joint inflammation. The cause of RA is unknown, and there is no known cure. Although RA can attack any joint, the wrists and knuckles are almost always involved, with the knees and feet often affected as well. Over time, RA inflammatory processes can gradually digest cartilage and bone in affected joints. Other physical symptoms commonly associated with RA include pain, fatigue, muscle aches, and low-grade fever. RA also can damage other body systems, including the lungs, eyes, nervous system, and cardiovascular system. Although RA sometimes manifests and resolves within a few months, most individuals with RA experience a more chronic disease pattern, characterized by waxing and waning of severe symptoms, with progressive disfigurement and disability. RA is about two to three times more common in women that men, and the prevalence is greater in older people. There also appear to be ethnic/racial variations. For example, the estimated prevalence in Caucasian populations is 1% to 2%, whereas approximately two to three times as many Native Americans have RA.

BIOPSYCHOSOCIAL FACTORS AND RA

Biopsychosocial approaches in medicine focus on the interplay between physical factors (e.g., swollen painful joints in RA) and associated psychosocial factors such as an individual's mental health and levels of social support. RA is best viewed from a biopsychosocial perspective because it is expressed and experienced within a web of overlapping psychosocial factors.

PAIN

Many individuals with RA experience significant pain. Interestingly, most research suggests that RA-related pain is more closely associated with psychosocial factors than with disease-related variables. For example, high levels of emotional distress, poor coping, and low levels of social support have been more closely associated with increased pain than have measures of disease activity like number of swollen joints. However, relationships between pain and psychosocial variables can be complex. For example, emotional difficulties like depression may increase sensitivity to pain, but experiencing chronic RA pain also may increase the likelihood that individuals will become depressed. Also, whereas anxiety usually increases pain if an individual is at rest, high levels of anxiety in stressful distracting situations often decrease perceived pain levels.

Although psychosocial variables significantly influence RA-related pain, physiological factors also play an important role. For example, individuals with chronic pain sometimes notice that perceived pain may "spread" beyond parts of the body clearly affected by disease activity. In fact, research suggests that intense persistent pain signals can change the message patterns between affected parts of the body and the spinal cord/brain, thereby expanding the range of stimuli that cause pain sensations. Also, because pain signals appear to be hardwired into parts of the brain associated with negative emotions like anger and anxiety, individuals experiencing chronic pain may be more inclined to experience these negative emotions, independent of psychosocial factors.

FATIGUE

Fatigue also is a troublesome problem for many individuals with RA. Rates of fatigue have been found to be 80% and higher among individuals with RA, and even though fatigue is not a diagnostic criterion for RA, over 50% of individuals with RA have reported that fatigue is the most problematic aspect of their disease. As with pain, a growing body of research suggests that fatigue may be relatively independent from standard measures of disease activity, and is more strongly associated with psychosocial variables like higher levels of pain and depression and lower levels of social support.

NEGATIVE AFFECT

Not surprisingly, many individuals with RA experience a range of negative affect (i.e., emotions like depression and anxiety). Estimated rates of clinically significant depression and anxiety among individuals with RA range between about 15% to 45%. Some data indicate that middle-aged and younger individuals are more prone to depression and anxiety than older individuals with RA. In any case, mood disturbance is strongly associated with increased pain, increased functional impairment, and overutilization of medical services. Also, although measures of disease activity are associated with psychological distress, other variables like pain severity, neuroticism, daily stressors, work demands, and functional ability appear to be better predictors of anxiety and depression.

STRESS

The multifaceted concept of "stress" is important to a biopsychosocial understanding of RA. One meaning of the term *stress* refers to situational factors that act as stressful stimuli. As discussed above, RA often produces pain and psychological distress, which are, in themselves, significant stressors. Having RA also can create a number of other stressors, including reductions in home and work-related activities, and, correspondingly, financial hardship secondary to

decreased earnings and increased health care costs. Finally, approximately half of individuals with RA report problems in the areas of social interaction and communication with others. Perhaps not surprisingly, higher perceived levels of positive social support tend to buffer the adverse effects of environmental stressors, whereas lower levels of social support have been associated with increased physical disability and depression.

Although stressors have not been reliably associated with the onset of RA, minor stressors and daily hassles have been associated with exacerbation of symptoms in already established RA. Somewhat paradoxically, some evidence suggests that major life stressors like the death of a family member can be associated with decreases in disease activity. The effects of diverse types of stressors on RA disease activity may be a consequence of differential activation of stress-related physiological systems.

Although a variety of physiological systems are involved in stress responses, two are particularly relevant to the current discussion: (1) the hypothalamo-pituitary-adrenal (HPA) axis, which produces cortisol, a hormone that generally down-regulates immune functioning, and (2) the sympathetic adrenal-medullary (SAM) system, which produces adrenaline and noradrenaline and generally activates immune functioning. Several lines of evidence suggest that in RA, the HPA axis is hypoactive, whereas the SAM system may be hyperactive. This could explain why acute stressors tend to exacerbate RA disease symptoms, in that they increase immune functioning, thereby intensifying the autoimmune action of RA. In contrast, chronic stress situations may prompt a strong enough release of cortisol to down-regulate immune functioning and, somewhat paradoxically, improve RA disease symptoms.

COGNITIVE AND COPING FACTORS

The relationship between RA and two cognitive factors, learned helplessness and self-efficacy, has been well studied. Helplessness refers to a state where individuals believe they lack viable ways to eliminate or alleviate sources of stress. Because RA symptoms can wax and wane unpredictably, patients with RA may be particularly susceptible to helplessness. In any case, individuals with RA reporting high levels of helplessness are more likely to report higher pain levels, greater depression, and greater functional impairment. Self-efficacy tends to be more behavior specific, and refers to the confidence individuals have regarding their own ability to perform specific goal-directed tasks. For example, individuals with low self-efficacy are less likely to persist and comply with treatment regimens, regardless of their beliefs about the potential helpfulness of the intervention. In RA, increases in self-efficacy have been associated with decreased depression, pain, and disease activity, and increased treatment adherence.

Coping refers to behaviors aimed at managing internal or external demands with available resources. Important distinctions include the difference between problem-focused versus emotion-focused coping, as well as passive versus active coping. Generally, emotion-focused and passive coping approaches have been found most maladaptive for individuals with RA. For example, passive strategies characterized by catastrophizing (e.g., making a mountain out of a mole hill) or hoping that things will just get better have been associated with greater pain and psychological distress, and poorer functional outcome.

WORK DISABILITY

Rheumatic disease is the leading cause of work loss and the second leading cause of work disability payments, and roughly 25% to 50% of individuals with RA are disabled after one decade of the disease. A number of risk factors for RA-related work disability have been identified, including poor disease status, increasing time off work, less education, less social support, and depression.

BIOPSYCHOSOCIAL CONSIDERATIONS AND RA TREATMENT

The foregoing section highlights the interconnected biopsychosocial aspects of RA. For example, one can readily conceive of a situation where RA produces painful joints, which limits function, which fosters depression, which in turn promotes work disability, which exacerbates martial problems, which further increases disease activity. Fortunately, these biopsychosocial interconnections also point to effective treatment approaches.

Pharmacological management of RA is usually geared toward control of underlying disease processes with disease-modifying antirheumatic drugs such as hydroxychloroquine and methotrexate, as well as pain management with medications like nonsteroidal anti-inflammatory drugs (e.g., ibuprofen and naproxen). Many individuals with RA respond adequately to such treatment. However, these interventions are not sufficient for many other patients. Thus, effective management of RA often requires appropriate and individualized attention to psychosocial variables. Increasing evidence suggests that multimodal approaches (i.e., those that combine medical, cognitive-behavioral interventions, and exercise under the auspices of appropriate professionals) are the most effective treatments for individuals with RA who do not respond adequately to conservative biomedical interventions.

Comprehensive and action-oriented interventions like cognitive-behavioral therapies (CBTs) have been associated with a variety of positive outcomes, including decreased pain, depression, and anxiety, and increased self-efficacy, function, and work levels. These treatment gains tend to be long term (i.e., over 12 months) for many individuals, particularly among those who continue to practice coping skills on a regular basis. Key components of this approach include three basic elements: (1) education/rationale for treatment (e.g., explaining pain theories and the interrelationships between psychosocial factors and RA), (2) coping skills training (e.g., relaxation training, explanation of effective pacing strategies, and cognitive restructuring), and (3) relapse prevention (e.g., emphasizing the importance of continued practice of new behavioral skills and learning to identify early signs of relapse like increased pain or depression).

Most CBTs for RA are delivered in classroom-type settings at hospitals or medicine clinics. However, newer delivery systems such as telephone counseling and mail-delivered self-management programs also have been associated with a variety of positive outcomes, including improved psychological functioning, increased functioning, and improvements on disease parameters. Also, emotional disclosure of stressful events via journaling has been associated with improved psychological functioning and disease status parameters in individuals with RA. As suggested above, multimodal management of RA frequently includes exercise interventions. Many individuals with RA have low levels of physical fitness, and this contributes to a variety of problems, including excess fatigue, low functional status, low pain threshold, sleep disturbances, and depression. Fortunately, increased physical fitness in young and old individuals with RA often improves range of motion, muscle strength, general conditioning, and functional abilities, and reduces pain, fatigue, and depression, without exacerbating disease severity.

—*Bruce A. Huyser and*
Jerry C. Parker

See also CHRONIC DISEASE MANAGEMENT; CHRONIC PAIN MANAGEMENT

Further Reading

Fries, J. F. (1995). *Arthritis: A take care of yourself health guide for understanding your arthritis* (4th ed.). Reading, MA: Perseus.

Henkel, G., & Pincus, T. (2000). *The Arthritis Foundation's guide to good living with rheumatoid arthritis*. Atlanta, GA: Arthritis Foundation.

Huyser, B. A., & Parker, J. C. (1998). Stress and rheumatoid arthritis: An integrative review. *Arthritis Care and Research, 11,* 135-145.

Klippel, J. H., & Crofford, L. (Eds.). (2001). *Primer on the rheumatic diseases* (12th ed.). Atlanta, GA: Arthritis Foundation.

Minor, M. A. (1996). Rest and exercise. In S. T. Wegener, B. L. Belza, & E. P. Gall (Eds.), *Clinical care in the rheumatic diseases* (pp. 73-78). Atlanta, GA: American College of Rheumatology.

S

SCHOOL-BASED HEALTH PROMOTION

School-based health promotion refers to activities that occur in schools and on school grounds that facilitate student and school staff adoption of healthful behaviors and healthful lifestyle choices. School-based health promotion is not just about teaching students what they should do to be healthy; rather, it includes providing environments where making the healthy choice is the easy and normative choice for students. School health promotion includes not just health education but also provision of healthy foods offered throughout the school, daily physical education that is fun and includes all students, a tobacco- and drug-free campus, a social environment where healthy choices are modeled and reinforced by students and adults in the school, and policies that create psychological, social, and physical environments that support health and wellness in students and school staff.

School-based health promotion is very important as the health behaviors of youth affect their health as youth as well as their risk for future chronic diseases. Next to families, schools are the most important community institution for enhancing and protecting youth health. Not only do the vast majority of youth attend school, but schools also provide the social, normative, and physical environments wherein youth health behaviors are learned, practiced, modeled, and solidified.

School health promotion is an important part of comprehensive or coordinated school health. Comprehensive school health is a model where health and nutrition services, health education, and healthy school environments, including health promotion for students and staff, occur with the support and involvement of parents and the larger community as an integrated system. While the realization of fully comprehensive school health is yet elusive, there is evidence that multicomponent programs using elements of comprehensive school health and health promotion can make significant changes in student health behaviors.

EVOLUTION OF SCHOOL-BASED HEALTH PROMOTION PROGRAMS

The modern school health era began in 1850 with the publication of the Shattuck report drawing attention to the role that schools play in communicable disease. For the first time ever, schools were recognized as convenient public institutions in which to provide health care, specifically vaccinations, to youth as well as being potential sites for the spread of infectious diseases. At the beginning of the 20th century, school nurses were involved in reducing the spread of disease in schools, treating minor ailments at school, communicating with parents, conducting medical inspections of students, and making referrals to physicians.

School health began to inch toward health promotion after World War I. Beyond preventing communicable disease, schools were recognized as good places to educate youth on the importance of healthy behaviors, including brushing teeth, eating a healthy diet, playing outdoors daily, sleeping with the windows open, and bathing at least once a week! Nutritional deficiencies seen in draft inductees in World War II led to the institutionalization of the federally sponsored National School Lunch Act, designed to use surplus agricultural commodities and funds to provide nutritious lunches for schoolchildren. School health was slowly moving from an emphasis on taking care of sick children in schools to an emphasis on preventing disease and promoting wellness by encouraging and promoting healthy behaviors (Allensworth, Lawson, Nicholson, & Wyche, 1997).

In the 21st century, much is new, but much is the same in school health. Certainly, communicable diseases are still a concern in schools and school nurses still provide some of the same services as they did at the beginning of the 20th century. New health concerns of youth are helping to shape school-based health promotion, however, and expanding its scope from detecting and treating acute illnesses to preventing illness and promoting health. Results from the 1997 Youth Risk Behavior Survey (YRBS) of students in Grades 9 through 12 (a survey administered nationally by the Centers for Disease Control and Prevention) spotlight some of the health issues that schools address in health promotion activities (Bogden, 2000). According to the survey, less than 30% of students had eaten the recommended five or more servings of fruits or vegetables during the day before the survey and nearly half of the females surveyed and a quarter of the males surveyed had not participated in vigorous physical activity for at least 20 minutes on at least 3 days of the week before the survey.

These behavioral trends in tandem with the dramatic rise in youth obesity in the past 30 years have brought attention to the role that schools play in feeding children and providing them with opportunities to be physically active (Troiano & Flegal, 1998). The 1997 YRBS data also revealed that more than one third of high school students were current smokers, one half of all students had at least one drink in the past 30 days, and one third had five or more drinks in one sitting. Sixteen percent of the students had sniffed glue or inhaled aerosol sprays to become intoxicated. Student use of tobacco, alcohol, and other drugs has resulted in the call for health education to help students learn the dangers of those substances and the social skills needed to resist social pressure to initiate use.

The YRBS also showed that nearly half of all high school students had sexual intercourse at least once in their lifetime and 16% had four or more sex partners. More than one quarter of male high school students

had carried a weapon (e.g., a knife, gun, or club) in the past 30 days and nearly half had been in a physical fight in the past 12 months (Bogden, 2000). School health has expanded to address these health issues as well. Some schools now offer parenting classes and varying options of sex education; conflict resolution classes have been adopted as school curricula in some states.

Health behaviors of youth may have both immediate and delayed consequences; sexual activity, drug use, and violent behaviors obviously have potential negative sequelae in the short term. While not as alarming, the existence of other proximal consequences of unhealthy behaviors are supported by data that suggest that students who engage in healthier behaviors such as eating breakfast and being physically active have lower absenteeism rates at school and come to school better prepared to learn (Bogden, 2000).

Other health behaviors, such as smoking, dietary behaviors, and physical activity, were previously considered as risk behaviors for youth only to the extent that the less healthful behavior was maintained into adulthood. The vast majority of adult smokers begin smoking before they are 18 years old, putting them at risk for cardiovascular disease and cancer. Students who learn to prefer diets high in fat, sodium, and calories and low in fruits, vegetables, and fiber when they are young, and do not change their diet as they mature, put themselves at risk for cardiovascular disease, diet-related cancers, and other chronic diseases (Committee on Diet and Health, 1989). Students who are not physically active as youth may find it hard to begin to be active as adults, perpetuating a cycle of inactivity borne from the difficulty in starting to be active when one is not physically fit.

While the implications of chronic disease risk for adult morbidity are still very relevant, the nation is facing an epidemic of childhood obesity with rates more than doubling in the past 30 years (Troiano & Flegal, 1998). For the first time ever, non-insulin-dependent (Type 2) diabetes in youth is emerging. Some studies have reported a 10-fold increase in the incidence of Type 2 diabetes in children (Dabelea, Pettitt, Jones, & Arsianian, 1999). While the causes of childhood obesity and non-insulin-dependent diabetes are very complex, most experts agree that diet and activity levels play a very important role. It is estimated that tobacco, diet, physical activity, drugs and alcohol, sex, and intentional and unintentional injuries account for 70% of adolescent morbidity and mortality (Allensworth et al., 1997), making health promotion efforts in youth a national priority.

The U.S. Department of Health and Human Services (DHHS) determines and publishes health directives or goals for the nation on a regular basis. These goals address the priority areas for reducing the nation's morbidity and mortality costs. The most recent of these directives is Healthy People 2010 (DHHS, 2000). The Healthy People 2010 goals include goals both at the individual and the institutional levels. For example, included in Healthy People 2010 are the following nutrition-related goals targeting change at the individual level: (1) Reduce the proportion of children and adolescents who are overweight or obese, and (2) increase the proportion of persons age 2 years and older who consume at least two daily servings of fruit. Goals are also written targeting changes at the institutional or school level. For example, goals for the delivery of school physical education classes include the following: (1) Increase the proportion of adolescents who participate in daily school physical education, and (2) increase the proportion of adolescents who spend at least 50% of school physical education class time being physically active (DHHS, 2000). Goals found in Healthy People 2010 reflect the recognition that health promotion involves more than positive behaviors of individuals, it also involves creating more healthful institutions and communities.

In the new millennium, schools serve as an important venue for improving the health and the health behaviors of youth. Schooling is the only universal entitlement for youth in the United States. Not only do most of America's children attend school, making school the most convenient and efficient place to disseminate information and skills for positive health behaviors, it is also the only organized institution that engages the four major systems of influences— family, friends or peers, school, and community (Allensworth et al., 1997). The inclusion of these four systems of influence in a single community institution provides the capacity to affect change not only through the traditional means of health education, teaching students health-related knowledge and skills for making healthy choices, but also through positively influencing normative beliefs and expectations of family, other adults in the lives of youth and peers, and establishing policies and creating school environments that reinforce and facilitate healthy choices.

Schools have the opportunity not only to educate by what is taught in the classroom but also to create environments where healthy choices are modeled by peers and school staff, where healthy behaviors can be reinforced, and where the school environment facilitates, encourages, and models healthy choices. In other words, schools are an important place to both talk the talk and walk the walk for positive youth health behaviors.

ELEMENTS OF SCHOOL-BASED HEALTH PROMOTION

School-based health promotion has most commonly been considered as part of a comprehensive school health program. The vision of comprehensive school health programs has been evolving over the past century. For the majority of the 20th century, three components made up a school health program: (1) health instruction, focusing on a health education curriculum; (2) health service, focusing on prevention, identification, and remediation of student health problems; and (3) a healthful environment, focusing on the physical and psychological setting.

The Centers for Disease Control and Prevention (CDC), Division of Adolescent and School Health, has been a leader in developing a vision of comprehensive school health and in providing schools and communities with tools to help create healthier schools. In the 1980s, the CDC introduced its vision of comprehensive school health, which includes eight components: (1) health education; (2) physical education; (3) health services; (4) nutrition services; (5) health promotion for staff; (6) counseling, psychological, and social services; (7) healthy school environment; and (8) parent and community involvement. Advocates of the eight-component comprehensive school health model discuss the need to integrate these components and to involve interdisciplinary teams of school, family, student, and community stakeholders to accomplish goals (Allensworth et al., 1997; Marx, Wooley, & Northrop, 1998).

The CDC has also attempted to further the mission of creating healthier schools and healthier children through publishing and disseminating CDC guidelines, or position papers. To date, four guidelines have been released, one for preventing the spread of AIDS, and the others dealing with tobacco, school nutrition, and physical activity (CDC, 1988, 1994, 1996, 1997). The guidelines present the rationale for health promotion in the content area and present recommendations for curricular, policy, environmental, and family school involvement. The recommendations in the four reports are intended to help policymakers at the school, state, and national levels meet national health objectives and education goals through school-based health promotion programs tailored to meet local needs.

The vision of comprehensive or coordinated school health programs has generated much discussion in the school health community; however, realization of such programs has been quite elusive. In the mid-1990s, an Institute of Medicine expert panel was convened to study comprehensive school health programs in Grades K-12. It defined comprehensive school health promotion as

> an integrated set of planned, sequential, school-affiliated strategies, activities, and services designed to promote the optimal physical, emotional, social, and educational development of students. The program involves and is supportive of families and is determined by the local community based on community needs, resources, standards, and requirements. It is coordinated by a multidisciplinary team and accountable to the community for program quality and effectiveness. (Allensworth et al., 1997, p. 60)

The emphasis of this definition is on community and family involvement, multiple interventions, integration of activities, and collaboration across disciplines.

In fact, truly comprehensive and integrated school health programs are rare. Even the best programs include only some of the components and evidence of integration of components is sparse. Challenges to implementing quality school health promotion programs as noted by the Institute of Medicine report include (1) difficulty in the dissemination of recommendations and guidelines from the national to the local level; (2) lack of involvement of critical community stakeholders for the design, implementation, and support of school health promotion efforts; (3) lack of interdisciplinary collaboration and communication; and (4) inability of schools to deliver medical services commonly dispensed through the private sector.

The largest challenge for comprehensive school health or strong school-based health promotion programs may be the lack of stable and adequate funding for schools. When financial resources are inadequate, schools have limited options to remedy the situation. Some of those options include cutting back on health promotion programming and health services; another option involves subsidizing income through sales of food not included in the federally supported reimbursable meals or entering into pouring rights contracts with soft drink companies. These contracts usually involve payments to schools in exchange for the school's agreement to exclusively offer the company's products in vending machines and at school events. Approximately 200 school districts in 33 states had "pouring rights" contracts with soft drink companies by early 2000. A Colorado school district entered into an $8 million, 10-year agreement with Coke that included cash bonuses to the district for exceeding sales targets (Nestle, 2002). Obviously, such agreements add challenges to creating a healthful school food environment.

If the connection between health and learning is not understood or appreciated by the nation, state, school district, principal, parents, or taxpayers, funding for school health services and school health promotion will suffer. Recognition of the links between health and student success and well-being as well as involvement and commitment of stakeholders in the community will be essential for the realization of vital and effective school health programs (Marx et al., 1998).

CHILD AND ADOLESCENT TRIAL FOR CARDIOVASCULAR HEALTH (CATCH): AN EXAMPLE OF A SCHOOL-BASED HEALTH PROMOTION PROGRAM

The Child and Adolescent Trial for Cardiovascular Health (CATCH) was a school-based health promotion research trial conducted in the 1990s to assess the effectiveness of a multicomponent health promotion program in reducing cardiovascular risk factors in elementary-age children. Ninety-six schools and more than 5,000 students in four states were involved in the research conducted in elementary schools with children in third to fifth grades (Luepker et al., 1996). The CATCH intervention targeted five channels for health promotive change: health curriculum in Grades 3 to 5, families of third to fifth graders, physical education (PE) classes, the school cafeteria, and school policies for tobacco-free schools (Perry et al., 1997).

The CATCH health curriculum used behaviorally based lessons designed to encourage students to eat foods lower in total fat, saturated fat, and sodium; to be more physically active; and to resist the initiation of tobacco use. The lessons included simple snack preparation, provided skill-building practice by asking students to generate solutions to challenges for being active, and practice social skills to resist peer pressure to try tobacco. All lessons were designed to be interactive, experiential, and fun and were taught by classroom teachers trained to deliver the CATCH lessons.

Half of the schools receiving the CATCH intervention also had a family component. Families received take-home packets with homework and activities that supported and reinforced the behavioral messages in the CATCH classroom curriculum. In addition, in Grades 3 and 4, families attended a Family Fun Night at the school where students performed an aerobic dance routine, healthy snacks were served, and carnival-type booths and games reinforced the heart-healthy messages.

CATCH PE worked with school PE specialists to modify classes so that students would spend more time in moderate to vigorous activity during class and less time being inactive. The emphasis was on including all students in all activities, reducing competition as an emphasis, and enhancing student enjoyment of being active. In schools where PE was offered for less than 90 minutes per week, classroom teachers were trained to deliver CATCH PE as part of their classroom activities.

CATCH Eat Smart involved training and working with school food service personnel to reduce the total fat, saturated fat, and sodium that were offered in school meals by modifying recipes, food purchasing patterns, and food preparation. CATCH also worked to help schools and school districts implement policies for tobacco-free schools. The CATCH curriculum and family components focused on affecting individual or family motivation, skills, sense of competence, and perceptions of the barriers and benefits of heart-healthy behaviors. CATCH PE, Eat Smart, and policy approaches for tobacco-free schools focused on changing the school environment to increase students' exposure to healthy food, activity, and smoke-free options and to provide positive role modeling and normative support for heart-healthy choices (Perry et al., 1997).

The effectiveness of the CATCH intervention was determined by comparing change in 40 schools randomized into the control condition with 56 schools randomized into the intervention or treatment condition between baseline and the end of the intervention.

The student-level indicators included some physiological assessments such as serum cholesterol, blood pressure, and body composition as well as behavioral assessments including dietary intake, physical activity levels, and tobacco use behaviors. In addition, the health-related knowledge and attitudes were assessed in the students participating in the study. The effectiveness of the school- or environmental-level aspects of the intervention were evaluated by assessing activity levels during PE class and the school lunch menus and recipes for total fat, saturated fat, and sodium content before and after the CATCH intervention, comparing intervention and control schools.

At the end of the 3-year intervention period, there were no statistically significant changes in the physiological measures taken. However, students who were enrolled in CATCH schools showed statistically significant decreases in their intake of dietary fat and saturated fat as compared to students in the control schools and reported participating in significantly more vigorous physical activity during the day. Likewise, students in the CATCH intervention schools had statistically significantly more positive scores on scales measuring knowledge and health behavior attitudes (Luepker et al., 1996).

Positive results were also seen at the school or environmental level. CATCH intervention schools increased the amount of time that students were involved in moderate to vigorous and vigorous physical activity during PE class as compared to nonintervention CATCH schools. Schools participating in Eat Smart significantly reduced the amount of energy, total fat, and saturated fat offered to students in school lunch. Before the CATCH intervention, the average fat content of school meals as offered had 39% of the energy from the meals coming from total fat. At the end of the intervention period, CATCH intervention schools had reduced that amount to 32% of energy from total fat, nearly reaching the nationally recommended amount, which is 30% of energy from total fat.

Health behaviors learned, practiced, and modeled while students were in Grades 3 to 5 were maintained as demonstrated in a follow-up CATCH study. Students' dietary, activity, and smoking behaviors were assessed after they left their CATCH schools and moved into middle school. Even in the absence of the CATCH intervention program, eighth grade students who had participated in CATCH intervention activities during their elementary years still ate significantly less total fat and saturated fat and reported higher levels of physical activity as compared to students who attended CATCH control schools (Nader et al., 1999).

CATCH used elements of a coordinated school health promotion program to affect students' eating, physical activity, and tobacco use behaviors. It involved five of the eight components of comprehensive school health, with the exception of health services, health promotion for school staff, and counseling, psychological, and social services. CATCH showed that students can adopt and maintain healthier eating and activity behaviors when learning occurs in a school environment that supports healthy behavioral choices. CATCH also showed that schools can change the way that they operate when their awareness is raised and they receive training and support for making healthful changes.

—*Leslie Lytle*

See also HEALTH PROMOTION AND DISEASE PREVENTION

Further Reading

Allensworth, D., Lawson, E., Nicholson, L., & Wyche, J. (Eds.). (1997). *Schools and health: Our nation's investment.* Washington, DC: National Academy Press.

Bogden, J. F. (2000). *Fit, healthy, and ready to learn: A school health policy guide, Part I: Physical activity, healthy eating, and tobacco-use prevention.* Alexandria, VA: National Association of State Boards of Education.

Centers for Disease Control and Prevention. (1988). Guidelines for effective school health education to prevent the spread of AIDS. *Morbidity and Mortality Weekly Report, 37,* 1-14.

Centers for Disease Control and Prevention. (1994). Guidelines for school health programs to prevent tobacco use and addiction. *Morbidity and Mortality Weekly Report, 43,* 1-18.

Centers for Disease Control and Prevention. (1996). Guidelines for school health programs to promote lifelong healthy eating. *Morbidity and Mortality Weekly Report, 45,* 1-41.

Centers for Disease Control and Prevention. (1997). Guidelines for school and community programs to promote lifelong physical activity among young people. *Morbidity and Mortality Weekly Report, 46,* 1-36.

Committee on Diet and Health; National Research Council. (1989). *Diet and health: Implications for reducing chronic disease risk.* Washington, DC: National Academy Press.

Dabelea, D., Pettitt, D. J., Jones, K. L., & Arsianian, S. A. (1999). Type 2 diabetes mellitus in minority children and adolescents: An emerging problem. *Endocrinology and Metabolism Clinics of North America, 28,* 709-729.

Luepker, R. V., Perry, C. L., McKinlay, S. M., Nader, P. R., Parcel, G. S., Stone, E. J., Webber, L. S., Elder, J. P., Feldman, H. A., Johnson, C. C., Kelder, S. H., & Wu, M. (1996). Outcomes of a field trial to improve children's dietary patterns and physical activity: The Child and Adolescent Trial for Cardiovascular Health (CATCH). *Journal of the American Medical Association, 275,* 768-776.

Marx, E., Wooley, S. F., & Northrop, D. (Eds.). (1998). *Health is academic: A guide to coordinated school health programs.* New York: Teachers College Press.

Nader, P. R., Stone, E. J., Lytle, L. A., Perry, C. L., Osganian, S. K., Kelder, S., Webber, L. S., Elder, J. P., Montgomery, D., Feldman, H. A., Wu, M., Johnson, C., Parcel, G., & Luepker, R. V. (1999). Three-year maintenance of improved diet and physical activity: The CATCH cohort. *Archives of Pediatrics and Adolescent Medicine, 153*(7), 695-704.

Nestle, M. (2002). *Food politics: How the food industry influences nutrition and health.* Berkeley: University of California Press.

Perry, C. L., Sellers, D. E., Johnson, C., Pedersen, S., Bachman, K. J., Parcel, G. S., Stone, E. J., Luepker, R. V., Wu, M., Nader, P. R., & Cook, K. (1997). The Child and Adolescent Trial for Cardiovascular Health (CATCH): Intervention, implementation, and feasibility for elementary schools in the United States. *Health Education and Behavior, 24*(6), 716-735.

Troiano, R. P., & Flegal, K. M. (1998). Overweight children and adolescents: Description, epidemiology, and demographics. *Pediatrics, 101,* 497-504.

U.S. Department of Health and Human Services. (2000, January). *Healthy People 2010* (Conference edition, in two vols.). Washington, DC: Author.

SELF-EFFICACY

The recent years have witnessed a change in the health field from a disease model to a health model. It is just as meaningful to speak of levels of vitality and healthfulness as of degrees of impairment and debility. Viewed from this perspective, health is measured not only in terms of life span and mortality and disability rates but in years of healthy life. The quality of health is heavily influenced by lifestyle habits. By exercising control over several health habits, people can live longer and healthier, and slow the process of aging. The structuring of health promotion should begin with goals, not means. If health is the goal, psychosocial approaches provide an important means to it.

This entry analyzes the application of social cognitive theory to health promotion and disease prevention (Bandura, 1997). This theory identifies a core set of determinants, specifies the mechanism through which they produce their effects, and provides guides on the optimal ways of implementing them. The core determinants include knowledge of health risks and benefits of different health practices, perceived self-efficacy that one can exercise control over one's health habits, outcome expectations in the form of expected costs and benefits for different health habits, the health goals people set for themselves and the concrete plans and strategies for realizing them, and perceived facilitators and the social and structural impediments to the changes they seek.

Knowledge of health risks and benefits is one contributing factor. If people lack knowledge of how their lifestyle habits affect their health, they have little reason to put themselves through the agony of changing the injurious habits they enjoy. Knowledge of health risks and benefits creates the precondition for change. But additional self-influences are needed for most people to overcome the impediments to adopting new lifestyle habits and maintaining them.

Beliefs of personal efficacy play a central role in social cognitive theory. Perceived efficacy refers to people's beliefs in their capabilities to exercise control over their own functioning and over events that affect their lives. Efficacy belief is the foundation of human motivation and action. Unless people believe they can produce desired effects by their actions they have little incentive to act or to persevere in the face of difficulties. Whatever else may serve as guides and motivators, they are rooted in the core belief that one has the power to produce desired changes by one's actions.

Health behavior is also affected by the outcomes people expect their actions to produce. Outcome expectations can take three major forms. One set of outcomes includes the physical pleasures and the aversive physical effects the behavior produces. Behavior is also partly regulated by the social reactions it evokes. The social approval and disapproval the behavior produces are the second major class

of outcomes. People adopt personal standards and regulate their behavior by their self-reactions. They do things that give them self-satisfaction and self-worth, and refrain from behaving in ways that breed self-dissatisfaction. This third class of outcomes concerns the positive and negative self-evaluative reactions to one's health behavior.

Personal goals, rooted in a value system, provide further self-incentives and guides for health habits. Goals may be long-term ones that set the course of personal change or short-term ones that regulate effort and guide action in the here and how.

Personal change would be easy if there were no impediments or barriers to surmount. The facilitators and obstacles people see to changing their behavior are other determinants of health habits. Some of the impediments are personal ones that deter performance of healthful behavior. Others are social obstacles and still others are rooted in how human services are structured socially and economically.

CAUSAL STRUCTURE

Self-efficacy is a key determinant because it affects health behavior both directly and by its influence on these other determinants. Efficacy beliefs determine goals and aspirations. The stronger the efficacy, the higher the goal challenges people set for themselves and the firmer their commitment to them. Efficacy beliefs shape the outcomes people expect their efforts to produce. Those who are assured in their efficacy expect favorable outcomes. Those who expect deficient performances of themselves expect their efforts to bring poor results. Efficacy beliefs also determine how obstacles and impediments are viewed. People of low efficacy are easily convinced of the futility of effort in the face of difficulties. Those of high efficacy view impediments as surmountable through perseverant effort and improvement of self-management skills. Figure 1 presents the paths of influence in the causal model. Perceived self-efficacy affects health behavior both directly and by its impact on goals, outcome expectations, and perceived facilitators and impediments.

SELF-MANAGEMENT MODEL FOR HEALTH PROMOTION

Habit change is not achieved through an act of will. It requires development of self-regulatory skills.

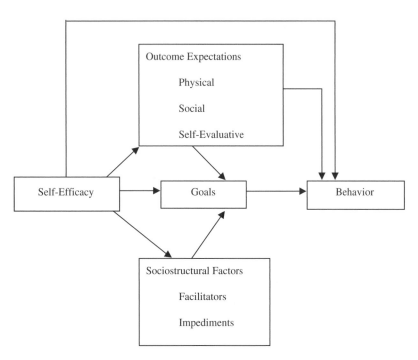

Figure 1   Paths of Influence Through Which Key Social Cognitive Factors Regulate Motivation and Health Behavior

Self-regulation operates through a set of psychological subfunctions that must be developed and mobilized for self-directed change (Bandura, 1986). Neither good intentions nor desire alone has much effect if people lack skills for exercising influence over their own motivation and behavior.

People cannot alter their health if they do not monitor their health status and health habits. Therefore, success in self-regulation partly depends on keeping close track of one's health-related behavior. Self-monitoring is the first step in efforts to improve one's health but, in itself, such information provides little basis for self-directed influence.

People motivate themselves and guide their behavior by the goals, aspirations, and challenges they set for themselves. Goals motivate by enlisting self-commitment to the activity. The effectiveness of goals depends on how far into the future they are projected. Long-range goals specify the destination, but they are too distant to serve as current motivators. There are too many competing influences for distant futures to regulate current behavior. People need to set short-term goals to get themselves to stick to the undertaking. Subgoal attainments build self-efficacy and strengthen motivation. People also need to learn how

to create incentives for themselves and to enlist social supports to sustain their efforts.

DeBusk and his colleagues have devised a self-management system combining self-regulatory principles with computerized implementation that promotes habits conducive to health and reduces those that impair it (Bandura, 1997; DeBusk et al., 1994). The system is founded on knowledge of the major subfunctions of self-regulation and their self-efficacy underpinning.

A few health habits have a major impact on the quality of health. To stay healthy, people must exercise, reduce dietary fat, refrain from smoking, keep blood pressure down, and develop effective ways of managing stressors. For each health habit, individuals are provided with detailed guides on how to achieve and maintain behavior conducive to health. A single program implementer, assisted by the computerized system, can oversee the behavioral changes of hundreds of participants concurrently. Figure 2 portrays the structure of the self-management system. Participants monitor the behavior they seek to change. They set short-range, attainable subgoals to motivate and guide their efforts. They receive detailed feedback of progress as further motivators for self-directed change.

At selected intervals, the computer generates and mails to participants individually tailored guides for self-directed change. These guides provide attainable subgoals for progressive change. The participants send performance cards to the implementer on the changes they have achieved and their perceived efficacy for the next cycle of self-directed change. Efficacy ratings identify areas of difficulty that foretell likely relapse unless participants are taught how to manage them effectively. The computer-generated feedback portrays graphically the progress patients are making toward each of their subgoals and shows their month-to-month changes, and also suggests strategies on how to surmount the identified difficulties.

In preventive applications of this self-management system, people lower risk factors for disease by altering their health habits under the guidance of a single implementer. The self-management system is also

Self-Regulatory Delivery System

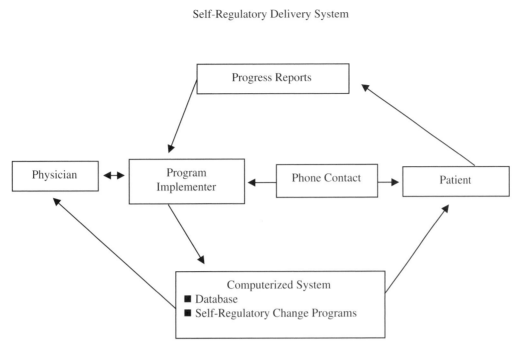

Figure 2 Computer-Assisted System for Self-Management of Health Habits

In this stepwise approach, the level and type of interactive guidance is tailored to people's self-management capabilities and motivational preparedness to achieve desired changes. The self-management system lends itself well to calibrating the amount of interactive guidance needed to attain desired changes. People of higher self-efficacy and positive outcome expectations can succeed with minimal interventions that provide sufficient structured guidance to accomplish the changes they seek.

successful in promoting lifestyle changes in individuals who are beginning to suffer medical problems. Coronary artery disease, which poses high risk of heart attacks, is but one example (Haskell et al., 1994). In long-term follow-up, those receiving medical care by their physicians showed no change or a slight worsening of their condition. In contrast, those aided in self-management of health habits achieved large reductions in risk factors. They lowered their intake of saturated fat, lost weight, lowered their bad cholesterol and raised their good cholesterol, exercised more, and increased their cardiovascular capacity. This system can also alter the physical progression of disease. Those receiving the self-management program had 47% less buildup of plaque on artery walls. They also had fewer coronary events, fewer hospitalizations for coronary heart problems, and fewer deaths.

The effectiveness of the self-management system has also been compared with the standard medical postcoronary care to reduce morbidity and mortality in patients who have already suffered a heart attack. The self-regulatory system has been shown to be more effective in reducing risk factors and increasing cardiovascular functioning than the standard medical care.

The social utility of the self-management system can be enhanced by a stepwise implementation model.

Individuals who harbor self-doubts about their efficacy make half-hearted efforts to change their health habits and are quick to give up when they run into difficulties. They need additional support and guidance by interactive means to see them through tough times. Much of the guidance can be provided through tailored print or telephone consultation. Individuals who believe that their health habits are beyond their control need a great deal of personal guidance in a stepwise mastery program. Graduated successes build belief in their ability to exercise control over health habits and bolster their staying power in the face of difficulties and setbacks.

The self-management system to health promotion combines the high individualization of the clinical approach with the large-scale applicability of the public health approach. The system is well received for several reasons. It is individually tailored to people's needs. It provides them with continuing personalized guidance and informative feedback that enables them to exercise considerable control over their own change. It is a home-based program that does not require any special facilities, equipment, or attendance at group meetings that usually have high dropout rates. It is not constrained by time and place. It can serve large numbers of people simultaneously and provide them with valuable health-promoting services at low cost.

In previous applications, the computer is used mainly as a tool to guide self-directed change through enabling instruction, goal setting, and feedback of progress. Linking the interactive aspects of the self-management system to the Internet can vastly expand its reach and availability. Online interactivity can further boost the health promotive power by providing a ready means of strategic guidance and for enlisting social support when needed. The amount and form of personalized guidance can be tailored to recipients' needs. Much needed productivity gains in risk reduction and health promotion can be realized by creatively coupling the knowledge of self-regulation with the disseminative and instructive power of computer-assisted implementation.

PUBLIC HEALTH CAMPAIGNS

Societal efforts to get people to adopt healthful practices rely heavily on persuasive communications in public health campaigns. These population-based approaches pick off the easier cases in the stepwise model. For the most part, these are people with a high sense of self-management efficacy and expectations that personal changes will improve their health. Meyerowitz and Chaiken (1987) examined four alternative mechanisms through which health communications could alter health habits: transmission of factual information about the determinants of health and disease, fear arousal over the prospect of disease, change in risk perception, and enhancement of perceived self-efficacy. They found that health communications fostered adoption of preventive health practices primarily by their effects on perceived self-efficacy. These findings indicate that efforts to enhance the effectiveness of public health campaigns to promote health require a shift in emphasis from trying to scare people into health to empowering them with the tools and self-beliefs of efficacy to exercise control over their health habits.

Analyses of how community-wide media campaigns change health habits similarly reveal that both the preexisting and developed levels of perceived self-efficacy play an influential role in the adoption and social diffusion of health practices (Maibach, Flora, & Nass, 1991; Rimal, 2000). The stronger the preexisting perceived self-efficacy, and the more the media campaigns enhanced people's self-regulative efficacy, the more they adopted the recommended practices. It is the individuals with a high sense of efficacy who translate health knowledge into healthful practices. Many people change detrimental health habits on their own. For example, more than 40 million people have quit the smoking habit on their own, even though nicotine is one of the most addictive drugs. Longitudinal studies show that heavy smokers who quit on their own had a stronger sense of efficacy at the outset than did continuous smokers and relapsers (Carey & Carey, 1993).

The absence of performance trials with enabling and supportive feedback places limits on the power of one-way health communications. The revolutionary advances in electronic technology provide the means to enhance the reach and productivity of health promotion programs. On the input side, health communications can now be personally tailored to relevant attributes, such as sociodemographic status, efficacy beliefs, outcome expectations, and perceived facilitators and impediments. Personalized communications are viewed as more relevant and credible, are better remembered, and are more effective in influencing health behavior than general health messages. The benefits of individualization will, of course, depend on the predictive value of the tailored factors. Development of good measures for key social cognitive determinants of health will provide informative guides for tailoring strategies.

Individualized interactivity, on the behavioral adaptation side, further enhances the impact of health promotion programs. Interactive computer-assisted feedback provides the means for informing, motivating, and guiding people in their efforts to make lifestyle changes. The enabling personalized feedback can be adjusted to participants' efficacy level, the unique impediments in their lives, and the progress they are making.

There is another way in which the power of population-based approaches to health promotion can be substantially augmented. There is only so much that large-scale health campaigns can do on their own, regardless of whether they are tailored or generic. As previously noted, there are two pathways through which health communication can alter health habits, the direct pathway and the socially mediated pathway, which links participants to informal social networks and community settings that provide ongoing guidance and support for desired changes.

The social linking function of media presentations is illustrated in worldwide applications of serial television dramas to stem the soaring population growth and the environmental devastation it produces (Bandura, 2002). The story lines model family planning, women's equality, beneficial health practices, and a variety of effective life skills. Epilogues connect viewers to enabling and supportive social systems. These dramatic serials raise people's efficacy to exercise control over their family lives, enhance the status of women, and bring families to family planning clinics where they receive extensive guidance. Dramatic segments that center on modeling safer sexual practices eliminate cultural misbeliefs about HIV transmission, increase adoption of condom use, and reduce the number of sexual partners.

Psychosocial programs for health promotion will be increasingly implemented via interactive Internet-based systems. Individuals at risk for health problems typically shun preventive or remedial health services. But they will pursue online assistance because it is readily accessible and convenient, and it provides a feeling of anonymity. For example, young women at risk of eating disorders reduce dissatisfaction with their weight and body shape and alter disordered eating behavior through interactive Internet-delivered behavioral guidance (Taylor, Winzelberg, & Celio, 2001). In the electronically mediated pathways, the impact of population-based approaches is augmented by linking people to interactive online systems that provide ongoing individualized guidance for personal change. Such systems can also promote supportive connectedness to others mastering similar problems.

SOCIALLY ORIENTED APPROACHES TO HEALTH

The quality of health of a nation is a social matter, not just a personal one. Health promotion, therefore, requires changing the practices of social systems that affect health rather than just changing the habits of individuals. The central focus is on enablement of people to work together to influence social, political, and environmental practices to promote public policies conducive to health. Such social efforts are aimed at raising public awareness of health hazards, educating and influencing policymakers, mobilizing public support for policy initiatives, and devising effective strategies for improving health conditions. People's beliefs in their collective efficacy to accomplish social change play a key role in the policy and public health approaches to health promotion and disease prevention (Bandura, 1997).

While collective efforts are made to change unhealthful social practices, people need to improve their current life circumstances over which they have some control. The approaches that work best promote community self-help through collective enablement. Consider a community effort to reduce infant mortality resulting from unsanitary conditions in poor neighborhoods (McAlister, Puska, Orlandi, Bye, & Zbylot, 1991). The community was fully informed of the impact of unsanitary conditions on children's health through the local media, churches, schools, and neighborhood meetings conducted by influential persons in the community. The residents were taught how to install plumbing systems, sanitary sewerage facilities, and refuse storage. They were shown how to secure the funds needed from different local and government sources. This self-help program, which provided needed resources and enabling guidance, greatly improved sanitation and markedly reduced infant mortality.

To contribute significantly to the betterment of human health by psychosocial means requires broadening the perspective on health promotion and disease prevention beyond the individual level. This calls for a more ambitious socially oriented agenda of research and practice. The impact of psychosocial programs on human health can be further amplified by making creative use of evolving interactive technologies that expand the scope and strength of health promotion efforts.

—Albert Bandura

See also CHRONIC DISEASE MANAGEMENT; ECOLOGICAL MODELS: APPLICATION TO PHYSICAL ACTIVITY; ECOSOCIAL THEORY; HEALTH PROMOTION AND DISEASE PREVENTION

Further Reading

Bandura, A. (1986). *Social foundations of thought and action: A social cognitive theory*. Englewood Cliffs, NJ: Prentice Hall.

Bandura, A. (1997). *Self-efficacy: The exercise of control*. New York: W. H. Freeman.

Bandura, A. (2002). Environmental sustainability by sociocognitive deceleration of population growth. In P. Schmuch & W. Schultz (Eds.), *The psychology of sustainable development* (pp. 209-238). Dordrecht, the Netherlands: Kluwer.

Carey, K. B., & Carey, M. P. (1993). Changes in self-efficacy resulting from unaided attempts to quit smoking. *Psychology of Addictive Behaviors, 7*, 219-224.

DeBusk, R. F., Miller, N. H., Superko, H. R., Dennis, C. A., Thomas, R. J., Lew, H. T., Berger, W. E., III, Heller, R. S., Rompf, J., Gee, D., Kraemer, H. C., Bandura, A., Ghandour, G., Clark, M., Shah, R. V., Fisher, L., & Taylor, C. B. (1994). A case-management system for coronary risk factor modification after acute myocardial infarction. *Annals of Internal Medicine, 120,* 721-729.

Haskell, W. L., Alderman, E. L., Fair, J. M., Maron, D. J., Mackey, S. F., Superko, H. R., Williams, P. T., Johnstone, I. M., Champagne, M. A., Krauss, R. M., & Farquhar, J. W. (1994). Effects of intensive multiple risk factor reduction on coronary atherosclerosis and clinical cardiac events in men and women with coronary artery disease. *Circulation, 89,* 975-990.

Maibach, E., Flora, J., & Nass, C. (1991). Changes in self-efficacy and health behavior in response to a minimal contact community health campaign. *Health Communication, 3,* 1-15.

McAlister, A. L., Puska, P., Orlandi, M., Bye, L. L., & Zbylot, P. (1991). Behaviour modification: Principles and illustrations. In W. W. Holland, R. Detels, & E. G. Knox (Eds.), *Oxford textbook of public health: Vol. 3. Applications in public health* (2nd ed., pp. 3-16). Oxford, UK: Oxford University Press.

Meyerowitz, B. E., & Chaiken, S. (1987). The effect of message framing on breast self-examination attitudes, intentions, and behavior. *Journal of Personality and Social Psychology, 52,* 500-510.

Rimal, R. N. (2000). Closing the knowledge-behavior gap in health promotion: The mediating role of self-efficacy. *Health Communication, 12,* 219-237.

Taylor, C. B., Winzelberg, A., & Celio, A. (2001). Use of interactive media to prevent eating disorders. In R. Striegel-Moor & L. Smolak (Eds.), *Eating disorders: New direction for research and practice* (pp. 255-270). Washington, DC: American Psychological Association.

SELF-REPORTED HEALTH

Self-reported health can be defined as the individual's personal evaluation of overall health. Many terms are used to describe this measure of health, such as self-reported health, self-rated health, self-assessed health, self-perceived health, self-appraisal of health, subjective health, perceived health status, general health rating, and general health perception.

Self-reported health differs from other health measures because the individual is asked to integrate all aspects of health without specific reference to the different components of health, such as physical, mental, social, or functional health, and without being prompted in one direction or another. Each individual may integrate different aspects of health depending on cultural, demographic, socioeconomic, and individual factors.

This simple-looking measure composed of one question has been found to be a very powerful measure of health when trying to understand health and social aspects of individuals and societies. When developing the measure it was intended to be used as a proxy for other more objective but more difficult to collect health measures. Soon it was obvious that self-reported health appears to add information to that obtained from objective measures of specific health components. Since its development, it has been used for (1) describing and following the health of populations, (2) screening populations to identify high-risk groups and risk factors, (3) studying variables affecting health, and (4) studying variables affected by health.

The advantage of the measure is in its ability to predict future health outcomes and in its simplicity, the data are easily collected in a questionnaire.

DEVELOPMENT OF THE MEASURE

The use of self-reported health began mainly in studies of the elderly, but later the use broadened to include middle-aged and younger populations. Lately, this measure has also been used in research of adolescents. Today, in different countries this measure is an intrinsic part of many studies and national surveys.

The use of this measure started in the 1950s when researchers developed a one-item question and a multi-item question to rate general perception of health (Ware, Davies-Avery, & Donald, 1978). The Health Perception Questionnaire (HPQ) was developed during the 1970s with 32 items divided into eight scales, and it was used in the Health Insurance Study. However, most of the research during the past 30 years regarding self-perception of health uses the one-item question. At first there was a need to validate the new measure and see if the measure actually represents the health of the individual. Already in the 1960s and 1970s, self-reported health was found to be strongly associated with and predictive of survival and other health outcomes; this gave a great boost to the use of self-reported health.

During the past 50 years, a lack of consensus has been observed regarding the terms used and the wording of the questions and the categories (answers) regarding the one-item question (self-reported health).

Wording of the Measure

Differently worded questions have been used to prompt the individual's evaluation of overall health, and these have changed over the years. Moreover, different answering systems to the question have been provided.

Two general concepts of the question exist. The first is a general request for overall evaluation of health, with wordings such as

1. In general (all in all) would you say your health is excellent, very good, good, fair, or poor?

2. How would you characterize your health overall?

3. How is your health in general?

4. How would you rate your health (at the present time) (these days) right now?

The second type is a comparative question, with wordings such as

1. Compared with others your age (and sex) would you say your health is . . .

2. How would you rate your health compared to others your age?

3. Is your health better, worse, about the same as it was 10 years ago?

The methods of scoring the question vary too. Between four and seven categories can be provided with wording such as *excellent, very good, good, fair*, and *poor*, or *very good, pretty good, not so good*, and *poor*. Comparative categories exist, too, such as *better, same, worse*. These questions have been translated to many different languages. The most frequently used question is the noncomparative general question.

Not much attention has been given to the differences in wording, and the assumption has been that the influences of linguistic variations in the questions were small. The variations in wording of the question, however, may contribute to the discrepancies between various studies in the literature. Moreover, analysis of

the differences between the two types of questions (comparative and noncomparative) may provide useful information about how people evaluate their health.

Lately, many questionnaires include both types of questions, the general type and the comparative type, enabling the analysis of the differences between the two types of questions. A certain percentage of people tend to give a different answer to the two questions; for example, older people tend to rate their health as better compared to people their age and younger people tend to rate it as worse compared to people their age (Baron-Epel & Kaplan, 2001).

HOW DO PEOPLE EVALUATE THEIR HEALTH?

Self-reported health represents an overall summary of different aspects of one's health. The process by which respondents construct their judgment is affected by different components of health and is processed in various ways depending on the individual. Culture, values, and beliefs also play a role in the evaluation of subjective health. This complex process of judging one's health consists of a few steps, such as collection of objective and subjective information relevant to the individual's health, deciding on the priority of the different aspects of health, integration and evaluation of the information, comparing this evaluation to the individual's social surroundings, and making a final judgment.

Generally, there seem to be three different issues influencing the evaluation of subjective health, the first is the actual health, objective and subjective; the second is the cultural surroundings in which the individual lives; and the third is the comparisons the individual performs in order to judge subjective health.

More specifically, knowledge, information, and perceptions that the individual has about many factors, such as physical illness or diseases, mental health, general feeling, pain, disabilities, tiredness, medications, medical treatments, social factors, and health behaviors, may play a role in the self-evaluation of health.

Research indicates that factors influencing how individuals respond to the question about their self-rated health can be grouped into three broad categories. The first includes emotional aspects or perceived "feelings" of health, general feeling, and emotional feelings. The second category includes all biomedical issues, such as diseases, medication, and pain. The third category relates to functional issues, such as inability or difficulty in performing certain activities. The influence of each component may vary in different populations; older people were found to report functional issues as more influential than younger people, and those reporting suboptimal self-reported tiredness and pain as more influential. Younger people seem to relate more to health behaviors they perceive as having an effect on health (Kaplan & Baron-Epel, 2003).

Cultural and environmental surroundings have an influence on the subjective evaluation of health. For example, individuals living in a community with many diseases and no health care system may perceive their health as optimal even though in the same situation in a healthier community this perception would be different. This can be related also to the comparative factor within the measure. People with more education and better medical facilities may have better skills with which to evaluate their health compared to people in less advantaged communities. Culture may influence sensitivity to symptoms, interpretation of their severity and significance, and behaviors adopted to deal with health (prevention and treatment). Moreover, in certain communities beliefs that are part of the culture may influence the verbal expression of ill health. In some cultures, people may express in general worse health and in others they may express better health depending on their perception of the expectations of their society. Therefore, comparing this measure between different cultures with different beliefs and attitudes about health can be very problematic (Wiseman, 1999).

Comparing one's health to others or other times may also play a role even when not asked to compare one's health to other factors.

The individual performs a spontaneous comparison of health to others that can be explained using the sociological reference group theory, which assumes that self-reported health depends on the individual's comparison group. Generally, this comparison exists spontaneously in a high percentage of individuals. Elderly people more often than young people compare their health to their age peers without being prompted to do so. It has been found that patients with Parkinson's disease seem to select others of their own age rather than others with the same disease for this comparison. Older people with poor self-reported health also spontaneously compare themselves more often to people their age compared to people in good health. Each

individual may try to find ways to evaluate health in a more positive way without being prompted in a certain direction.

DETERMINANTS OF SELF-REPORTED HEALTH

Many longitudinal and cross-sectional studies analyzed the factors determining self-reported health. Cross-sectional surveys indicate associations between self-reported health and other factors, and longitudinal studies may indicate prediction and even causality. All the determinants mentioned were shown to be associated independently or to be independent predictors of self-reported health after adjusting for other factors that are associated with self-reported health. However, there is not always an agreement across studies on the effect of these determinants. In many of the cases, prediction and causality are assumed even though not demonstrated.

The strongest predictors of self-reported poor health are self-reported diseases or disease history, number of diseases, somatic and psychological symptoms, and medication. These medical factors are thought to have a causal effect on self-reported health.

Self-reported health has been found to depend also on demographic and socioeconomic factors, such as age, sex, income, education, social class, and place of residence. Generally, a higher percentage of women and older people report poor health, and a lower percentage of better-educated people report poor health. It has been found that low literacy is strongly associated with poor self-reported health, and the association is stronger than the association with years of schooling. This research was performed in developed countries and therefore it may not be possible to generalize these findings to other populations in less developed countries (see Ross & Van Willigen, 1997). People with lower income and those living in rural areas were also found to report poorer health. Social class predicts the worsening of self-reported health in follow-up studies. Work environment and lifestyle factors can explain a high percentage of this variation. Working conditions and lifestyle may contribute to or cause ill health in the long run; self-reported health is an expression of this ill health. It is important to note that not all these determinants have the same effect on both sexes.

Functional limitations or disabilities are also an important determinant of self-reported health. However, not all types of disability have the same effect on self-reported health. It seems that in men disability in mobility and basic activities of daily living (ADLs) did have an effect on self-reported health, whereas disability in instrumental activities of daily living (IADLs) had no effect.

Most of the health measures studied in association with self-reported health were negative measures or absence of limitations; however, positive indicators of health may also play a role in determining self-reported health. In women, mobility measured as speed of walking and difficulty in walking was found to be associated with lower self-reported health. Measures such as speed during everyday activities, energy levels or feeling of energy, positive mood, social support, and active functioning had an independent effect on self-reported health.

Self-reported health is affected by depression, poor adjustment to the environment, distress, and mood (negative and positive), all representing mental health. Individuals reporting high levels of distress, for example, more frequently report lower levels of self-reported health.

Personal traits, such as locus of control and perceived control, may also have an effect on the evaluation of health.

Individuals with better social networks, social support, and family relationships have a higher chance of reporting positive self-reported health. The quality and quantity of social support (e.g., intimacy, reciprocity, number of social contacts) all are associated with self-reported health.

Lately, the research interest in the association between individuals' social surroundings and their self-reported health seems to be rising. For example, regional income inequality, measured by the Gini index, was found to be associated with worse self-reported health, especially among those with the lowest income. This may also depend on the type of area the individual lives in, mainly urban compared to rural areas. In non-metropolitan areas and rural areas, the association between self-reported health and inequality seems to be much stronger. These social factors remain after allowing for variation in individual-level factors.

In a follow-up study, poverty area residence was a strong predictor of decline in self-reported health. In another study, neighborhood environment, measured by the Care Need Index (CNI), was found to be associated with self-reported health: Respondents living in deprived neighborhoods reported poorer health after adjusting for other variables. Social capital, defined as the extent of interpersonal trust, norms of reciprocity, and density of civic associations (terms that facilitate cooperation for mutual benefit), was found to be associated with self-reported health; low social capital is associated with poor health. All in all, the characteristics of the community in which the individual lives seem to be associated with self-reported health (Kawachi, Kennedy, & Glass, 1999).

Specific social groups may show a different pattern of associations with self-reported health. For example, immigration status was also associated with low self-reported health; however, the concept of self-reported health may depend on the level of acculturation.

Nearly all the research was performed with middle-aged and elderly people, moreover, the same factors determine lower levels of self-reported health in adolescents, health problems, disability, age, being a woman, lower income, smoking, and higher BMI (body mass index).

The amount of variance in self-reported health that can be explained by a long list of health status correlates rarely exceeds 40%. This demonstrates the independence of the self-reported health measure and the fact that we do not yet fully understand all the factors contributing to the subjective evaluation of health.

THE PREDICTIVE VALUE OF SELF-REPORTED HEALTH

Research interests in self-reported health have grown considerably since follow-up studies found that self-reported health predicts a number of future health outcomes. The most important outcome is survival or mortality, and much research in the past 25 years has been directed that way (Idler & Benyamini, 1997). Self-reported health can predict mortality or survival in longitudinal studies. The first study reporting this ability to predict mortality was published in 1963, and thereafter many studies showed that the survival chances for those reporting optimal self-reported health were higher than those reporting poor health. Populations have been followed up for different periods of time from 2 years up to more than 20 years, depending on the age of the population.

Extremely consistent findings emerge from these studies. Most of the research on the prediction of survival or mortality has been performed in the older populations. The prediction of survival by self-reported health persists also for populations of middle-aged people, younger populations, and people with specific diseases or risk factors such as smoking. The prediction of survival was tested also in many communities around the world with the same findings implicating the generalization of the prediction. However, there are specific groups of people in which this prediction may not be valid. For example, in immigrants, the prediction of mortality may depend on the level of acculturation; thus, in those not yet acculturated, self-reported health is not a good predictor of survival. Instead it may express the stress of acculturation and not the overall health that predicts mortality.

Self-reported health and survival were studied together with measures that are known to be associated with survival, such as demographic variables, data from medical records, self-reported chronic diseases, measures of functioning, medication use, health care utilization, height, weight, blood pressure, other physical measures, cognitive function, health behaviors, and social networks or support. In most of the studies, self-reported health holds an independent effect when all covariates are entered into the statistical model. After adjusting for these variables and others, using statistical regression models, the self-reported health measure added to the understanding of the variation in survival. The adjusted odds ratio reported in most studies ranges from about 1.5 to about 3 for the survival of those reporting better health compared to those reporting poor health. Therefore, self-reported health adds information beyond the known mortality risk factors.

Univariate association between survival and self-reported health are observed both in men and women. However, the prediction of survival seems to be different in men compared to women after adjustment for other variables, although these differences are not consistent. All studies show a strong prediction of mortality in men for those reporting poor health after adjusting for other variables. However, in women, in most studies, when adjusting for other variables, the association between self-reported health and survival or mortality diminishes. In women, some studies show that socioeconomic factors, physical health status, and disability can explain the relationship between self-reported health and survival. This may imply a difference in the way women evaluate their health compared to men. It has been suggested that in older people women's evaluation of health incorporates factors not related directly to mortality, such as negative affect, emotional distress, and disruptive but non-life-threatening diseases (such as musculoskeletal problems), together with factors related to mortality, whereas in men the major factors taken into account when evaluating health are life-threatening issues. Older women may incorporate into their health evaluation the distress from events in other lives surrounding them as they are more involved in the lives of those around them, and these do not have an impact on the individual's mortality.

Self-reported health has been found to predict other health-related variables less dramatic than mortality. In follow-up studies, poor self-reported health predicted functional limitations, disability, receiving disability pension, future morbidity, hip fracture, recovery from illness, future physician rating of health, and institutionalization in the elderly. Self-reported health was also a predictor of long-term use of health services including visiting a general practitioner and community nurse, home help support, hospitalization, and increased medication use.

In follow-up studies, poor self-reported health predicted high levels of distress (low mental health) and together with the fact that distress adds to low self-reported health, these findings point to a downward spiral reaction. Distress may cause poor self-reported health, which leads over time to more poor self-reported health. Self-reported health can serve as a useful tool for identifying individuals at risk for subsequent health problems that may be preventable.

Four possible interpretations have been proposed for the relationship between self-reported health and adverse health outcomes (Idler & Benyamini, 1997). The first suggests that self-reported health is a holistic overall estimation of health that incorporates all aspects of health—physical, mental, social, and more—and that this is not possible when measuring specific aspects of health. Only the individual can make this overall summation of health. This may even include symptoms of undiagnosed diseases, judgment of severity of current diseases, and family history. The second interpretation can be called the "trajectory" interpretation in which the individual not only reports current level of health status but also anticipates future decline in health. The third explanation suggests that perceptions of one's health affect health behaviors, therefore affecting health in the long run. People with poor self-reported health will not adopt preventive behavior, screening practices, or self-care and will not adhere to medication and treatment, therefore enhancing morbidity and mortality. The fourth explanation suggests that the individual, when evaluating health, incorporates the availability of external and internal resources that can help in preventing the decline in health. To date, there is no preferred interpretation to explain the relationship between self-reported health and health outcomes.

FUTURE USE AND RESEARCH OF SELF-REPORTED HEALTH

The findings presented provide support for using self-reported health as a proxy or holistic measure of health in other studies where health is a nondependent variable that can explain other phenomena. Self-reported health can be regarded as a measure representing more than the medical aspects of health, and as such it can be a powerful overall measure to use in research. Self-reported health serves as a proxy for health in studies that look at factors that may be affected by health but in which health is not the main interest. As such, self-reported health serves to control for health in statistical models. For example, it was found that tiredness in daily activities at age 70 was an independent predictor of mortality after controlling or adjusting for self-reported health.

Moreover, self-reported health enables us to understand additional factors affecting health. These data support the idea that medical diagnosis cannot cover all aspects of health, and there may be subjective aspects that affect health in the long run. Uncovering these additional personal aspects should not be overlooked when trying to understand the overall picture of health.

To date, most researchers are tempted to conceptualize self-reported health as a causal factor in health outcome measures such as survival. However, there is no concrete evidence to consider self-reported health as a causal factor in health outcomes. This concept of causality could bring on interventions to try to change self-reported health where there is no evidence that this would bring positive results. The difference between causality and prediction should be explored further in the future.

—*Orna Baron-Epel*

See also SOCIAL CAPITAL AND HEALTH; SOCIOECONOMIC STATUS AND HEALTH

Further Reading

Baron-Epel, O., & Kaplan, G. (2001). General subjective health status or age-related health status: Does it make a difference? *Social Science & Medicine, 53*, 1373-1381.

Idler, E. L., & Benyamini, Y. (1997). Self-rated health and mortality: A review of twenty-seven community studies. *Journal of Health and Social Behavior, 38*, 21-37.

Kaplan, G., & Baron-Epel, O. (2003). What lies behind the subjective evaluation of health status? *Social Science & Medicine, 56*(8), 1669-1676.

Kawachi, I., Kennedy, B. P., & Glass, R. (1999). Social capital and self-rated health: A contextual analysis. *American Journal of Public Health, 89*, 1187-1193.

Ross, C. E., & Van Willigen, M. (1997). Education and the subjective quality of life. *Journal of Health and Social Behavior, 38*, 277-297.

Ware, J. E., Davies-Avery, A., & Donald, C. A. (1978). *Conceptualization and measurement of health for adults in the health insurance study: Vol. 5. General health perceptions.* RAND Corporation Report R-1987/5-HEW. Santa Monica, CA: RAND.

Wiseman, V. L. (1999). Culture, self-rated health and resource allocation decision-making. *Health Care Analysis, 7*, 207-223.

SEXUALLY TRANSMITTED DISEASES: PREVENTION

The American public health system has been reluctant to address sexual health issues openly because of the stigma associated with sexually transmitted diseases (STDs). This is embedded in wider cultural taboos about sexual health issues, such as sex education and teen pregnancy prevention. Annually, there are 12 million new cases of STDs, of which 3 million are in adolescents. In fact, among the top 10 diseases subject to mandatory reporting by U.S. authorities in 1995, 5 of them were STDs.

EPIDEMIOLOGY AND TYPES OF STDS

The relative estimated incidence of common STDs in 1994 is chlamydia, 4 million; gonorrhea, 800,000; syphilis, 101,000; genital herpes, 200,000 to 500,000; and trichomoniasis, 3 million. However, Americans underestimate their risk for acquiring an STD. In a 1993 survey, 84% of women surveyed were not concerned about acquiring an STD, including 72% of women between 18 and 24 years of age, even though 78% of those women reported having multiple partners over their lifetime (EDK Associates, 1994). The results of another study of individuals selected because they are at high risk for acquiring an STD provides further corroboration that Americans are not realistic about their perception of risk for STDs: 77% of the women and 72% of the men stated that they were not worried about getting an STD (EDK Associates, 1995).

There are 25 infectious organisms divided into three types that are transmitted through sexual activity: (1) bacteria (e.g., *Neisseria gonorrhoeae*, *Chlamydia trachomatis*, *Treponema pallidum* [syphilis]); (2) viruses (e.g., HIV, Types 1 and 2 [AIDS]; herpes simplex virus, hepatitis B virus); and (3) protozoan (e.g., *Trichomonas vaginalis*).

The STD health consequences range from mild acute illness to serious problems associated with reproductive health (e.g., infertility, ectopic pregnancy, stillborns, chronic pelvic pain), liver disease, cancer, neurological damage, and even death. Women are more vulnerable to serious consequences from STDs because they are often asymptomatic, which delays the diagnosis and treatment of curable STDs.

MODEL OF INFECTIOUSNESS

To understand the role of behavior change in preventing the further spread of STDs, it is helpful to examine the May and Anderson (1987) model of the reproductive rate of an STD:

$$Ro = BcD.$$

The reproductive rate of transmission (*Ro*) is assessed by the measures of infectivity or transmissibility (*B*), interaction rates between susceptibles and infectors (*c*), and duration of infectiousness (*D*). All of the factors on the right hand side of this formula can be influenced by individual behavior change. The degree of infectivity can be decreased by increasing condom use or by delaying the initiation of sexual activity. The infection rate can be influenced by decreasing the number of new partners or being monogamous. Duration of infections can be affected by seeking early treatment for STD treatment (Fishbein, 1997).

THEORIES OF BEHAVIOR CHANGE

To address the behavior change required to address the factors in the model of infectiousness, it is important to understand why people put themselves at risk for STDs and any other adverse health outcomes and what motivates them to reduce their risky behavior. Three theories predict individual behavior change and have had a profound impact on the development of STD prevention programs: (1) the health belief model (Rosenstock, Strecher, & Becker, 1994), (2) the social cognitive theory (Bandura, 1994), and (3) the theory of reasoned action (Fishbein, Middlestadt, & Hitchcock, 1991).

Five theorists convened by the National Institute of Mental Health for a workshop reviewed the common variables in these and other behavior change theories. There was consensus that there are eight common variables central to predicting behavior change. Three of these are necessary and probably sufficient: (1) intentions to perform a given behavior, (2) skills and abilities necessary to perform the behavior, and (3) the presence or absence of environmental constraints that would prevent someone from performing the behavior. Specifically, if a person intends to use a condom during every sexual act, has the skills to use a condom correctly, and has access to condoms when needed, there is an extremely high probably that the behavior will be executed.

STD PREVENTION STRATEGIES

In designing STD prevention programs, multiple strategies have been used that reduce the risk of acquiring an STD:

- *Increase use of latex condoms or other barrier methods.* Consistently using latex condoms is the best way to avoid contracting most STDs, although they are not as effective with herpes.
- *Delaying sexual initiation.* If adolescents delay initiation of sexual behavior this can be very important in preventing early acquisition of STD infections. Young women in menarche are more susceptible to some STDs because of the lack of maturity of the cervix.
- *Reduce number of partners.* The greater the number of partners, the more likely an individual is to be exposed to a partner who is positive for one or more STDs.

- *Avoid risky partners.* Risky partners are more likely to have multiple partners, use injection drugs, not use condoms, and be positive for one or more STDs.
- *Refrain from sexual encounters during outbreaks or while contagious.* Even if a partner is positive for herpes, a person can be protected by not having contact during those periods. While a person is receiving treatment for an STD, if the couple is abstinent, then they can avoid passing the same STD to each other.
- *Reduce use of vaginal douching.* Women who douche frequently are at higher risk for later complications of STDs, such as pelvic inflammatory disease.
- *Regularly seek health care.* Early treatment can limit the time that someone is infectious and prevent some of the negative health consequences of having an STD.

TYPES OF STD PREVENTION PROGRAMS

The three primary goals of both individual and population-based interventions are to prevent exposure to an STD, prevent acquisition of infection once exposed, and prevent transmission of the infection to others.

Behavioral Interventions

To prevent further transmission and acquisition of STDs, the behavior of individuals must be changed. Individual behavior change can be affected by evidence-based (scientifically proven) interventions delivered at multiple levels: (1) individual, (2) couples, (3) family, (4) community, and (5) societal (policy and media) (Pequegnat & Stover, 2000).

It is also critical that the intervention be based on a theory to ensure that modifiable risk and protective processes are targeted by the intervention to affect the outcome. Interventions that are delivered at the five levels use different theoretical approaches. For example, individual and couples interventions have been based on social cognitive theory and are effective because they focus on perceptions of risk, skills building, and enhancing negotiation skills. The structural ecological model has been used effectively with families to restructure relationships within the family to enhance social support dynamics. The theory of diffusion of innovation posits that in every community there are popular opinion leaders who can be trained to deliver prevention messages during conversations with friends and neighbors that will result in change in social norms about engaging in lower-risk behaviors (e.g., consistently using condoms) and ultimately in incidence of STDs (Kelly, 1999; Kelly et al., 1991; Rogers, 1983).

Prevention scientists must also consider the developmental level of the target population and match the intervention to the life experience of the target group. For example, an intervention aimed at preadolescents who are not sexually active should be prevention messages delivered by the parents encouraging delay of initiation of sexual behavior. Prevention programs for sexually active adolescents may also be delivered by parents, but it is also important to address the social norms and perception of behavior by peers in order to support safer HIV-related behaviors. An intervention designed for adults would focus on consistent condom use with all partners.

Abstinence and Delay of Sexual Initiation

Some prevention programs have been developed for adolescents to maintain abstinence and prevent them from initiating sexual activity. Many of these programs are designed to be delivered to parents, who then deliver the prevention messages to their children (Pequegnat & Szapocznik, 2000). Other programs with similar goals have been delivered in schools. While many of these programs focus on preventing STDs, they may also result in pregnancy prevention.

Prophylaxis

The only efficacious vaccine currently available is for hepatitis B. Although the hepatitis B vaccine has been available for more than a decade, few people have been vaccinated because a selective vaccination strategy was initially adopted and there has been little public information about the vaccine. Vaccines for herpes simplex virus are in clinical trials, and vaccines for other STDs are in various stages of development.

Clinical Care Screening for Asymptomatic STDs

In addition to interventions designed to prevent STDs through behavior change or vaccines, there are interventions to reduce the duration of the infection. Many people are asymptomatic for STDs and therefore clinical screening programs are essential to identify individuals who are positive for an STD so they do not transmit to their partners. Some opportunities for screening occur when people are seeking health services for medical clearance to play sports, seeking contraception and family planning services, having an annual health checkup, or having a health examination for life insurance. These health care visits may be optimal times because individuals are more likely to be receptive to STD prevention messages because they are already seeking health care.

Early Treatment for Symptomatic STDs

Prevention campaigns that encourage health-seeking behavior for STD symptoms are important.

Early treatment for symptomatic people is essential to contain the contagion of STDs and prevent complications for STDs in infected individuals.

The STD treatment guidelines published by the Centers for Disease Control and Prevention (CDC; 1993) provide the current standards for therapy of STDs. A problem with treatment is the failure to adhere to the full course of medication. To address this problem, effective single-dose therapy for several STDs (e.g., chancroid, gonorrhea, syphilis, trichomoniasis) have been developed and single-dose therapy for chlamydia infection has recently become available. These single-dose regimens have been shown to be as effective as multiple-dose regimens (Zenilman, 1996). However, single-dose therapies can be significantly more expensive than standard multiple-dose medications.

Many viral STDs (e.g., HIV infection, genital herpes, hepatitis B virus infection) are being diagnosed as suppressible (not curable) infections with new therapies. These treatments suppress viral replication and thereby reduce transmission and may be considered to be a viable approach for preventing STDs.

Partner Notification and Treatment

A partner notification program was initiated for syphilis after penicillin became widely available in the 1940s. This worked well for syphilis because there is a long incubation period (approximately 3 weeks but can be between 10 and 90 days from exposure to onset of symptoms) so it was possible to treat incubating syphilis.

When this approach was expanded to include the referral of partners exposed to other STDs, the strategy had to be changed because the incubation period for gonorrhea (usually a week or less) and chlamydia (1 to 2 weeks) is too brief to prevent incubation. Therefore, the rationale for partner notification became locating and treatment of asymptomatic infected female partners of symptomatic men and on providing early treatment to prevent complications. Partner notification followed by partner treatment, therefore, is considered to be a strategy that benefits the individual patient, his or her partner, and the community as a whole.

When the model was applied to HIV/AIDS, there were other concerns because the incubation period is so long that it makes partner notification more difficult, the disease is very stigmatized, and there are not curative therapies. However, early intervention with anti-retroviral therapy and prophylaxis against opportunistic infections may be more beneficial if there is patient adherence.

SUMMARY

While there are efficacious STD prevention and treatment programs, there are multiple barriers to successfully implementing them effectively in public health agencies. Individual factors, such as high-risk sexual behavior, misperception of risk, and lack of skills needed to negotiate and use condoms, increase risk of STDs. Factors that prevent persons from seeking health care for STDs, including lack of perception of risk, misinformation, lack of knowledge about STDs, and the social stigma of STDs, must be addressed by the public health system. Although newer laboratory tests have improved the screening and diagnosis process, expense and accessibility to these tests are major barriers to clinical diagnosis and treatment. Because of the variety of barriers that influence the risk for STDs, it is clear that both biomedical and behavioral interventions must be integrated in a national STD prevention campaign.

—*Willo Pequegnat*

See also AIDS AND HIV: PREVENTION OF HIV INFECTION; HEALTH PROMOTION AND DISEASE PREVENTION

Further Reading

Bandura, A. (1994). Social cognitive theory and exercise of control over HIV infection. In R. J. DiClemente & J. L. Peterson (Eds.), *Preventing AIDS: Theories and methods of behavioral interventions* (pp. 25-29). New York: Plenum.

Centers for Disease Control and Prevention. (1993). Sexually transmitted diseases treatment guideline. *Morbidity and Mortality Weekly Report, 42* (No. RR-14), 56-66.

Centers for Disease Control and Prevention. (1996). Ten leading nationally notifiable infectious diseases—United States, 1995. *Morbidity and Mortality Weekly Report, 45*, 883-884.

EDK Associates. (1994). *Women and sexually transmitted diseases: The danger of denial.* New York: Author.

EDK Associates. (1995). *The ABCs of STDs.* New York: Author.

Fishbein, M. (1997). *Theoretical models of HIV prevention. NIH Consensus Development Conference: Interventions to prevent HIV risk behaviors* [Program and Abstracts]. Bethesda, MD: National Institutes of Health.

Fishbein, M., Bandura, A., Triandis, H. C., Kanfer, F. H., Becker, M. H., Middlestadt, S. E., & Eichler, A. (1992). *Factors influencing behavior and behavior change: Final report—Theorist's workshop.* Rockville, MD: National Institute of Mental Health.

Fishbein, M., Middlestadt, S. E., & Hitchcock, P. J. (1991). Using information to change sexually transmitted diseases-related behaviors: An analysis based on the theory of reasoned action. In N. J. Wasserheti, S. O. Aral, & K. K. Holmes (Eds.), *Research issues in human behavior and sexually transmitted diseases in the AIDS era.* Washington, DC: American Society for Microbiology.

Kelly, J. A. (1999). Community-level interventions are needed to prevent new HIV infections. *American Journal of Public Health, 89*, 299-301.

Kelly, J. A., St. Lawrence, J. S., Diaz, Y. E., Stevenson, L. Y., Hauth, A. C., & Brasfied, T. L. (1991). HIV risk behavior following intervention with key opinion leaders of a population: An experimental community level analysis. *American Journal of Public Health, 81*, 168-171.

May, R. M., & Anderson, R. M. (1987). Transmission dynamics and HIV infection. *Nature, 326*, 137-142.

NIH Consensus Panel. (2000). National Institutes of Health Consensus Development Conference Statement, February 11-13, 1997. *AIDS, 14*(2), S85-S96.

Pequegnat, W., & Stover, E. (2000). Behavioral prevention is today's AIDS vaccine! *AIDS, 14*(2), S1-S7.

Pequegnat, W., & Szapocznik, J. (2000). *Working with families in the era of AIDS.* Thousand Oaks, CA: Sage.

Rogers, E. E. (1983). *Diffusion of innovations.* New York: Free Press.

Rosenstock, I. M., Strecher, V. J., & Becker, M. H. (1994). The health belief model and HIV risk behavior change.

In R. J. DiClemente & J. L. Peterson (Eds.), *Preventing AIDS: Theories and methods of behavioral interventions* (pp. 5-24). New York: Plenum.

Zenilman, J. (1996). Gonococcal susceptibility to antimicrobials in Baltimore, 1988-1994. What was the impact of ciprofloxcin as first-line therapy for gonorrhea? *Sexually Transmitted Diseases, 23*, 213-218.

SICKLE CELL DISEASE: PSYCHOSOCIAL ASPECTS

Sickle cell disease (SCD) is an inherited disease that is found in people of African descent as well as those whose ancestry is from certain groups in India, the Middle East, and the Mediterranean. Its presence in Latin America is related to the intermingling of gene pools between people of African origin and the indigenous populations.

SCD is understood on a molecular, cellular, and clinical basis. The molecular problem is an abnormal structure of the hemoglobin molecule that causes the molecules to aggregate into well-ordered bundles within the red blood cells instead of remaining in solution as is usually the case. This abnormal aggregation or polymerization of hemoglobin molecules causes numerous abnormalities on the cellular level. The red cells' shapes are distorted by the presence of the polymers. There is physical disruption of the cell membrane causing both abnormal binding of the red cells to blood vessel walls and leakage of water and electrolytes from the cells. The red cells cause vaso-occlusion in the smallest blood vessels throughout the body, and are destroyed much more quickly than normal cells.

The immediate consequences of the cellular abnormality are anemia, because of the increased destruction, and pain and organ damage, due to vaso-occlusion. The clinical problems that result include fatigue and decreased exercise tolerance; episodes of acute, severe pain; sequestration of red cells in liver and spleen; and cumulative damage to organs, especially bones, kidneys, liver, lungs, and brain. There is also increased susceptibility to infection, particularly in children, who also have growth delay and the late onset of puberty.

There is a wide range of clinical severity in SCD, with some children having initial symptoms of pain in infancy and others not experiencing pain or other complications until school years or later. Pain, which occurs in episodes of sudden onset, is the hallmark of the disease. This is acute, severe pain that can occur in any part of the body; the onset of pain episode is completely unpredictable. Most pain can be managed at home, using a combination of nonpharmacological measures such as heat, massage, rest, and distraction, along with medications. Nonsteroidal anti-inflammatory agents, acetaminophen and lower-strength opioid medications, are commonly used by patients at home. When these fail, medical attention is usually sought. Parenteral opioids are then given in a clinic, emergency room (ER), or inpatient setting. A major barrier to effective treatment of pain crises is lack of understanding on the part of ER personnel resulting in inadequate pain relief and unsympathetic care. Many individuals with SCD have no alternatives to ERs for treatment of pain episodes.

Other acute complications that occur in SCD are acute chest syndrome, a pneumonia-like illness that can be quite serious or even fatal; splenic sequestration, which causes a life-threatening worsening of anemia; acute, severe infections such as meningitis or bacteremia; and stroke. The chronic conditions, which are now are being seen more frequently as people with SCD survive longer, include bone disease, renal insufficiency and failure, hepatic insufficiency, decline in pulmonary function, and leg ulcers. Despite the many potential problems associated with the disease, a majority of affected individuals have relatively few problems.

MEDICAL TREATMENT

Medical treatment for acute pain episodes, as noted above, is primarily achieved with analgesics and anti-inflammatory agents at home. In hospitals, the most commonly used agents are parenteral morphine and meperidine, although there is an effort to greatly reduce or eliminate the use of meperidine because of the risk of significant toxicity with more than very short-term use. Morphine provides good analgesia when given appropriately, although the adverse effects of itching, oversedation with respiratory depression, nausea, and constipation have to be monitored and treated as necessary. Ensuring adequate hydration and oxygenation, and treating concomitant infections, are important adjuncts to analgesia. Emotional support and sympathetic nursing care are extremely important.

Transfusions are used for selected problems such as some instances of acute worsening of anemia, acute chest syndrome with respiratory insufficiency, acute stroke and secondary stroke prevention, some cases of pulmonary hypertension, and preparation for major surgery. Depending on the indication, the transfusions are either simple or exchange transfusions.

Preventive care for children with SCD includes the daily administration of penicillin to children under 5 years for the prevention of invasive pneumococcal infections, and yearly transcranial doppler exams of the intracranial arteries to assess for stroke risk. The standard childhood vaccines are of great importance; in addition, these children should receive influenza vaccine yearly, and continue to receive the older 23 valent pneumococcal vaccine as well as the newer conjugated pneumococcal vaccine, which is now standard pediatric care.

Hydroxyurea is now widely used in SCD. Chronic administration of this drug causes an increase in fetal hemoglobin production, and other less well understood effects that combine to ameliorate the course of the disease. It reduces the rate of painful crises, hospitalizations, and acute chest events and the requirement for transfusion all by 40% to 50%. In use for about 10 years in SCD, an increased rate of malignancy has not been observed; there is some evidence that it is associated with a lower death rate in those who use it. Although it has not yet been approved by the Food and Drug Administration in children, it is being used with similar effects as seen in adults.

Bone marrow transplantation using stem cells from an unaffected, matched sibling donor has a success rate of about 85% in children with SCD. These children are cured; their red cells contain normal hemoglobin. This has been performed in more than 100 children in the United States and in a slightly smaller number in Europe. There has not been great success in transplanting adults with SCD.

Research into new treatments is being carried out in a number of centers in the United States and abroad. Areas of investigation include new drug therapies, gene therapy, lessening the toxicity of stem cell transplantation, nutritional therapy, genetic investigation for better prognostication, and interventions for specific complications of the disease.

Although progress is being made in the medical care of people with SCD, there is still a great deal of disability and suffering that is associated with the disease. The psychological burden of a chronic disease is significant at all ages, and psychosocial assessment and the provision of support and advocacy has long been part of comprehensive sickle cell medical care.

ACADEMIC AND PSYCHOSOCIAL SEQUELAE OF SICKLE CELL DISEASE

One of the most commonly cited consequences of SCD for children is impaired academic functioning as reflected in lower teacher evaluations, sub-par achievement, and grade retention (Barbarin, Whitten, & Bonds, 1994). Distraction due to pain, and interruption due to hospitalization, may place children at risk for poor academic performance. In addition, Brown, Armstrong, and Eckman (1993) suggest that subtle neurological deficits associated with cerebral vascular accidents affect cognitive processes and higher-order cognitive abilities and later impede learning and academic achievement. However, studies that control for socioeconomic status and other demographic features find no effect of SCD on IQ,[1] performance on standardized tests of reading and math, or grade retention (Midence, McManus, Fuggle, & Davies, 1996; Richard & Burlew, 1997).

Although children with SCD experience social and psychological stressors as sequelae of the disease, evidence of academic and psychological impairment is minimal once the effects of socioeconomic disadvantage are controlled. Although children with SCD are rated as less sociable and less well accepted than non-ill peers, no differences are found on indicators of emotional well-being such as depression and self-concept (Midence et al., 1996; Noll, Vanatta, & Koontz, 1996). The relationship between SCD is strong for adolescents but not young children (Barbarin, 1999; Lemanek, Horwitz, & Ohene-Frempong, 1994). In addition to problems with social functioning, adolescents with SCD face special difficulty in making the transition to independence. This may be because SCD is commonly accompanied by episodes in which one is almost helpless, as well as the other barriers experienced by chronically ill children and adolescents.

For adults, the sequelae of SCD include the experience of fear, guilt, loss of morale, and zest for life and a higher risk for marital dysfunction and chronic problems with employment, anxiety, and fear regarding body deterioration, and a lack of assertiveness in social situations (Barrett et al., 1988; Belgrave & Molock, 1991). Anxiety is provoked by the complete unpredictability of the onset of pain, and the intensity of pain often causes individuals to fear that they will die during the crisis.

In work life, persons with SCD experience physical limitations such as decreased capacity for strenuous activity and lowered tolerance for extreme temperatures, high altitudes, dangerous toxins, and infectious environments. In addition to the limitations that restrict what a person with SCD can perform at work, there are a few other issues. Once having obtained a job, they often are fired because of absences due to illness. This is also an issue for the parents of children with SCD who miss work to take care of their sick child. In low-skill jobs there is little tolerance for sick days. Also, when one is paid by the hour, missing work means missed pay. Employability may be further compromised by the same social factors such as racial discrimination that affects employment of African Americans who do not have SCD (Utsey, 1991).

Then there is the issue of disability, which presents a complex dilemma for adults with SCD. Some individuals have qualified as being disabled simply by virtue of having SCD, while some have documented disabling conditions; of those who have disabling conditions, some work and others do not. Some children have qualified to have Supplemental Security Income grants and therefore approach adulthood with the label of *disabled* already in place. This almost certainly affects their self-image, life goals, and ambitions. This financial grant, small as it is, combined with difficulty in obtaining and maintaining employment often is a disincentive to do anything to shake off that label, even when the individual may be capable of working.

Life expectancy and quality for persons with SCD have improved measurably over the past decade. With good health care and preventive interventions, many live to old age. However, the psychosocial challenges of social stigma, anxiety, and poverty continue to make life difficult. Thus, the need for strong programs of socioemotional support is as great as ever.

—Oscar A. Barbarin, Rupa Redding-Lallinger, and Marcelle Christian Holmes

See also CHRONIC DISEASE MANAGEMENT; CHRONIC PAIN MANAGEMENT

Note

1. There is definite abnormal neuropsych performance by children with SCD who have had clinical strokes in

comparison to those with SCD who have "silent" lesions in CNS and those with normal CNS imaging (see Armstrong et al., 1996, *Pediatrics, 97,* 864-870).

Further Reading

Barbarin, O. (1999). Do parental coping, involvement, religiosity and racial identity mediate children's psychological adjustment to sickle cell disease? *Journal of Black Psychology, 25,* 391-426.

Barbarin, O., Whitten, C., & Bonds, S. (1994). Estimating rates of psychosocial problems in urban and poor children with sickle cell anemia. *Health and Social Work, 19,* 112-119.

Barrett, D., Wisotzek, I. E., Abel, G. G., Rouleau, J. L., Plat, A. F., Pollard, W. E., & Eckman, J. R. (1988). Assessment of psychosocial functioning of patients with sickle cell disease. *Southern Medical Journal, 81,* 745-750.

Belgrave, F., & Molock, S. (1991). The role of depression in hospital admissions and emergency treatment of patients with sickle cell disease. *Journal of the National Medical Association, 83,* 777-781.

Brown, R. T., Armstrong, F. D., & Eckman, J. R. (1993). Neurocognitive aspects of paediatric sickle cell disease. *Journal of Learning Disabilities, 26,* 33-45.

Haynes, J., Manci, E., & Voelkel, N. (1994). Pulmonary complications. In S. H. Embury, R. P. Hebbel, N. Mohandas, & M. Steinberg (Eds.), *Sickle cell disease: Basic principles and clinical practice* (pp. 623-631). New York: Raven.

Lemanek, K. L., Horwitz, W. L., & Ohene-Frempong, K. (1994). A multi-perspective investigation of social competence in children with sickle cell disease. *Journal of Pediatric Psychology, 19,* 443-456.

Lemanek, K. L., Moore, S. L., Gresham, F. M., Williamson, D. A., & Kelley, M. L. (1986). Psychological adjustment of children with sickle cell anemia. *Journal of Pediatric Psychology, 11,* 397-410.

Midence, K., McManus, C., Fuggle, P., & Davies, S. (1996). Psychological adjustment and family functioning in a group of British children with sickle cell disease: Preliminary empirical findings and a meta-analysis. *British Journal of Clinical Psychology, 35,* 439-450.

Noll, R. B., Vanatta, K., & Koontz, K. (1996). Peer relationships and emotional well-being of youngsters with sickle cell disease. *Child Development, 67,* 423-436.

Richard, H. W., & Burlew, A. K. (1997). Academic performance among children with sickle cell disease: Setting minimum standards for comparison groups. *Psychological Reports, 81,* 27-34.

Shafer, F. E., & Vichinsky, E. (1994). New advances in the pathophysiology and management of sickle cell disease. *Current Opinion in Hematology, 1,* 125-135.

Stefanatou, A., & Bowler, D. (1997). Depiction of pain in the self-drawings of children with sickle cell disease. *Child Care, Health, and Development, 23,* 135-155.

Utsey, S. O. (1991). Vocational rehabilitation and counseling approaches with sickle cell anemia. *Journal of Applied Rehabilitation Counseling, 22,* 29-31.

Walco, G. A., & Dampier, C. D. (1990). Pain in children and adolescents with sickle cell disease: A descriptive study. *Journal of Pediatric Psychology, 15,* 643-658.

SLEEP DISORDERS: BEHAVIORAL TREATMENT

Because thoughts, feelings, and actions can all have an impact on the quality of a night's sleep, sleep may be considered a behavior that is in part under conscious control of an individual. Psychology specializes in helping individuals modify their thoughts, feelings, and actions using a variety of techniques based on well-known principles. Behavioral sleep medicine is a field that has recently come into existence and focuses on the identification and treatment of those psychological factors that contribute to the development and/or maintenance of sleep disorders (Stepanski & Perlis, 2000). Behavioral sleep medicine specialists are typically psychologists who have completed a Ph.D. in clinical psychology or a related psychological area with appropriate training; the most advanced are board certified in sleep medicine. The behavioral treatment of sleep disorders focuses on the assessment and treatment of the complaint of insomnia, providing adjunctive therapy for sleep disorders that result in excessive daytime sleepiness, assessment and treatment of pediatric sleep disorders, and improving adherence with pharmacological and nonpharmacological treatments for sleep disorders.

THE SLEEP DISORDERS

The most widely recognized sleep disorder classification system is the International Classification of Sleep Disorders (American Sleep Disorders Association, 1997). Sleep disorders are classified into dyssomnias (sleep disorders that produce either insomnia or excessive sleepiness), parasomnias (undesirable physical phenomena that occur predominantly during sleep), and those associated with medical or psychiatric disorders. Dyssomnias are the most common sleep disorders. Examples of dyssomnias that cause sleepiness include sleep apnea and narcolepsy; an example of a dyssomnia that causes insomnia is psychophysiological insomnia. Sleep apnea alone accounts for about 80% of all sleep disorder diagnoses.

Sleep disorders are prevalent in the United States, yet most individuals with sleep complaints have not been fully evaluated by a sleep professional. A National Sleep Foundation poll conducted in 2002 found that nearly one third of randomly selected Americans reported that their sleep quality was fair or poor. More than one half of the respondents reported having experienced at least one of four symptoms of insomnia at least a few nights per week. And over one third reported that they were so sleepy during the day that it interfered with their daily activities a few days per month or more. In fact, fully three fourths of respondents experienced at least one symptom of a sleep disorder a few nights per week or more. Perhaps the most important finding of the poll was that only a small fraction of those respondents who reported symptoms of any sleep disorder talked to a health care professional about the sleep complaint. In short, symptoms of sleep disorders are common in the United States and most of those with a sleep disorder have not been appropriately tested.

When someone is suspected of having a sleep disorder, they are typically referred to an accredited sleep disorders clinic. Accredited sleep disorders centers are those clinics that have met rigorous standards and passed a strict evaluation from the American Academy of Sleep Medicine. Sleep disorders are diagnosed and treated by many different health care professionals, including general practitioners and specialists in neurology, pulmonary medicine, psychiatry, psychology, pediatrics, and dentistry as well as other fields. Larger sleep centers have several of these specialists on staff who will consult with each other on the appropriate diagnosis and treatment for any one individual. For example, a patient who complains of insomnia could be started on a sleep-promoting medication by a neurologist or psychiatrist while a behavioral sleep medicine specialist begins to help the patient learn how thoughts, feelings, and actions are contributing to sleep difficulties.

Typically, the patient will undergo an interview with a sleep professional and then have his or her sleep monitored while sleeping in the center. Electroencephalography, electro-oculography, and electromyography allow the recording of brain activity, eye movements, and chin muscle activity, respectively, so that the stage of sleep may be identified. Other parameters that may be recorded include airflow, breathing effort, oxygen level, body position, leg movements, heart rate, and snoring level. Sleep consists of non-rapid eye movement (NREM) sleep and rapid eye movement (REM) sleep. NREM sleep consists of Stages 1 through 4, with Stage 1 being transitional sleep and Stages 3 and 4 consisting of "deep" sleep, which is considered the most restful. About 50% of the night is spent in Stage 2 sleep. REM sleep is the stage during which dreaming takes place and occurs about every 90 minutes during sleep. People cycle through these stages in characteristic ways. Sleep disorders often result in a disruption of these sleep stages; for example, sleep apnea results in many frequent awakenings from sleep such that a disproportionate amount of time is spent in Stages 1 and 2, which leads to inadequate sleep and subsequent excessive daytime sleepiness. Narcolepsy is characterized by entering REM sleep rather than Stage 1 sleep.

GOOD SLEEP HYGIENE

The foundation of all behavioral treatments of sleep disorders rests on the "good sleep hygiene" habits listed in Table 1. Some or all of these recommendations can play a role in the reviewed sleep disorders. However, these good sleep habits alone typically are not sufficient for the appropriate treatment of sleep disorders. A behavioral sleep medicine specialist will help identify the two or three most important behaviors to change and develop a treatment plan to implement these changes, in conjunction with the patient. These habits can be classified according to health practices (i.e., diet, exercise, and substance abuse) and environmental influences (i.e., light, noise, temperature, and mattress).

BEHAVIORAL TREATMENT FOR INSOMNIA

Insomnia is a complaint of insufficient sleep and is not a disorder itself. There are three types of primary insomnia including psychophysiological insomnia, idiopathic insomnia, and sleep-state misperception and several types of secondary insomnia including insomnia associated with psychiatric disorders or insomnia

Table 1   Good Sleep Hygiene Habits

1. Sleep only when sleepy or drowsy. If unable to fall asleep or stay asleep, leave the bedroom and engage in quiet activity elsewhere. Return to bed when—and only when—sleepy.
2. Avoid caffeine within 4 to 6 hours of bedtime and avoid the use of nicotine close to bedtime or during the night.
3. Do not drink alcoholic beverages within 4 to 6 hours of bedtime.
4. Get regular exercise each day. Refrain from strenuous exercise at least 4 hours before bedtime.
5. Establish regular bedtimes and uptimes, even on days off work and on weekends.
6. Avoid looking at the alarm clock at night.
7. Avoid napping during the daytime. If daytime sleepiness becomes overwhelming, limit nap time to a single nap of less than 1 hour, no later than 3 p.m.
8. Develop sleep rituals.
9. While a light snack before bedtime can help promote sound sleep, avoid large meals.
10. Minimize light, noise, and extremes in temperature in the bedroom.

associated with medical disorders. Sleep-state insomnia is a condition whereby the patient's complaint is not corroborated by polysomnographic recording. Psychophysiological insomnia is considered a learned insomnia; for example, a patient may not be able to fall asleep within a reasonable amount of time in his or her own bed, yet fall asleep quickly when in a hotel room. Idiopathic insomnia is typically diagnosed when no known cause can be identified. These types of insomnia can be classified according to whether they are transient, acute, or chronic.

Spielman and colleagues (Spielman, Caruso, & Glovinsky, 1987) developed a useful theoretical framework to help understand the complex interactions among the many factors that may be involved in the complaint of insomnia. *Predisposing* factors include those factors (including emotional, cognitive, or behavioral) that promote insomnia but are insufficient alone to cause insomnia without the presence of other factors. For example, individuals who are worriers would be considered to be at higher risk for insomnia. *Precipitating* factors are often identifiable events that precede insomnia (e.g., something major such as death of a loved one or minor such as sleeping in an unfamiliar bed). *Perpetuating* factors are behaviors that help to maintain sleeplessness once it has begun and are typically learned during episodes of insomnia. These include irregular sleep habits (e.g., monitoring the clock) that might lead to performance anxiety. Performance anxiety occurs when an individual puts extra pressure on himself or herself to fall asleep, which usually has the effect of delaying sleep onset.

Behavioral treatments are aimed at reducing factors that perpetuate insomnia. Techniques include relaxation techniques, stimulus control therapy, sleep restriction therapy, and cognitive-behavioral therapy. Relaxation therapy helps to reduce physiological tension and is typically used in conjunction with other treatment techniques. Stimulus control therapy attempts to break the learned association between the feeling of being awake in one's sleep environment by teaching one to (1) be in the bedroom only when drowsy or asleep and (2) not to engage in behaviors incompatible with sleep in the bedroom (e.g., paying bills or dealing with problems). Sleep restriction therapy attempts to help one increase the drive for sleep by partially depriving sleep. A schedule of strict bedtimes and uptimes is prescribed to help consolidate sleep and decrease the amount of time spent awake during the night. Cognitive-behavioral therapy (CBT) focuses on helping to change unrealistic beliefs or irrational fears about sleep. CBT is the most widely studied approach and typically incorporates each of the described techniques.

How effective are behavioral interventions for insomnia? Several meta-analyses have been published comparing behavioral treatment of insomnia with pharmacological treatment (Morin, Culbert, & Schwartz, 1994; Murtagh & Greenwood, 1995; Smith et al., 2002). They found that behavioral treatment of insomnia produced reliable and durable changes in the sleep of patients and that behavioral treatments produced similar short-term outcomes as that of pharmacotherapy. Pharmacotherapy for insomnia is thought to be limited for use over the long term because it may result in tolerance, dependence, or rebound insomnia upon discontinuation. Behavioral treatment of insomnia has the benefit of few, if any, side effects. Stimulus control and sleep restriction are the most effective single behavior therapy procedures, whereas sleep hygiene education and relaxation alone do not appear to be effective but are important adjunct treatments.

ADJUNCTIVE THERAPIES FOR SLEEP DISORDERS ASSOCIATED WITH EXCESSIVE DAYTIME SLEEPINESS

Behavioral sleep medicine specialists can play an important role in providing adjunctive behavioral treatments for sleep disorders associated with excessive sleepiness.

Obstructive sleep apnea is a sleep disorder characterized by repeated cessations of breath at night, which result in sleep fragmentation, lowered oxygen saturation levels, excessive daytime sleepiness, and cardiovascular consequences. Obstructive sleep apnea is often worsened when sleeping in the supine position. Behavioral treatments geared toward encouraging sleep in the nonsupine position (1) may provide a simple and effective primary treatment for mild to moderate obstructive sleep apnea in some patients and (2) can improve the effectiveness of other treatments for apnea (e.g., by increasing the efficacy of continuous positive airway pressure devices).

Narcolepsy is a sleep disorder characterized by an uncontrollable urge to fall asleep that is associated with muscle weakness. Narcolepsy is composed of four key symptoms: excessive daytime sleepiness; cataplexy (sudden loss of voluntary muscle control, usually triggered by emotions such as laughter, surprise, fear or anger); hypnagogic hallucinations (vivid, realistic, often frightening dreams); and sleep paralysis (a temporary inability to move). Behavioral sleep medicine practitioners play an important role in the management of narcolepsy by helping to schedule daytime naps (Mullington & Broughton, 1993). By scheduling naps, patients with narcolepsy can have a reduced incidence of cataplexy and improved daytime functioning, thereby improving their overall quality of life.

Finally, adjunctive behavioral treatment for sleep disorders may involve treating psychiatric symptoms and/or disorders that are associated with primary sleep disorders. For example, patients with insomnia may have anxiety symptoms, and obstructive sleep apnea patients may have depressive symptoms that cognitive-behavioral treatment can help ameliorate.

PEDIATRIC SLEEP DISORDERS

Several pediatric sleep disorders are amenable to behavioral treatments including nocturnal enuresis, limit-setting sleep disorder, and sleep onset association disorder (Ferber, 1985). Detailed behavioral sleep medicine treatments have been described for nocturnal enuresis including the "bell and pad" technique (Houts, Liebert, & Padawer, 1983) and for bedtime refusal problems including extinction procedures (Adams & Rickert, 1989; France & Hudson, 1990).

ADHERENCE TO MEDICAL TREATMENT

Evidence is accumulating that shows the effectiveness of behavioral treatments in treating medical adherence issues with sleep disorders. For example, continuous positive airway pressure treatment (CPAP) for sleep apnea is cumbersome and can be a difficult treatment to adjust to and use over the long term. Modifiable factors associated with adherence include perceived self-efficacy, social support, and education. Self-efficacy refers to the belief that an individual can engage in the desired behavior or perform the desired task. Cognitive-behavioral treatments focusing on perceived self-efficacy, social support, and education can increase adherence rates modestly. Patients who have phobic or anxious reactions to using CPAP are appropriate candidates for systematic desensitization procedures. Systematic desensitization is an effective cognitive-behavioral treatment that attempts to substitute an anxious response with a pleasurable response.

CONCLUSIONS

1. Sleep disorders are common, and most individuals in the United States have not discussed their sleep problem with their physician or been fully evaluated.

2. Behavioral treatments for sleep disorders are playing an increasingly important role in sleep disorders centers.

3. Comparative data suggest that CBT is associated with effects equal to that of pharmacotherapy in the short term, and greater, longer-lasting benefits than pharmacotherapy in the long term. Motivated, adherent patients are important to achieving these treatment gains.

—Carl J. Stepnowsky Jr.

Further Reading

Adams, L. A., & Rickert, V. I. (1989). Reducing bedtime tantrums: Comparison between positive routines and graduated extinction. *Pediatrics, 84,* 756-761.

American Sleep Disorders Association. (1997). *International Classification of Sleep Disorders, revised: Diagnostic and coding manual.* Rochester, MN: Author.

Ferber, R. (1985). *Solve your children's sleep problems.* New York: Simon & Schuster.

France, K. G., & Hudson, S. M. (1990). Behavior management of infant sleep disturbance. *Journal of Applied Behavior Analysis, 23,* 91-98.

Houts, A. C., Liebert, R. M., & Padawer, W. (1983). A delivery system for the treatment of primary enuresis. *Journal of Abnormal Child Psychology, 11,* 513-519.

Morin, C. M., Culbert, J. P., & Schwartz, S. M. (1994). Nonpharmacological interventions for insomnia: A meta-analysis of treatment efficacy. *American Journal of Psychiatry, 151,* 1172-1180.

Mullington, J., & Broughton, R. (1993). Scheduled naps in the management of daytime sleepiness in narcolepsy-cataplexy. *Sleep, 16,* 444-456.

Murtagh, D. R., & Greenwood, K. M. (1995). Identifying effective psychological treatments for insomnia: A meta-analysis. *Journal of Consulting and Clinical Psychology, 63,* 79-89.

National Sleep Foundation. (2002). *Sleep in America poll.* Washington, DC: Author.

Smith, M. T., Perlis, M. L., Park, A., Smith, M. S., Pennington, J., Giles, D. E., & Buysse, D. J. (2002). Comparative meta-analysis of pharmacotherapy and behavior therapy for persistent insomnia. *American Journal of Psychiatry, 159,* 5-11.

Spielman, A. J., Caruso, L. S., & Glovinsky, P. B. (1987). A behavioral perspective on insomnia treatment. *Psychiatric Clinics of North America, 10,* 541-553.

Stepanski, E. J., & Perlis, M. L. (2000). Behavioral sleep medicine: An emerging subspecialty in health psychology and sleep medicine. *Journal of Psychosomatic Research, 49,* 343-347.

SMOKING AND HEALTH

People smoke in order to obtain a "hit" with nicotine. The reward from smoking occurs when nicotine, absorbed into the general circulation from the lungs, meets nicotine receptors in the brain. Smoking tobacco in the form of cigarettes provides a very efficient drug delivery system for nicotine. The problem is that more than 4,000 other compounds enter body tissues, many of them extremely toxic. Smoking is the most common cause of preventable death worldwide. In developed countries where the smoking epidemic took hold early, roughly a quarter of male deaths and about 7% of female deaths are due to smoking (Peto, Lopez, Boreham, Thun, & Heath, 1994). Elsewhere information on tobacco and health is less reliable, but it is estimated that there are currently around 4 million deaths a year worldwide due to smoking.

As the effects of growing numbers of smokers in countries such as China become apparent, attributable deaths are bound to rise, perhaps as high as 10 million a year by the middle of the 21st century. But we know the problem is preventable. Smoking and diseases due to smoking are both waning in many countries. For example, tobacco consumption per head of population has been halved in the past 25 years in New Zealand. From its peak in the 1960s, the smoking death rate has fallen by almost 50% in middle-aged men in the United Kingdom.

This entry describes patterns of smoking worldwide, summarizes the ways in which smoking causes ill health, and reviews what is known about interventions to prevent tobacco-induced diseases and premature deaths.

WHO SMOKES?

Cigarettes are by far the most common form of smoked tobacco worldwide, although in some regions hand-rolled cigarettes, bidis, cigars, and pipes are also popular. Roughly a billion people are regular smokers (about 30% of the world adult population). Men are more likely to smoke than women although recent surveys in some countries show that smoking by young women and girls is rapidly becoming more common. With relatively few exceptions, the addiction to nicotine begins in adolescence and most current adult smokers were regular smokers by their 18th birthday. Otherwise, the pattern varies widely. For example, among men, there is more than a twofold difference in smoking prevalence between sub-Saharan Africa, the region with the lowest prevalence, and East Asia, with the highest. Smoking among women is still uncommon in South Asia (about 1-4%) although increasing, but prevalence is over 20% in Latin America and the Caribbean.

In most high-income countries, smoking is becoming less common, chiefly due to an increasing number of smokers successfully quitting. In low-income countries, prevalence ratios are still rising, especially among men. Differences in smoking prevalence are apparent within most countries by socioeconomic status and ethnicity. The most common pattern is higher smoking prevalence in less advantaged social groups. However, this is not universal—in some parts of the world, particularly where the rise in smoking prevalence is relatively recent, the social gradient in smoking is either flat or indicates that more advantaged groups are trend-setters. Over and above socioeconomic differences, higher smoking levels are commonly observed among minority ethnic groups.

HOW DOES SMOKING AFFECT HEALTH?

Early reports on the health risks of smoking, in Germany before 1940 and subsequently in the United Kingdom and the United States, concentrated on lung cancer. This caught the attention of researchers because it is an uncommon condition in nonsmoking populations, with a distinctive and severe clinical presentation. The increased risk due to smoking depends on amount smoked, pattern of smoking (inhaling or not), and duration of smoking. It is not clear whether the risk for women differs from that for men, for the same smoking history. Cigarette composition very likely affects the risk of cancer and other health problems, but the details are not fully understood. However, because of increased or "compensatory" smoking, users of low-tar and low-nicotine cigarettes are probably not at an appreciably lower risk of cancer or other problems such as heart and lung disease.

Since the first reports on lung cancer, the list of conditions associated with smoking has increased considerably. The only cancers known to occur less commonly in smokers are endometrial cancer (in postmenopausal women) and possibly, thyroid cancer. These effects may be due to the antiestrogenic actions of smoke constituents. Otherwise, there is strong evidence of cancers caused by smoking ranging from cancer of the mouth, larynx, and esophagus to cancers of the large bowel, kidney, and bladder.

Smoking is associated also with more than 20 non-malignant diseases and health problems. In high-income countries, more deaths result from vascular diseases caused by smoking than all cancers combined. The increased risk for a smoker is relatively less than for lung cancer because other causes of heart disease (such as high blood pressure and cholesterol) are widespread. But heart disease and stroke are the predominant causes of death in many parts of the world, so they contribute the bulk of smoking deaths. The mechanisms by which smoking affects vascular disease are being gradually unraveled, and it appears they include both "early" effects on the lining of blood vessels and relatively "late" effects on clotting and platelet function.

Smoking damages the reproductive system of both males and females. In men, low sperm counts, damaged sperm, and impotence are common findings. In women, there are increased risks of delay in conceiving, permanent infertility, and increased incidence of cervical cancer. There is a risk of more frequent preterm delivery if mothers smoke during pregnancy, and a higher proportion of low birth weight babies. Infants of smoking mothers have a worse health experience and more admissions to hospital during the first year of life. Smoking increases substantially the risk of heart and vascular disease associated with oral contraceptive use, and among older women, is associated with low bone density and hip fracture.

Passive smoking, breathing in other people's smoke (second-hand smoke), has long been regarded as a source of annoyance, but was first identified as a hazard to health in the 1972 Office of the Surgeon General's report. Very strong harmful effects are found in children, who are more than twice as likely to suffer chest infections and other serious respiratory problems if their parents smoke. Adult nonsmokers exposed to smoke in the home or at work also have a much increased risk of bronchitic symptoms (such as cough, phlegm, and wheeze), illness episodes with time off work, and increased health care costs. Nonsmoking adults with second-hand smoke exposures are more likely to develop lung cancer and coronary heart disease. For any individual, the risks associated with passive smoking are of course less than those due to active smoking, but large numbers of nonsmokers are exposed, resulting in a large burden of illness. The fact that the exposure is involuntary has given the health effects of passive smoking particular prominence in tobacco control.

Despite the wealth of studies on the topic, there remain important unanswered questions about the effects of smoking on health. Further work is needed on how the findings in countries such as the United States and the United Kingdom can be extrapolated to settings with quite different social and health profiles. Recent studies in low-income countries have shown that smoking tends to amplify their common causes of death, such as chronic lung disease and tuberculosis in China and India. As the epidemic progresses, however, cancers and heart disease will also become important in developing countries.

Ways in which smoking interacts with other risk factors are not well understood but are important in understanding the present distribution of disease and projecting future trends. For example, lower heart disease rates in heavy-smoking Asian populations compared to the West have raised the question of whether dietary factors may modify some of the effects of smoking. There is a great deal of interest also in the question of genetic susceptibility, focusing particularly on variants in the genes responsible for activating and detoxifying chemical carcinogens found in cigarette smoke. Some studies suggest that some genetic variations do increase susceptibility to the effects of active and passive smoking. However, the work is in its early stages.

HOW DO WE REDUCE THE DAMAGE CAUSED BY SMOKING?

Just as malaria prevention depends on control of the mosquito as the disease vector, so the prevention of smoking-related conditions depends on curbing the activities of the tobacco industry, principally the recruitment of young people of all ages to nicotine addiction. This is a formidable task. The tobacco industry spends many times the public health budgets of most countries to attract adolescents and young adults to use its products. In 1998, for instance, in the United States alone, the industry spent $18 million a day marketing cigarettes. The efforts of the industry extend beyond public advertising. Court action by states' attorneys general in the United States in the 1990s aimed to recover Medicaid expenditures. It also made public millions of previously confidential industry documents, and these describe in detail ways in which the industry has sought to undermine research and obstruct health policies that threaten its commercial interests (Glantz, Slade, Bero, Hanauer, & Barnes, 1996). Unless these activities of industry are countered, efforts to prevent disease will very likely have limited success. Restrictions on advertising, sponsorship, and other forms of industry promotion make up the first step toward a comprehensive tobacco control program.

Educational interventions to discourage new smokers include face-to-face programs (such as those included in school curricula) and mass media activities. Both kinds of activity have been shown to reduce uptake, especially if part of a wide-based and sustained program that engages parents and communities. But the effect is generally short term, which is not surprising since educational activities of this kind generally operate in the face of environmental factors that are powerful promoters of smoking. Pervasive advertising and sponsorship, exemplified by strategic product placement in popular films, shape young people's understanding of tobacco and their attitudes toward the use of tobacco products.

Another consideration is the availability of tobacco products. Measures known to reduce the supply to minors include setting a minimum age for purchase of cigarettes, licensing and training vendors, restricting locations of vending machines, and ensuring there is visible enforcement of such legislation. Comprehensive and enforceable legislation is an essential component of tobacco control.

Clinical interventions to increase smoking cessation include simple advice to quit, intensive education and counseling, and treatment of nicotine addiction with different types of nicotine replacement therapy. On its own, advice has a small effect, but may reach a large number of smokers, especially when provided by family doctors or other health professionals who have contact with a large proportion of the population. Among all preventive activities in medical practice (including screening for cancers and treatment of high blood pressure), smoking cessation is the most cost-effective. Intensive educational interventions increase the quit rate but reach many fewer smokers. Treatment of nicotine addiction also improves outcomes, especially when combined with counseling, though at increased cost, including possible side effects.

It is unclear whether the redesign of cigarettes to create "safer" products has much to offer disease prevention. In the past, low-tar and low-nicotine cigarettes were promoted as safer alternatives, but there is no evidence to support these claims. Little is known about the health effects of the many additives introduced into cigarettes to improve taste and combustion properties and absorption of nicotine. On the basis of the consumers' right to know what they are purchasing, there are strong grounds for requiring full disclosure of contents and toxicity of all the constituents of cigarettes. It is telling that tobacco is not covered by legislation concerned with safety of food, drugs, and other potentially hazardous substances—an anomaly that may be due in part to the long history of tobacco use, but is largely a consequence of sustained political pressure from the industry.

Restrictions on smoking in workplaces and in public settings reduce the exposure of nonsmokers to second-hand smoke. Studies have shown that these restrictions also cut the consumption of tobacco by smokers and increase cessation rates. Smoke-free environments have achieved wide acceptance, among smokers as well as nonsmokers, in many countries including the United States, Australia, and New Zealand. Exposure to second-hand smoke in the home, the major hazard for the most vulnerable group, children, is less susceptible to control by regulation.

Price has a strong influence on demand for tobacco products, especially among adolescents and young adults. Consequently, taxation is regarded as an important component of tobacco control. Sources of contention include effects on equity (since the tax affects mostly heavy-smoking, low-income groups) and over whether tax revenue matches the public costs of tobacco use. Revenue replacement, not necessarily the most important reason for taxing tobacco, depends on how ill health due to smoking is costed. However, the World Bank estimates that there is a large net loss from tobacco use worldwide.

CONCLUSIONS

The challenge is twofold: first, to reduce the frequency of tobacco-induced diseases in the population overall, and second, to reduce inequalities in ill health caused by tobacco. The two goals may require different strategies, since whole-population interventions do not always work well for subgroups. For example, if smoking cessation programs are provided solely through mainstream health services, this is likely to disadvantage minority groups that find it difficult to access these services for cultural, economic, or social reasons. Similar arguments apply to tobacco control at an international level: The goal ideally is to reduce consumption without increasing disparities between countries. Greatest savings in the medium term will be achieved by increasing quit rates while benefits of reducing initiation to nicotine addiction will not become apparent until the second half of this century.

Comprehensive tobacco control programs offer the greatest potential for reducing smoking and preventing disease, due to the combined effects of education, regulation, economic incentives, and support for cessation. A good fit with the local context is key to the successful implementation of health promotion, but at the same time the most powerful forces promoting tobacco use are transnational companies. This means that tobacco control must include a mix of local and international activity. An international focus is particularly important since almost 90% of the increase in tobacco-attributable deaths between 1990 and 2020 will occur in low-income countries.

A global strategy for the prevention of the tobacco epidemic is now in progress under the World Health Organization's Framework Convention for Tobacco Control (FCTC). It has the tacit support of the 194 member countries of the World Health Assembly, but within this group there are many vested interests that seek to water down or derail the process.

—*Alistair Woodward and
Anthony Hedley*

See also CANCER AND SMOKING; HEART DISEASE AND SMOKING; SMOKING AND NICOTINE DEPENDENCE; SMOKING AND NICOTINE DEPENDENCE: INTERVENTIONS

Further Reading

Doll, R., Peto, R., Wheatley, K., Gray, R., & Sutherland, I. (1994). Mortality in relation to smoking: 40 years observations on male British doctors. *BMJ, 309,* 901-911.

Glantz, S. A., Slade, J., Bero, L. A., Hanauer, P., & Barnes, D. E. (1996). *The cigarette papers.* Berkeley: University of California Press.

Mackay, J., & Eriksen, M. (2002). *The tobacco atlas.* Geneva: World Health Organization.

Peto, R., Lopez, A. D., Boreham, J., Thun, M., & Heath, C. (1994). *Mortality from smoking in developed countries, 1950-2000: Indirect estimates from national vital statistics.* Oxford, UK: Oxford University Press.

World Health Organization. (1997). *Tobacco or health: A global status report.* Geneva: Author.

SMOKING AND NICOTINE DEPENDENCE

Cigarette smoking is now well accepted as the leading cause of preventable death in the United States. The latest statistics reveal that about 3 million smokers worldwide die annually from smoking and that the rapid increase in smoking in developing countries will cause this annual toll to rise to about 10 million by the year 2030. Several hundred million adults who are current smokers are expected to die from smoking, most often from chronic diseases of the heart and lungs. And one in five deaths in the United States is smoking related. Even among nonsmokers, exposure to secondhand smoke causes an estimated 3,000 deaths per year. Although the harmful health effects from smoking are widely known, only an estimated 3% of smokers successfully quit each year, less than 10% of those who attempt smoking abstinence. Thus, the current and future public health impact of smoking warrants greater effort being paid to understanding and treating nicotine dependence.

THE CASE THAT NICOTINE IS ADDICTIVE

Much of the debate regarding why people continue smoking in spite of its negative health consequences centers around the argument of whether or not, like other drugs of abuse, nicotine is addictive. When we talk about the addictiveness of a drug, we are referring to the ability of that substance to produce dependence. This is also termed *abuse liability*. No single task can accurately determine the addictiveness of a drug; rather, it is a preponderance of evidence across various criteria that leads to conclusions regarding a drug's abuse liability. Therefore, we consider three hallmark criteria for determining a drug's addictiveness as they apply to nicotine: (1) self-administration, (2) persistent inability to quit, including continued use despite known harmful consequences, and (3) concordance of use patterns between nicotine and "classic" drugs of abuse.

Self-administration is defined as the extent to which a drug is consumed more frequently than "placebo," or a concurrently available and similar substance that does not contain a drug. In a series of studies that dramatically increased attention on the influence of nicotine, researchers demonstrated that smokers would respond more on a choice lever to receive intravenous infusions if the infusions contained nicotine than if they contained only saline. Past studies have also shown that manipulating the amount of nicotine in cigarettes generally produces alterations in smoking behavior that appear intended to maintain a certain amount of nicotine intake. For example, decreasing the amount of nicotine per cigarette tends

to produce an increase in smoking behavior. That is, people smoke more, drag harder, and so on, when availability of nicotine is reduced in their cigarettes. However, increasing nicotine availability per cigarette decreases smoking behavior. This demonstrates that smokers self-regulate the amount of nicotine they ingest, not necessarily the number of cigarettes they smoke or puffs they take. Further evidence, albeit indirect, of the importance of nicotine in maintaining smoking behavior comes from the failure of nonnicotine cigarette brands to be successful in the marketplace. This fact mirrors the interesting experimental observation that complete removal of nicotine from cigarettes results in "extinction," or a nearly complete cessation of smoking behavior, in nonhuman primates trained to smoke tobacco.

Self-administration of nicotine from cigarettes is so persistent that smokers continue to smoke despite its known harm. Statistics illustrating the harmful effects of smoking and its links to various diseases are readily available. Indeed, since 1965 the Office of the Surgeon General has required that all cigarette packages contain a warning about the negative health consequences that may result from smoking. Regardless, 25% of all Americans continue to smoke, down only moderately from a prevalence of about 40% in 1965. However, perhaps even more compelling as evidence that smokers continue to smoke in spite of known negative consequences are the findings from past research demonstrating that 49% of women with a diagnosis or recurrence of lung cancer return to daily smoking, similar to the 50% of smokers who relapse following surgery for lung cancer. Clearly, even those who are undeniably aware of the negative consequences of smoking and have the most salient health reasons to quit continue to smoke.

Finally, how does nicotine compare with other self-administered drugs of abuse? Although nicotine use is in some ways very different from other drugs, epidemiological research has shown that the proportion of "ever users" of a drug who subsequently become dependent on that drug is greater for nicotine (32%) than for any other, including alcohol, heroin, or cocaine (15%, 23%, and 17% respectively). Furthermore, many if not most users of alcohol, marijuana, and other drugs are "casual users," able to consume these drugs infrequently or in moderation, and often able to stop their use with little difficulty. On the other hand, "nondependent" use of cigarettes characterizes fewer than 10% of smokers, with the vast majority of smokers meeting criteria for nicotine dependence and unable to stop its use. With regard to cessation rates, the likelihood and time course of relapse back to smoking after quitting appear very similar to relapse back to alcohol, heroin, or other drug use after treatment. At least 80% of all smokers either have tried to quit or have not tried but want to quit, yet fewer than 10% will be successful in any given year. Even with intensive behavioral counseling, pharmacological assistance, or both, success rates for smoking treatment programs rarely exceed 30%. This means that more than two thirds of those trying to quit smoking fail even with substantial professional assistance.

Considering the preponderance of evidence, nicotine easily meets the hallmark criteria for determining drug addictiveness. Clearly, individuals self-administer nicotine more frequently than nondrug substances, they continue to smoke even in the face of known health consequences, and the persistence of use and difficulty quitting is at least as great with smoking as with other drugs of abuse.

NOVEL MEANS OF DELIVERING NICOTINE

When one accepts that nicotine is addictive, the seemingly contradictory notion arises that if nicotine is addictive, why are people addicted to cigarettes but not nicotine-containing products like the patch or gum? The answer to this question lies in the speed with which cigarettes, versus patch or gum, deliver nicotine to the brain. Smoking a cigarette delivers nicotine to the brain within 20 seconds, as rapidly as intravenous infusion. This quick uptake of nicotine following a puff is key to the reinforcing effects of cigarette smoking. On the other hand, therapeutic forms of nicotine, such as the patch and gum, generally deliver nicotine to the brain within several minutes or hours. These methods of nicotine delivery fail to be addictive, mainly because of the slow speed with which they deliver nicotine to the brain, which renders the drug less reinforcing.

EFFECTS OF NICOTINE

Having determined that people readily self-administer nicotine, have trouble keeping their use at low levels, and repeatedly fail in attempting to quit, the next question of course is, Why? Nicotine has a number of relatively modest, acute behavioral and subjective effects, depending, not surprisingly, on dose and speed of uptake. Generally speaking, human research has shown that nicotine often increases subjective measures associated with drug "liking," "head rush," and "euphoria." However, it is important to reiterate that these effects are generally observed only with nicotine delivery systems producing rapid uptake of nicotine into the brain, like cigarettes, intravenous infusion, and nasal spray, and that the same doses delivered by slower means, like patch or gum, produce minimal or even aversive effects. These subjective effects of nicotine likely stem from the influence of nicotine on increasing brain levels of dopamine, norepinephrine, and acetylcholine, among other neurochemicals associated with pleasure systems in the brain.

While positively reinforcing effects of nicotine, such as acute responses, may help explain why people get started smoking in the first place, nicotine also provides negatively reinforcing effects in more experienced smokers that may explain its remarkable persistence, as noted previously. Following brief abstinence from smoking (e.g., overnight), most regular smokers experience characteristic tobacco withdrawal signs and symptoms, including restlessness, dysphoria, fatigue, difficulty concentrating, tension, impaired psychomotor function, jitteriness, irritable mood, and cough. Nicotine intake via smoking, and to a lesser extent by nicotine replacement products, reverses this withdrawal, thereby providing additional reinforcement to continue smoking. This negative reinforcement, coupled with the positively reinforcing effects of nicotine, provides some understanding of the strong persistence of tobacco smoking.

CONTRIBUTIONS OF CUES TO SMOKING REINFORCEMENT

Although the negative reinforcing properties of nicotine withdrawal might play a key role in the continuation of smoking behavior, past research has demonstrated that withdrawal from nicotine does not appear to be the sole cause of many smokers' inability to quit or their continuation of use. This seems particularly true when one considers that most smokers who achieve prolonged abstinence (> 1 month), beyond the time when withdrawal has abated, return to smoking.

Several theories purport that learning, or conditioning, might be one of the alternative factors responsible for both the perpetuation of smoking behavior and the initiation of relapse. That is, aside from the effects of nicotine per se, environmental events commonly paired with nicotine intake can become cues able to strongly influence nicotine or smoking self-administration in animals and humans. Indeed, there is a wealth of research demonstrating that smokers react to cues linked with past smoking behavior. Take, for example, a smoker's daily smoke break at work as a cue. A smoker might learn to associate break time, the environment where it takes place, and, undoubtedly, his or her cigarettes with smoking (classical conditioning), or learn that smoking offers a much needed reprieve from hard work (operant conditioning). Through repeated pairing of one's break time with smoking, exposure to this cue/environment alone leads to strong reactivity such as subjective craving, physiological changes, and drug-seeking behavior. This conditioning holds fast, so that even long after the smoker has quit, these cues might serve to motivate smoking behavior.

INDIVIDUAL DIFFERENCES

The risk of becoming a smoker and the difficultly in quitting might also be linked to individual differences, particularly related to comorbid psychiatric diagnoses. Nicotine dependence rates are exceptionally high among individuals diagnosed with such illnesses as depression, schizophrenia, and alcoholism. This finding has led to contemporary research examining the mechanisms that might be associated with elevated levels of dependence among clinical populations. These studies examine the possibility that nicotine may serve additional "palliative" functions in these populations, over and above the dependence-producing effects noted previously. For example, nicotine may help alleviate negative mood or focus attention, functions that may be very reinforcing in those with depression or impulsive disorders. Moreover, genetic research has shown that nicotine dependence is highly heritable (inherited), to about the same degree as alcoholism. Thus, specific genetic factors may influence the degree to which nicotine intake is reinforcing in individuals, affecting the likelihood of subsequent onset of dependence and/or inability to quit. In addition, considerable research continues to examine variations in nicotine response as a function of personality traits, sex, family history, and combined abuse of other substances. Overall, these associations are leading researchers toward a clearer understanding of the underlying mechanisms of nicotine dependence and use, as well as the role individual differences might play in these processes.

IMPLICATIONS FOR TREATMENT

Contemporary approaches to treating nicotine addiction have largely taken advantage of advances in pharmacotherapy, or medication approaches to treatment. The most popular of these is nicotine replacement therapy (NRT). NRTs, such as the patch and gum, were designed to maintain individual nicotine levels through nonaddictive, less harmful means of drug administration. The premise of this treatment centered around the belief that not having to contend with strong physiological withdrawal while attempting to refrain from smoking cigarettes would make quitting much easier. During NRT, ex-smokers are stepped down gradually, reducing nicotine intake over several weeks rather than all at once, as is the case with going cold turkey. Presumably, this method eliminates acute withdrawal, which makes giving up nicotine and smoking more bearable.

Although this pharmacological approach to treatment has aided many smokers in quitting, it has failed to be the panacea of smoking cessation. The most common reason NRTs fail is that they have little or no impact on reducing smokers' reactivity to salient drug cues. As introduced earlier, smokers' reactivity to cues associated with past smoking can serve to initiate lapse or even relapse to smoking following abstinence. A second, often overlooked, reason NRT fails is that smokers get incomplete or erroneous instructions on how to use such products. Without proper instructing, either because of a failure to read instructions and follow them correctly, or negligence on the part of care workers to offer it, smokers often misuse NRTs, leading to underdosing and/or inflated expectations about the benefits of NRTs. Last, studies have shown that NRTs and counseling (e.g., cognitive-behavioral approaches) are equally effective in increasing smoking cessation rates. However, treatments incorporating both techniques are significantly more effective than either alone. Therefore, it is clear that consideration of both the physiological and psychological components of nicotine addiction must be addressed within treatment for cessation attempts to be most successful.

SUMMARY

Over the past 20 years, scientific studies have clearly established the link between smoking and negative health consequences, as well as the addictive nature of nicotine. Here we have reviewed the hallmark criteria by which the abuse liability of all drugs are evaluated, and demonstrated why nicotine can be classified as an addictive substance. We have also made the case that nicotine addiction can be best understood through consideration of not only its physiological properties but in light of individual differences and the influence of conditioned cues as well. Past research has demonstrated that each of these factors might play a key role in the continuation of smoking as well as the inability of many smokers to quit. In fact, treatments that address both physiological and psychological factors have been shown to be most effective in helping smokers quit, thus further supporting the importance of adopting this joint approach in both understanding and treating nicotine addiction.

—*Cynthia A. Conklin and*
Kenneth A. Perkins

See also HEART DISEASE AND SMOKING; SMOKING AND HEALTH; SMOKING AND NICOTINE DEPENDENCE: INTERVENTIONS

Further Reading

Conklin, C. A., & Tiffany, S. T. (2002). Applying extinction research and theory to cue-exposure addiction treatments. *Addiction, 97,* 155-167.

Perkins, K. A. (1999). Nicotine self-administration. *Nicotine and Tobacco Research, 1,* S133-S137.

Stolerman, J. P., & Jarvis, M. J. (1995). The scientific case that nicotine is addictive. *Psychopharmacology, 117,* 2-10.

SMOKING AND NICOTINE DEPENDENCE: INTERVENTIONS

Cigarette smoking is the leading preventable cause of illness, death, and disability in the United States, causing more than 430,000 deaths in the United States each year. Despite the enormous health consequences associated with smoking, 48 million adult Americans continue to smoke cigarettes (Centers for Disease Control and Prevention [CDC], 1999).

Nicotine, the psychoactive substance in tobacco, is a highly addictive substance that may control significant aspects of a person's behavior. It shares a number of common factors with the other recognized euphoriants (i.e., cocaine, opiates, alcohol), producing effects on mood and feeling states, acting as a reinforcer for animals, leading to drug-seeking behavior with deprivation, and showing similar patterns of persistence in the face of evidence that it is highly damaging to health (Fagerstrom, 1991). As with other addicting substances, individual variability in the intensity of the dependence is wide, and although a large number of smokers successfully quit on their own, many others can benefit from a variety of available interventions ranging from self-help to brief counseling to intensive treatment.

Following is a description of an approach to determining readiness for quitting, current treatment strategies available to the smoker and clinician for assisting the smoker to stop, and special problem areas in smoking treatment that need to be addressed. The approaches are based on the evidence-based Agency for Healthcare Research and Quality (AHRQ) *Treating Tobacco Use and Dependence* guideline (Fiore et al., 2000) and the "American Psychiatric Association Practice Guideline for the Treatment of Patients With Nicotine Dependence" (Hughes, Fiester, Goldstein, Resnick, Rock, & Ziedonis, 1996). Also discussed is the nicotine-dependent patient who presents with special clinical problems, such as the patient with alcoholism or serious psychiatric problems, in particular depression.

ASSESSING MOTIVATION AND READINESS TO QUIT

Nicotine dependence is a chronic, relapsing disorder, often requiring five to seven attempts before maintained abstinence is achieved. Stopping smoking is therefore a long-term process of change that takes place in stages over time. Individuals typically proceed through the following stages of change: (1) precontemplation, (2) contemplation, (3) preparation, (4) action, and (5) maintenance (DiClemente et al., 1991). Different stages of change require different degrees of help and interventions on the part of the clinician.

Approximately 40% of smokers are not thinking about stopping smoking and are said to be in the *precontemplation* stage of change (Velicer et al., 1995). These smokers may be unaware of the risks of smoking, unwilling to consider making a change, or discouraged regarding their ability to quit. Many psychiatric patients fall into this stage of change. For the precontemplator, the clinician's goal is to raise doubt in the person's mind about whether he or she wants to continue smoking by increasing the patient's perception of the risks and problems associated with his or her current behavior and the potential benefits of quitting. Another 40% of smokers express ambivalence regarding stopping smoking. These smokers are in the *contemplation* stage of change. They report thinking about quitting and seek information about smoking and stopping, but are not ready to commit to quit and express uncertainty regarding their desire or ability to stop.

The final 20% of current smokers are ready to stop smoking in the next month and are in the *preparation* stage of change. Many of these individuals have made a serious quit attempt in the past year or have taken steps toward stopping, such as telling others of their intent to quit, cutting down on the number of cigarettes smoked, or imagining themselves as nonsmokers. The clinician's goal with the smoker in the preparation stage is to help the individual determine the best course of action to take and develop the strategies and skills needed to make a successful quit attempt. Individuals in the *action* and *maintenance* stages of change are no longer smoking. Particularly in the action stage they are at risk for relapse and the best approach with them is to work on relapse prevention.

MODES OF INTERVENTION DELIVERY

Smoking interventions can be delivered through a variety of modalities, as reflected in the *Best Practices for Comprehensive Tobacco Control Programs* document produced by the CDC (1999). The CDC recommends identification, advice, and provision of brief counseling to smokers within the course of routine care, as well as making available to the smoker a full range of self-help materials, cessation aids, and services including pharmacological aids, behavioral counseling (group and individual), and follow-up visits. Since only a small minority of even motivated smokers will attend intensive treatment programs, self-help interventions have increased in popularity over the past several years. Self-help includes the use of booklets and manuals, audiotapes, videos, Internet, or hotlines or seeking the help of friends, colleagues, or family.

The value of brief counseling has been demonstrated, particularly when accompanied by the use of pharmacological aids such as nicotine replacement therapy (NRT) or bupropion, and when some type of follow-up occurs, either in person or by telephone

(Fiore et al., 2000). Clinicians conducting brief counseling can supplement their intervention with a wide range of self-help materials and audiotapes now available. A stepped-care approach can be used in which, for example, less dependent smokers or smokers who are ready for action may benefit from brief counseling while a more dependent smoker or one who needs more intensive help can be referred to a smoking treatment specialist or a treatment group.

Intensive treatment programs are available mostly in outpatient settings, through telephone counseling, and through the few inpatient treatment programs that exist. For more intensive individual or group treatment, weekly contact for approximately 4 weeks and then biweekly contact for another 4 weeks is a reasonable frequency and one that provides the tapering of contact necessary for the patient to internalize control. For the more dependent smoker or one who has other psychiatric problems, a longer and more intensive intervention may be necessary.

Smokers who are ready to make a quit attempt can be helped by clinicians who provide assistance ranging from very brief (5 minutes) to very intensive interventions. At any intensity, developing a quit plan and arranging follow-up to support the individual through the quitting process are recommended. In an individual treatment plan, the physiological, psychological, and social aspects of the patient's dependence need to be taken into consideration. The treatment plan should include the evidence-based strategies identified by the AHRQ clinical practice guideline (Fiore et al., 2000) and summarized in Table 1.

Professional Treatment

Addressing Physiological Dependence

Nicotine replacement therapy and bupropion are effective treatments for nicotine dependence and can be used by smokers who are interested in quitting, unless contraindicated. The Fagerstrom Test for Nicotine Dependence (FTND) is an excellent tool for assessing level of dependence. If a smoker reports having had significant withdrawal symptoms during prior quit attempts, has a pattern of relapsing within a few hours or days, and scores high on the FTND, nicotine dependence probably plays an important role in maintaining his or her smoking behavior. For all smokers, and especially highly dependent persons, nicotine fading, nicotine replacement therapy, or nonnicotine medication (bupropion) could be used.

Table 1   Strategies for Assisting Smokers Who Are Ready to Quit

Action	*Strategies for Implementation*
1. Help the patient develop a quit plan	*Set a quit date*, preferably within the next week.
	Tell family, friends, and coworkers of intent to quit and request understanding and support.
	Anticipate challenges to planned quit attempt, particularly during the critical first few weeks, including nicotine withdrawal symptoms, and prepare to address them.
	Remove cigarettes from environment.
2. Provide practical counseling (problem solving/skills training)	*Abstinence:* Total abstinence is essential. "Not even a single puff after the quit date."
	Past quit experience: Review to identify high-risk situations and what helped and hurt.
	Anticipate triggers or challenges: Discuss challenges/triggers and how patient will successfully address them.
	Alcohol: Consider limiting or abstaining from alcohol during the quitting process as alcohol is highly associated with relapse.
	Other smokers in the household: Encourage patient to quit with housemates or ask that they not smoke in their presence.
3. Provide intratreatment social support	Provide a *supportive clinical environment* while encouraging the patient in his or her quit attempt, clearly stating the clinic staff's availability to assist the patient.
4. Help patient obtain extratreatment social support	Encourage the patient to *ask spouse/partner, friends, and coworkers to support* his or her quit attempt.
5. Recommend the use of pharmacotherapy, unless contraindicated	Recommend the use of *nicotine replacement therapy or nonnicotine pill, bupropion* (see section on pharmacotherapy).
6. Provide supplementary materials	Provide patient with *self-help materials* appropriate to his or her age, culture, race, and educational level.
7. Schedule follow-up contact, either in person or via telephone	*Follow-up* should occur within the first week after the quit date.
	If abstinent at follow-up, congratulate success, address problems encountered and challenges anticipated, and monitor pharmacological aids used.
	If smoking occurred, review circumstances leading to smoking, elicit recommitment to total abstinence, address problems encountered and challenges anticipated, review pharmacological aid use and problems, and consider referral to more intensive, specialized treatment.

SOURCE: Adapted from Fiore et al. (2000). This document is in the public domain and may be used without special permission.

Nicotine Fading

Nicotine fading (Foxx & Brown, 1979) has two components: brand switching to a lower-nicotine-level cigarette and gradual reduction of number of cigarettes smoked. Switching to brands with lower nicotine levels one or more times over several weeks, in combination with reducing the number of cigarettes smoked by about one half per week, can reduce withdrawal symptoms in the person who smokes heavily. However, the evidence does not support brand switching alone. In fact, if smokers use compensation techniques such as vent blocking, puffing more frequently, or inhaling more deeply when smoking lower-nicotine cigarettes, their nicotine yield will be considerably higher than that suggested by the Federal Trade Commission ratings. Smokers should be cautioned about this possibility and advised to keep such compensation behaviors to a minimum during the nicotine fading process. On the other hand, unlike the myth that a smoker needs to quit "cold turkey," there does not appear to be a significant difference in cessation rates between quitting cold turkey compared to gradually reducing the number of cigarettes smoked

(Fiore et al., 2000): therefore, patient preference should determine the approach selected. If nicotine fading is used, it should be combined with behavioral management strategies such that "lower need" cigarettes are eliminated first and awareness of the function of each cigarette is increased.

Pharmacotherapy

Five pharmacological aids have been approved by the Food and Drug Administration for use in the treatment of nicotine dependence. These pharmacotherapies fall into two general categories: nicotine replacement therapies and a nonnicotine pill (bupropion). It is important to emphasize to smokers that pharmacotherapies are not "magic bullets." Rather, they are used to help minimize or dampen withdrawal symptoms while smokers work to break the conditioned connections between smoking and the activities and emotions of their daily lives, and to develop coping skills to replace the many functions of smoking. Table 2 provides a summary of all five pharmacological aids currently recommended as first-line medications.

The purpose of the four nicotine replacement therapies is to prevent or minimize the symptoms of withdrawal or cravings by replacing some of the nicotine that would otherwise be obtained from smoking. This allows the individual to focus on the behavioral and emotional aspects of stopping smoking. All four forms of nicotine replacement therapy have been found to be equally efficacious, approximately doubling quit rates compared to placebo. In most studies, concomitant supportive or behavior therapy has produced substantially higher quit rates than either behavior therapy or nicotine replacement alone.

Bupropion HCl SR is an atypical antidepressant believed to work on the neurochemistry of addiction by enhancing dopamine levels and affecting the action of norepinephrine in the brain, both neurotransmitters believed to be involved in nicotine dependence (Ascher et al., 1995). As with the nicotine replacement therapies, bupropion has been found to consistently double quit rates compared to placebo.

Addressing Psychological Dependence: Cognitive and Behavioral Interventions

Cognitive and behavioral interventions for smoking have been developed from cognitive and behavioral treatment techniques used to treat a wide range of behavioral and addictive disorders and have been found to typically double quit rates compared to control groups (Fiore et al., 2000). The cognitive-behavioral approach intertwines assessment and intervention. First, past quit attempts are reviewed to identify the reasons why the quit attempts were made, what methods the smoker used (e.g., cold turkey, tapering, pharmacological aids), problems experienced (including withdrawal symptoms), strategies that helped, and what led to relapse. The key is to assist the patient in reframing past efforts to stop smoking as learning experiences and to apply what was learned to the current quit attempt. Second, current smoking patterns are assessed. In what situations and in response to what feelings or emotions does the patient most feel like smoking? These are "high need" cigarettes. Asking the smoker to rate the level of need for each cigarette smoked on a scale of 1 (*low need*) to 5 (*high need*) is often helpful. Once anticipated problems and triggers are identified through review of past quit attempts and assessment of current smoking patterns, the patient can be helped to develop specific cognitive-behavioral coping strategies to address these problems and triggers.

Preventing Relapse and Maintaining Change

A major difficulty in smoking cessation, as with other substance abuse behaviors, is maintenance of the changed behavior. As many as 70% of those who stop smoking relapse within a year, with the strongest predictor of relapse being a slip within a relatively brief period of time (average between 18 and 60 days of cessation) (Ockene et al., 2000). Up to 65% of persons who quit smoking on their own relapse within the first week after cessation (Hughes & Hatsukami, 1992). Relapse prevention includes being aware of any slip that occurs, that is, taking a puff or more of a cigarette, and catching it before it becomes a relapse. Intensive relapse prevention interventions should be delivered when an individual experiences problems in maintaining abstinence, tailored to the specific problems encountered.

SPECIAL PROBLEM AREAS

Smoking Cessation and Weight Gain

Although the average weight gain for sustained quitters of 5-6 kilograms (Froom, Melamed, & Benbasal, 1998) does not present a medical risk equal

Table 2   First-Line Medications for Treating Nicotine Dependence

Product	Nicotine Patches[1]	Nicotine Gum[1]	Nicotine Inhaler	Nicotine Spray	Bupropion SR
Brand names	Nicotrol CQ Nicoderm Generic (various store brands)	Nicorette Generic (various store brands)	**Nicotrol Inhaler**	**Nicotrol NS**	**Zyban, Wellbutrin**[2]
Product strengths	7 mg, 14 mg, 21 mg per patch (for typical systems that deliver 17, 32, 52 mg per day of nicotine)	2 mg (for avg smokers < = 24 cigs/day) 4 mg (for heavy smokers > 24 cigs/day)	10 mg/cartridge	10 mg/ml	150 mg
Amount of nicotine delivered[3]	*16-hr patch:* 15 mg/day *24-hr patch:* 7 mg/day, 14 mg/day, 21 mg/day	Up to 0.8 mg per 2-mg piece Up to 1.5 mg per 4-mg piece	Up to 2 mg per cartridge	0.5 mg 2 sprays	N/A
Special directions for use	Apply to nonhairy part of body	Alternately chew and park for 20 minutes; nicotine absorbed through oral mucosa when gum is parked; avoid acidic beverages	Take frequent puffs over 20 minutes; nicotine absorbed through oral mucosa; avoid acidic beverages	Two sprays in each nostril	None
Dosing intervals and maximum doses	*16-hr patch:* 16 hrs on; 8 hrs off *24-hr patch:* Replace every 24 hrs (option to remove at bedtime)	1 piece every 1 to 2 hours and as needed for craving Maximum: 24 pieces per day	Multiple puffs on a cartridge every 1-2 hours or as needed 6-16 cartridges per day Maximum: 16 cartridges per day	1-2 doses/hr (1 dose = 2 sprays or 1 per nostril)	150 mg/day (days 1-3) 150/twice per day (after day 3)
Time to peak plasma level	5-10 hrs	20-30 mins	15 mins	5-7 mins	3 hrs
Manufacturer's recommended tx duration[4]	*16-mg patch:* 6 weeks *24-hr patch:* Initial: 21 mg for 4 weeks; taper: 14 mg and 7 mg for 2 weeks each	Initial: 6 weeks Taper: 6 weeks	Initial: Up to 12 weeks Taper: 12 weeks	Initial: Up to 8 weeks Taper: 4-6 weeks	7-12 weeks Maintenance: Up to 6 months
Adverse reactions (treatment of reaction)	50% experience mild irritant skin reactions (rotate and use steroid cream, rare allergic skin reaction; vivid dreams, sleep disturbances while on the patch 24 hrs (remove at bedtime)	Mouth soreness, hiccups, dyspepsia, and jaw ache (usually mild and transient; correct technique)	40% experience mouth and throat irritation (may resolve with regular use); dyspepsia	Local transient irritation in the nose and throat, watery eyes, sneezing and cough	Dry mouth; insomnia (avoid bedtime dose); shakiness

(Continued)

Table 2 (Continued)

Absolute contraindications	Previous hypersensitivity reaction to any of the products (i.e., serious allergic reaction)
	Heart attack within 6 weeks or unstable angina
	Heart attack within 6 weeks; unstable angina; serious heart arrhythmia; uncontrolled hypertension; active peptic ulcer disease for all NRT

	Severe eczema or other skin diseases that may be exacerbated by the patch	Severe TMJ disease or other jaw problems; dentures	Allergy to menthol	Active rhinitis; active sinusitis	History of seizure; current or prior dx of bulimia or anorexia nervosa; concurrent or recent use of MAO inhibitors
Relative contraindications/ precautions	Moderate or severe hepatic or renal impairment for all products				
	Active hyperthyroidism; peripheral vascular disease for all NRT				
	Hot work environment (reduced patch adhesion); mild-moderate skin disease	Any jaw problem that affects gum chewing; dental appliances affected by gum	Oral or pharyngeal inflammation	Asthma; nasal polyps	Agitation; anxiety, insomnia; history of head trauma or other risk factor for seizure
Pregnancy category[5]	D	C	D	D	B

1. Available without prescription
2. Zyban is brand name for bupropion SR marketed for smoking cessation with support materials; Wellbutrin is brand name for bupropion SR marketed for depression.
3. Typical cigarette delivers 1-3 mg of nicotine.
4. Manufacturer recommendations based on duration of treatment in initial clinical trials. Many independent trials of NRT suggest treatment for 8 weeks is as effective as longer treatments for most, but shorter and longer intervals are reasonable depending on individual smoker.
5. Pregnancy categories:

B: *No evidence of risk in humans.* Adequate, well-controlled studies in pregnant women have not shown increased risk of fetal abnormalities despite adverse findings in animals, or, in the absence of adequate human studies, animal studies show no fetal risk. The chance of fetal harm is remote, but remains a possibility.

C: *Risk cannot be ruled out.* Adequate, well-controlled human studies are lacking, and animal studies have shown a risk to the fetus or are lacking as well. There is a chance of fetal harm if the drug is administered during pregnancy; but the potential benefits may outweigh the potential risks.

D: *Positive evidence of risk.* Studies in humans, or investigational or postmarketing data, have demonstrated fetal risk. Nevertheless, potential benefits from the use of the drug may outweigh the potential risk. For example, the drug may be acceptable if needed in a life-threatening situation or serious disease for which safer drugs cannot be used or are ineffective.

to smoking a pack of cigarettes a day, weight gain is an issue that is important to many people and provides a common reason for starting, continuing, and returning to smoking. Several factors have been implicated in weight gain, including an increase in metabolism from nicotine intake (Perkins, 1992), which may cause increased weight while quitting even without increased caloric intake and change in preference for sweets while smoking. These biological factors, in combination with the use of food as a behavioral substitute, make it important to address weight gain explicitly in most treatment programs. However, to date there has been no published empirically tested treatment that successfully addresses weight gain while quitting. Dieting while quitting increases the rate of relapse (Ockene et al., 2000).

Smoking Cessation and Alcohol

Tobacco use and alcohol abuse are moderately to strongly related (Istvan & Matarazzo, 1984). Among identified alcoholic persons, the incidence of smoking has been 80% to 90% in all studies; alcoholic persons also are more likely to smoke heavily (Bien & Burge, 1990; Bobo, 1989). Consequently, most patients seen in an alcohol treatment program will be smokers, many of them at a level that is acutely health endangering, thereby underscoring the need to treat nicotine dependence in this patient population.

Data obtained from individuals in substance abuse treatment suggests that it is difficult to quit smoking while undergoing substance abuse treatment but that working on smoking cessation does not increase relapse to alcohol use (Kalman, 1998). In fact, it has been found that in some instances smoking cessation is associated with a decreased relapse back to alcohol use. The American Psychiatric Association practice guidelines for the treatment of patients with nicotine dependence (Hughes et al., 1996) recommends that the timing of smoking cessation in relationship to alcohol abuse treatment should be determined by the patient.

Smoking Cessation and Psychiatric Disorders

Increasing attention is being paid to the role of smoking in psychiatric disorders in regard both to the role of the CNS effects of nicotine and to the apparent special value of smoking to psychiatric patients (Glassman, 1993). Several studies show a much higher prevalence of smoking in psychiatric populations (i.e., 50-90%), particularly in those with depression (Covey, Glassman, & Stetner, 1998) and schizophrenia (Glassman, 1993). The evidence is less clear regarding the increased prevalence in those with anxiety disorders. Some psychiatric patients may be actively self-medicating through their use of cigarettes.

Although research is beginning to document the effects of smoking in psychiatric populations, little empirical evidence is available regarding the treatment of nicotine dependence in such patients. In the psychiatric patient for whom smoking cessation is critical for medical reasons, a comprehensive intervention plan is indicated including the treatment components outlined earlier in this entry. In particular, behavior therapy focused on the development of coping and social skills is important and adjustment of medication may be needed, either in an attempt to decrease continued dependence on self-medicating with nicotine or in response to possible interaction effects.

SUMMARY

Clear, evidence-based clinical practice guidelines are available to assist the clinician in treating nicotine dependence. As a chronic, relapsing disorder, stopping smoking requires a long-term process of change. The assessment of an individual's motivation or readiness to quit allows the clinician to tailor intervention accordingly. It is recommended that brief counseling be provided to all smokers within the context of routine care and that a full range of cessation aides and services be made available. These include self-help materials, pharmacological aids, group and individual cognitive and behavioral counseling, and follow-up. Special attention should be given to smokers who present with concerns regarding weight gain and those with alcohol and psychiatric disorders.

—*Judith K. Ockene and Lori Pbert*

See also HEART DISEASE AND SMOKING; SMOKING AND HEALTH; SMOKING AND NICOTINE DEPENDENCE; SMOKING PREVENTION AND TOBACCO CONTROL AMONG YOUTH

Further Reading

Ascher, J., Cole, J., Colin, J.-N., Feighner, J., Ferris, R., Fibiger, H., Golden, R., Martin, P., Potter, W., Richelson, E., et al. (1995). Bupropion: A review of its mechanism of antidepressant activity. *Journal of Clinical Psychiatry, 56,* 395-401.

Bien, T., & Burge, R. (1990). Smoking and drinking: A review of the literature. *International Journal of Addictions, 25*, 1429-1454.

Bobo, J. (1989). Nicotine dependence and alcoholism epidemiology and treatment. *Journal of Psychoactive Drugs, 21*(3), 323-329.

Centers for Disease Control and Prevention. (1999a, March). *Best practices for comprehensive tobacco control programs.* Atlanta, GA: U.S. Department of Health and Human Services, Centers for Disease Control and Prevention, National Center for Chronic Disease Prevention and Health Promotion, Office on Smoking and Health.

Centers for Disease Control and Prevention. (1999b). Cigarette smoking among adults—United States, 1997. *Morbidity and Mortality Weekly Report, 48*, 993-996.

Covey, L., Glassman, A., & Stetner, F. (1998). Cigarette smoking and major depression. In M. Gold & B. Stimmel (Eds.), *Smoking and illicit drug use* (pp. 35-46). Binghamton, NY: Haworth Medical Press.

DiClemente, C., Prochaska, J., Fairhurst, S., Velicer, W., Velasquez, M., & Rossi, J. (1991). The process of smoking cessation: An analysis of precontemplation, contemplation, and preparation stages of change. *Journal of Consulting and Clinical Psychology, 59*(2), 295-304.

Fagerstrom, K. (1991). Towards better diagnoses and more individual treatment of tobacco dependence. Special issue: Future directions in tobacco research. *Brit J Addiction, 86*(5), 543-547.

Fiore, M., Bailey, W., Cohen, S., Dorfman, S., Goldstein, M., Gritz, E., Heyman, R., Holbrook, J., Jaen, C., Kottke, T., Lando, H., Mecklenburg, R., Mullen, P., Nett, L., Robinson, L., Stitzer, M., Tommasello, A., Villejo, L., & Wewers, M. (2000, June). *Treating tobacco use and dependence* [Clinical practice guideline]. Rockville, MD: U.S. Department of Health and Human Services, Public Health Service, Agency for Healthcare Research and Quality.

Foxx, R., & Brown, R. (1979). Nicotine fading and self-monitoring for cigarette abstinence or controlled smoking. *Journal of Applied Behavior Analysis, 12*, 111-125.

Froom, P., Melamed, S., & Benbasal, J. (1998). Smoking cessation and weight gain. *Journal of Family Practice, 46*(6), 460-464.

Glassman, A. (1993). Cigarette smoking: Implications for psychiatric illness. *American Journal of Psychiatry 150,* 546-553.

Hughes, J., Fiester, S., Goldstein, M., Resnick, M., Rock, N., & Ziedonis, D. (1996). American Psychiatric Association practice guideline for the treatment of patients with nicotine dependence. *American Journal of Psychiatry, 153*(Suppl. 10), S1-S31.

Hughes, J., Goldstein, M., Hurt, R., & Shiffman, S. (1999). Recent advances in the pharmacotherapy of smoking. *Journal of the American Medical Association, 281*, 72-76.

Hughes, J., & Hatsukami, D. (1992). The nicotine withdrawal syndrome: A brief review and update. *International Journal of Smoking Cessation, 1*, 21-26.

Istvan, J., & Matarazzo, J. (1984). Tobacco, alcohol and caffeine use: A review of their interrelationships. *Psychological Bulletin, 95*, 301-326.

Kalman, D. (1998). Smoking cessation treatment for substance misusers in early recovery: A review of the literature and recommendations for practice. *Substance Use and Misuse, 33*, 2021-2047.

Ockene, J., Emmons, K., Mermelstein, R., Perkins, K., Bonollo, D., Voorhees, C., & Hollis, J. (2000). Relapse and maintenance issues for smoking cessation. *Health Psychology, 19*(Suppl. 1), 17-31.

Perkins, K. (1992). Metabolic effects of cigarette smoking. *Journal of Applied Physiology, 72*, 401-409.

Velicer, W., Fava, J., Prochaska, J., Abrams, D., Emmons, K., & Piere, J. (1995). Distribution of smokers by stage in three representative samples. *Preventive Medicine, 24*, 401-411.

Wack, J., & Rodin, L. (1982). Smoking and its effects on body weight and the systems of caloric regulation. *American Journal of Clinical Nutrition, 35*, 366-380.

SMOKING PREVENTION AND TOBACCO CONTROL AMONG YOUTH

The prevention of cigarette smoking and other forms of tobacco use is among the world's leading public health priorities. Tobacco use continues to be the leading preventable cause of death in the United States. Smoking and spit tobacco use begins early in life; currently, about one third of high school-age adolescents in the United States use tobacco. Adolescence is the critical time period for prevention and early cessation efforts, given both the highly addictive nature of the substance and that the vast majority of smokers begin smoking before the age of 18. If interventions can keep youth tobacco free through adolescence, the chances of their initiating smoking after high school are much smaller.

Numerous studies have also found that adolescents who smoke are more likely to use other drugs. The social, psychological, and biological factors that contribute to an individual's use of tobacco are similar to the factors that contribute to the use of other drugs. Cigarette smoking is also correlated with other high-risk behaviors, such as violence and unprotected sex. These added risks underscore the need for effective smoking prevention programs, as it may be possible to delay or prevent the other behaviors by preventing tobacco use.

The need for effective tobacco prevention in youth derives from some important health consequences of adolescent tobacco use. Cigarette smoking during adolescence appears to reduce the rate of lung growth and inhibits full lung function. Adolescents who smoke are more likely to be less physically fit than nonsmokers and are more likely to experience shortness of breath and other respiratory problems. Smoking during adolescence also sets the stage for threats to adult health, as health problems associated with smoking are a function of duration and amount of use. If smoking begins during adolescence, the duration of the habit is longer and long-term health outcomes are more serious. Smoking during adolescence leads to an increased risk of early atherosclerotic lesions. Spit tobacco use directly contributes to periodontal disease and can cause oral cancer even among youth. Overall, tobacco use during adolescence has a deleterious health impact on young people, accelerating as they develop and grow into adults.

INFLUENCES

For the development of effective interventions, it is necessary to examine environmental, psychological, and behavioral variables that affect adolescent tobacco use. Such variables may be relatively distal or proximal to actual smoking behavior. Distal factors do not always have a direct or immediate impact on smoking, nor is their causal pathway necessarily well known. Proximal influences in contrast may demonstrate an immediate and obvious influence, but in turn may be caused by or mediate the impact of the distal factors. Influences must be examined not only in terms of regular smoking outcomes but also in the context of movement along a continuum of smoking uptake, from not considering smoking, to not smoking but being susceptible to the possibility of being offered a cigarette in the future, to less and then more frequent experimentation, and finally, to regular smoking.

Socioeconomic status, for example, comprises an important distal predictor of adolescent substance use. Children from single-parent homes or poor families are more likely to initiate smoking during adolescence. Mass media may also be influential in adolescent tobacco use. Cigarette advertising appears to have an indirect effect on legitimizing tobacco use, while concurrently directly affecting adolescents' perceptions of smoking prevalence, the esteem in which smoking is held, and attitudes about the function of smoking. Since these cognitive factors represent psychosocial risks for smoking, advertising may have a direct impact on the initiation of tobacco use.

Yet more proximal to the uptake of smoking are physical and social environmental factors such as the availability of cigarettes and peer influence to smoke. If someone in the household smokes, adolescents have cigarettes easily available to them. It has also been found that if a youth's friends smoke, he or she is more likely to smoke as well, a product of both peer pressure and availability factors. Peer groups influence expectations, reinforce smoking behavior, provide cues for experimentation, and provide the actual cigarettes.

Other proximal intrapersonal risk factors associated with tobacco use include low self-image, low self-esteem, lack of self-confidence, and insufficient knowledge about tobacco use. These factors contribute to an inability to say no to peers. A lack of self-confidence may represent a reflection of low self-esteem and low self-image. If adolescents do not feel that they have the ability to refuse a cigarette and still be liked by their peers, they are more likely to succumb to peer pressure to smoke. Insufficient knowledge about tobacco use also contributes to initiation. If one is not aware that smoking is harmful or has incorrect knowledge about its addictive capabilities, that person is more likely to accept a cigarette. If subjective norms lead adolescents to believe that there are more people smoking than is actually the case, they will be more likely to initiate smoking. Subjective norm effects hold true for availability as well: Those who perceive that cigarettes are easily obtained are more likely to begin using tobacco than those who perceive more difficulty in obtaining cigarettes. Therefore, the salient influences to smoke may derive not only from the actual environment but also from the adolescent's perception of that environment.

Behavioral risk factors associated with adolescent tobacco use include general risk-related behaviors, such as poor academic achievement and low school involvement. Individuals with poor grades and low school involvement are more likely to have low self-esteem and feelings of self-worth, which, in turn, make them more vulnerable to tobacco and other substance use.

Immediately proximal to the onset of tobacco use are interpersonal skill deficits, specifically, a lack of ability to refuse the offer of a cigarette or other substance from a peer in a socially adept manner. Most risk factors for initiation of smoking are interrelated with each other. Therefore, it is a combination of these factors that must be taken into account when designing interventions to properly address the process of smoking initiation.

Exposure to environmental tobacco smoke (ETS) not only may influence youth to smoke but at the same time comprises a direct threat to their health as well as that of all others who are exposed. The Environmental Protection Agency (EPA) has concluded that exposure to tobacco smoke causes lung cancer as well as coronary heart disease, causes serious respiratory problems in children, and can lead to death. Secondhand smoke has also been classified as a Group A carcinogen by the EPA. Thus, the importance of policies that are geared at decreasing ETS cannot be underestimated.

The tobacco industry from its inception has been quick to take advantage of the power of media and advertising. Given the association between cigarette advertising and smoking among youth, antitobacco efforts have also been quick to act and create policies that have severely restricted the industry's ability to advertise through certain means of communication. For example, the universally recognized "Marlboro Man" cowboy saw his last appearance on television in 1971, when all tobacco commercials were banned from American television. The 1980s saw the birth of Joe Camel, a cartoon character designed to promote Camel cigarettes. Although Joe Camel was forced from the scene, the tobacco industry continues to find other avenues through which it can effectively continue to target youth such as through brand placement and the depiction of cigarette smoking in movies.

INTERVENTIONS

In a literature review, Lantz and her colleagues categorize current smoking prevention and control strategies as applied to youth tobacco consumption. These categories (many of which relate to adult consumption and prevalence as well) include (1) school-based educational interventions (or classroom-like programs offered in the community), (2) school policies, (3) community interventions, (4) mass media and anti-tobacco advertising campaigns, (5) tobacco advertising and marketing restrictions, (6) restrictions regarding youth access to tobacco and on the sale of tobacco products, (7) tobacco excise taxes, (8) restrictions on smoking and penalties for possession and use, (9) vendor penalties, and (10) interventions with high-risk youth and early-cessation programs.

School-Based Educational Interventions

School-based educational interventions traditionally focus on cognitive and affective responses among youth, in attempts to influence knowledge, beliefs, attitudes, intentions, and subjective norms related to smoking. In general, these approaches appear to be ineffective when not accompanied by direct behavior change efforts. A second typical educational intervention evolved more recently, emphasizing peer pressure resistance or "social inoculation." Brief interventions center around social inoculation activities, which through role-plays teach refusal skills for resisting prompts to smoke. These role-plays are placed in the context of realistic mock situations, in which peers or others play the part of the friend, sibling, or adult trying to convince the participant to try a cigarette. Social inoculation programs have been shown to be at least somewhat effective in reducing smoking onset.

Teachers, older youth (including college students), or same-age peers typically lead school-based interventions. Peer-led interventions have often been touted as being more effective than teacher-led interventions; however, training and deploying same-age peers can present significant logistical problems. Therefore, older high school or even college students may be recruited to perform the function of the peer leader, as they have sufficient maturity to accept this responsibility but at the same time are still sufficiently young to be able to relate to students typically of middle school age.

Current school-based programs typically involve most or all of the following components: behavioral skills (especially refusal skills) development, behavioral contracting, media pressure and health education, social influences and normative education, peer interaction and instruction, the development of self-confidence and self-esteem, stress management, community involvement, and cessation tips for those already smoking. A typical sixth-grade curriculum will include lessons on health effects, values clarification, decision making, health consequences, behavioral alternatives, refusal skills, and encouraging adults to quit. In seventh grade, this would evolve to norm perceptions and false perceptions, dangerous industry and retail practices, equating cigarettes to smokeless tobacco, the role of peer pressure and how to deal with it, making choices, saying no without being left out, and extensive role-plays. Eighth-grade classes might emphasize cessation, social activism, and reaching out to younger relatives and friends to keep them away from cigarettes. Lessons are augmented by handouts and videos that complement and extend the information presented by the peer leaders or teachers.

Multiple-year school-based interventions, extending throughout the middle school years and even into high school (and thereby capturing the adolescent at different developmental stages), may be more effective than single-year interventions. These longer interventions allow for multiple themes to be addressed (e.g., social inoculation, media, politics, and the tobacco industry), and adjust for developmental change in the target population as they move through these years of higher risk.

School Policies and Penalties for Possession and Use

Educational efforts alone are probably insufficient to realize an adequate prevention effect. Fairly recently, a variety of communities and states have initiated efforts to place penalties on the books for underage individuals carrying or using tobacco products in school or generally in public. Typically, youth are ticketed or fined for possession or use. Relatedly, strong school policies that proscribe smoking, in place with smoking prevention efforts, may prove effective in lowering schoolwide prevalence.

Community Interventions

Schools are not established primarily for the purposes of health promotion and substance use prevention. In fact, pressures to improve standardized test scores, provide extracurricular activities, and at the same time offer an extensive and varied curriculum make schools increasingly reluctant to designate classroom time for tobacco education. Some community

programs have circumvented this barrier by either conducting programs with community-based groups of youth (e.g., YMCA/YWCA, religious groups, Scouts) or delivering prevention interventions through brief phone calls to students. In the latter scenario, students are introduced to the project in the school and then told they will receive several smoking prevention newsletters and be contacted by a peer counselor. This older youth calls periodically following the mailing of the newsletter with information such as that presented above, such as encouraging the younger student to make a commitment not to smoke, and problem solving any difficult social pressures that are being encountered. Calls are typically made during latchkey hours (i.e., unsupervised periods at home, typically before parents arrive home from work), which are times of a higher probability of smoking and other high-risk behaviors.

Community interventions have many parallels with school-based interventions, but more typically involve families, school administration, churches, businesses, media, social service and health agencies, government, and law enforcement. These approaches assume a broader, ecological view of the smoking onset problem and how to confront it. The community environment may influence smoking or its prevention through the availability of cigarettes and spit tobacco, laws and social norms, and media and societal messages (e.g., thetruth.com antitobacco messages via the Internet; and conversely, tobacco product placement and the depiction of smoking in movies). Community-based interventions offer the prospect of reaching a larger audience, complemented by school-based and other tobacco control programs that increase the frequency with which the nonsmoking message is received by the target audience. Students participating in school programs may actually be encouraged to write letters to local newspapers, elected officials, and retailers, and in other ways demonstrate their antitobacco attitudes to the community. School-based or classroom-like programs and community interventions may have a synergistic effect in communities, which benefit from both of them.

Tobacco Advertising Restrictions

As the tobacco industry continues to strategize about how to promote its product to youth, it is necessary that public health professionals ensure that policies are being constantly created to counteract each and every new move. For example, the Joe Camel campaign caused such an uproar that its usage was eventually banned, as this cartoon character was seen to be deliberately created to target youth. In California, R.J. Reynolds Tobacco Company was fined for specifically targeting kids in magazines, and was also specifically ordered to stop marketing to youth.

As researchers have demonstrated the effectiveness of tobacco advertising in increasing youth curiosity about and attraction to using tobacco products, calls to restrict or ban advertising have increased. However, bans may not achieve the intended effectiveness, because cigarettes can still be promoted via placement in movies, at sporting events, and in other formats and venues popular among youth. Recently, the European Union realized a very important step in the fight against tobacco by banning advertisements in magazines, in newspapers, on the radio, and via the Internet. Tobacco companies are also prohibited from sponsoring events like Formula One motor racing. Recommended but not required are bans on billboard advertisements and the use of brands and logos on clothing and other consumer materials. Barring court challenges, member countries are to enact these regulations no later than January 2005.

Mass Media Campaigns

A variety of studies have shown mass media campaigns to be effective in decreasing tobacco use onset and increasing antitobacco attitudes. This has especially been shown to be the case if such efforts are accompanied by other potentially powerful interventions such as taxation or school interventions. Media messages that advocate social change in which youth are exhorted to be aware of the manipulation that the tobacco industry is trying to realize in promoting smoking to them may be especially attractive to youth.

Recent advertising campaigns have been deployed to counter tobacco advertising and to increase the attention to and attractiveness of the nonsmoking/antitobacco spots. These campaigns may comprise important complements to the overall tobacco control effort (e.g., increasing excise taxes, developing and enforcing sales policies).

"The Truth" exemplifies recent effective media campaigns targeting youth smoking. The Truth has framed the issue of youth smoking not by telling young people not to smoke, but rather by informing them about general tobacco-related issues and helping them make their own decisions. The Truth claims that their goal is not to end smoking, but rather to tell the "truth about how it really is." One of its main objectives is to inform young people about the hidden practices of the tobacco industry, how cigarettes and spit tobacco get marketed, the nature of addiction, and tobacco's impact on health. Launched in 1999 by the American Legacy Foundation, The Truth ads now appear in a variety of media, including television, radio, magazines, and the Internet (thetruth.com).

Stopping the Sale of Tobacco to Youth

The Symar Amendment of 1991 establishes that all states in the United States must enforce laws that restrict the sale of tobacco to youth, and must demonstrate success in reducing youth access. This amendment has led to a variety of complementary interventions to restrict youth access and enforce existing laws, such as sting operations that employ underage confederates to attempt cigarette purchases in targeted convenience stores, gas stations, and other tobacco retail outlets. If "successful" in their effort, these teens inform the sales clerk that he or she is breaking the law by offering to sell the product. When clerks refuse to sell, they and the store managers are reinforced for their compliance. Such efforts apparently are effective in reducing illegal tobacco sales, at least in those stores specifically targeted by sting operations. Complementary media efforts may be required to communicate the program's purpose to nontargeted stores, such as by providing positive publicity to those stores that complied with the law.

Although restricting youth purchasing of cigarettes is important, it must also be shown that such restrictions actually decrease the amount of youth smoking. Community-wide efforts to limit sources of sales through development of new policies by community officials, and the enforcement of existing policies by working with retailers, can be effective in at least slowing the onset of smoking. Nevertheless, youth still have other avenues for obtaining cigarettes, including through "social sources," that is, the cigarettes they receive from friends, brothers and sisters, or even parents.

Cigarette Prices and Tobacco Excise Taxes

Cigarette taxes in many parts of the United States are still quite low compared to many European and

Canadian standards. Although youth who already smoke may continue to spend money on cigarettes regardless of the price, continuing to increase the unit price to them will result in a decrease of consumption and even convince some not to take up the habit in the first place.

The primary method for increasing tobacco product prices is through tobacco excise taxes. Tobacco excise taxes comprise specific state and local government taxes on cigarette products. Until about 15 years ago, such taxes were seldom seen as a method of tobacco control. However, following the 1988 Proposition 99 voter-initiated tax increase in California, through which the excise tax was increased $0.25 per pack and a sharp reduction in tobacco purchasing was quickly evident, public health officials have increasingly advocated the use of such "sin taxes." Excise taxes may be especially effective if the revenue is dedicated to additional antitobacco education and policy development. The U.S. Surgeon General's office now advocates increased tobacco prices to promote prevention and cessation efforts.

Smoking Cessation

A sole focus on primary prevention ignores the fact that addiction and health damage may be prevented among the many adolescents who already experiment or regularly smoke. Cessation interventions for adolescents who are already smoking on a daily or otherwise frequent basis have gained increasing attention over the past few years. Smoking cessation rates among motivated adolescents enrolled in formal programs may approach those of adults. The American Lung Association's NOT on Tobacco (NOT) Program provides one example of a promising smoking cessation effort. Specifically for adolescents, NOT includes ten 50-minute sessions offered weekly over consecutive weeks. NOT comprises a "total health approach" to smoking cessation, with a focus on motivation, smoking history, addiction, consequences of smoking, preparing for quitting, preventing relapse, dealing with ongoing social pressure to smoke, and increasing healthy physical activity levels and nutrition change.

Adult smokers who receive regular advice from their physicians to quit smoking will evidence modest but important improvements in their cessation rates over those who do not receive such advice. Recently, experts have begun to argue that adolescents should receive similar advice for cessation, since many teen smokers, especially daily users, desire to give up the habit. The office environment can support such efforts through chart marking, waiting room literature and signs, and identifying a smoking cessation coordinator. Nurses and other allied health professionals can also complement the advice and follow-up on referrals to make sure that teen smokers get the help that they need to quit. The nicotine patch and other pharmacological adjuncts may be important elements of cessation, although the effectiveness of this approach for teens has yet to be proven. Nevertheless, interventions for teen smokers should be modified depending on how far the habit has progressed, from light experimentation to heavy smoking.

Direct Restrictions

In addition to restrictions on sale by banning vending machines or exiling them to adult-only venues (e.g., bars), recent efforts have emphasized reduction in self-service displays of tobacco. Some communities have banned billboard advertisement and other forms of marketing tobacco near school grounds. Over the years, the implementation of laws that restrict smoking in certain public places comprise some of the great achievements in the war against tobacco in terms of prevention, cessation, and exposure of nonsmokers. In 1994, the Pro-Children's Act was passed by the federal government to prohibit smoking in all facilities where federally funded children's services are provided. The use of tobacco products is now banned from airplanes, school grounds, some government-owned facilities, and some work places, all of which have reduced the threat of environmental tobacco smoke. "Clean air" laws in many states and communities ban smoking inside a building in which others may be exposed, or at least banish it to a ventilated smoking-break room. Past studies have shown that such indoor smoking bans can be effective in reducing on-site smoking and increasing the smoking cessation rates. Restrictions of smoking in public places may also reduce cigarette smoking among young people.

FUTURE DIRECTIONS

Prevention efforts remain central to halting the worldwide tobacco pandemic. Lantz and others recommend greater emphasis on the following intervention components:

Aggressive media campaigns. Multiple-year efforts to reduce demands for smoking and increase anti-tobacco industry attitudes through hard-hitting media spots designed specifically for youth may be a fairly effective intervention approach, or at least one that complements other effective interventions. Ideally, such campaigns would highlight the connections between the industry and the national, regional, and local political processes that they influence.

Cessation efforts. For decades, tobacco control efforts have emphasized prevention for youth rather than cessation, assuming that such cessation efforts were either not recommended because regular smokers were already fairly committed to their habit or conversely that adolescent experimenters could quit easily. Nevertheless, a substantial majority of teens who regularly consume tobacco wish to quit and have not, indicating that a mild to strong addiction has already set in. A strong emphasis, therefore, is needed on helping these teens quit, thereby substantially improving their health and quality of life.

Changing the environment. Prevention and cessation efforts, no matter how well meaning, often involve "blaming the victim" activities that put the onus of change on children or youth themselves. By eliminating cigarette advertising, restricting access to tobacco, and communicating an antitobacco attitude through media and cultural messages, environments may become increasingly less conducive to the uptake of the tobacco habit. Limiting access by banning vending machines and making over-the-counter sales less convenient will reduce commercial sources, while media need to be directed to convince adult smokers to eliminate social source availability. The enactment and enforcement of laws to restrict tobacco sales to youth and the continued propagation of clean indoor air statutes will also communicate directly to the youth that society is headed in a non-smoking direction.

Maintaining an orientation to data. The public often is unaware of youth tobacco use. Data on local and national prevalence polls, sales to minors, and cigarette versus spit tobacco use; sporting events, movies, and other entertainment media that promote brands and smoking behavior; and even information about what politicians receive funding from the tobacco industry can be used to mobilize public opinion for prevention.

Although prevention efforts have enjoyed some success, teen smoking prevalence remains stubbornly high. In spite of increased restrictions, tobacco products remain highly available to youth. Whatever retail sources of tobacco have been diminished, social sources have seemed to make up for less access from the commercial sector. Clearly, consistent, tenacious, and ever-expanding efforts are required to truly achieve broad-based prevention.

—John P. Elder, Sandra Larios,
and Esmeralda M. Iñiguez

See also HEALTH PROMOTION AND DISEASE PREVENTION; HEART DISEASE AND SMOKING; SMOKING AND HEALTH; SMOKING AND NICOTINE DEPENDENCE: INTERVENTIONS

Further Reading

Forest, J. L., Murry, D. M., Wolfson, M., et al. (1998). The effects of community policies to reduce youth access to tobacco. *American Journal of Public Health, 88,* 1193-1198.

Institute of Medicine. (1994). *Growing up tobacco free: Preventing nicotine addiction in children and youth.* Washington, DC: National Academy Press.

Kaufman, N. J., Castrucci, B. C., Mowery, P. D., Gerlach, K. K., Emont, S., & Orleans, T. (2002). Predictors of change on the smoking uptake continuum among adolescents. *Archives of Pediatrics and Adolescent Medicine, 156,* 581-587.

Lantz, P., Jacobson, P., Warner, J., Wasserman, J., Pollack, H., Berson, J., & Ahlstrom, A. (2000). Investing in youth tobacco control: A review of smoking prevention and control strategies. *Tobacco Control, 9,* 47-63.

Sussman, S., Dent, C. W., Burton, D., Stacy, A. W., & Flay, B. R. (1995). *Developing school-based tobacco use prevention and cessation programs.* Thousand Oaks, CA: Sage.

U.S. Department of Health and Human Services. (1994). *Preventing tobacco use among young people. A report of the surgeon general.* Atlanta, GA: Public Health Service, Centers for Disease Control and Prevention, Office on Smoking and Health. (No S/N 017-001-00491-0)

SOCIAL CAPITAL AND HEALTH

The concept of social capital was originally developed in sociology and political science to describe the resources available to individuals through their membership in community networks. In contrast to financial capital, which resides in people's bank accounts, or human capital, which is embodied in individuals' investment in their education and job training, social capital inheres in the structure and quality of social relationships between individuals. Coleman (1990) identified several forms of social capital, including levels of trust within a social structure, "appropriable" social organizations, norms and sanctions, and information channels. Appropriable social organizations are groups established by individuals to address a particular problem, which can be subsequently appropriated to solve other problems of collective action. For example, a group of residents in a neighborhood might volunteer to establish a community policing association. Besides monitoring and preventing the occurrence of crime in the area, the same association is now potentially available to improve the quality of life of residents in other respects, for example, organizing to prevent the closure of local fire stations, or lobbying municipal authorities to fix broken street lights.

Although the precise definition of social capital is contested and continues to evolve, most versions encompass two dimensions: the structural and the cognitive. The *structural component* of social capital includes the extent and intensity of associational links and activity in society (e.g., as measured by the density of civic associations, measures of informal sociability, and indicators of civic engagement). The *cognitive component* includes people's perceptions of trust, reciprocity, and sharing (Harpham, Grant, & Thomas, 2002). An additional distinction is commonly made between *bonding* and *bridging* social capital. Bonding capital refers to the social connections that exist within a group structure, while bridging capital refers to the social connections that link diverse communities and groups within a society (Putnam, 2000).

MEASUREMENT OF SOCIAL CAPITAL

Compared to other forms of capital (financial, human), social capital is less tangible, and hence more difficult to measure. Two approaches to measuring social capital include direct social observation, and aggregating responses from social surveys. Because social capital can assume a variety of forms (levels of trust, norms and sanctions, density of civic

associations), the measurement of this construct calls for the use of a variety of approaches.

Direct social observation can include the use of experimental methods, such as the "letter drop experiment," in which stamped, addressed envelopes are deliberately dropped on street corners to determine the proportion of letters that are subsequently picked up by strangers and mailed to the addressee (an experimental indicator of reciprocity). More commonly, empirical studies have resorted to the use of more proxy measures, such as aggregated responses to social survey items inquiring about the extent of interpersonal trust between citizens (e.g., percentage of respondents in a community who agree that "most people can be trusted"), or the density of membership in a range of civic associations including church groups, sports groups, hobby groups, fraternal organizations, labor unions, and so on.

There is some debate over the extent to which the concept of social capital represents "old wine in new bottles." For instance, community psychologists have an established tradition of working with concepts such as "sense of community," "community competence," and "neighboring," all of which appear to tap into aspects of social capital (Lochner, Kawachi, & Kennedy, 1999). Moreover, an extensive literature in health psychology and social epidemiology has dealt with apparently related constructs such as social networks, social support, and social integration. One important distinction that can be drawn between the concepts of social capital, on the one hand, and social networks/social support, on the other hand, is that the former is often explicitly conceptualized and measured at the group level. In other words, social capital is considered a property of the collective (neighborhood, region, state).

A crucial question is whether aggregated responses to survey items (e.g., concerning trust between neighborhood residents) genuinely represent a contextual influence, or whether they are confounded by the demographic, social, and economic attributes of individual respondents that systematically correlate with their perceptions of social capital. Evidence suggests that aggregated survey responses can indeed capture genuine contextual differences. A multilevel analysis of the Community Survey of the Project on Human Development in Chicago Neighborhoods found that even after controlling for demographic (age, sex, race, marital status) and socioeconomic (income, educational attainment) factors at the individual level, significant neighborhood differences remained in perceptions of trust, substantiating the notion of social capital as a true contextual construct (Subramanian, Lochner, & Kawachi, 2003).

SOCIAL CAPITAL AND POPULATION HEALTH

Social capital has been linked to economic development, the smooth functioning of democracies, and the prevention of crime, among other benefits (Putnam, 2000). More recently, the notion of social capital has been extended to the population health field to explain variations in the health achievement of societies.

Indicators of social capital are not routinely available on administrative data sets (such as the government census), hence researchers have resorted to the use of secondary sources to tap indicators of social capital, such as the density of membership in civic associations from social surveys, and national opinion poll data on interpersonal trust and perceptions of reciprocity between citizens.

Following the example of the political scientist Robert Putnam (2000), U.S. researchers have analyzed state-level data on interpersonal trust, norms of reciprocity, and membership in voluntary associations from the National Opinion Research Center's General Social Surveys. When correlated with state-level health indicators, these social capital variables explained a significant proportion of the cross-sectional variations in mortality rates across states of the United States (Kawachi, Kennedy, & Prothrow-Stith, 1997). For instance, the level of mistrust (the proportion of residents in a state who agreed that "most people would take advantage of you") was shown to be strikingly correlated with average age-adjusted mortality rates ($r = 0.79$, $p < .001$). Lower levels of trust were associated with higher rates of most major causes of death, including heart disease, cancers, infant mortality, and violent deaths, including homicide. A one standard deviation increase in trust was associated with about a 9% lower level of overall mortality. Similar associations were found between death rates and other indicators of social capital, including norms of reciprocity (the proportion of residents agreeing that "most of the time, people try to be helpful"), as well as per capita membership in a variety of civic associations. The association of social capital indicators with mortality remained after accounting for state differences in median income and poverty rates.

Social capital is associated with not only mortality rates but more general indicators of health status as well. Using data from 167,259 respondents in the Centers for Disease Control and Prevention's Behavioral Risk Factor Surveillance System (BRFSS), a strong correlation was found between mistrust and the proportion of residents in each state who rated their own health as being only "fair or poor," as opposed to "excellent, very good, or good" ($r = 0.71$, $p < .0001$) (Kawachi, Kennedy, & Glass, 1999). These associations persisted after control for individual-level factors that could account for poor health status. After taking account of individual-level differences in variables such as health insurance coverage, personal income, educational attainment, race/ethnicity, cigarette smoking, and obesity, residence in a low social capital area was still associated with about a 40% excess risk of reporting poor health.

In another study also using BRFSS data, independent effects were observed for mistrust, even after controlling for other contextual effects such as income inequality and median income, in addition to adjusting for individual socioeconomic status (Subramanian, Kawachi, & Kennedy, 2001). Empirical evidence from other countries, such as Sweden and Finland, have suggested links between community social capital and lower prevalence of high-risk health behaviors, as well as mental health problems.

In addition to health outcomes at the state level, social capital has been examined in relation to neighborhood-level outcomes. A study based on the 343 neighborhoods of Chicago city found that the degree of social cohesion in a neighborhood (assessed, e.g., by the extent to which residents said their neighbors could be trusted), combined with their willingness to intervene for the public good, was a significant predictor of juvenile delinquency, crime victimization, and homicide rates (Sampson, Raudenbush, & Earls, 1997). In the same study, neighborhood variations in trust, reciprocity, and group membership were significantly correlated with overall and cause-specific mortality rates (including cardiovascular disease mortality rates), even after control for levels of socioeconomic deprivation (Lochner et al., 2003).

Recent investigations on whether community levels of trust influence health outcomes after controlling for individual perceptions of the trustworthiness of other members of the community have revealed a complex pattern of interactions between individual perceptions and community aggregate levels of trust. A multilevel analysis of the 2000 Social Capital

Benchmark Survey (conducted in 40 U.S. communities) showed that while controlling for individual trust perception rendered the main effect of community social trust statistically insignificant, a complex interaction effect was also observed, such that the health-promoting effect of community social trust was significantly greater for individuals expressing higher trust of others. On the other hand, for individuals expressing mistrust of others, higher community levels of trust were associated with an effect in the opposite direction, that is, living in higher-trust communities was associated with worse health status for low-trust individuals (Subramanian, Daniels, & Kawachi, 2002).

MECHANISMS LINKING SOCIAL CAPITAL TO HEALTH OUTCOMES

The precise mechanisms underlying the connection between social capital and health remain to be teased out, but a great deal of evidence from epidemiology suggests that social support is an important determinant of longevity and quality of life (Kawachi & Berkman, 2000). Leaving aside the obvious point that access to mutual support can enhance individual well-being (e.g., through the ability to buffer the effects of stress—such as borrowing cash or arranging child care in a medical emergency), there are other, plausible mechanisms by which social capital may influence health outcomes. These mechanisms, reviewed by Kawachi and Berkman, include

a. a community's ability to enforce healthy norms (also referred to as "collective efficacy"), such as through collective action to introduce smoking restrictions in public places via local ordinances;

b. collective action to garner health-promoting services and amenities (e.g., lobbying to improve access to recreational facilities, such as bike paths); and

c. diffusion of innovation through information channels (e.g., enhanced knowledge and community awareness of innovations, such as new forms of cancer screening).

THE DOWNSIDES OF SOCIAL CAPITAL

For all the potential benefits of social capital, it is not a panacea for health promotion. Like any form of capital (such as financial capital), social capital can be used for desirable as well as undesirable ends. Strong social ties *within* a particular group or community

(strong "bonding" social capital) may coexist with conflict *between* that social group and outside social groups. For instance, in India, a high level of social cohesion within Hindu and Muslim communities is not sufficient to prevent ethnic conflict. Strong *bridging* forms of social capital—represented by networks of civic engagement that bring Hindu and Muslim urban communities together, as exemplified by integrated business organizations, trade unions, and political parties—are necessary to prevent the outbreak of ethnic violence (Varshney, 2002). Some forms of association, such as criminal gangs and the Mafia, may provide social capital to its members, but do very little to foster social cohesion in the rest of society.

In addition, social connectedness is not universally or necessarily associated with beneficial health outcomes. If group norms encourage deleterious behaviors (such as within networks of injection drug users), being connected to such groups will not promote health. Communities characterized by strong social bonds may also imply certain restrictions on individual freedom, as well as pressures to conform and to reciprocate social support. Given the gendered pattern of caregiving in most societies, women in particular can often end up shouldering the burden of providing the social support to community members. The excessive obligations to provide support to others can become a source of stress. Finally, some critics have accused the concept of social capital of fostering a victim-blaming attitude, in which communities end up being blamed for insufficient bonding and mutual support. These valid criticisms emphasize the care that is warranted in advocating the strengthening of social capital as a health promotion strategy.

—*Ichiro Kawachi and
S. V. Subramanian*

See also ECOSOCIAL THEORY; INCOME INEQUALITY AND HEALTH; SOCIAL INTEGRATION, SOCIAL NETWORKS, AND HEALTH; SOCIOECONOMIC STATUS AND HEALTH

Further Reading

Coleman, J. S. (1990). *Foundations of social theory.* Cambridge, MA: Harvard University Press.

Harpham, T., Grant, E., & Thomas, E. (2002). Measuring social capital within health surveys: Key issues. *Health Policy and Planning, 17*(1), 106-111.

Kawachi, I., & Berkman, L. F. (2000). Social cohesion, social capital, and health. In L. F. Berkman & I. Kawachi

(Eds.), *Social epidemiology* (pp. 174-190). New York: Oxford University Press.

Kawachi, I., Kennedy, B. P., & Glass, R. (1999). Social capital and self-rated health: A contextual analysis. *American Journal of Public Health, 89,* 1187-1193.

Kawachi, I., Kennedy, B. P., & Prothrow-Stith, D. (1997). Social capital, income inequality and mortality. *American Journal of Public Health, 87,* 1491-1498.

Lochner, K., et al. (2003). Social capital and neighborhood mortality rates in Chicago. *Social Science and Medicine, 56,* 1797-1805.

Lochner, K., Kawachi, I., & Kennedy, B. P. (1999). Social capital: A guide to its measurement. *Health and Place, 5,* 259-270.

Putnam, R. D. (2000). *Bowling alone: The collapse and revival of American community.* New York: Simon & Schuster.

Sampson, R. J., Raudenbush, S. W., & Earls, F. (1997). Neighborhoods and violent crime: A multilevel study of collective efficacy. *Science, 277,* 918-924.

Subramanian, S. V., Daniels, K., & Kawachi, I. (2002). Social trust and self-rated poor health in U.S. communities: A multilevel analysis. *Journal of Urban Health, 79*(4, Suppl. 1), S21-S34.

Subramanian, S. V., Kawachi, I., & Kennedy, B. P. (2001). Does the state you live in make a difference? Multilevel analysis of self-rated health in the U.S. *Social Science and Medicine, 53,* 9-19.

Subramanian, S. V., Lochner, K., & Kawachi, I. (2003). Neighborhood differences in social capital in the U.S.: Compositional artifact or a contextual construct. *Health and Place, 9,* 33-44.

Varshney, A. (2002). *Ethnic conflict and civic life.* New Haven, CT: Yale University Press.

SOCIAL INTEGRATION, SOCIAL NETWORKS, AND HEALTH

Over the past 25 years, there have been dozens of articles and now books on issues related to social networks and social support. It is now widely recognized that social relationships and affiliation have powerful effects on physical and mental health for a number of reasons (Berkman & Glass, 2000; Cohen, Underwood, & Gottlieb, 2000; Seeman, 1996).

When investigators write about the impact of social relationships on health, many terms are used loosely and interchangeably including *social networks, social support, social ties,* and *social integration.* This entry discusses (1) theoretical orientations from diverse disciplines that are fundamental to advancing research in this area, (2) findings related to mortality, (3) a set of definitions of networks and aspects of networks and support, and (4) an overarching model that integrates multilevel phenomena.

THEORETICAL ORIENTATIONS

There are several sets of theories that form the bedrock for the empirical investigation of social relationships and their influence on health. The earliest theories came from sociologists such as Émile Durkheim, as well as from psychoanalysts such as John Bowlby, who first formulated attachment theory. A major wave of conceptual development also came from anthropologists including Bott, Barnes, and Mitchell as well as quantitative sociologists such as Fischer, Laumann, Wellman, and Marsden, who, along with others, have developed social network analysis. This eclectic mix of theoretical approaches coupled with the contributions of epidemiologists form the foundation of research on social ties and health.

Durkheim's contribution to the study of the relationship between society and health is immeasurable. Perhaps most important is the contribution he has made to the understanding of how social integration and cohesion influence suicide. Durkheim's primary aim was to explain how individual pathology was a function of social dynamics. In light of recent attention to "upstream" determinants of health, Durkheim's work reemerges with great relevance today.

John Bowlby, one of the most important psychiatrists in the 20th century, proposed theories suggesting that the environment, especially in early childhood, played a critical role in the genesis of neurosis. Bowlby proposed that there is a universal human need to form close affectional bonds. Attachment theory, proposed by Bowlby, contends that the attached figure creates a secure base from which an infant or toddler can explore and venture forth. The strength of Bowlby's theory lies in its articulation of an individual's need for secure attachment for its own sake, for the love and reliability it provides, and for its own "safe haven." Primary attachment promotes a sense of security and self-esteem that ultimately provides the basis on which the individual will form lasting, secure, and loving relationships in adult life.

Social Network Theory: A New Way of Looking at Social Structure and Community

During the mid-1950s, a number of British anthropologists found it increasingly difficult to understand the behavior of either individuals or groups on the basis of traditional categories such as kin groups, tribes, or villages. Barnes and Bott developed the concept of "social networks" to analyze ties that cut across traditional kinship, residential, and class groups to explain behaviors they observed such as access to jobs, political activity, or marital roles. The development of social network models provided a way to view the structural properties of relationships among people.

Network analysis "focuses on the characteristic patterns of ties between actors in a social system rather than on characteristics of the individual actors themselves and use these descriptions to study how these social structures constrain network member's behavior" (Hall & Wellman, 1985, p. 26). Network analysis focuses on the structure and composition of the network, and the contents or specific resources that flow through those networks. The strength of social network theory rests on the testable assumption that the social structure of the network itself is largely responsible for determining individual behavior and attitudes by shaping the flow of resources that determines access to opportunities and constraints on behavior.

HEALTH, SOCIAL NETWORKS, AND INTEGRATION

From the mid-1970s through the present, there has been a series of studies consistently showing that the lack of social ties or social networks predicted mortality from almost every cause of death. These studies have been done in the United States, Europe, and Asia. These studies most often captured numbers of close friends and relatives, marital status, and affiliation or membership in religious and voluntary associations. These measures were conceptualized in any number of ways as assessments of social networks or ties, social connectedness, integration, activity, or embeddedness. Whatever they were named, they uniformly defined embeddedness or integration as involvement with ties spanning the range from intimate to extended.

In the first of these studies from Alameda County, California (Berkman & Syme, 1979), men and women who lacked ties to others (in this case, based on an index assessing contacts with friends and relatives, marital status, and church and group membership) were 1.9 to 3.1 times more likely to die in a 9-year follow-up period than those who had many more contacts.

Another study, in Tecumseh, Michigan (House, Robbins, & Metzner, 1982), showed a similar strength of positive association for men, but not for women, between social connectedness/social participation and mortality risk over a 10- to 12-year period. An additional strength of this study was the ability to control for some biomedical predictors assessed from physical examination (e.g., cholesterol, blood pressure, and respiratory function).

Similar results from several more studies have been reported from studies in the United States and three from Scandinavia. Investigators working on a study from Evans County, Georgia, found risks to be significant in older White men and women even when controlling for biomedical and sociodemographic risk factors although some racial and gender differences were observed. In Sweden, two studies reported significantly increased risks among socially isolated adults. Finally, in a study of 13,301 men and women in eastern Finland, Kaplan and associates (1988) have shown that an index of social connections predicts mortality risk for men but not for women, independent of standard cardiovascular risk factors.

Studies of older men and women confirm the continued importance of these relationships into late life (Seeman et al., 1993). Furthermore, two studies of large cohorts of men and women in a large health maintenance organization (HMO) and 32,000 male health professionals (Kawachi et al., 1996) suggested that social networks are, in general, more strongly related to mortality than to the incidence or onset of disease.

Two recent studies of Danish men (Penninx et al., 1997) and Japanese men and women (Sugisawa, Liang, & Liu, 1994) further indicated that aspects of social isolation or social support are related to mortality. Virtually all of these studies found that people who are socially isolated or disconnected to others are between 2 and 5 times the risk of dying from all causes compared to those who maintain strong ties to friends, family, and community.

Social networks and support have been found to predict a very broad array of other health outcomes from survival post-myocardial infarction to disease progression, functioning, and the onset and course of infectious diseases.

A CONCEPTUAL MODEL LINKING SOCIAL NETWORKS TO HEALTH

Although the power of measures of networks or social integration to predict health outcomes is indisputable, the interpretation of what the measures actually measure has been open to much debate. Hall and Wellman have appropriately commented that much of the work in social epidemiology has used the term *social networks* metaphorically since rarely have investigators conformed to more standard assessments used in network analysis. This criticism has been duly noted and several calls have gone out to develop a second generation of network measures.

A second wave of research developed in reaction to this early work and as an outgrowth of work in health psychology that turned the orientation of the field in several ways. These social scientists focused on the qualitative aspects of social relations (i.e., their provision of social support or, conversely, detrimental aspects of relationships) rather than on the elaboration of the structural aspects of social networks.

Most of these investigators follow an assumption that what is most important about networks is the support functions they provide. While social support is among the primary pathways by which social networks may influence physical and mental health status, it is *not* the *only* critical pathway (Berkman & Glass, 2000). Moreover, the exclusive study of more proximal pathways detracts from the need to focus on the social context and structural underpinnings that may importantly influence the types and extent of social support that is provided.

To have a comprehensive framework in which to explain these phenomena, it is helpful to move "upstream" and return to a more Durkheimian orientation to network structure and social context. It is critical to maintain a view of social networks as lodged within those larger social and cultural contexts that shape the structure of networks. In fact, some of the most interesting work in the field today relates social affiliation to social status and social and economic inequality.

Conceptually, social networks are embedded in a macro-social environment in which large-scale social forces may influence network structure, which, in turn, influences a cascading causal process beginning with the macro-social to psychobiological processes to affect health. In this framework, social networks are embedded in a larger social and cultural context in which upstream forces are seen to condition network structure. Serious consideration of the larger macro-social context in which networks form and are sustained has been lacking in all but a small number of studies and is almost completely absent in studies of social network influences on health.

Networks may operate at the behavioral level through at least four primary pathways: provision of social support, social influence, in social engagement and attachment, and access to resources and material goods. These psychosocial and behavioral processes may influence even more proximate pathways to health status including (1) direct physiological responses; (2) psychological states including self-esteem, self-efficacy, and depression; (3) health-damaging behaviors such as tobacco consumption or high-risk sexual activity, and health promoting behavior such as appropriate health service utilization and exercise; and (4) exposure to infectious disease agents such as HIV, other sexually transmitted diseases (STDs), or tuberculosis.

The following sections review the four primary pathways by which networks may influence health. The reader is referred to Berkman and Glass (2000) for a lengthier review.

The Assessment of Social Networks

Social networks might be defined as the web of social relationships that surround an individual and the characteristics of those ties (Fischer et al., 1977). Burt (1982) has defined network models as describing "the structure of one or more networks of relations within a system of actors." Network characteristics cover.

- Range or size (number of network members)
- Density (the extent to which the members are connected to each other)
- Boundedness (the degree to which they are defined on the basis of traditional structures such as kin, work, neighborhood)
- Homogeneity (the extent to which individuals are similar to each other in a network)

Related to network structure, characteristics of individual ties include

- Frequency of contact
- Multiplexity (the number of types of transactions or support flowing through ties)

- Duration (the length of time an individual knows another)
- Reciprocity (the extent to which exchanges are reciprocal)

Downstream Social and Behavioral Pathways

Social Support

Moving downstream, we now come to a discussion of the mediating pathways by which networks might influence health status. Most obviously, the structure of network ties influences health via the provision of many kinds of support. This framework immediately acknowledges that *not all* ties are supportive and that there is variation in the type, frequency, intensity, and extent of support provided. For example, some ties provide several types of support while other ties are specialized and provide only one type. Social support is typically divided into subtypes, which include emotional, instrumental, appraisal, and informational support. Emotional support is related to the amount of "love and caring, sympathy and understanding and/or esteem or value available from others" (Thoits, 1995). Emotional support is most often provided by a confidant or intimate other, although less intimate ties can provide such support under circumscribed conditions.

Instrumental support refers to help, aid, or assistance with tangible needs such as getting groceries, getting to appointments, phoning, cooking, cleaning, or paying bills. House identifies instrumental support as aid in kind, money, or labor. Appraisal support, often defined as the third type of support, relates to help in decision making, giving appropriate feedback, or help deciding which course of action to take. Informational support is related to the provision of advice or information in the service of particular needs. Emotional, appraisal, and informational support are often difficult to disaggregate and have various other definitions (e.g., self-esteem support).

Perhaps even deeper than support are the ways in which social relationships provide a basis for intimacy and attachment. Intimacy and attachment have meaning not only for relationships that we traditionally think of as intimate (e.g., between partners, parents and children) but for more extended ties. For instance, when relationships are solid at a community level, individuals feel strong bonds and attachment to places (e.g., neighborhood) and organizations (e.g., voluntary and religious).

Social Influence

Networks may influence health via several other pathways. One pathway that is often ignored is based on social influence. Shared norms around health behaviors (e.g., alcohol and cigarette consumption, health care utilization) might be powerful sources of social influence with direct consequences for the behaviors of network members. These processes of mutual influence might occur quite apart from the provision of social support taking place within the network concurrently. For instance, cigarette smoking by peers is among the best predictors of smoking for adolescents. The social influence that extends from the network's values and norms constitutes an important and underappreciated pathway through which networks affect health.

Social Engagement

A third and more difficult-to-define pathway by which networks may influence health status is by promoting social participation and social engagement. Participation and engagement result from the enactment of potential ties in real-life activity. Getting together with friends, attending social functions or church, participating in occupational or social roles, and participating in group recreation are all instances of social engagement. Thus, through opportunities for engagement, social networks define and reinforce meaningful social roles including parental, familial, occupational, and community roles, which, in turn, provides a sense of value, belonging, and attachment. Several recent studies suggest that social engagement is critical in maintaining cognitive ability (Bassuk, Glass, & Berkman, 1999) and reducing mortality (Glass, Mendes de Leon, Marottoli, & Berkman, 1999).

In addition, network participation provides opportunities for companionship and sociability. Rook (1990) argued that these behaviors and attitudes are not the result of the provision of support per se, but are the consequence of participation in a meaningful social context in and of itself. One reason measures of social integration or "connectedness" may be such powerful predictors of mortality over long periods of follow-up is that these ties give meaning to an individual's life by virtue of enabling him or her to participate in it fully, to be obligated (in fact, often to be the provider of support), and to feel attached to his or her community.

Person-to-Person Contact

Another behavioral pathway by which networks influence disease is by restricting or promoting exposure to infectious disease agents. In this regard, the methodological links between epidemiology and networks are striking. What is perhaps most remarkable is that the same network characteristics that can be health promoting can at the same time be health damaging if they serve as vectors for the spread of infectious disease. Efforts to link mathematical modeling applying network approaches to epidemiology are in their infancy and have started to appear over the past 10 years.

The contribution of social network analysis to the modeling of disease transmission is the understanding that in many if not most cases, disease transmission is not spread randomly throughout a population. Social network analysis is well suited to the development of models in which exposure between individuals is not random but rather is based on geographic location, sociodemographic characteristics (age, race, gender), or other important characteristics of the individual such as socioeconomic position, occupation, and sexual orientation. Furthermore, because social network analysis focuses on characteristics of the network rather than on characteristics of the individual, it is ideally suited to the study of diffusion of transmissible diseases through populations via bridging ties between networks, or uncovering characteristics of ego-centered networks that promote the spread of disease.

Access to Material Resources

Surprisingly little research has sought to examine differential access to material goods, resources, and services as a mechanism through which social networks might operate. This, in our view, is unfortunate given the work of sociologists showing that social networks operate by regulating an individual's access to life opportunities by virtue of the extent to which networks overlap with other networks. In this way, networks operate to provide access or to restrict opportunities in much the same way the social status works. Perhaps the most important among studies exploring this tie is Granovetter's (1973) classic study of the power of "weak ties" that on the one hand, lack intimacy, but on the other hand, facilitate the diffusion of influence and information, and provide opportunities for mobility.

This entry has identified five mechanisms by which the structure of social networks might influence disease patterns. While social support is the mechanism most commonly invoked, social networks also influence health through additional behavioral mechanisms including (1) forces of social influence, (2) levels of social engagement and participation, (3) the regulation of contact with infectious disease, and (4) access to material goods and resources. To date, the evidence linking aspects of social relationships to health outcomes is strongest for general measures of social integration, social support, and social engagement. However, these mechanisms are not mutually exclusive. In fact, it is most likely that in many cases they operate simultaneously.

CONCLUSION

The aim in this entry was to integrate some classical theoretical work in sociology, anthropology, and psychiatry with the current empirical research under way on social networks, social integration, and social support. Rather than review the vast amount of work on health outcomes, which is the subject of several excellent recent papers, the entry developed a conceptual framework that might guide work in this field in the future.

—*Lisa F. Berkman*

NOTE: This entry is adapted from L. F. Berkman and T. Glass, "Social Integration, Social Networks, Social Support and Health," in L. F. Berkman and I. Kawachi (Eds.), *Social Epidemiology*, 2000, New York: Oxford University Press.

See also ALAMEDA COUNTY STUDY; CAREGIVING AND STRESS; SOCIAL CAPITAL AND HEALTH; SOCIAL OR STATUS INCONGRUENCE; SOCIOECONOMIC STATUS AND HEALTH; SUPPORT GROUPS AND HEALTH

Further Reading

Bassuk, S., Glass, T., & Berkman, L. (1999). Social disengagement and incident cognitive decline in community-dwelling elderly persons. *Annals of Internal Medicine, 131,* 165-173.

Berkman, L., & Syme, S. (1979). Social networks, host resistance, and mortality: A nine-year follow-up of Alameda County residents. *American Journal of Epidemiology, 109,* 186-204.

Berkman, L. F., & Glass, T. (2000). Social integration, social networks, social support and health. In L. F. Berkman & I. Kawachi (Eds.), *Social epidemiology* (pp. 137-173). New York: Oxford University Press.

Burt, R. S. (1982). *Toward a structural theory of action.* New York: Academic Press.

Cohen, S., Underwood, S., & Gottlieb, B. (2000). *Social support measures and intervention.* New York: Oxford University Press.

Fischer, C. S., Jackson, R. M., Steuve, C. A., Gerson, K., Jones, L. M., & Baldassare, M. (1977). *Networks and places.* New York: Free Press.

Glass, T., Mendes de Leon, C., Marottoli, R., & Berkman, L. (1999). Population based study of social and productive activities as predictors of survival among elderly Americans. *BMJ, 319,* 478-483.

Granovetter, M. (1973). The strength of weak ties. *American Journal of Sociology, 78,* 1360-1380.

Hall, A., & Wellman, B. (1985). Social networks and social support. In S. Cohen & S. L. Syme (Eds.), *Social support and health* (pp. 23-41). Orlando, FL: Academic Press.

House, J., Robbins, C., & Metzner, H. (1982). The association of social relationships and activities with mortality: Prospective evidence from the Tecumseh Community Health Study. *American Journal of Epidemiology, 116,* 123-140.

Kaplan, G., Salonen, J., Cohen, R., Brand, R., Syme, S., & Puska, P. (1988). Social connections and mortality from all causes and cardiovascular disease: Prospective evidence from eastern Finland. *American Journal of Epidemiology, 128,* 370-380.

Kawachi, I., Colditz, G. A., Ascherio, A., Rimm, E. B., Giovannucci, E., Stampfer, M. J. et al. (1996). A prospective study of social networks in relation to total mortality and cardiovascular disease in men in the U.S.A. *Journal of Epidemiology and Community Health, 50,* 245-251.

Penninx, B. W., van Tilburg, T., Kriegsman, D. M., Deeg, D. J., Boeke, A. J., & van Eijk, J. T. (1997). Effects of social support and personal coping resources on mortality in older age: The Longitudinal Aging Study, Amsterdam. *American Journal of Epidemiology, 146,* 510-519.

Rook, K. S. (1990). Social relationships as a source of companionship: implications for older adults psychological well being. In B. R. Sarason, T. G. Sarason, & G. R. Pierce (Eds.), *Social support: An interactional view* (pp. 221-250). New York: John Wiley.

Seeman, T. (1996). Social ties and health: the benefits of social integration. *Annals of Epidemiology, 6,* 442-451.

Seeman, T., Berkman, L., Kohout, F., LaCroix, A., Glynn, R. & Blazer, D. (1993). Intercommunity variation in the association between social ties and mortality in the elderly: A comparative analysis of three communities. *Annals of Epidemiology, 3,* 325-335.

Sugisawa, H., Liang, J., & Liu, X. (1994). Social networks, social support and mortality among older people in Japan. *Journal of Gerontology, 49,* S3-S13.

Thoits, P. (1995). Stress, coping, and social support processes: where are we? What next? *Journal of Health and Social Behavior* [Extra issue], pp. 53-79.

SOCIAL MARKETING

Social marketing is a systematic process to change behavior. The simplest way to intuitively understand social marketing and its importance is its relations to commercial marketing. The premise is, "Why can't people be persuaded to change behaviors that benefit themselves and society the same way they would be persuaded to purchase a product or service?" Social marketing is a viable "population" means to address an assumption that all people are entitled to equitable health and well-being, a protected environment, and communities that welcome their participation. It has been applied to a wide variety of health and societal issues.

DEFINITIONS

Social marketing. There are several definitions of social marketing and all share the following six elements: (a) application of commercial marketing principles for the purpose of pro-social benefits; (b) translation of marketing knowledge and scientific evidence into effective interventions; (c) utilization of a philosophy or principles where the consumer is foremost and all strategies begin with the consumer, behavior change is the bottom line, and benefits outweigh costs; (d) adoption of social messages to voluntarily change beliefs, values, attitudes, and behaviors of individuals within target audiences; (e) integration of marketing concepts called the 4 *P*s (product, price, place, and promotion) to promote an idea appealing to segments of the population or target groups that have been identified based on data; and (f) application of an ongoing process that includes planning; development, testing, and refinement;

implementation; and evaluation. In simplest terms, social marketing applies marketing principles and is a strategy that requires application of the 4 *P*s that are blended based on the exchange of costs and benefits to motivate a targeted group to change behaviors that benefit the individual and society.

Commercial social marketing. Another type of social marketing is commercial social marketing. Commercial social marketing is a for-profit company or organization that offers a good or service to increase sales, but also has a pro-social benefit to the individual and society. An example is a commercial vendor offering strategies for weight reduction. The similarities between social and commercial social marketing are that both ascribe to the same six elements (a-f) as noted above. The *consumer* in both cases is paramount, and both concentrate on changing behaviors that result in pro-social outcomes.

Health communication. There are forms of health communication that have been mistaken for social marketing. One example is social advertising. Social advertising focuses only on one concept of social marketing, which is known as "promotion" (explained in more detail below). Social advertising uses advertising campaigns to inform and influence public beliefs, values, attitudes, and behaviors. Social advertising may or may not be developed with the consumer's wants and needs in mind. Although social advertising is an important part of social marketing, social advertising is insufficient unto itself. Social marketing requires the use and blending of a finite set of social marketing concepts and not relying on any single one.

HISTORY AND IMPORTANCE

G. D. Wiebe, from the field of commercial marketing, originally raised the issue in 1952 of marketing social causes like commercial products when he asked, "Why can't you sell brotherhood like you sell soap?" The question today is, "Why can't we sell healthy lifestyle practices or behavior change like sleek cars?" What makes these notions titillating is if objects that are common and have no utilitarian value such as the "Pet Rock" in the 1970s and the "Pocket Stones" in 2000 can make million-dollar profits, then surely, it could be reputed that if marketing strategies were applied to products of social importance, efficacy would be similar. However, the public may perceive products of social importance as less valuable or useful than even the Pet Rock or Pocket Stones, making the application of social marketing principles even more essential to behavior change professionals.

It was not until the early 1970s that social marketing became eminent when Philip Kotler and Gerald Zaltman coined the term. In 1971, their article "Social Marketing: An Approach to Planned Social Change" appeared in the *Journal of Marketing* and discussed the premise that commercial marketing principles and techniques might be effectively applied to promote socially relevant behaviors. Early adopters of the concept focused on social advertising and not social marketing.

Ironically, even though social marketing was conceptualized in the United States, much of social marketing application has occurred in other countries such as Canada (Ottawa), Scotland, and South Africa. Only within the past two decades has the United States shown serious interest in applying social marketing. In 1997, Lefebvre and Rochlin reported to the Institute of Medicine of the National Academy of Sciences that there was a need in the United States for social marketing research in critical areas, including collection and analysis of consumer data to include classifying and selecting audience segments, and channels and design of appealing messages.

The importance of social marketing is the use of a marketing strategy to "tip the balance" so benefits outweigh barriers. The benefit and cost exchange may be perceived by the consumer as negatively balanced because usually the request is change of a habitual and recalcitrant behavior that has offered immediate positive reinforcement such as overeating, drinking, smoking, inactivity, and sexual behaviors. If these behaviors were ameliorated, health outcomes might be delayed and less satisfying. Therefore, the consumer might perceive the product (new behavior) as undesirable or having low appeal. Social marketing holds promise for shifting this balance so that consumers perceive the new behavior as having a greater value than the cost.

KEY TERMS

Integral to social marketing is a development, implementation, and evaluation process that respects the perspectives, interests, and desires of the target audience. Concepts investigated using this process include the following: (a) audience segmentation,

(b) marketing 4 *P*s, and (c) marketing mix. These terms and the process are explained below:

Development, implementation, and evaluation process. A multistage process used in social marketing is illustrated as a circle including as many as six stages where data are regularly collected. Data are collected during each stage because the primary objective is to meet the needs, interests, and wants of the target audience with continuous input from them. Specific activities for the first stage of planning and strategy selection include reviewing available data, identifying existing activities and gaps, writing goals and objectives, gathering new data, determining target audiences, establishing an audience tracking system, assessing resources, drafting communication strategies, and writing a program plan and timetable. Activities for the second stage of selecting channels and materials involves choosing the communication channels, considering public service media, identifying messages and materials, and deciding whether to produce new materials. The third stage of developing materials and pretesting involves developing and testing message concepts, creating draft materials, pretesting, and making changes based on the results of the pretesting. Fourth-stage activities for program implementation consist of preparing to introduce the intervention, conducting process evaluations, collaborating with partners, and reviewing and revising the intervention. Activities for the fifth stage of assessing effectiveness comprise deciding on the evaluation design, selecting/developing evaluation measures, and conducting outcome and impact evaluations. The last stage of feedback to refine the program entails refining the intervention if needed and communicating the efficacy of the intervention.

These six stages have been simplified to three phases: (a) preproduction/prepromotion, (b) media development and testing, and (c) application and evaluation. Preproduction/prepromotion includes Stages 1 and 2 in the "pinwheel," media development and testing includes Stage 3, and application and evaluation are represented by Stages 4-6.

Audience segmentation. Audience segmentation is a process of subdividing a population into homogeneous (similar) segments or target audiences who are more like each other than members of other or larger groups. The purpose is to better describe and understand a target audience and to predict behaviors in order to formulate tailored messages and programs to meet specific needs. Audience segmentation can be conceptualized as a population divided according to a "nested hierarchy," where decreasingly smaller similar segments are derived from larger more dissimilar ones.

Individuals can be divided into segments as follows: (a) similarity or sharing of antecedent characteristics that influence the behavior in question, and (b) exposure to similar preferred or trusted communication channels. Segmenting audiences can be based on demographic, socioeconomic, geographic, psychological, biological, and physiological characteristics and media correlates to develop and tailor messages and campaigns to the specific wants, needs, and perspectives of a particular segment. Another means of segmenting audiences is the use of constructs or variables from various marketing and behavioral theoretical models. Data can be collected by investigators or through secondary data sources. Secondary data are data collected by another researcher, and are often available at the local, state, regional, and national levels. Data also can be used that result in the marketing mix.

*Marketing 4 *P*s.* The marketing 4 *P*s are product, price, place, and promotion. In commercial marketing, the product refers to goods and services. There are many examples of goods (cars, appliances, and electronic equipment) and services (hair styling, lawn care, and automotive repair). In social marketing, the product is behavior change. Examples of social marketing products are using a condom during sexual activity, obtaining a mammogram to detect breast cancer, enrolling in an alcohol prevention program, and modifying one's lifestyle to reduce cardiovascular risk.

Product can be divided into three levels: core, actual, and augmented. Core product is the benefit to the individual and society from a pro-social activity. The benefit may be related to health promotion, illness and injury prevention, environmental protection, or community involvement. An example of a benefit related to health promotion and illness/injury prevention is regular exercise resulting in improved general health and musculoskeletal fitness to avoid falls. Actual product is the specific behavior(s) necessary to achieve the core product. An example might be 30 minutes of brisk walking 3 to 5 days/week. Augmented product is the additional interpersonal and situational influences that support engaging in the behavior. An example of augmented product is a map of walking trails in a community or walking with a friend.

Another conceptualization of product includes positive and negative core and tangible product. This conceptualization adds negative core product to core, actual, and augmented. Negative core product is the negative or undesirable effect of engaging or participating in the behavior. An example is muscle soreness following initiation of physical activity.

Price is the cost the consumer associates with the new behavior. The number of price categories varies, but some are monetary, time, psychological, physical, and opportunity. Monetary is financial investment; time is temporal units required; psychological is emotions (such as anxiety, guilt, and embarrassment); physical is pain and suffering; and opportunity is giving up pleasure, comfort, and the security required to engage in the behavior. An essential concept related to price is exchange. Exchange means that the product must be worth the price. In other words, the new behavior must be worth more to the individual than what it costs the person.

Place is where and when the behavior will occur. Place includes access, convenience, and pleasantness associated with engaging in the new behavior while making the existing or competing behavior less convenient or pleasant. Place can be divided into the categories of personal and nonpersonal. Personal place may refer to individuals or professionals who make the task of engaging in the behavior easier and more pleasant, for example, a personal trainer who provides individualized instruction about how to exercise safely. Nonpersonal place may refer to the location and appeal that make the task of engaging in the behavior more accessible and attractive, for example, engaging in physical activity in an appealing exercise facility that is nearby.

Promotion is persuasion that the product (positive benefits of the behavior) is greater than the price (negativism toward the behavior). Promotion involves selecting the following: (a) content or actual "best" words and "ideal" images; (b) incentives, rewards, or benefits for taking action (e.g., health benefits, reduced price, coupons, rebates, gifts); (c) effective communication channel(s) either by mass communication (e.g., television, radio, billboards, newspapers, magazines, governmental signage), selective communication (e.g., letters, direct mail, flyers, brochures, posters, special events, telemarketing, Internet), and/or personal communication (e.g., face-to-face meetings, telephone conversations, workshops, seminars, training sessions); (d) a

spokesperson who is credible and appealing to the target audience; and (e) the timing or when to initiate the campaign (e.g., designated health month, week, or day; period of heightened awareness), duration/frequency of the campaign, and communication channels (reach).

Marketing mix. This term equates to taking into account and integrating or blending information of the 4 *P*s. These blended data form the basic core or building blocks for designing an intervention tailored and targeted to a specific audience segment. The marketing mix is used to produce the desired behavioral response in the target audience.

INTEGRATION WITH THEORIES/FRAMEWORKS

Incorporating various behavioral theories can enhance social marketing throughout the development, implementation, and evaluation processes. Theoretical constructs can be used to help clarify the needs, interests, and wants of the target audience. An example of a behavioral theory that has been integrated into each of the 4 *P*s is the theory of planned behavior (e.g., value/expectancies integrated into *p*roduct and barriers into *p*rice). Other theories/ frameworks that have been used in conjunction with social marketing are operationalizing the 4 *P*s based on marketing theory, and conceptualizing the marketing message as a "minimal intervention" and focusing on recruitment to programs as central issues based on the stepped approach model. Other theories and theoretical constructs that might be used to supplement or enhance the marketing 4 *P*s include social cognitive theory and the construct of self-efficacy, the health belief model, transtheoretical model of behavior change, diffusion of innovation, communication of persuasion, and extended parallel process model.

In pursuit of a "master" theory, several of the aforementioned theories might be integrated within a social marketing perspective. When integrating a theory or theories into social marketing, the emphasis should always be on audience segmentation, the 4 *P*s, and the marketing mix. All of the social marketing constructs should be considered in all stages of the pinwheel.

EXAMPLES OF APPLICATIONS, OUTCOMES, AND REACH

Select examples of interventions are presented that exemplify the use of social marketing, as it is described above. Representative applications have been to increase breast cancer screening use of at-risk women from diverse ethnic origins; breastfeeding among women enrolled in the National Women, Infants, and Children Program; and student attendance at a university alcohol prevention program. In all cases, Stages 1 and 2, formative data collection procedures, included questionnaires, in-depth interviews, and focus groups. In addition, all programs used the 4 Ps in their assessment of demographics and psychographics (e.g., barriers, facilitative factors, knowledge, attitudes, and beliefs). Also the 4 Ps were used for Stage 3 in developing materials, which were pretested for the identified specific audience segments. Stage 4, implementation, occurred according to the pretesting results. Stages 5 and 6 should involve appropriate assessments of efficacy and program refinement.

A detailed heuristic illustration of application of social marketing using the six stages is provided related to promoting breast cancer screening services. Stage 1 involved a literature review to identify the target audience and data collection needs and methods. Qualitative and quantitative data were used to identify women's perceptions about mammography. These data were used to segment the audience to target older, low-income women and to identify benefits and costs of using mammography screening and channels and spokespersons for promotion. Behavioral objectives for audience segments were written. Meetings were held with community informants to develop a marketing plan based on the 4 Ps.

Results of Stage 2 identified female physicians and breast cancer survivors as spokespersons for all promotional materials. A mix of channels was considered that included television, radio, educational pamphlets, posters, and discount coupons. Television was used to create the program's image, and radio was used to provide more detailed information about the need for screening and how to access services. All materials emphasized annual mammograms, early detection, and serenity.

Stage 3 resulted in colorful materials depicting women 50 years and older representing diverse backgrounds. Materials were pretested in three pilot sites. Two of three themes, annual mammography and serenity, were considered to have the most potential impact. Stage 4 introduced the program in three sites. Process evaluation was suggested to include tracking the number of phone calls, collecting demographic data of telephone inquirers, and field notes to document compliance and barriers to implementing the program. Stage 5 was suggested as the number of women who scheduled a mammogram, were satisfied with the program, and intended to schedule future mammograms. Stage 6 was not reported but would include examining process data to improve the program and its implementation.

The reach of social marketing is both national and international. Academies, agencies, organizations, and institutions throughout the world use social marketing. For example, social marketing is used by the National Cancer Institute (http://www.nci.nih.gov/); National Heart, Lung, and Blood Institute (http://www.nhlbi.nih.gov/health/prof/heart/other/whhw.pdf; World Health Organization (http://www. who.int/en/); Population Services International (www.psiwash.org); Centers for Disease Control and Prevention (http://www.cdc.gov); Health Canada (http://www.hc-sc.gc.ca/hppb/socialmarketing); and the U.S. Environmental Protection Agency (http://www.epa.gov/opcustsv/selbyppt/tsld014.htm). Examination of reach indicates use in agriculture, environment, health, and industry. Social marketing is widely used and applied to promote behavior change.

SUMMARY

Social marketing has appeal because it is comprehendible and understandable based on its origin and success in commercial marketing. Social marketing is historically recognized as a set of principles from commercial marketing that includes three basic elements and a development, implementation, and evaluation process. Social marketing uses a "bottom-up" process with guidance derived from the target audience rather than the typical "top-down" approach where others make decisions about what is needed and wanted by the target audience. Social marketing is notorious for recognizing that each person will make the ultimate decision about engaging in a behavior. Social marketing begins and ends with the target audience, the people whose behavior is to be influenced. Therefore, a thorough understanding of the needs, wants, and perceptions of the various segments of the target audience is essential.

The bottom line for judging the success of social marketing is behavior change and not satisfaction with the intervention, attitude changes, knowledge gained, and behavioral intentions unless they lead to the desired behavioral outcome. Social marketers are fanatically consumer centered and outcome oriented. Social marketers rely extensively on data and constant feedback from the target audience so they can develop insights into their needs, wants, and perceptions. These insights then lead to development of an acceptable exchange of value in which both the target audience in the social marketer satisfy their wants and needs by the exchange. Both parties must be satisfied for the exchange and social marketing to be a success in changing behaviors. Future applications of social marketing principles are encouraged to further comprehend, refine, and strengthen social marketing as a viable component of a total effort to resolve many of the health and social issues confronting society.

—*David R. Black and*
Carolyn L. Blue

See also COMMUNITY-BASED PARTICIPATORY RESEARCH; HEALTH COMMUNICATION; HEALTH LITERACY; HEALTH PROMOTION AND DISEASE PREVENTION; KEY INFORMANTS; TAILORED COMMUNICATIONS; THEORY OF REASONED ACTION

Further Reading

Andreasen, A. R. (1995). *Marketing social change: Changing behavior to promote health, social development, and the environment.* San Francisco: Jossey-Bass.

Kotler, P., Roberto, N., & Lee, N. (2002). *Social marketing: Improving the quality of life* (2nd ed.). Thousand Oaks, CA: Sage.

National Cancer Institute. (n.d.). *Clear & simple: Developing effective print materials for low-literate readers.* Retrieved August 28, 2002, from http://oc.nci.nih.gov/services/clear_and_simple/home.htm

U.S. Department of Health and Human Services. (1989). *Making health communication programs work* (NIH Publication No. 89-1493). Office of Cancer Communications, National Cancer Institute. Rockville, MD: Author.

SOCIAL OR STATUS INCONGRUENCE

Although many of us believe ourselves and our lives to be exemplary with respect to the consistency in our thoughts and behaviors, much of human social life and belief is fraught with inconsistencies, contradictions, and contested meanings. The effects of these inconsistencies on human health have been investigated for the past 50 years. In this contribution, research on both social or status incongruence (also referred to as status inconsistency) and cultural consonance (which measures cultural incongruities) will be reviewed and summarized.

SOCIAL OR STATUS INCONGRUENCE

The hypothesis that discrepancies or inconsistencies in status might be related to health outcomes is derived from more general theories of socioeconomic differences and health. The general perspective on socioeconomic status implicit in most research derives from Max Weber's perspective on status. In this view, individuals in complex societies are ranked according to a number of criteria, including their relationship to the labor market (as assessed by occupation), their skills that can be marketed (as assessed by education), and the degree to which they are rewarded in the market for those skills (as assessed by income). Individuals can be ranked on these dimensions separately or according to some summary measure including all three. Generally speaking, the higher an individual's socioeconomic rank, the better his or her health status.

The question can be posed, however, regarding *nonvertical* dimensions of socioeconomic status. This question was first raised by Everett C. Hughes in 1944 in an article that examined how differences or discrepancies or inconsistencies in status for individuals might be problematic. Keeping in mind that he was writing before the modern civil rights movement, the ideal type that Hughes used for his analysis is instructive. He offered the case of an African American physician in the United States. On the one hand, physicians hold positions of both considerable esteem and considerable economic power. On the other hand, African Americans, as a result of systemic racism in this society, occupy a position with much lower status.

Hughes suggested that there would be considerable frustration and uncertainty in mundane social interaction for an African American physician, because at times he or she might receive the deference due the high status of physician while at others times being the object of racist interactions. This would lead to a lack of predictability in social interaction. At the same time, assuming that his or her sense of self would be significantly shaped by achievements in educational and occupational status, it would be a stressful and frustrating experience to offer one presentation of self in social interaction (i.e., the successful physician), only to have others respond in terms of a disvalued status (i.e., ethnicity).

This example summarizes the basic hypothesis regarding status incongruence. Researchers generalized Hughes's argument to include all differences along status dimensions. In other words, it was hypothesized that an individual whose occupational status was quite different from his or her educational status would experience the same uncertainties and frustrations that Hughes described. Within social epidemiological research in the 1950s and 1960s, especially in sociology but also in epidemiology, researchers examined closely the relationship between inconsistencies in status (along the traditional dimensions of socioeconomic status) and various health outcomes. These included studies of mental health, rheumatoid arthritis, overall mortality, and especially, coronary artery disease (see Vernon & Buffler, 1988).

Generally speaking, status incongruence was found to be associated with an increased risk of adverse health outcomes. Also during this time, the term *status inconsistency* was proposed to apply to intraindividual discrepancies in status (e.g., the PhD who sells shoes for a living), while the term *status incongruence* was proposed to apply to discrepancies in status within a family unit, especially between husbands and wives (e.g., the PhD married to an auto mechanic). A number of studies showed that these interindividual discrepancies in status between husbands and wives in the United States were associated with adverse health outcomes. Although this terminology was proposed and an understanding of the literature requires that the variety of uses of terms be understood, in this entry the term status incongruence will be used to refer to the intraindividual concept.

Despite the theoretical and empirical yield of the idea of status incongruence, research on the topic in sociology and social epidemiology slowed considerably in the late 1960s and early 1970s, as a result of a series of papers by Hubert M. Blalock (summarized in Whitt, 1983). Status incongruence had typically been operationalized as some kind of difference term, indicating the degree of difference on a status dimension for an individual. Sometimes this was a directional term, that is, the degree to which one dimension exceeded another. At other times no direction was indicated, that is, the absolute difference between the status dimensions was calculated.

In either case, status incongruence would be used as a variable without reference to an individual's overall socioeconomic status. Blalock argued quite persuasively that examining the discrepancies in status made sense only after the vertical effects of status had been taken into account. In other words, since overall socioeconomic status was known to influence health, examining nonvertical effects made sense only after the vertical effects had been removed. What became apparent, however, was that there was no valid statistical procedure for separating vertical and nonvertical effects *in a single model*; that is, an effect of the vertical dimension and an effect of the nonvertical dimension could not be simultaneously estimated. In all existing research on status incongruence, the effect attributed to status incongruence could have been merely typical socioeconomic status effects masquerading as a discrepancy effect.

While Blalock's critique slowed research on status incongruence in some fields of study, the basic theoretical sense of the concept continued to guide research in other areas. In anthropology in the 1950s and 1960s, a great deal of research was taking place on acculturation (or the degree to which individuals in traditional societies adopted beliefs and behaviors introduced from other, usually more modernized, societies) and health. Mostly these were linear models suggesting that the greater the degree of acculturation, the greater the stress and risk of adverse health outcomes (see Dressler, 1999, for a review). There were several papers, however, that suggested a status incongruence effect. One of the major changes occurring in any community undergoing culture change is a shift in material lifestyles. Higher status comes to be associated with the ability to consume material goods associated with middle-class lifestyles in Europe and North America. Several authors suggested, although did not test directly, the idea that the attempt to satisfy these material aspirations could be stressful if individuals did not have resources (which might include access to paid employment or education qualifications) to make possible the acquisition of that lifestyle.

These ideas from anthropology were then integrated with the status incongruence hypothesis in a series of studies (Dressler, 1993). The association of higher status with the ability to attain a middle-class material lifestyle (which includes the acquisition of consumer goods such as manufactured furniture, appliances, and stereos as well as behaviors such as watching television, traveling, and reading books and magazines) appears to occur in virtually all societies undergoing modernization or culture change. Changing dimensions of status are not particularly problematic, except that these changes can occur much more rapidly than the economic expansion necessary to provide the access to the paid employment, which, in turn, makes possible the acquisition and maintenance of such a lifestyle. Therefore, virtually by definition, there will be individuals aspiring to such a lifestyle whose economic resources are not congruent with that lifestyle. This is an explicit directional hypothesis, in which the degree to which lifestyle aspirations exceed economic resources is thought to be stressful, but not the reverse.

At about the same time, a methodological solution to the dilemma posed by Blalock in the testing of discrepancy effects appeared in the literature. It was shown that if one assumed that the vertical dimension of status could be estimated using a sum of the separate status variables, then it was possible to estimate a discrepancy effect (Whitt, 1983). One could have, in essence, two variables: the sum of two status dimensions that operationalized the overall vertical effect, and a signed difference between two status dimensions estimating the discrepancy effect. Using this model, effects of what was referred to as "lifestyle incongruity" were found on arterial blood pressure in St. Lucia, Mexico, Brazil, and the African American community in the rural southern United States, as well as on depressive symptoms in the African American community and on disordered glucose metabolism among the Mississippi Choctaw.

Furthermore, the effect turned out not to be a simple matter of economic stresses, although that certainly would be a part of it. But where perceived economic stress was directly measured and controlled for, lifestyle incongruity continued to have an independent effect on health. Furthermore, the effect of lifestyle incongruity was moderated by the perceived availability of social support. This led to the argument that in fact the genesis of the stress associated with incongruities in status was probably in social interaction. Like Hughes's Black physician, an individual aspiring to a higher material lifestyle would be in essence projecting a sense of self into mundane social interaction, a self perception involving one's belief in one's ability to participate in what is basically a

middle-class lifestyle; however, others may respond in mundane social interaction less in terms of status defined by a mutable lifestyle, and more in terms of more fixed status characteristics like occupational or educational status. The person with high status incongruence, then, may fail to receive confirmation of his or her self perception in mundane social interaction, the result being frustration, stress, and ultimately, poorer health outcomes.

The lifestyle incongruity hypothesis has been replicated by a number of researchers in a variety of settings, including studies of blood pressure and mental health in adults, and of cell-mediated immune status in adolescents. These studies have also found that the effects of lifestyle incongruity can be moderated by a number of factors, including household structure, social support, and community characteristics.

One aspect of this research worth noting is that the anthropological studies have moved away from using the conventional status dimensions of survey sociology in favor of the measurement of status in terms more ethnographically authentic. That is, while the importance of the traditional dimensions of status is without question in influencing one's life chances, measures of status such as lifestyle capture the way that status is performed in mundane social interaction.

CULTURAL CONSONANCE

Incongruence along other dimensions has been explored as well. Cassel, Patrick, and Jenkins (1960) some years ago offered what they called the "cultural incongruity" hypothesis. They were particularly interested in what happened to migrants from rural areas to urban areas, although the same reasoning can be applied to culture change occurring within any community. They offered the following hypothesis: The migrant to a novel setting carries with her a particular understanding of how the world works, in every sense (i.e., what it means to work, how marriages are constituted, how families treat themselves and their neighbors, how to worship—everything). She is confronted, however, with a system for which her understanding may not work. The novel and dominant culture of the new setting must be learned for everyone else's behavior to be understood, and indeed for her to behave in ways that are understandable to others. She must, in other words, adapt to the new setting. Even if she is successful, such adaptation can be stressful and costly, and the cost of adaptation is written on the body in terms of what we call health. Cassel et al. argued that the less successfully the migrant culturally adapts to the new setting, the higher her risk of disease.

Unfortunately, Cassel and his associates had neither the theoretical nor the methodological tools to move this research forward. Recently, however, methods have been developed to make it possible to test these ideas directly. These studies employ the concept of "cultural consonance" to describe the discrepancy between an individual's behavior within some cultural domain, and the behaviors that are culturally valorized within that domain (Dressler & Bindon, 2000). The measurement of these factors has been made possible by the development of procedures that can be used to determine when in fact there are strongly shared (and hence cultural) models of appropriate beliefs and behaviors in some domain of culture. Then, the degree to which individuals deviate from that shared model can be measured using epidemiological survey techniques. In research both in the United States and in Brazil, it has been shown that there are indeed broadly shared cultural models both of valued lifestyles and of preferred patterns of access to social support. A higher degree of consonance or congruence with the culturally valued models for individuals is associated with lower levels of perceived stress, depressive symptoms, and arterial blood pressure. Furthermore, all of these associations are independent of conventional measures of socioeconomic status and social integration.

The cultural consonance hypothesis is again consistent with the basic ideas that Hughes proposed more than a half century ago. Conventional expectations regarding how life is to be lived are encoded in mental representations that we call cultural models. Many of these cultural models are widely shared, some are highly contested. Where they are widely shared, there are expectations, stemming both from the individual, regarding himself or herself, and from others in the social field, regarding the appropriate range of behaviors for any given individual. When, usually as a result of restricted access to economic resources, an individual is unable to act on these widely shared expectations regarding behavior, he or she is likely to experience frustration, uncertainty in social interaction, and a general sense that life lacks coherence. This can be a profoundly stressful experience that, when continued over a long period of time, can lead to poor health.

SUMMARY

The status incongruence hypothesis and the cultural congruity hypothesis have been extremely productive with respect to research in social epidemiology. Similarly, there is recent evidence that cultural consonance can be associated with health behaviors such as the decision to use health promotion/disease prevention services and level of participation in treatment support groups for chronic disease. Future studies should explore the broader health implications of these inconsistencies and uncertainties in the social and cultural dimensions of everyday life.

—*William W. Dressler*

See also Cultural Factors and Health; Ecosocial Theory; Health Disparities; Income Inequality and Health; Neighborhood Effects on Health and Behavior; Social Integration, Social Networks, and Health; Socioeconomic Status and Health; Stress, Appraisal, and Coping

Further Reading

Cassel, J. C., Patrick, R., & Jenkins, C. D. (1960). Epidemiological analysis of the health implications of culture change. *Annals of the New York Academy of Sciences, 84*, 938-949.

Dressler, W. W. (1993). Social and cultural dimensions of hypertension in Blacks: Underlying mechanisms. In J. G. Douglas & J. C. S. Fray (Eds.), *Pathophysiology of hypertension in Blacks* (pp. 69-89). New York: Oxford University Press.

Dressler, W. W. (1999). Modernization, stress and blood pressure: New directions in research. *Human Biology, 71*, 583-605.

Dressler, W. W., & Bindon, J. R. (2000). The health consequences of cultural consonance: Cultural dimensions of lifestyle, social support and arterial blood pressure in an African American community. *American Anthropologist, 102*, 244-260.

Hughes, E. C. (1944). Dilemmas and contradictions of status. *American Journal of Sociology, 50*, 353-359.

Vernon, S. W., & Buffler, P. A. (1988). The status of status inconsistency. *Epidemiologic Reviews, 10*, 65-86.

Whitt, H. P. (1983). Status inconsistency: A body of negative evidence or a statistical artifact? *Social Forces, 62*, 201-233.

SOCIAL SUPPORT AND HEALTH.
See SOCIAL INTEGRATION, SOCIAL NETWORKS, AND HEALTH

SOCIOECONOMIC STATUS AND HEALTH

Socioeconomic status (SES), traditionally assessed by income, education, and occupation, reflects individuals' material and social resources. Various theories of social stratification emphasize different aspects of SES and suggest different types of measurement. However, virtually all measures of SES are related to morbidity and mortality, suggesting that SES is a pervasive and robust influence on health.

WHAT IS THE ASSOCIATION OF SES AND HEALTH?

In industrialized countries, SES is related to health at all levels of the socioeconomic hierarchy. It is not simply that those in poverty experience poorer health than those with more income; even individuals well above the poverty level have poorer health than those who are relatively more affluent. At an individual level, the health burden of socioeconomic disadvantage is most acute for the very poorest. At a population level, because a far greater proportion of people are in the middle of the SES distribution than at the extremes, a substantial proportion of health effects related to socioeconomic factors are occurring to those who are not in extreme poverty. Although the association of SES and health extends up to the top of the SES hierarchy, for some health outcomes (e.g., infant mortality), the association is stronger at the bottom than at the top. Thus, while health benefits still accrue as SES improves up to the very top, the marginal benefits of higher SES may diminish at upper levels.

The monotonic relationship of SES and health has been demonstrated with each of the main components of SES. With regard to occupation, the Whitehall studies of British civil servants found that higher occupational grade was associated with lower mortality, not only comparing the lowest-grade civil servants to the highest but also comparing midlevel civil servants to those at the highest levels (Marmot et al., 1991). As noted above, studies of income also reveal lower mortality as income increases, although there is a steeper drop in mortality

associated with increasing income among those with the least income (Adler et al., 1994). Benefits of education also accrue to health not simply from high school graduation but also from college graduation and from graduate degrees (Elo & Preston, 1996), although these benefits may not be equally enjoyed by men and by women and by all racial/ethnic groups.

Given the association of SES with mortality, it is not surprising that SES is also related to morbidity. Incidence and prevalence of most diseases increase as SES decreases. The association is especially strong for cardiovascular disease, arthritis, diabetes, chronic respiratory diseases, and cervical cancer (Adler & Ostrove, 1999). Incidence of mental diseases is also greater among lower-SES populations (Kessler et al., 1994). Among the mental diseases, SES is most closely associated with schizophrenia, substance use, and anxiety disorders. There are a few diseases that show the opposite pattern and are more common among higher-SES individuals. Most notable are breast cancer and malignant melanoma. These associations are partially accounted for by SES-related differences in risk-related behaviors: delayed childbearing with regard to breast cancer and recreational tanning with regard to melanoma.

WHAT ACCOUNTS FOR THE ASSOCIATION OF SES AND HEALTH?

There is no single factor accounting for the association of SES and health. Several pathways have been identified as summarized below.

Physical conditions. Lower-SES individuals are subject to a range of health-damaging conditions. Less affluent populations have greater exposure to adverse living conditions including crowding, poor sanitation, peeling lead paint, substandard housing, proximity to dumpsites, and greater air pollution (Evans & Kantrowitz, 2002). The environmental justice movement has raised awareness of such differential exposure. Environmental justice has been adopted by government agencies, including the Environmental Protection Agency, and has led to policy and zoning reform to ensure a more equal burden of environmental risk.

Physical exposures also occur in the workplace. Lower-SES occupations more often involve manual labor that may place workers at risk for injury and involve greater exposure to toxins. Material conditions, such as car and house ownership, have also been linked to better health and appear to make an independent contribution to morbidity and mortality above and beyond the standard SES measures (Macintyre, Ellaway, Der, Ford, & Hunt, 1998).

Access to health care. Those who are poorer, unemployed, and less educated are less likely to have access to high-quality health care. In the United States, private health insurance is tied to employment, and a substantial segment of the population is uninsured. The uninsured have less access to preventive services, screening and early diagnosis, and high-quality care (Committee on the Consequences of Uninsurance, 2002). Even among those who have access to the same system of health care (e.g., members of health maintenance organizations [HMOs]), lower SES continues to be linked to poorer health outcomes. Knowledge of how to utilize the health system to get higher-quality care (which is likely to be greater among those with more education) may play a role in this association. However, it may also be due to conditions outside of the health care system linked to SES that are affecting outcomes.

Health behaviors. Health behaviors are estimated to be responsible for over 40% of premature mortality (McGinnis, Williams-Russo, & Knickman, 2002). Behaviors that are most responsible for premature mortality are smoking, sedentary lifestyle, diet, sexual risk behaviors, and substance use. Rates of these health-risking behaviors increase the lower one's income, education, and/or occupational status. For example, 52% of men with less than a high school education smoke cigarettes compared to 43% of high school graduates and 29% of college graduates (National Center for Health Statistics, 1998).

In addition to behavioral contributions to the onset of disease, SES-related behaviors may affect the course of disease. Treatment for many diseases and conditions requires close adherence to prescribed regimens. For example, the course of diabetes is greatly affected by dietary intake and monitoring of blood glucose. Diabetics with less education have been found to show poorer adherence, and differences in adherence largely account for the association of education and course of disease. Similar findings emerge with regard to adherence to antiretroviral therapy among HIV-positive patients (Goldman & Smith, 2002).

Psychosocial responses. Higher SES is associated with greater protection from adverse health effects of stress. Both acute and chronic stress are reported more frequently among those lower on the SES hierarchy.

Possessing more resources, whether from higher education, income, or occupational status, may help people avoid situations that are stressful and also help them cope more effectively with those that they do encounter. It is easier to engage in active coping strategies, which are generally associated with better health, when one has more resources with which to address threatening situations. The wear-and-tear on the body of responding to more frequent and chronic exposures to stress heighten the risk of dysregulation of the HPA axis, which is central to the stress response and to the development of disease (McEwen, 2002).

More threatening and adverse environments associated with lower SES may engender psychological responses that increase the risk of disease. Hostility, anger, optimism/pessimism, sense of control, and social support, all of which are associated with disease risk, are also related to SES. Though few studies have directly tested whether these psychological variables mediate the impact of SES on disease, there are numerous studies showing that they are related, on the one hand, to SES and, on the other hand, to disease risk (Gallo & Matthews, 2003).

Health affects SES. While the predominant causal direction appears to be from SES to health, health may also affect SES. Individuals who are in poorer health may be less likely to achieve higher SES status. Children from poorer families are reported by their parents to have worse health (Case & Paxson, 2002). Poorer health in childhood can contribute to missed school and lower achievement. The impact of health on educational attainment is likely to be greatest from diseases that have their onset during childhood and adolescence (e.g., asthma, schizophrenia). In later life, those who become ill may be less likely to be able to work, affecting their income and occupational status (Smith, 1999).

HOW DOES SES RELATE TO RACE/ETHNICITY AND GENDER?

People of color in the United States generally have poorer health status than do White European Americans. For example, compared to Whites, African Americans have poorer overall health and higher rates of HIV/AIDS, diabetes, heart disease, cancer, and stroke (Williams, 1999). For some conditions, racial/ethnic group differences become nonsignificant once socioeconomic factors (e.g., income) are controlled for. For other conditions, racial/ethnic group differences remain even after controlling for SES.

These findings suggest that to some extent racial/ethnic health disparities are due to socioeconomic disadvantage but that unique experiences associated with minority status (e.g., experiences of discrimination, residential segregation) also play a role.

Associations of SES with health differ by gender as well as by race and ethnicity. The meaning of a given SES indicator may vary for men versus women and for Whites versus people of color, suggesting the importance of looking at SES influences on health within each group.

—*Nancy E. Adler*

See also CULTURAL FACTORS AND HEALTH; ECOSOCIAL THEORY; HEALTH DISPARITIES; INCOME INEQUALITY AND HEALTH; NEIGHBORHOOD EFFECTS ON HEALTH AND BEHAVIOR; SOCIAL INTEGRATION, SOCIAL NETWORKS, AND HEALTH; SOCIAL OR STATUS INCONGRUENCE

Further Reading

Adler, N. E., Boyce, T., Chesney, M., Cohen, S., Folkman, S., Kahn, R., & Syme, L. (1994). Socioeconomic status and health: The challenge of the gradient. *American Psychologist, 49*, 15-24.

Adler, N. E., & Ostrove, J. M. (1999). SES and health: What we know and what we don't. *Annals of the New York Academy of Sciences, 896*, 3-15.

Case, A., & Paxson, C. (2002). Parental behavior and child health. *Health Affairs, 21*(2), 164-178.

Committee on the Consequences of Uninsurance, Board on Health Care Services. (2002). *Care without courage: Too little, too late.* IOM report. Washington, DC: National Academy Press.

Elo, I. T., & Preston, S. H. (1996). Educational differentials in mortality: United States, 1979-85. *Social Science and Medicine, 42*(1), 47-57.

Evans, G. W., & Kantrowitz, E. (2002). Socioeconomic status and health: The potential role of environmental risk exposure. *Annual Review of Public Health, 23*, 303-331.

Gallo, L. C., & Matthews, K. A. (2003). Understanding the association between socioeconomic status and physical health: Do negative emotions play a role? *Psychological Bulletin, 129*(1), 10-51.

Goldman, D. P., & Smith, J. P. (2002). Can patient self-management help explain the SES health gradient? *Proceedings of the National Academy of Sciences of the United States of America, 99*(16), 10929-10934.

Kessler, R. C., McGonagle, K. A., Zhao, S., Nelson, C. B., Hughes, M., Eshelman, S., Wittchen, H. U., & Kendler, K. S. (1994). Lifetime and 12-month prevalence of *DSM-III-R:* Psychiatric disorders in the United States. *Archives of General Psychiatry, 51*, 8-19.

Macintyre, S., Ellaway, A., Der, G., Ford, G., & Hunt, K. (1998). Do housing tenure and car access predict health because they are simply markers of income or self-esteem? A Scottish study. *Journal of Epidemiology and Community Health, 52*, 657-664.

Marmot, M. G., Davey Smith, G., Stansfeld, S., Patel, C., North, F., Head, J., White, I., Brunner, E., & Feeney, A. (1991). Health inequalities among British civil servants: The Whitehall II Study. *Lancet, 337*, 1387-1393.

McEwen, B. S. (2002). Research to understand the mechanisms through which social and behavioral factors influence health. In L. F. Berkman (Ed.), *Through the kaleidoscope: Viewing the contributions of the behavioral and social sciences to health* (pp. 31-35). Washington, DC: National Academy Press.

McGinnis, J. M., Williams-Russo, P., & Knickman, J. R. (2002). The case for more active policy attention to health promotion. *Health Affairs, 21*(2), 78-93.

National Center for Health Statistics. (1998). *Health, United States.* Retrieved from www1.oecd.org/std/others1.html

Ostrove, J. M., & Adler, N. E. (1998). Socioeconomic status and health. *Current Opinion in Psychiatry, 11*, 649-653.

Smith, J. (1999). Healthy bodies and thick wallets: The dual relationship between health and socioeconomic status. *Journal of Economic Perspectives*, pp. 145-166.

Williams, D. R. (1999). Race, socioeconomic status, and health: The added effects of racism and discrimination. In N. E. Adler, M. Marmot, B. S. McEwen, & J. Stewart (Eds.), *Socioeconomic status and health in industrial nations: Social, psychological, and biological pathways* (Vol. 896, pp. 173-188). New York: New York Academy of Sciences.

SPIRITUALITY AND HEALTH

For thousands of years, spirituality and health have been closely allied with each other, in concept and in practice. Historically, treatment was administered by religious and spiritual healers. However, with the Age of Enlightenment and the advent of modern medicine, diagnosis and treatment were separated from their spiritual context. Despite this initial separation between health and spirituality, in recent years, a rapprochement has been taking place. Empirical studies are revealing significant links between spirituality and health. And religious/spiritual and health care communities have begun to join forces in the prevention and treatment of illness and the promotion of health and well-being.

THE MEANING OF SPIRITUALITY

The term *spirituality* comes from the word *spirit* (to breathe). Although there is a lack of consensus about its precise meaning, there is general agreement that spirituality is a living, dynamic process that is oriented around whatever the individual may hold sacred. The sacred refers to concepts of God, the divine, and transcendence as well as other aspects of life that take on spiritual character and significance by virtue of their association with the divine. Thus, the sacred can also include material objects (e.g., crucifix), special times (e.g., the Sabbath), special places (e.g., cathedral), relationships (e.g., marriage), and psychological attributes (e.g., soul). Spirituality refers to the attempt to discover the sacred, hold on to the sacred, and, when necessary, transform the sacred.

In their search for the sacred, people may take a variety of spiritual pathways. These paths include traditional or nontraditional organized religious beliefs (e.g., God, afterlife, karma), practices (e.g., prayer, meditation, rituals), experiences (e.g., mysticism, conversion), and institutions (e.g., church attendance, Bible study). Pathways to the sacred may also take nonreligious forms, such as walking in the outdoors, listening to music, intimate relations with others, or participating in social action. The richness and complexity of spirituality is a reflection of the many different ways people can define the sacred in their lives and the many different pathways they can follow to discover and rediscover the sacred.

EMPIRICAL LINKS BETWEEN SPIRITUALITY AND HEALTH

A substantial body of research has examined the relationships between various dimensions of spirituality and health. Studies have shown that both organizational forms of spirituality (e.g., church attendance, religious affiliation) and more private expressions of spirituality (e.g., personal spiritual practices and beliefs, spiritual coping) are related to a variety of health dimensions. Despite the different methodologies used to examine the relationships among these complex constructs, in general, empirical studies

demonstrate that spirituality appears to have beneficial consequences with respect to physical and mental health.

A number of studies have found that greater frequency of attendance at religious services is associated with better health. For example, more frequent worship attendance has been tied to a lower risk of drug and alcohol abuse, sexual promiscuity, and suicidality. Moreover, greater frequency of worship attendance is predictive of a lower risk of mortality even after controlling for relevant demographic, health practice, and other potentially confounding variables. That is, people who attend religious services more frequently have a lower risk of dying, after accounting for other potentially relevant variables, such as age, gender, socioeconomic status, diet, and exercise. Thus, organized forms of spirituality appear to be associated with better health.

More private expressions of spirituality also have important implications for health. For example, personal spiritual practices such as prayer and meditation have typically been linked with better health. Prayer involves an attempt to commune with a supernatural, transcendent, divine presence. People who pray more frequently and describe mystical and positive religious experiences during prayer also report greater feelings of subjective well-being, such as purpose in life, general life satisfaction, and existential well-being. Furthermore, in some studies employing experimental designs using randomized control trials, prayer has demonstrated positive effects on health by reducing chronic pain, muscle tension, anger, and anxiety. Similarly, meditation, clearing the mind, and focusing on one thought as an approach toward transcendental consciousness has been associated with lower levels of anxiety, hostility, depression, and dysphoria and higher levels of positive affect and self-actualization. In intervention studies, people who employ meditation techniques show reduced rates of metabolism. Meditation has also been proven to be an effective treatment for alcoholism, smoking, and illicit drug use.

Spiritual beliefs are another personal form of spiritual expression that have been associated with health benefits. Empirical studies have linked the belief in an afterlife to less depression and death anxiety, lower risk of suicide, and greater recovery from bereavement. Similarly, the belief in a loving God shows generalized health benefits and appears to be particularly valuable to people dealing with specific stressful situations. Among people facing a variety of major life stressors, religious coping methods that reflect a perceived closeness to God have been associated with better self-rated health and better psychological adjustment. Thus, the belief in a loving God appears to promote health in general and in response to specific stressful situations.

Despite the apparent benefits of spirituality for health, certain aspects of spirituality, such as spiritual struggles, may be a source of considerable strain and distress. Spiritual struggles represent efforts to conserve or transform a spirituality that has been threatened or damaged. Examples of spiritual struggles include anger at God, difficulty forgiving God, feelings of alienation or punishment from God, interpersonal religious conflicts and discontent with family, congregation members, and clergy, and religious doubts, fear, or guilt. Although spirituality generally serves as a protective resource for many people, a growing number of studies demonstrate that spiritual struggles are not uncommon among diverse groups, including medically ill elderly patients, mental health outpatients, college students, adolescents, and people undergoing a variety of life stressors.

Empirical studies have shown that spiritual struggles typically have negative implications for health. For example, various types of spiritual struggles have been associated with psychological distress, anxiety, depression, lower self-esteem, trait anger, posttraumatic stress disorder symptoms, callousness, poorer mental health, and less happiness and life satisfaction. In longitudinal studies, spiritual struggles with the divine have been predictive of poorer recovery among rehabilitation patients and greater risk of mortality among medically ill elderly patients, even after controlling for other potentially important confounding variables.

EXPLANATIONS FOR THE LINKS BETWEEN SPIRITUALITY AND HEALTH

Science, with its reliance upon direct observation of behavior, cannot determine whether God exists and intervenes in human affairs to promote health and well-being. However, scholars have offered a variety of plausible worldly explanations for the relationship between spirituality and health. One explanation for the beneficial relationship is that spirituality operates through physiological mechanisms. For example, it has been suggested that spirituality may promote health through the relaxation response. The relaxation response is a self-induced altered state of consciousness that results in an integrated hypothalamic function, increased plasma noradrenaline levels, and generalized decreased sympathetic nervous system activity. Various spiritual practices (e.g., prayer, meditation) may induce the relaxation response. Preliminary research also suggests that spirituality may affect health through changes in immunological functioning. For example, certain spiritual practices and beliefs have been associated with lower serum cortisol levels and better immune functions among samples of the elderly and persons who are HIV-positive or have AIDS.

Another explanation for the salutary function of spirituality is that spirituality encourages healthy behaviors. For example, a number of empirical studies have demonstrated that people who are more religious are less likely to smoke cigarettes, abuse alcohol and drugs, engage in premarital sex, have multiple sexual partners or extramarital affairs, engage in crime and delinquency, and more likely to wear seat belts. Thus, spirituality may promote health by discouraging risky behaviors and encouraging healthy behaviors.

Psychological explanations have also been offered to account for the relationship between spirituality and health. Spirituality offers meaning, direction, and a sense of coherence. Furthermore, when negative life events are experienced, spirituality enables people to appraise negative events from a different vantage point. Crises become an opportunity for growth, transformation, or intimacy with God. In this regard, spirituality provides hope and may serve as a buffer for negative emotions. Similarly, spirituality may serve as a catalyst for positive emotions. For example, spirituality may enhance feelings of self-esteem and empowerment as people associate themselves with an all-loving, omnipotent God who cares for them and loves them unconditionally.

Scholars have also suggested that spirituality affects health through social means. For example, spirituality offers tangible social support, such as access to information, goods, and services. In addition, spirituality and religious involvement provide various opportunities for companionship and friendship, emotional support, a sense of connectedness, and intimacy. Interpersonal relationships based upon shared religious values and beliefs may lead to a strong sense of affirmation and a secure attachment to others. Thus, spirituality may promote health by enhancing both the quantity and quality of social resources available to people.

Despite the compelling character of such worldly explanations, as yet, empirical studies have not been able to fully account for the links between spirituality and health through physiological, behavioral, psychological, and social means. The possibility remains that there is something distinctive or unique about spirituality that exerts special effects on health. For example, spiritual coping methods (e.g., spiritual support from God, positive spiritual appraisals, spiritual discontent) may offer unique ways of understanding and dealing with life stressors. And psychospiritual virtues (e.g., forgiveness, gratitude, humility), grounded in spiritual values and worldviews, may create healthy attitudes toward oneself and the world that relate, in turn, to healthy lifestyles.

While reasonable explanations have been offered for the beneficial relationship between spirituality and health, the explanation for the harmful roles of spirituality are less clear. It is possible that harmful forms of spirituality may also exert their deleterious effects through physiological, behavioral, psychological, social, and distinctly spiritual means. For example, harmful forms of spirituality may compromise immunological functioning. Particular spiritual beliefs or practices may discourage people from seeking necessary health care or complying with medical treatment recommendations. Religious doubts, fear, and guilt may elicit negative emotions. Interpersonal religious conflicts or discontent with family, clergy, or congregations may result in social alienation. And anger at God, difficulty forgiving God, feelings of alienation or punishment from God, or spiritual discontent may result in a loss of purpose, meaning, or sense of coherence. With more sophisticated empirical studies, explanations for the potentially harmful roles of spirituality will become clearer.

SPIRITUALLY SENSITIVE PREVENTION, INTERVENTION, AND PROMOTION

For a number of years, relationships between religious and health care communities have been strained and one-sided. While religious professionals frequently refer people to the health care system, these acts are rarely reciprocated. The bifurcation between religious and health care communities is further evidenced by the relative lack of collaborative and integrated programs. There are, however, exceptions to this rule, such as 12-step programs that incorporate spirituality into treatment.

More recently, we are beginning to see some new collaborative efforts between religious and health care communities. For example, a growing number of church-based health prevention and health promotion programs have been established. Some low-cost health promotion clinics have been set up in high-access community churches. Other initiatives include church-based programs aimed at reducing cardiovascular risk through behavioral interventions, and educational and promotion programs focusing on cervical cancer, hypertension, nutrition and physical exercise, AIDS, sexuality, drug use, and mental illness. In addition to these church-based health programs, spiritually integrated forms of psychotherapy are rapidly developing. Spiritual practices (e.g., prayer and meditation) are being incorporated into treatment, spiritual issues (e.g., forgiveness, acceptance, serenity) are being addressed in psychotherapy, and behavioral treatments are being used to enhance spirituality.

Collaborative efforts between spiritual and health care communities are still in their infancy. Empirical studies are needed to demonstrate the effectiveness of these spiritually sensitive health-related programs. Nevertheless, these collaborative efforts represent important beginning steps toward the integration of modern scientific health care techniques with established spiritual beliefs and practices, and a return of prevention, diagnosis, and treatment to their original holistic context.

—*Kenneth I. Pargament
and Gene G. Ano*

Further Reading

Ellison, C. G., & Levin, J. S. (1998). The religion-health connection: Evidence, theory, and future directions. *Health Education and Behavior, 25,* 700-720.

Koenig, H. G., McCullough, M. E., & Larson, D. B. (2001). *Handbook of religion and health.* New York: Oxford University Press.

Miller, W. R. (Ed.). (1999). *Integrating spirituality into treatment: Resources for practitioners.* Washington, DC: American Psychological Association.

Pargament, K. I. (1997). *The psychology of religion and coping: Theory, research, and practice.* New York: Guilford.

Resnicow, K., Jackson, A., Wang, T., De, A. K., McCarty, F., Dudley, W. N., et al. (2001). A motivational interviewing intervention to increase fruit and vegetable intake through Black churches: Results of the Eat for Life trial. *American Journal of Public Health, 91*, 1686-1693.

STRESS, APPRAISAL, AND COPING

It is widely accepted that everyone experiences stress and that stress has deleterious effects on mental and physical health. While it is true that just about everyone experiences stress, it is not true that it always has deleterious health effects. This observation is probably as old as recorded history. Over the past 40 years, it has become the central interest of a number of psychologists working in the areas of cognitive, health, and clinical psychology.

The systematic process of developing and testing hypotheses regarding stress and its effects on health depends on having a theory. In 1966, Richard Lazarus published a landmark book, *Psychological Stress and the Coping Process*, that presented a cognitive theory of stress. This book and its successor, *Stress, Appraisal, and Coping*, published in 1984, laid the foundation for much of the research on psychological stress that has occurred since then.

At the heart of this cognitive theory of stress are two concepts—appraisal and coping—that together help explain why people vary in their judgments as to what is stressful, their emotional responses to the stress, and their coping responses. These processes are contextual; they are shaped by both the person and the environment at a given time. They are also dynamic in that both appraisal and coping change as a situation unfolds.

APPRAISAL

Appraisal is an evaluation of a situation that determines the quality and intensity of a stress response. The appraisal process helps account for differences between individuals' responses with respect to the same event, and it helps account for differences in responses within individuals over time. Stress and coping theory defines two kinds of appraisal, primary appraisal, which is the evaluation of the personal significance of a situation, and secondary appraisal, which is an evaluation of the options for coping.

Primary appraisal is influenced by the person's values, beliefs, and goals, which determine the personal significance or the meaning of a given situation. A dent in the fender of a car will be more stressful for a person who prizes that car than for a person for whom the car is merely a means of transportation. The threat of a layoff will be more stressful for a person who is the single head of a household than for a person whose income is not critical for a family's well-being.

Secondary appraisal is often cast in terms of personal control—is there something the person can do to control the situation, or is it a situation the person has to accept? This appraisal is often complex. For example, there may be something that can be done to change the outcome of a situation, but to exercise that option may cause conflict elsewhere. This is often the case when money is needed to solve a problem. The money may be needed for more than one purpose. To use it to deal with the immediate problem—say, pay a bill—may mean that another bill goes unpaid.

Together, primary and secondary appraisal determine whether the situation is perceived as stressful—as a harm or loss, a threat, or a challenge. The greater the personal significance and the less adequate the options for coping, the more intense the appraisal of harm, loss, or threat. The appraisals of harm, loss, or threat are accompanied by negatively toned emotions such as fear, anger, worry, or sadness. Challenge refers to the possibility of mastery or gain. It is included as a stress appraisal because challenge always contains the possibility of failure. It is accompanied by positively toned emotions such as eagerness and excitement, as well as negatively toned emotions such as fear.

At the most fundamental level, appraisal has adaptive significance. A failure to appraise a real danger realistically can result in great harm to the individual. Conversely, the failure to evaluate a benign situation realistically will lead to inappropriate responses that can cause difficulty.

COPING

Coping refers to the changing thoughts and behaviors that people use to manage the underlying problem and regulate the emotional response in situations that are appraised as stressful. This is a contextual definition in that coping is a response to the appraised demands—both internal and external—of the situation at hand. The definition also implies that coping is a dynamic process that changes as the appraisal of the person-environment relationship changes over time.

Furthermore, the definition makes no assumptions as to what constitutes good or bad, adaptive or maladaptive coping. A given coping strategy, such as information seeking, may be adaptive in a situation where there is time and a purpose to be served, but it may be maladaptive in a situation where a quick response is necessary. Similarly, a strategy for managing fear such as meditation may be useful when there is nothing that needs to be done immediately, but it could be maladaptive in the case where immediate action is necessary.

Dimensions

A number of coping dimensions are described in the literature, including one group that has to do with controlling the environment versus controlling oneself: primary control (controlling the environmental problem) and secondary control (controlling one's response to the problem); assimilative (altering the environment) and accommodative (altering oneself); and mastery and meaning. Another group has to do with approach and avoidance, for example, vigilance versus cognitive avoidance. Probably the most commonly used dimensions are those suggested by Lazarus and Folkman: problem-focused coping, which is used to manage underlying problems, and emotion-focused coping, which is used to manage distress.

Regardless of the ways in which they are identified, coping dimensions tend to be interdependent as a stressful encounter unfolds. For example, sometimes it is necessary to engage in emotion-focused coping before proceeding with problem-focused coping, as when a person experiences anxiety just before giving a public address and does some deep-breathing before going to the podium. Sometimes problem-focused coping is used to reduce distress, as when a person makes up a "to-do" list (a problem-focused technique) as a way of reducing anxiety about being overloaded with work. For this reason, people usually use a complex array of coping strategies over the course of an encounter. Greater emphasis is given to problem-focused, vigilant, instrumental, or approach strategies when the situation is appraised as potentially controllable. Greater emphasis is given to emotion-focused, palliative, or avoidant coping in situations that are appraised as not within the individual's personal control.

More recently, several coping researchers identified a gap in the coping literature having to do with coping strategies that are used to generate and sustain positive emotion. Interest in this type of coping was motivated by findings that people often experience positive emotions during periods of intense stress. Sometimes these emotions are the result of experiences of mastery and competence, sometimes they come from finding some kind of benefit or meaning in adversity. Concepts such as "stress-related growth," "benefit-finding and benefit reminding," and "meaning-focused coping" have entered the coping literature. The measurement of these kinds of coping promises to broaden our understanding of how individuals manage to get through very difficult times.

Measurement

A number of measures of coping have made their way into the literature. For the most part, these are self-report measures that are consistent with the conceptualization of coping as complex, contextual process involving thoughts and actions to manage problems and regulate distress. Subjects are typically asked to focus on a specific stressful event that is relevant to the research at hand. Sometimes the event was recently experienced (e.g., a layoff or an argument with a spouse), sometimes it is ongoing (e.g., preparing for an exam, waiting for a biopsy result), and sometimes it is in the form of a researcher-originated vignette. Subjects indicate the extent to which they used or are using the coping strategies listed on the checklist, such as gathering information, distracting oneself from the problem, expressing one's feelings, trying to minimize significance, or avoidance through the use of alcohol or drugs. Often factor analyses are conducted to identify specific types of coping, such as problem solving, escape avoidance, distancing, and seeking emotional support. The internal consistency of subscales of coping tends to be in the range of $a = .6–.8$, which is lower than psychologists are accustomed to seeing in established measures. The accepted reason for this level of internal consistency is that if a given strategy from a particular scale (such as problem solving) works, people are unlikely to use the other strategies from that same scale. Among the most widely used of the self-report measures are the COPE by Carver, Scheier, and Weintraub (1989), the Coping Responses Inventory by Moos (1997), and the Ways of Coping by Folkman and Lazarus (1988).

Checklist measures of coping have important limitations, including biases and distortions associated with retrospective approaches, and their inability to capture temporal ordering. New technologies that have become available facilitate the assessment of coping in real time on a daily basis. Subjects are given a general list of types of coping. For each type of coping that the subject indicated he or she used, the subject is to describe exactly what he or she did. Often this type of research is conducted with palm-held computers or personal digital assistants (PDAs).

HOW DO APPRAISAL AND COPING AFFECT HEALTH?

Stress can affect health in a number of ways. It can have a direct effect through repeated or prolonged activation of the physiological stress response. Although the physiological stress response is adaptive in the short term because it serves to mobilize energy and ready the body to respond physically to the stress (the fight-or-flight response), prolonged or repeated activation of the stress response can have a host of negative consequences including suppressed immune function, increased blood pressure, and endocrine dysregulation, which can increase risk for cardiovascular and other disorders.

Appraisal plays a role in this process because the appraisal determines whether a particular event will be seen as stressful at all (and therefore determines whether the physiological stress response will occur). Two people experiencing the same objective event may have very different physiological reactions because one appraises the situation as a threat and experience the physiological stress response, and the other appraises it as benign and there is no physiological perturbation. Effective coping can shorten the duration of the stress response, and ineffective coping can prolong it. For example, imagine two cars stuck in a traffic jam. The individual in the first car screams at the other drivers, honks her horn, makes obscene gestures, and tries to drive on the shoulder to get ahead. She is clearly trying a number of coping responses, none of which is likely to make the traffic jam resolve more quickly. The second driver calls ahead to her appointment to let them know she has been delayed and decides to take this opportunity to listen to the book on tape she's been meaning to get to. Rather than trying to exert control over the traffic jam, she focuses on things that she can do.

Although they experienced the same objective stressor, the first driver is likely to have a more costly physiological response than the second driver. If the first driver typically appraises and copes with daily stress in this way, the damage is likely to become more serious over time.

Some coping responses are, in and of themselves, health damaging or health promoting. For example, although smoking or drinking in response to stress may decrease levels of negative emotions, each can have deleterious effects on physical health in the long run. On the other hand, some individuals exercise or meditate in response to stress and these practices can have beneficial effects on health.

Health care seeking in response to a symptom is one pathway through which appraisal and coping play a role after a health problem has occurred. At about the same time that Lazarus was developing his cognitive theory of stress, Howard Leventhal independently developed an appraisal model, the "common sense model of illness representation," concerned specifically with health threats. The appraisal of a health threat revolves around five attributes of an illness representation: its identity (e.g., disease label), the time line (e.g., does the cue signal an acute, chronic, or cyclic condition), the causal attribute (e.g., does the cue occur after a heavy meal, after exercising), the controllability (e.g., its responsiveness to intervention), and the imagined consequences (e.g., personal experience, economic hardship). The same illness representations also evoke emotional responses through a parallel and associated process. The cognitive and emotional processes lead to coping responses to deal with the illness and with the distress associated with its appraisal.

—*Susan Folkman and Judith Tedlie Moskowitz*

See also CAREGIVING AND STRESS; EMOTIONS: NEGATIVE EMOTIONS AND HEALTH; JOB STRAIN AND HEALTH; STRESS-BUFFERING HYPOTHESIS; WORK-RELATED STRESS AND HEALTH

Further Reading

Affleck, G., & Tennen, H. (1996). Construing benefits from adversity. *Journal of Personality, 64,* 900-922.

Carver, C. S., Scheier, M. F., & Weintraub, J. K. (1989). Assessing coping strategies: A theoretically based approach. *Journal of Personality and Social Psychology, 56,* 267-283.

Folkman, S., & Lazarus, R. S. (1988). *The Ways of Coping.* Palo Alto, CA: Mind Garden.

Folkman, S., & Moskowitz, J. (2000). Positive affect and the other side of coping. *American Psychologist, 55,* 647-654.

Lazarus, R. S., & Folkman, S. (1984). *Stress, appraisal, and coping.* New York: Springer.

Leventhal, H., Nerenz, D. R., & Steele, D. J. (1984). Illness representations and coping with health threats. In A. Baum, S. E. Taylor, & J. E. Singer (Eds.), *Handbook of psychology and health* (pp. 219-252). Hillsdale, NJ: Lawrence Erlbaum.

Moos, R. H. (1997). Coping Responses Inventory. In C. P. Zalaquett & R. J. Wood (Eds.), *Evaluating stress: A book of resources* (pp. 51-65). Lanham, MD: Scarecrow.

Taylor, S. E., & Brown, J. D. (1994). Positive illusions and well-being revisited: Separating fact from fiction. *Psychological Bulletin, 116,* 21-27.

Tedeschi, R. G., Park, C. L., & Calhoun, L. G. (Eds.). (1998). *Posttraumatic growth: Positive changes in the aftermath of crisis.* Mahwah, NJ: Lawrence Erlbaum.

Tennen, H., Affleck, G., Urrows, S., Higgins, P., & Mendola, R. (1992). Perceiving control, construing benefits, and daily processes in rheumatoid arthritis. *Canadian Journal of Behavioral Science, 242,* 186-203.

Zeidner, M., & Endler, N. S. (Eds.). (1996). *Handbook of coping.* New York: John Wiley.

STRESS: BIOLOGICAL ASPECTS

THE STRESS RESPONSE

The stress response refers to how the different physiological systems of the body respond to a stressor. A stressor can be either physical, such as the demands imposed on the body by the physical exertion of exercise, or psychological or mental, such as the stress we may experience in our day-to-day lives. These include a student taking an exam, meeting work deadlines, and being stuck in traffic; even winning a lottery ticket can be experienced by some people as a stressor. It is important to keep in mind that not all people experience the same event as stressful. That is, it is more our reaction that determines whether it is stressful rather than any necessarily inherent nature of the event or experience itself.

The stress response as we know it is rooted in an ancient part of our body's physiological responses known as the fight-or-flight response. In this sense, the response first evolved as a mechanism for survival.

It is only when this same response is turned on chronically that it can exert deleterious effects on our physical and mental health.

This section reviews how the major physiological systems of the body are affected by acute and chronic stress.

Nervous System

The brain regulates body functions at all times. The hypothalamic-pituitary-adrenal axis together with the autonomic nervous system controls the stress response. The hypothalamic-pituitary-adrenal axis consists of the hypothalamus (base of the brain), pituitary gland (below the hypothalamus), and adrenal gland (over the kidneys). The hypothalamus releases corticotropin-releasing factor, which stimulates the pituitary gland to release adrenocorticotropic hormone. Adrenocorticotropic hormone in turn stimulates the adrenal gland to release steroids called glucocorticoids (e.g., cortisol). Cortisol acts as a key regulator of the body's stress response. There is a negative feedback system that regulates cortisol levels. When cortisol levels rise, a negative feedback signal to the hypothalamus inhibits further release of corticotropin-releasing hormone. This essential ability of the negative feedback system to limit the production of cortisol is impaired in individuals with a history of chronic emotional/physical stress. Excessive and sustained cortisol secretion has been linked to a host of diseases such as hypertension, depression, and osteoporosis.

The autonomic nervous system is the other part of the nervous system that controls the stress response. The autonomic nervous system consists of two components, a sympathetic nervous system and a parasympathetic nervous system. The two systems work in opposition whereby the activation of one is accompanied by the suppression of the other. The sympathetic nervous system is activated during stress and mediates the fight-or-flight response in which two chemical messengers, epinephrine and norepinephrine, are released from the nerve endings and from the adrenal glands.

What happens to our different body systems during stress is mainly, but not exclusively, regulated by epinephrine, norepinephrine, and glucocorticoids. It is now known that chronic stress may be a precipitating or at least an aggravating factor in many diseases through its effects on different biological systems as is outlined below.

Metabolism

In response to stress, a mobilization of energy is necessary to deliver nutrients to the muscles that need it the most. Repeated or continuous activation of this system causes depletion of energy stores and increased fatigue, as a simple first consequence. A more drastic consequence of continuous activation may be diabetes mellitus, a disease characterized by an elevation of blood sugar levels. Hormones of the stress response cause glucose and fatty acid mobilization into the bloodstream and also block insulin secretion, causing glucose to accumulate in the blood. Moreover, epinephrine, norepinephrine, and glucose act on fat cells throughout the body to make them less sensitive to insulin (i.e., insulin resistance). The elevated blood sugar levels adversely affect the eyes, kidneys, nerves, and heart. In nondiabetics, chronic stress causes elevation of blood sugar levels with an increased possibility of vascular damage. In diabetics, chronic stress can exacerbate the existing insulin resistance and further disturb metabolic control.

Cardiovascular System

In response to stress, the activation of the sympathetic nervous system leads to an increase in the rate and force of contraction of the heart accompanied by contraction of the peripheral blood vessels. This causes an increase in blood pressure. This response is designed to divert blood to the muscles that need it the most as part of the fight-or-flight response. However, in the case of repeated or chronic stressors, the increase in blood pressure increases the force with which blood moves through the blood vessels thus resulting in damage and scarring of their inner layer. Subsequently, fatty acids, glucose, platelets, and foam cells (a type of white blood cells) are deposited in the scarred inner layer of the blood vessels. This process leads to the narrowing and hardening of the blood vessels, that is, atherosclerosis.

Myocardial ischemia occurs when the blood vessels feeding the heart have become clogged by atherosclerosis. In this case, the heart itself becomes deprived of the oxygen and glucose it needs for normal functioning, and myocardial ischemia ensues. A most drastic consequence of myocardial ischemia is sudden cardiac death. Acute stress can lead to sudden cardiac death by causing ventricular fibrillation on top of an already ischemic heart.

Cardiovascular disease is the No. 1 killer in the United States today. There is certainly individual variation in the susceptibility to cardiovascular disease. Behavioral factors such as diet and exercise play a role in this individual variability. Among other behavioral factors that influence one's susceptibility to this debilitating illness is the way an individual tends to respond to stress.

Immune System

Stress, whether physical or psychological, acute or chronic, leads to major changes in the number and characteristics of the immune cells that circulate in the blood. Immune system responses to stress have been linked to different disease processes such as atherosclerosis, infectious diseases, cancer, and depression. Stress increases an individual's susceptibility to an infection mainly through its effects on lymphocytes (white blood cells that normally fight off infectious agents). Glucocorticoids secreted in response to stress cause shrinkage of the thymus gland in which lymphocytes are formed, thus decreasing the formation of lymphocytes. They also inhibit the release of certain cytokines (chemical messengers secreted by immune cells), thus causing the circulating lymphocytes to become less responsive. This is in addition to the sympathetic nervous system hormones secreted during stress, which also suppress immunity, and can lead to an increase in one's susceptibility to infections.

Accordingly, research has provided evidence for a link between psychological stress and disease progression including HIV infection. There is also accumulating evidence of a link between immune system responses to stress and tumor development and/or progression. One mechanism is through the reduction in the number or activity of natural killer cells (the immune cells that prevent tumors from spreading) that accompanies stress. The association between stress and cardiovascular disease is also mediated through an immunological pathway. The first stages of atherosclerosis are of an inflammatory nature, thus the immune system is also a link between stress and some forms of cardiovascular disease.

Gastrointestinal System

Stress effects on the gastrointestinal system may manifest in the form of peptic ulcers or functional gastrointestinal disorders such as functional dyspepsia or irritable bowel syndrome. Functional gastrointestinal disorders can be caused by changes in gastric motility due to psychological stress. Stress management techniques have been found to be effective in reducing symptoms in patients with functional dyspepsia and irritable bowel syndrome.

A more severe consequence of stress is peptic ulcer formation. The vast majority of peptic ulcers are associated with gastric *Helicobacter pylori* infections. However, only a fraction of Helicobacter pylori-infected subjects develop an ulcer. Psychological stress is an important cofactor in the process of ulcer formation through a drop in immunity, which increases the likelihood of a Helicobacter pylori infection. Stress also decreases the blood flow to the gut (blood is diverted to other muscles that need it more during stress), leading to decrease in the oxygen supply to the stomach walls. This leads to small infarcts in the stomach wall, and it is these necrotic lesions in the gut that are the building blocks for peptic ulcers. Moreover, prostaglandins normally repair small ulcers that form in the gut. However, the secretion of glucocorticoids in response to stress leads to a decrease in prostaglandin synthesis and loss of this repair ability.

In addition to the direct consequences of stress on gastric acid secretion, behavioral changes in smoking, drinking, or dietary habits that may occur in response to being under stress may also play a role in the effect of stress on peptic ulcer formation.

Reproductive System

Stress affects sexual function and fertility in both males and females. This effect is exerted primarily through a chain of events that leads to a decrease in testosterone formation in males and estrogen in females. In addition, erections in males are caused by the parasympathetic nervous system. The decreased parasympathetic nervous system activation during stress leads to sexual dysfunction such as difficult erections, impotence and premature ejaculation.

In females, the drop in reproductive hormone levels leads to loss of libido (sexual drive), irregular menstrual cycles, and in severe cases to anovulatory amenorrhea (cessation of ovulation and menstruation). Stress affects fertility in females through an increase in prolactin secretion, which interferes with progesterone activity and thus disrupts the maturation of the uterine wall and decreases the likelihood of implantation of a fertilized ovum. Moreover, the success of assisted reproductive techniques (e.g., in vitro fertilization) may also be affected by stress. It has been suggested that the rates of conception after in vitro fertilization are affected by psychological distress during the treatment cycle. Although rare, stress-induced abortion may also occur.

The increased sympathetic nervous system activation during stress causes an increase in epinephrine and norepinephrine release, and the result is a drop in blood flow through the uterus. This leads to a drop in blood pressure and heart rate in the fetus. If this scenario is repeated frequently, fetal death may occur due to hypoxia. Stress during pregnancy has also been linked to preterm birth and lower birth weight. After delivery, psychological stress may interfere with lactation. This occurs either through a decrease in milk synthesis or ejection due to stress-related inhibition of prolactin or oxytocin release or an increase in sympathetic nervous system activity.

Growth

In older adults, the increased glucocorticoids secretion that occurs in response to stress leads to a triad that increases the risk of osteoporosis. This triad consists of a blockage of the uptake of dietary calcium in the intestines, an increased excretion of calcium by the kidney, and acceleration of bone resorption.

In children, a rare condition termed *stress dwarfism* occurs due to severe emotional neglect or psychological abuse. Psychological stress in these children leads to a marked increase in glucocorticoids, which both blocks the secretion of growth hormone and decreases the sensitivity of the target cells to growth hormone. The elevated glucocorticoids also affect bone growth through the triad described above. The stunted growth in these children resumes upon removal of the stressor.

INDIVIDUAL VARIABILITY IN THE STRESS RESPONSE

Establishing the role of the mind in disease is complicated by the fact that cause-effect relationships are very hard to establish. The differences in individual responses to stress complicate this matter further. Interindividual variability in response to stress is determined by many factors including age, ethnicity, gender, coping style, psychological factors, and genetic factors, to name a few. In our modern society, stress-related diseases are on the rise. Behavioral research bears the task of continuing research on the relationship between mind and body and the subsequent effects on human health and disease.

BEHAVIORAL STRESS MANAGEMENT TECHNIQUES

On a more positive note, our responses to stress are not completely preset and out of our control. Stress management techniques teach individuals how to prevent, reduce, and cope with stress. Examples of such techniques are relaxation, hypnosis, cognitive restructuring, visualization, disclosure, conditioning, assertiveness training, biofeedback, and meditation. Stress management has been found to be successful in preventing the development of and reducing already established disease. In myocardial infarction patients, stress management was found to improve the quality of life and reduce morbidity. It has also been found to decrease blood pressure in patients with hypertension. In HIV disease, stress management training buffered illness-related psychological distress. In cancer patients, stress management intervention was found to influence immune responses of patients as well as the course of their illness.

—*Noha H. Farag and*
Paul J. Mills

See also ALLOSTATIS, ALLOSTATIC LOAD, AND STRESS;
ASTHMA AND STRESS; BLOOD PRESSURE, HYPERTENSION,
AND STRESS; CARDIOVASCULAR PSYCHOPHYSIOLOGY:
MEASURES; CARDIOVASCULAR REACTIVITY; GASTRIC
ULCERS AND STRESS; METABOLIC SYNDROME AND STRESS;
PEPTIC ULCERS AND STRESS; PSYCHONEUROIMMUNOLOGY;
PSYCHOPHYSIOLOGY: THEORY AND METHODS; WOUND
HEALING AND STRESS

Further Reading

Sapolsky, R. M. (2000). *Why zebras don't get ulcers.* New York: W. H. Freeman.

Schneiderman, N., McCabe, P., & Baum, A. (Eds.). (1992). *Perspectives in behavioral medicine: Stress and disease processes.* Hillsdale, NJ: Lawrence Erlbaum.

Turner, J. R., Sherwood, A., & Light, K. C. (Eds.). (1992). *Individual differences in cardiovascular response to stress.* New York: Plenum.

STRESS–BUFFERING HYPOTHESIS

Acute or chronic stressful experiences such as illness, life events, and developmental transitions often impose demands that we are unable to address. Such experiences are thought to put people at risk for psychological and physical disease and disorder. The provision or exchange of emotional, informational, or instrumental resources in response to others' needs is thought to facilitate coping with these demands and consequently be protective. This proposal is called the stress-buffering hypothesis—social resources (supports) will ameliorate the potentially pathogenic effects of stressful events. Although aid can be provided by professionals or in the context of formal "helping" groups, this entry focuses on support provided in informal relationships.

The stress-buffering hypothesis was formally proposed in 1976 by physician and epidemiologist John Cassel and psychiatrist Sidney Cobb. Both argued that those with strong social ties were protected from the potential pathogenic effects of stressful events. Cassel (1976) thought that stressors that placed persons at risk for disease were often characterized by confusing or absent feedback from the social environment. In contrast, the impact of the stressors was mitigated among individuals whose networks provided them with consistent communication of what is expected of them, assistance with tasks, evaluation of their performance, and appropriate rewards (Cassel, 1976). Similarly, Cobb (1976) thought that major life transitions and crises placed people at risk. He argued that those who interpreted communications from others signifying that they were cared for and valued and that they belonged to a network of mutual obligation were protected. He thought that this protection occurred because these perceptions facilitated coping and adaptation (see more recent discussion by Lakey & Cohen, 2000; Thoits, 1986).

Correlational studies testing the stress-buffering hypothesis have generally been supportive. Although this literature has primarily focused on psychological distress as an outcome (see Cohen & Wills, 1985; Schwartzer & Leppin, 1989), there are a few studies focusing on physical disease outcomes as well (e.g., Rosengren, Orth-Gomer, Wedel, & Wilhelmsen, 1993). Overall, work on stress-buffering indicates the importance of the "perceived availability" of support (e.g., Wethington & Kessler, 1986). In contrast, actually receiving support has often been correlated with negative outcomes, presumably because actual receipt indicates the need for support as well as its availability.

Research also suggests that the most effective support is not asked for, but is instead provided in the course of everyday social transactions (Barerra,

Sandler, & Ramsay, 1981; Eckenrode & Wethington, 1990; Pearlin & Scholler, 1978). We do not generally think of support provided by close friends and relatives as help and often are unaware of receiving it (Bolger, Zuckerman, & Kessler, 2000). Actually asking for help is a more complicated issue with the request raising issues of equity and relationship maintenance and quality (Fisher, Nadler, & Whitcher-Alagna, 1982). The idea is that our close relations should know we can use their support and respond without the need for a formal request for help.

How does social support provide protection from stressful events? Support may play a role at several points in the causal chain linking stress to health (Cohen, Gottieb, & Underwood, 2000; Gore, 1981; House, 1981). First, support may intervene between the stressful event and a stress reaction by attenuating or preventing a stress appraisal. More specifically, the perception that others can and will provide resources may redefine the harm potential of a situation and bolster one's perceived ability to cope with imposed demands, thereby preventing a situation from being appraised as highly stressful (Thoits, 1986). Second, support beliefs may reduce or eliminate the affective reaction to a stressful event, dampen physiological responses to the event, or prevent or alter maladaptive behavioral responses. The availability of persons to talk to about problems has also been found to reduce the intrusive thoughts that act to maintain chronic maladaptive responses to stressful events (Lepore, Silver, Wortman, & Wayment, 1996). Finally, support may intervene by reducing the stress reaction or by directly influencing physiological processes. Support may alleviate the impact of stress by providing a solution to the problem, by reducing the perceived importance of the problem, or by providing a distraction from the problem. It may also tranquilize the neuroendocrine system so that people are less stress reactive, or facilitate health-promoting behaviors such as exercise, proper nutrition, and rest (cf. Cohen & Wills, 1985; House, 1981).

Several different types of support have been delineated, and it is posited that these functions may be differentially useful for a range of stressors (Cohen & McKay, 1984; Cohen & Wills, 1985; Cutrona & Russell, 1990; Sandler, Miller, Short, & Wolchik, 1989). There are several typologies of support, but most include components of emotional (being cared for and valued), informational (information about the stressful events and coping with them), and material aid. The stress-support matching hypothesis (Cohen &

McKay, 1984; Cutrona & Russell, 1990) suggests that the potential benefit of a support type depends on which function will be most effective for a particular type of stressful event. Interestingly, evidence suggests that emotional support provides protection in the face of a wide range of stressful events, while other types of support seem to respond more specifically to specific needs elicited by stressful events (Cohen & Wills, 1985).

Consistent evidence is found for the buffering hypothesis when one ensures that certain methodological constraints are met (Cohen & Wills, 1985; Schwarzer & Leppin, 1989). For example, it is important that the study have a large sample size, a reasonable distribution of stress and support values, measures with acceptable psychometric properties, and nonconfounded stress and support measures. As mentioned earlier, effects are most consistently found with measures of perceived availability of support, especially emotional support.

A second relevant literature is the study of the effectiveness of social support interventions for helping people in the face of stressful events (Cohen et al., 2000). Collectively, these group and dyadic interventions are impressive because they reveal the many ways in which it may be possible to engineer support on behalf of people in highly diverse stressful circumstances. However, to date, there is more evidence on the feasibility of marshaling support than of its effectiveness. For example, two reviews of the outcomes of support groups for family caregivers of elderly persons paint a bleak picture with respect to the attainment of desired goals (Lavoie, 1995; Toseland & Rossiter, 1989). The same is true in the context of support groups for cancer patients (Fawzy et al., 1990; Helgeson & Cohen, 1996). The authors of these reviews provide reasonable explanations for the lack of clear evidence that we can help people under stress by providing support. Nevertheless, we have not as yet been able to translate the studies of support in naturalistic settings to effective artificial interventions.

—*Sheldon Cohen and*
Sarah Pressman

Further Reading

Barrera, M., Jr., Sandler, I. N., & Ramsay, T. B. (1981). Preliminary development of a scale of social support: Studies on college students. *American Journal of Community Psychology, 9,* 435-447.

Bolger, N., Zuckerman, A., & Kessler, R. C. (2000). Invisible support and adjustment to stress. *Journal of Personality and Social Psychology, 79,* 953-961.

Cassel, J. (1976). The contribution of the social environment to host resistance. *American Journal of Epidemiology, 104,* 107-123.

Cobb, S. (1976). Social support as a moderator of life stress. *Psychosomatic Medicine, 38,* 300-314.

Cohen, S., Gottlieb, B. H., & Underwood, L. G. (2000). Social relationships and health. In S. Cohen, L. G. Underwood, & B. H. Gottlieb (Eds.), *Social support measurement and intervention: A guide for health and social scientists* (pp. 1-25). New York: Oxford University Press.

Cohen, S., & McKay, G. (1984). Social support, stress and the buffering hypothesis: A theoretical analysis. In A. Baum, S. E. Taylor, & J. E. Singer (Eds.), *Handbook of psychology and health* (pp. 253-267). Hillsdale, NJ: Lawrence Erlbaum.

Cohen, S., & Wills, T. A. (1985). Stress, social support, and the buffering hypothesis. *Psychological Bulletin, 98,* 310-357.

Cutrona, C. E., & Russell, D. W. (1990). Type of social support and specific stress: Toward a theory of optimal matching. In B. R. Sarason, I. G. Sarason, & G. R. Pierce (Eds.), *Social support: An interactional view.* New York: John Wiley.

Eckenrode, J. E., & Wethington, E. (1990). The process and outcome of mobilizing social support. In S. Duck (Ed.), *Personal relationships and social support* (pp. 83-103). Newbury Park, CA: Sage.

Fawzy, F. I., Cousins, N., Fawzy, N. W., Kemeny, M. E., Elashoff, R., & Morton, D. (1990). A structured psychiatric intervention for cancer patients: 1. Changes over time in methods of coping and affective disturbance. *Archives of General Psychiatry, 47,* 720-725.

Fisher, J. D., Nadler, A., & Whitcher-Alagna, S. (1982). Recipient reactions to aid. *Psychological Bulletin, 91,* 27-54.

Gore, S. (1981). Stress-buffering functions of social supports: An appraisal and clarification of research models. In B. S. Dohrenwend & B. P. Dohrenwend (Eds.), *Stressful life events and their contexts* (pp. 202-222). New York: Prodist.

Helgeson, V., & Cohen, S. (1996). Social support and adjustment to cancer: Reconciling descriptive, correlational, and intervention research. *Health Psychology, 15,* 135-148.

House, J. S. (1981). *Work stress and social support.* Reading, MA: Addison-Wesley.

Lakey, B., & Cohen, S. (2000). Social support theory and measurement. In S. Cohen, L. G. Underwood, & B. H. Gottlieb (Eds.), *Social support measurement and intervention: A guide for health and social scientists* (pp. 29-52). New York: Oxford University Press.

Lavoie, J. P. (1995). Support groups for informal caregivers don't work! Refocus the groups or the evaluations? *Canadian Journal on Aging, 14,* 580-595.

Lepore, S. J., Silver, R. C., Wortman, C. B., & Wayment, H. A. (1996). Social constraints, intrusive thoughts, and depressive symptoms among bereaved mothers. *Journal of Personality and Social Psychology, 70,* 271-282.

Pearlin, I. I., & Scholler, C. (1978). The structure of coping. *Journal of Health and Social Behavior, 19,* 2-21.

Rosengren, A., Orth-Gomer, K., Wedel, H., & Wilhelmsen, L. (1993). Stressful life events, social support, and mortality in men born in 1933. *British Medical Journal, 307,* 1102-1105.

Sandler, I. N., Miller, P., Short, J., & Wolchik, S. A. (1989). Social support as a protective factor for children in stress. In D. Belle (Ed.), *Children's social networks and social supports* (pp. 277-307). New York: John Wiley.

Schwarzer, R., & Leppin, A. (1989). Social support and health: A meta-analysis. *Psychology and Health, 3,* 1-15.

Thoits, P. A. (1986). Social support as coping assistance. *Journal of Consulting and Clinical Psychology, 54,* 416-423.

Toseland, R. W., & Rossiter, C. M. (1989). Group interventions to support family caregivers: A review and analysis. *The Gerontologist, 29*(4), 438-448.

Wethington, E., & Kessler, R. C. (1986). Perceived support, received support, and adjustment to stressful events. *Journal of Health and Social Behavior, 27,* 78-89.

STRESS AND HEALTH. *See* **AIDS AND HIV: Stress; Allostatis, Allostatic Load, and Stress; Blood Pressure, Hypertension, and Stress; Cardiovascular Reactivity; Caregiving and Stress; Child Abuse, Child Neglect, and Health; Disasters and Health; Emotions: Negative Emotions and Health; Endogenous Opioids, Stress, and Health; Gastric Ulcers and Stress;**

Immune Responses to Stress; Job Strain and Health; John Henryism and Health; Low Birth Weight: Psychosocial Aspects; Metabolic Syndrome and Stress; Peptic Ulcers and Stress; Stress, Appraisal, and Coping; Stress: Biological Aspects; Stress-Buffering Hypothesis; Stress-Related Growth; Wound Healing and Stress

STRESS MANAGEMENT.

See Arthritis: Behavioral Treatment; Asthma: Behavioral Treatment; Biofeedback; Cancer: Psychosocial Treatment; Chronic Obstructive Pulmonary Disease: Psychosocial Aspects and Behavioral Treatments; Chronic Pain Management; Diabetes: Behavioral Treatment; Headaches: Psychological Management; Irritable Bowel Syndrome: Psychological Treatment; Sleep Disorders: Behavioral Treatment

STRESS-RELATED GROWTH

Stress-related growth refers to the positive changes that people report experiencing following stressful or traumatic life experiences. These positive changes are attributed to the stressful encounter and are made in response to it or arise from efforts to cope with it. While not everyone experiences stress-related growth, it is a very common outcome following stressful experiences. Stress-related growth has been documented after encounters with bereavement, combat, natural disasters, terrorist attacks, and life-threatening health crises such as HIV infection, myocardial infarction, and cancer. Stress-related growth can also occur following less severe stressors, such as developmental transitions (e.g., leaving home for college, romantic breakup).

It is important to note that experiencing stress-related growth does not mean that people did not suffer or experience adverse consequences as a result of the stressful situation, but seems to be a separate outcome of stressful encounters. Research studies sometimes refer to stress-related growth as "perceived benefits" or "thriving."

TYPES OF STRESS-RELATED GROWTH

Many different kinds of stress-related growth have been reported; these can be categorized in four domains: competencies, life philosophies, relationships with others, and lifestyle changes. Stress-related growth in competencies can involve increased confidence, coping skills, and knowledge. Stress-related growth in life philosophies can include increased awareness and insight as well as changes in one's life meaning and spirituality and a reordering of life values, goals, and priorities. Social stress-related growth includes positive changes in social relationships, such as deepened bonds with others, a widened social network, and improved communication. Stress-related growth can also involve making changes toward a healthier lifestyle, such as decreasing alcohol and drug use, quitting smoking, starting a new exercise program, and reducing stress.

THEORIES OF HOW STRESS-RELATED GROWTH OCCURS

Stress-related growth can occur suddenly, but usually occurs over time and is related to the ways that individuals respond to their stressful encounters. Stress-related growth is more likely to occur when experiences are highly stressful, because these experiences cause more disruption of individuals' beliefs and goals and require more coping efforts and change. Stress-related growth appears to arise through people's efforts to restore their beliefs and to bring their perceptions of aversive situations more in line with their goals. For example, a stressful encounter such as the untimely death of a loved one might disrupt an individual's sense that the world is a fair or just place and his or her own sense of invulnerability as well as making some goals unattainable. Over time, individuals are likely to recognize some positive aspects of the loss and the lessons that they learned through coping with it, even though the loss itself may remain quite painful.

Certain types of coping with stressful situations are related to higher levels of stress-related growth. Attempting to actively resolve the problem and to create meaning from it are particularly likely to lead to stress-related growth. Meaning can be made by talking about the situation with others and spending time thinking about it and its implications for one's life. Stress-related growth is a typical outcome of this meaning making, involving identifying the positive changes that have occurred internally, making positive changes in one's social relationships and lifestyle, or even making changes in life goals such as devoting one's energies to a larger social cause. Stress-related growth usually develops as a natural part of the coping process, but it can be facilitated by psychotherapy.

Individuals who are more religious or spiritual, more optimistic, and more extraverted, and who have more social support resources, are more likely to experience stress-related growth. Some studies show that women report higher levels of stress-related growth than men do.

RELATIONSHIP OF STRESS-RELATED GROWTH TO HEALTH AND WELL-BEING

Stress-related growth is often related to better physical health and psychological well-being following stressful experiences. In terms of psychological well-being, it appears that stress-related growth is often, but not always, related to better psychological adjustment following the stressful experience, such as less depressed mood and higher life satisfaction. The very fact that people believe that they have grown is also sometimes considered to reflect increased well-being.

Stress-related growth often occurs in the context of physical health crises. Those crises that are life-threatening, in particular, appear to create the type of distressing situation that leads people to reconsider their lives, reevaluate their situations, and search for meaning. Many people institute positive changes in their lives following these crises in all of the domains listed above. For example, heart attack patients sometimes make dramatic changes in their lifestyle as part of their growth, in response to their near-death experience and their renewed sense of life's fragility and need for better care. Stress-related growth is also commonly found in those with chronic illnesses, such as rheumatoid arthritis.

In addition to commonly occurring in the context of serious illness and commonly relating to better psychological adjustment to these illnesses, stress-related growth appears to at least sometimes be related to the physical health of individuals dealing with health crises. For example, a study of heart attack patients who shortly after their hospitalization reported experiencing stress-related growth were more likely to be alive and less likely to have had a recurrence of heart attack 7 years later, and a study of HIV-positive men found that stress-related growth was related to better immune functioning (CD4 levels), even after taking into account all known physiological indicators.

—*Crystal L. Park*

See also STRESS, APPRAISAL, AND COPING

Further Reading

Armeli, S., Gunthert, K. C., & Cohen, L. H. (2001). Stressor appraisals, coping, and post-event outcomes: The dimensionality and antecedents of stress-related growth. *Journal of Social and Clinical Psychology, 20,* 366-395.

Ickovics, J., & Park, C. L. (1998).Thriving: Broadening the paradigm beyond illness to health [Special issue]. *Journal of Social Issues, 54.*

Park, C. L., Cohen, L. H., & Murch, R. (1996). Assessment and prediction of stress-related growth. *Journal of Personality, 64,* 71-105.

Tedeschi, R. G., Park, C. L., & Calhoun, L. G. (Eds.) (1998). *Posttraumatic growth: Positive changes in the aftermath of crisis.* Mahwah, NJ: Lawrence Erlbaum.

Updegraff, J. A., & Taylor, S. E. (2000). From vulnerability to growth: Positive and negative effects of stressful life events. In J. H. Harvey & E. D. Miller (Eds.), *Loss and trauma: General and close relationship perspectives* (pp. 3-28). Philadelphia: Brunner-Routledge.

SUCCESSFUL AGING

Successful aging is a relatively new construct, growing out of the recognition that there are individual differences in both the rate and the manner in which individuals age. Some individuals in their 60s and 70s can run marathons and are cognitively sharp, while others in midlife are coping with disabling chronic illnesses such as diabetes and may be suffering the beginnings of cognitive decline. Similarly, some individuals are happy and enjoy good relations with family and friends, while others are isolated and lonely. Given that the study of successful aging is relatively new, there are as yet no fixed definitions, although there are different models in the literature. This entry reviews these models as well as the predictors of successful aging.

MODELS OF SUCCESSFUL AGING

Rowe and Kahn (1998) have proposed the most widely accepted model. Their three components of successful aging include the absence of disease, good cognitive and physical functioning, and an active engagement with life, which is characterized by good social relations and productive behavior. The model is hierarchical in that it assumes that these three components build on each other. That is, the absence of disease is the basis of good cognitive and physical functioning, which, in turn, can promote an active engagement with life.

Vaillant's (2002) model is similar, but has six criteria rather than three. Three of the criteria concern physical health: absence of any physician-diagnosed chronic illness by age 75, good self-rated health including no problems with instrumental activities of daily living (IADLs), and the length of undisabled life. The other three criteria are good mental health, good social support (including religious attendance), and satisfaction with life in a variety of different domains.

While intuitively appealing, these models have been criticized as simply extending the criteria for good midlife functioning to late life, and may be too stringent. Most individuals who live to very late life will develop chronic illness at some point, and many still consider themselves to be successfully aging. Perhaps successful aging is simply doing the best one can with whatever resources and vulnerabilities one has; the term *optimal aging* reflects this more pragmatic viewpoint.

These models of successful aging also may neglect special characteristics of old age. Tornstam (1994) observed that the old-old individuals, over the age of 80, exhibited something he called "gerotranscendence," which is characterized by a lessening reliance on external definitions of the self; a quiet, more contemplative attitude; and an enhanced perspective on the interconnectedness of life. This "Zen-like" state, as well as an increase in spirituality in very late life, has been also noted by Vaillant. Snowdon (2001) observed that older adults with sometimes very grave disabilities could draw on their sense of spirituality to maintain their emotional equilibrium and contribute what they could to their communities. Thus, the development of wisdom may be a marker for successful aging, even in those individuals with physical disabilities.

PREDICTORS OF SUCCESSFUL AGING

While genetics plays some role in the development of illness and disability in late life, maintenance of good health largely depends on lifestyle options we have and the choices that we make. A balanced diet, moderate exercise, and avoiding toxins such as cigarettes help to maintain cardiovascular health and avoid diseases such as diabetes that accelerate the aging process. Cardiovascular health may also be the key to maintaining good cognitive functioning, and cognitive exercises such as reading, doing puzzles, or being active in volunteer or professional work may also contribute to cognitive health.

Supportive social relations may be key to maintaining good mental health in late life. However, social losses increase with age, and older adults may be at heightened risk for depression. Older adults may have outlived spouses, siblings, friends, and even children, and disabilities may be accompanied by chronic pain and social isolation, if sensory or mobility problems make it difficult to socialize. Although the size of social networks may decrease with age, most older adults have strong ties with a few close family and friends. Volunteer work may help older adults to feel that they are productive members of their community, and religiousness or spirituality may also protect against depression in late life.

Personality and coping resources may also play an important role in successful aging. Individuals high in emotional stability may show little increase in symptoms with age, while those high in anxiety and hostility may develop chronic illnesses earlier. Vaillant found that good coping strategies or "mature defenses" were among the best predictors of successful aging. This includes the use of altruism, sublimation, suppression, and humor to cope with problems. Perhaps the ability to transform stressors into opportunities for growth may make it possible to age successfully, despite the disabilities and losses that may accompany old age.

—*Carolyn M. Aldwin*

See also SELF-EFFICACY; SELF-REPORTED HEALTH; SOCIAL INTEGRATION, SOCIAL NETWORKS, AND HEALTH; STRESS, APPRAISAL, AND COPING

Further Reading

Aldwin, C. M., & Gilmer, D. F. (2003). *Health, illness, and optimal aging: Biological and psychosocial perspectives.* Thousand Oaks, CA: Sage.

Baltes, M. M., & Carstensen, L. L. (1996). The process of successful aging. *Ageing and Society, 16*, 397-422.

Rowe, J. W., & Kahn, R. L. (1998). *Successful aging.* New York: Pantheon.

Snowdon, D. (2001). *Aging with grace: What the Nun Study teaches us about leading longer, healthier, and more meaningful lives.* New York: Bantam.

Strawbridge, W. J., Wallhagen, M. I., & Cohen, R. D. (2002). Successful aging and well-being: Self-rated compared with Rowe and Kahn. *The Gerontologist, 42*, 727-733.

Tornstam, L. (1994). Gero-transcendence: A theoretical and empirical exploration. In L. E. Thomas & S. A. Eisenhandler (Eds.), *Aging and the religious dimension* (pp. 203-225). Westport, CT: Auburn House.

Vaillant, G. E. (2002). *Aging well: Surprising guideposts to a happier life.* Boston: Little, Brown.

SUPPORT GROUPS AND HEALTH

Support groups consist of small groups of individuals who meet, usually on a regular basis, to discuss mutual problems. The most common reason for participation in a support group is for help in coping with a physical illness. Over the past two decades, the availability of support groups has grown exponentially. Support groups have been found to have both mental and physical health benefits. Increasingly, support groups are being viewed as an important adjunct to the care of the medically ill and their loved ones.

WHAT IS A SUPPORT GROUP?

A support group usually consists of individuals who have the same type of illness (or have some other stressor in common, such as bereavement) or it might consist of the family members, close friends, or caregivers of these individuals. A support group provides a setting where individuals can share their experiences with others who are coping with the same stressor. Support groups vary in size, but a typical support group ranges from 6 to 12 members.

As the name suggests, the main purpose of a support group is to provide support to the group members. There are three types of support that a group might provide: emotional, informational, and instrumental. Providing emotional support is perhaps a support group's defining feature. Participants are encouraged to express their emotions and concerns and to give as well as receive support from individuals who are facing similar circumstances. The assumption is that benefit occurs from expressing emotions and sharing concerns with individuals in similar situations as well as from receiving their concern, understanding, and caring. It also appears that members can receive as much benefit from providing support to others as they do from receiving it. This has been referred to as the helper-therapy principle.

Some support groups provide information and education about the illness either formally or informally. A support group might be structured such that a portion of time is allotted for the group leader or an outside expert to provide education or information. In an unstructured group format, either the group leaders or the members might provide informal education or information.

Instrumental support is when group members carry out practical activities to help one another, such as assisting with child care, running errands, or preparing a meal for a group member in need. This type of support may or may not occur and if it does occur it will take place outside of the support group meeting.

CHARACTERISTICS OF SUPPORT GROUPS

Target Population

Support groups can be formed for any type of illness, such as cancer, multiple sclerosis, alcoholism, and so on. Support groups can be formed for the caregivers of those who are ill, such as family members or other loved ones. They can be formed for individuals who have lost a loved one, or who are the victims of some adverse event such as childhood sexual abuse.

The target population can be either broadly or narrowly defined. Take cancer as an example. There are many different kinds of cancer, and there are different stages of the illness. Thus, one group might narrowly target women recently diagnosed with primary breast cancer. Another group might enlist a broader range of individuals including people of either gender who have lung cancer and at any stage of the illness. Or a group might include individuals with all types of cancer and any stage of the illness.

It is often most beneficial to include people whose illnesses are as similar as possible. The advantage is that they will have many experiences in common, which can lead to greater understanding and support. It is not always possible to have homogeneous groups especially in small communities or with rare illnesses. Even if the support group is not homogeneous to the type and stage of illness, the benefits of a heterogeneous group often far outweigh the disadvantages.

One advantage of a heterogeneous group is that it can provide a range of experiences and perspectives.

There are some circumstances in which it is not appropriate to have an individual join a support group. For example, individuals who are in crisis may need more than a group can offer, especially when the stressor is not related to the focus of the group. Sometimes it is possible to have such individuals receive individual therapy to help them manage the crisis. In that case, it might then be possible for them to effectively participate in a support group. Naturally, illness-related crises will occur in the life of a group. These types of crises are to be expected and dealing with them in group should be considered an important group task. The main consideration regarding crises is whether focusing on that person's crisis will derail the focus on the group because it is protracted (i.e., taking up extensive time over several sessions) and off-topic. Other contraindications for support groups include individuals who are hostile, antisocial, psychotic, unmotivated, cognitively impaired, or acutely suicidal.

Leadership

Support groups can be either peer led or professionally led. Leaders of peer-led groups usually have first-hand experience with the focus of that group. For example, a bereaved parent might facilitate a group for bereaved parents or a former breast cancer patient might lead a breast cancer support group. Peer-led groups are also called self-help groups. However, many so-called self-help groups are actually professionally led. Some professionally led groups may describe their group as self-help to emphasize their viewpoint that it is what the members get from each other that is most beneficial. Professionally led groups are facilitated by social workers, psychologists, psychiatrists, or other trained mental health professionals. The focus of these support groups is often greatly influenced by the facilitators. In peer-led groups, the focus is likely to be determined primarily by the group members. In professionally led groups, the facilitator may steer the group members toward focusing on emotional and psychological issues. In peer-led groups, the members might focus more on sharing information with one another.

Group Format and Structure

A support group might be open (allowing members to come and go as they desire), closed (where members are preselected and new members are not allowed to join), time limited (where the group has a predetermined number of sessions), or open-ended (where the group meets for an indefinite number of sessions). Typically, time-limited groups are also closed groups. Open-ended groups may be either open to members joining at any time or closed to new members but allowing new members to join as old members leave.

Before the advent of the Internet, support groups were almost universally face-to-face. In recent years, there has been a proliferation of Internet support groups. For those who have access to the Internet, online support groups offer a convenient means for participation. Online groups can be either synchronous (chat rooms) or asynchronous (bulletin boards), peer led or professionally led, open or closed, and time limited or open-ended.

A support group should allow time for mutual sharing. Some support groups consist entirely of mutual sharing. In such groups, the emphasis is on having members share their experiences and concerns, express emotions, and receive and offer emotional support and also can include the sharing of information. Sometimes support groups are more structured, offering education about the illness and teaching coping strategies, with less time allotted for mutual sharing.

MENTAL HEALTH BENEFITS OF SUPPORT GROUPS

There are many mental health benefits of participating in a support group. One key benefit is that participants feel less isolated. Feelings of isolation can occur for a variety of reasons. This can include feeling as though other people do not understand, feeling stigmatized, looking different from others, believing people are afraid of them or blame them for their illness, being too ill to maintain social activities, and so on. It has been shown that people seek social support for help in dealing with illnesses that are embarrassing, stigmatizing, or disfiguring and for dealing with the threat of death or costly medical treatment. Research has shown that reassurance or empathy from family or friends is not necessarily helpful because it can be experienced as an attempt to minimize their problem. However, similar responses from people who are in their situation can be experienced as highly supportive. Participating in a support group likely alleviates feelings of isolation by virtue of being with a group of people who both understand and share their experiences and concerns.

Support groups provide an opportunity for members to speak freely about their situation. It is not uncommon for people who are seriously ill or otherwise distressed to avoid talking about their distress with their loved ones. Often this is done so as to protect them. For example, seriously ill patients may avoid talking about their fears of dying because they do not want to upset their family. Furthermore, they may have concerns or issues with their family that they may not feel free to discuss with them. Ideally, a support group provides a venue where members can speak about all of their feelings and concerns without having to worry about protecting the other.

Another benefit of support groups is that group members learn from each other, either explicitly or implicitly. Members might tell each other about coping strategies that have worked for them or share information about treatment and treatment options. Group members gain hope by seeing how well others cope or by seeing members with a similar prognosis do better than expected. Members offer each other advice, encouragement, and support. They also serve as role models for each other, modeling both adaptive and sometimes less adaptive ways of coping. Learning active coping strategies is a common benefit of participating in a support group.

Learning more adaptive coping strategies can lead to an increase in self-efficacy—the belief in one's ability to handle new situations. This is especially important for individuals recently diagnosed with a medical illness. For instance, a group member might learn more adaptive strategies for dealing with a doctor and as a result feel better equipped to deal with his or her doctor in the future.

In general, research has shown that support groups can improve emotional adjustment, including general mood, depression, and anxiety. However, a meta-analysis of psychosocial interventions for cancer patients suggests that the benefits may vary depending on who leads the support group. Professionally led support groups have been shown to improve emotional and functional adjustment; whereas peer-led support groups have had more mixed results. However, research examining the benefits of peer-led groups is limited and more is needed before definitive conclusions are drawn.

EFFECTS OF SUPPORT GROUPS ON PHYSICAL HEALTH

There is evidence that support groups can positively affect physical health. Professionally led support groups have been found to reduce pain and enhance the response of the immune system, and there is some evidence that they may even prolong life. Increased survival has been demonstrated for breast cancer, malignant melanoma, and heart disease. However, not all studies have shown this benefit and consequently more research is needed to answer this question.

Research is also needed to examine the underlying mechanisms that may lead to a health benefit. One possibility is that support groups improve health behavior. For instance, increases in self-efficacy have been shown to positively affect health behavior. Another possibility is that support groups might lead to better treatment compliance. A third potential mediator is that support groups influence biological pathways of disease progression. Recent research on the stress hormone, cortisol, has found that it is positively affected by support groups and that there is a relationship between a dysregulation of cortisol and mortality. However, more research is needed to address this and related questions.

—*Catherine Classen*

See also Social Integration, Social Networks, and Health

Further Reading

Davison, K. P., Pennebaker, J. W., & Dickerson, K. P. (2000). Who talks? The social psychology of illness support groups. *American Psychologist, 55*(2), 205-217.

Meyer, T. J., & Melvin, M. M. (1995). Effects of psychosocial interventions with adult cancer patients: A meta-analysis of randomized experiments. *Health Psychology, 14*(2), 101-108.

Spiegel, D., & Classen, C. (2000). *Group therapy for cancer patients: A research-based handbook of psychosocial care.* New York: Basic Books.

T

TAILORED COMMUNICATIONS

As used most often in current intervention research, *tailoring* denotes the strategy of providing materials, messages, and/or activities that are matched to characteristics of each individual participant (Kreuter, Farrell, Olevitch, & Brennan, 2000; Kreuter, Strecher, & Glassman, 1999; Rimer & Glassman, 1998). In effect, each individual receives a different version of intervention content. The individual-level specificity of tailoring is often contrasted with "one size fits all" strategies in which all participants (presumably from a diverse population) receive the same intervention. Tailoring is also distinguished from the approaches of "targeting" and "personalization." With targeting, broadly defined subgroups are identified and each gets a different intervention, but all members of a subgroup receive the same intervention. Tailoring can then be directed to the individuals within a targeted group, using an additional set of variables. With personalization, intervention materials are labeled with the participant's name and perhaps other standard demographic identifiers to create the impression of addressing the participant individually, but it is primarily for image rather than changing the content itself.

The term *tailored communications* therefore refers to the channels and formats by which individualized information is delivered to intervention participants. A wide variety of options exist, used alone or in combination, including traditional print formats such as brochures, booklets, reminders, and tip sheets; person-to-person contacts such as telephone counselors, health care providers, and lay/peer advisers; and interactive technology-based strategies including kiosks, CDs, Web-based programs, handheld devices, and television. There are no prescribed best methods or formats for delivering tailored communications. The core requirement is flexibility to allow individualizing the messages based on selected characteristics of each member of the target population. Tailored communication therefore also assumes that some interaction occurs between the participant and the delivery channel/agent, to obtain/provide the information needed for tailoring. Given the requirements for interaction and individualization, some delivery methods are less amenable to tailoring, such as billboards, public service announcements, and mass media campaigns. Such strategies may be better used to target messages to groups within the total audience.

The technology for delivering tailored communications to large numbers of people is relatively recent and closely tied to the evolution of computers and information-management capacity. The basic principle of individualized intervention has been long known and well accepted in health promotion/health education. However, the feasibility of implementing an individualized intervention has been subject to concerns about the time requirements placed on staff, the capacity to perform the necessary assessments, the ability to have presence in participants' daily lives, and the ability to achieve consistent intervention delivery across multiple project staff and settings. Computer-based production of health communications offers the promise of addressing these concerns, with the additional benefit of allocating intervention resources efficiently by providing intervention messages/materials/activities only where there is apparent need.

At the core of tailored communications are algorithms (decision rules) that take an individual's data on a set of predefined variables (e.g., from a questionnaire, interview, or medical record) and produce a classification on each variable (e.g., high/middle/low; in quartiles; above or below a dichotomous cutpoint). The classification individuals receive on a variable in turn determines which version of a tailored communication they are given, drawn from a comprehensive "inventory" or "library" established by the interventionists. The messages for each person are then combined into the final intervention package that may also have some targeted content for their specific population subgroup. Therefore, the production of tailored communications requires the a priori specification of the variables that will be used, the cutpoints on each of those variables to create the discrete classifications, the messages that correspond to each classification for each variable, and the format in which a communication will be delivered (if an intervention is multimodal). Strictly speaking, it is not necessary to reduce continuous variables to discrete categories, but using the complete range of values on a continuous variable can present a substantial challenge for message construction because every value must have a corresponding message. The potential of tailoring rests heavily on its ability to respond to a wide range of combinations of personal characteristics. It is therefore common for tailored interventions to highlight their ability to individualize by calculating the total number of possible message combinations. For example, a project might tailor with nine variables, each of which is classified into four levels. On the assumption that a person's status on these variables are potentially independent, then the tailoring can accommodate 4^9 or 262,144 combinations (i.e., four levels for each of nine variables). Fundamentally, this is the same logic that underlies having more complex automobile license plates in a state like California, as opposed to a lower-population state like Rhode Island.

Tailoring has a strong empirical grounding and is an application of evidence-based health education. The variables used for algorithm decision rules, and the cutpoints that define the classifications for those variables, should be based on analyses showing statistically significant associations with the target health practice. The creation of tailored communications is therefore closely tied to research that identifies correlates (but preferably predictors) of the health practice being considered. Tailored communications by nature also require knowing the larger context within which the health practice will occur. Being able to specify

that context, described as the "focal point" for the intervention (Rakowski, 1999; Rakowski & Clark, 2002), is comprised by the target population, the health practice, the intervention setting, and the performance setting, and informs selecting the variables to be examined as potential correlates. The variables that are used in the algorithm, and the conceptual model(s) that guide their use, have been referred to as the "deep knowledge" of the tailored intervention (Velicer et al., 1993). Furthermore, the empirical foundation of tailoring is presumed to be most reliable when it is based on longitudinal predictive analyses, in contrast to cross-sectional correlational analyses. Even with longitudinal analyses, however, the usefulness of a variable for tailoring depends on the plausibility of the presumed causal linkage between that variable and the health practice.

Tailoring is developing its own specialized terminology. Communications can be "normative" or "ipsative" (Dijkstra & De Vries, 1999; Prochaska, DiClemente, Velicer, & Rossi, 1993). A normative communication compares the individual against a reference group; an ipsative communication compares the individual to their own status at a previous time. Interventions are often assembled by an "expert system" (Velicer et al., 1993), which is the collection of programming code that takes the raw data of input and produces the final tailored product. In addition, the steps of preparing tailored communications can involve a "tailoring matrix," "message concept booklets," "message blocks," "macro-tailoring," and "micro-tailoring" (Dijkstra & De Vries, 1999; Kreuter et al., 2000). For example, a tailored print communication might be provided as a unit of text, such as a four-sentence paragraph, whose content would differ across the levels of a tailoring variable (macro-tailoring). Tailoring may also be done even further at the level of phrases or words in sentences, within the paragraph for a given level of that variable (micro-tailoring). Similarly, tailoring matrices and message concept booklets are the practical aids used to help keep track of the potential complexity of the tailored intervention, and plan the content of the messages and materials.

Although tailoring is generally viewed as occurring at the level of the individual, there can be a gray area. An exchange of commentaries (Kreuter & Skinner, 2000; Pasick, 2001; Rimer, 2001) involved the concept of "cultural tailoring" and whether tailoring can also occur at a group level. The different opinions expressed in these commentaries are an understandable reflection of the interface between an emerging technology that nonetheless uses existing words as its labels (targeting, tailoring, individualizing) and research programs that may have different disciplinary bases. The hallmark of tailoring is precision, relative to the unit of intervention that is typically studied by an investigator.

Psychologically based interventions typically emphasize the individual level; other disciplines address groups as the unit. At the writing of this entry, psychologically oriented variables and principles have a strong presence in the literature of behavioral science generally, and tailoring in particular. The tailoring objective of individualized communications is very consistent with psychological perspectives about the bases of personal health practices. However, interventionists who have traditionally emphasized cultural and group-level influences on health practices might interpret "tailoring" and "individualization" to happen by precisely defining the group(s) with which they work (e.g., racial/ethnic groups, families, classrooms). For example, relative to the very wide diversity of cultural groups that exist, an intervention for a group defined by several variables that distinguished its members from the majority population might be considered tailored for that group in contrast to a "one size fits all" approach of intervening similarly with each cultural group.

It is important not to attribute a priori superiority to tailored versus targeted communications. The variables used in one investigation to define a subgroup for a targeted intervention might be used as the bases for tailoring individualized communications in another investigation. Also, a very precisely targeted intervention may produce better outcomes than a tailored intervention that generates individualized communications but is incompletely conceptualized. Tailoring and targeting are both strategies for producing and delivering communications, and therefore both are also intermediate outcomes along the way to the desired behavior change. It is therefore legitimate and necessary to study whether the products of a tailoring algorithm, in their own right, meet the intended objectives of individualization.

—*William Rakowski*

See also CANCER PREVENTION; HEALTH COMUNICATION; HEALTH LITERACY; HEALTH PROMOTION AND DISEASE PREVENTION; PHYSICAL ACTIVITY INTERVENTIONS

Further Reading

Dijkstra, A., & De Vries, H. (1999). The development of computer-generated tailored interventions. *Patient Education and Counseling, 36,* 193-203.

Kreuter, M., Farrell, D., Olevitch, L., & Brennan, L. (2000). *Tailoring health messages: Customizing communication with computer technology.* Mahwah, NJ: Lawrence Erlbaum.

Kreuter, M. W., & Skinner, C. S. (2000). Tailoring: What's in a name? *Health Education Research, 15,* 1-4.

Kreuter, M. W., Strecher, V. J., & Glassman, B. (1999). One size does not fit all: The case for tailoring print materials. *Annals of Behavioral Medicine, 21,* 276-283.

Pasick, R. J. (2001). Response to Kreuter and Skinner. *Health Education Research, 16,* 503-505.

Prochaska, J. O., DiClemente, C. C., Velicer, W. F., & Rossi, J. S. (1993). Standardized, individualized, interactive, and personalized self-help programs for smoking cessation. *Health Psychology, 12,* 399-405.

Rakowski, W. (1999). The potential variances of tailoring in health behavior interventions. *Annals of Behavioral Medicine, 21,* 284-289.

Rakowski, W., & Clark, M. A. (2002). The potential for health care organizations to promote maintenance and change in health behaviors among the elderly. In K. W. Schaie & H. Leventhal (Eds.), *Effective health behavior in the elderly.* New York: Springer.

Rimer, B. K. (2001). Response to Kreuter and Skinner. *Health Education Research, 15,* 503.

Rimer, B. K., & Glassman, B. (1998). Tailoring communication for primary care settings. *Methods of Information in Medicine, 37,* 171-177.

Velicer, W. F., Prochaska, J. O., Bellis, J. M., DiClemente, C. C., Rossi, J. S., Fava, J. H., et al. (1993). An expert system intervention for smoking cessation. *Addictive Behaviors, 18,* 269-290.

TELEVISION VIEWING AND HEALTH

Television's powerful influence on health and health-related behaviors has become a major health concern, particularly as television viewing has increased. The American population spends more time watching television than it spends in any other activity except sleep, work, and school, averaging more than 4 hours of television per day. Television viewing has been associated with increased aggressive behaviors, violence, lower academic performance, poor body self-image, poor nutrition, increased risk of obesity, and increased substance use and abuse. While recognizing the complexity in determining the causes of these problems, researchers have increasingly examined the role of television, not only as contributing to these problems but as a viable solution for intervention. Both the inactivity of watching television and the content of television programs and commercials adversely affect health.

In numerous studies among children and adults, obesity prevalence is associated with daily television viewing, while in longitudinal studies, television viewing patterns predict incidence or remission of obesity. Furthermore, preschool-aged children with a television set in their bedrooms not only watch more daily hours of television but have a higher rate of obesity. Television viewing contributes to obesity by replacing more physically active behaviors that would burn more calories and promoting increased dietary energy intake from increased snacking and/or eating or in response to food advertising. It is possible to reverse some of the negative effects of television viewing. Both clinical and population-based interventions that reduced television viewing led to relative decreases in adiposity (body fatness) and lower obesity rates.

There is an inverse relationship between the amount of television viewing and the degree of physical activity. Television viewing results in a lower metabolic rate in both obese and normal weight children compared with other sedentary activities such as sewing, reading, writing, or resting. Prolonged time in front of the television has also been associated with an increased risk of Type 2 diabetes.

A significant proportion of television commercials are for foods, and most of these advertisements are for high-calorie, high-sugar, or high-fat foods of poor nutritional quality. Exposure to televised food commercials influences food preferences, promotes between-meal snacking, and contributes to increased dietary fat intake and total energy intake in both children and adults. Families that dine with the television on during meals have less nutritional dietary patterns. They consume fewer fruits, vegetables, and dairy products, drink more soda, and eat more fast-food items than families in which television viewing and eating are separate activities. In televised programs, obesity occurs far less frequently among characters than in the general population. Furthermore, television characters rarely perform healthy behaviors, such as exercising or eating a balanced diet, yet they tend to look healthy. Consequently, television contributes to the creation of misleading impressions between the relationship of behavior and health.

According to the American Academy of Pediatrics Committee on Public Education, next to the family, television may be the most important source of information for children and a principle factor influencing their development. This is of increasing concern, considering that over 1,000 studies and reviews show that significant exposure to television violence increases the likelihood of aggressive behavior in children and desensitizes them to violence. More important, an intervention that reduced the amount of television viewing resulted in a substantial reduction in children's aggressiveness and violent actions. Although television is promoted as an educational tool, studies show that an adult mediator or teacher is required to reinforce the concepts presented and for measurable learning to occur. Learning from television is passive rather than active, and watching more than 1 to 2 hours per day of television viewing has a negative effect on children's academic performance, especially reading scores.

Television advertisements encourage the use of drugs, alcohol, and tobacco by using unrealistic associations with positively valued activities such as romance and sociability. Furthermore, behaviors such as drinking and smoking portrayed in television shows, movies, and music videos are very influential on the health-related decisions of viewers. Despite cigarette advertising being banned from television since 1969, there has been a substantial increase in the frequency of smoking by characters in movies and television. Characters portrayed on television are more likely to smoke on screen than their real-life counterparts with similar demographic characteristics.

Television viewing also compromises sexual health and may contribute to America having the highest rates of sexually transmitted diseases and pregnancy among adolescents in the Western world. Among the 14,000 sexual references, innuendoes, and behaviors portrayed on television, only 1% of these exposures dealt responsibly with human sexuality. In a U.S. study of adolescent girls, the pregnant teens, compared to the pregnant teens, watched more soap operas before becoming pregnant and were less likely to think that their favorite soap opera characters would use birth control. Another study showed that teenagers who watch soap operas overestimated the prevalence of sexually active teenagers and extramarital affairs and underestimated the risk of contracting sexually transmitted diseases. This is not surprising, since the sexual content of soap operas has more than doubled between 1980 and 1989. Soap opera sex is 24 times more common between unmarried partners than between spouses, and birth control is almost nonexistent.

In general, the more time individuals spend viewing television, the unhealthier they seem to be. With the growth of cable and digital television, more programs will be available and television viewing is likely to increase in the coming years. Thus, the impact of television on health and health-related practices cannot be ignored. As awareness of the negative health impacts associated with television viewing increases, parents are being encouraged to monitor their children's television viewing and other media exposure. The American Academy of Pediatrics recommends that parents limit their children's television viewing to no more than 1 to 2 hours per day of high-quality shows, that children under the age of 2 be discouraged from viewing any television, and that television sets be kept out of children's bedrooms. As a way to increase awareness of the adverse effects associated with television viewing, local community programs, promoting a week without television and encouraging alternative activities, are being implemented nationwide. In addition, programs to teach media literacy to older children, adolescents, and parents are being developed to help protect against the harmful influences of television viewing. Finally, some groups have advocated for policies such as restricting advertising, especially advertising targeted at young children.

—Barbara A. Dennison and
Kristina Laskovski

See also Obesity: Causes and Consequences; Obesity in Children: Physical Activity and Nutritional Approaches; Obesity in Children: Prevention; Physical Activity and Health; Violence Prevention

Further Reading

American Academy of Pediatrics, Committee on Public Education. (2001). Children, Adolescents, and Television. *Pediatrics, 2,* 423-426.

Strasburger, V. C. (1997). "Sex, drugs, rock 'n' roll," and the media—Are the media responsible for adolescent behavior? *Adolescent Medicine, 8,* 403-414.

TV Turnoff Network. (2002). Retrieved October 15, 2002, from www.tvturnoff.org

Winn, M. (1985). *The plug-in drug: Television, children, and the family.* New York: Viking.

THEORY OF PLANNED BEHAVIOR

First proposed by Icek Ajzen in 1985, the theory of planned behavior (TPB) is today perhaps the most popular model for the prediction of social behavior. It has its foundation in Martin Fishbein and Icek Ajzen's theory of reasoned action, which was developed in response to observed lack of correspondence between general social attitudes and actual behavior. Fishbein and Ajzen formulated the principle of compatibility, which stipulates that predictive validity is only obtained when attitude and behavior are assessed at equivalent levels of generality or specificity. General attitudes toward racial or ethnic groups, policies, or institutions fail to predict specific behaviors directed at these objects because of a lack of compatibility. By turning the focus from general attitudes toward the object of a behavior to attitudes toward the behavior itself, the principle of compatibility became a cornerstone of the theories of reasoned action and planned behavior. However, the TPB goes beyond attitude to consider other influences on behavior as well.

THE THEORETICAL MODEL

According to the theory, human social behavior is guided by three kinds of considerations: beliefs about the behavior's likely positive and negative outcomes (behavioral beliefs), beliefs about the normative expectations of others (normative beliefs), and beliefs about the presence of factors that may facilitate or impede performance of the behavior (control beliefs). In their respective aggregates, behavioral beliefs produce a favorable or unfavorable attitude toward the behavior; normative beliefs result in perceived social pressure to perform or not to perform the behavior, or subjective norm; and control beliefs give rise to a sense of self-efficacy or perceived behavioral control. An expectancy-value formulation describes the effects of beliefs on attitudes, subjective norms, and perceptions of behavioral control. In the case of behavioral beliefs, the evaluation of each anticipated outcome contributes to attitude in direct proportion to the person's subjective probability that the behavior produces the outcome in question. Similarly, motivation to comply with each normative referent contributes to the subjective norm in direct proportion to the person's subjective probability that the referent thinks the person should perform the behavior; and the perceived power of each control factor to impede or facilitate performance of the behavior contributes to perceived behavioral control in direct proportion to the person's subjective probability that the control factor is present.

In combination, attitude toward the behavior, subjective norm, and perceived behavioral control lead to the formation of a behavioral intention. The relative weight or importance of each determinant of intention will vary from behavior to behavior and from population to population. However, as a general rule, the more favorable the attitude and subjective norm, and the greater the perceived behavioral control, the stronger the person's intention to perform the behavior in question. Finally, people are expected to carry out their intentions when the opportunity arises.

Intention is thus assumed to be an immediate antecedent of behavior. However, successful performance of a behavior depends not only on a favorable intention but also on a sufficient level of behavioral control, that is, on the possession of requisite skills, resources, opportunities, and the presence of other supportive conditions. Because many behaviors pose difficulties of execution, the TPB also relies on perceived behavioral control in the prediction of behavior. To the extent that perceived behavioral control is veridical, it can serve as a proxy of actual control and can, together with intention, be used in the prediction of behavior.

Beliefs play a central role in the theory of planned behavior. Accessible behavioral, normative, and control beliefs—elicited in a free-response format—are assumed to determine prevailing attitudes, subjective norms, and perceptions of behavioral control, and they thus serve as the fundamental explanatory constructs in the theory. Other variables, such as personality traits, gender, education, intelligence, motivation, or values are assumed to influence behavior indirectly by their effects on underlying beliefs.

The theory of planned behavior assumes that human social behavior is reasoned or planned in the sense that it takes account of a behavior's likely consequences, the normative expectations of important referents, and factors that may impede performance of the behavior. Although the beliefs people hold may sometimes be inaccurate, unfounded, or biased, their attitudes, subjective norms, and perceptions of behavioral control are thought to follow spontaneously and reasonably from these beliefs, produce a corresponding behavioral intention, and ultimately result in behavior that is consistent with the overall tenor of the beliefs. However, this does not necessarily presuppose a deliberate, effortful retrieval of information and construction of attitudes prior to every enactment of a behavior. After at least minimal experience with the behavior, attitude, subjective norm, and perceived behavioral control are assumed to be available automatically as performance of the behavior is contemplated.

Successful application of the TPB is predicated on two conditions. First, the measures of attitude, subjective norm, perceived behavioral control, and intention must observe the principle of compatibility, that is, they must be compatible with each other and with the measure of behavior in terms of the action involved, the target at which the action is directed, and the context and time of its enactment. Second, attitude, subjective norm, perceived behavioral control, and intention must remain relatively stable over time. Any changes in these variables prior to observation of the behavior will tend to impair their predictive validity.

EMPIRICAL SUPPORT

The theory of planned behavior has been applied in research on a myriad of social behaviors, including investment decisions, high school dropout, mountain climbing, driving violations, recycling, class attendance, voting in elections, extramarital affairs, antinuclear activism, playing basketball, choice of travel mode, tax evasion, and a host of other activities related to protection of the environment, crime, recreation, education, politics, religion, and virtually any imaginable sphere of human endeavor. It has found its most intense application, however, in the health domain, where it has been used to predict and explain such varied behaviors as drinking, smoking, drug use, exercising, blood donation, dental care, fat consumption, breast self-examination, condom use, weight loss, infant sugar intake, getting medical checkups, physician referrals, protection of the skin from the sun, living kidney donation, and compliance with medical regimens.

The results of these investigations have, by and large, confirmed the theory's structure and predictive validity, especially when its constructs were properly operationalized. Even without this caveat, the TPB has fared very well. Meta-analytic reviews of close to 200 data sets in a variety of behavioral domains have found that the theory accounts, on average, for about 40% of the variance in intentions, with all three predictors—attitude toward the behavior, subjective norm, and perceived behavioral control—making independent contributions to the prediction, and that intentions and perceptions of behavioral control explain about 30% of the behavioral variance. Effects of similar magnitude have been documented in the domain of health and safety, where meta-analytic reviews have focused on studies of addiction, clinical screening, driving, eating, exercising, HIV/AIDS prevention, and oral hygiene.

The TPB has also served as a useful tool for analyzing the transition from one stage of behavior to another in the context of the transtheoretical stages of change model. Attitudes, subjective norms, perceptions of behavioral control, and intentions are found to increase directly with stage of change, from precontemplation through contemplation, preparation, action, and maintenance.

Given its predictive validity, the TPB can serve as a conceptual framework for interventions designed to influence intentions and behavior. Thus far, only a small number of investigators have attempted to apply the theory in this fashion. The results of these attempts have been encouraging. Interventions directed at one or more of the theory's predictors have been found to increase use of public transportation among college students and to raise the effectiveness of job search behavior of unemployed individuals. In the health domain, interventions based on the theory of planned behavior have been found effective in promoting testicular self-examination and inducing alcoholics to join a treatment program.

FROM INTENTIONS TO BEHAVIOR

As noted earlier, for the theory of planned behavior to afford accurate prediction, intentions must remain relatively stable. Empirical evidence supports this expectation, showing that the intention-behavior relation declines with instability in intentions over time. More important, however, the theory also assumes that people will act on their intentions under appropriate circumstances. This expectation has frequently been challenged, beginning with R. T. LaPiere's classic study in which ready acceptance of a Chinese couple in hotels, motels, and restaurants contrasted sharply with stated intentions not to accept "members of the Chinese race" in these same establishments. Similar discrepancies have been revealed in investigations of health behavior where it is found that large proportions of participants fail to carry out their intentions to use condoms, to undergo cancer screening, to exercise, to perform breast self-examination, to take vitamin pills, to maintain a weight-loss program, and so forth.

A variety of factors may be responsible for observed failures of effective self-regulation, yet a simple intervention can often do much to reduce the gap between intended and actual behavior. When individuals are asked to formulate a specific plan—an implementation intention—indicating when, where, and how they will carry out the intended action, the correspondence between intended and actual behavior increases dramatically. Behavioral interventions that focus on implementation intentions have been shown to produce very high rates of compliance with such recommended practices as cervical cancer screening and breast self-examination.

CRITIQUES

Although popular and successful—or perhaps because of it—the TPB has not escaped criticism. One type of critique has challenged the unitary nature of the theory's major constructs. Thus, it has been argued that intentions are cognitive representations not only of behavioral plans but also of expectations regarding likely behavior; that attitudes contain affective as well as evaluative reactions to the behavior; that subjective norms, in addition to injunctive expectations, also subsume descriptive norms; and that perceived behavioral control includes self-efficacy as well as perceived controllability of the behavior.

A second type of criticism is directed at the theory's structure, that is, the relations among the theoretical constructs. It has been suggested that attitudes may have a direct effect on behavior, bypassing intentions, or that attitudes, subjective norms, and perceptions of behavioral control may interact with intentions to influence behavior.

Still other concerns have to do with the theory's sufficiency—the proposition that attitudes, subjective norms, and perceptions of behavioral control are sufficient to predict intentions and behavior. Investigators have suggested a number of variables that might be added to the theory to improve its predictive validity. Among the proposed additions are desire and need; affect and anticipated regret; personal and moral norms; past behavior; and self-identity, that is, the extent to which people view themselves as the kind of person who would perform the behavior in question.

Finally, investigators have challenged the theory's reasoned action assumption or, more precisely, they have argued that reasoned action may represent only one mode of operation, the controlled or deliberate mode. According to Russell Fazio's MODE model, reasoned action occurs when people are motivated and capable of retrieving their beliefs, attitudes, and intentions in an effortful manner. When they lack motivation or cognitive capacity to do so, they are said to operate in the spontaneous mode where attitudes must be strong enough to be activated automatically if they are to guide behavior.

An alternative critique of the TPB's reasoned action assumption relies on the well-known phenomenon that, with repeated performance, behavior becomes routine and no longer requires much conscious control for its execution. Some have suggested that as a result of this process of habituation, initiation of the behavior becomes automatic and control over the behavior is transferred from conscious intentions to critical stimulus cues. The finding that frequency of past behavior is often a good predictor of later behavior and, indeed, that it has a residual impact on later behavior over and above the influence of intention and perceived behavior control has been taken as evidence for automaticity in social behavior.

—*Icek Ajzen*

See also THEORY OF REASONED ACTION; THEORY OF TRIADIC INFLUENCE; TRANSTHEORETICAL MODEL OF BEHAVIOR CHANGE

Further Reading

Ajzen, I. (1991). The theory of planned behavior. *Organizational Behavior & Human Decision Processes, 50*, 179-211.

Ajzen, I., & Fishbein, M. (1980). *Understanding attitudes and predicting social behavior.* Englewood Cliffs, NJ: Prentice Hall.

Armitage, C. J., & Conner, M. (2001). Efficacy of the theory of planned behavior: A meta-analytic review. *British Journal of Social Psychology, 40*, 471-499.

Fazio, R. H. (1990). Multiple processes by which attitudes guide behavior: The MODE model as an integrative framework. In M. P. Zanna (Ed.), *Advances in experimental social psychology* (Vol. 23, pp. 75-109). San Diego, CA: Academic Press.

Gollwitzer, P. M. (1999). Implementation intentions: Strong effects of simple plans. *American Psychologist, 54*, 493-503.

LaPiere, R. T. (1934). Attitudes vs. actions. *Social Forces, 13*, 230-237.

THEORY OF REASONED ACTION

The theory of reasoned action (TRA) is a general theory of behavior that was developed largely in response to the repeated failure of traditional attitude measures to predict specific behaviors. First introduced in 1967 by Martin Fishbein, the theory was further developed by Fishbein and Icek Ajzen (see, e.g., Fishbein & Ajzen, 1975; Ajzen & Fishbein, 1980). In an atmosphere where it was assumed that behavioral prediction was difficult (if not impossible), the theory began with the premise that behavior could be predicted simply by asking a person whether he or she was or was not going to perform that behavior. Not surprisingly, people turned out to be very good predictors of their own behavior. Thus, according to the theory, performance or nonperformance of a given behavior is primarily determined by the strength of a person's intention to perform (or to not perform) that behavior, where intention is defined as the subjective likelihood that one will perform (or try to perform) the behavior in question.

In addition to forming intentions to perform specific behaviors (e.g., to jog 20 minutes every day, to always use a condom for vaginal sex with my spouse), people may also form intentions to engage in behavioral categories (e.g., to exercise, to practice safe sex) and to reach certain goals (e.g., to lose weight, to stay healthy). Unlike the strong relation between intentions to engage in a given behavior and behavioral performance, however, there is no necessary relation between intentions to engage in a behavioral category and performance of any single behavior in that category or between intentions to reach a goal and goal attainment. Thus, the TRA recognized that only intentions to engage in volitionally controlled behaviors will consistently lead to accurate behavioral predictions. Although this has been viewed as a limitation of the theory, most socially relevant behaviors are largely under volitional control.

PREDICTING INTENTIONS

The intention (I) to perform a given behavior (B) is, in turn, viewed as a function of two basic factors: the person's attitude toward performing the behavior (i.e., one's overall positive or negative feeling about personally performing the behavior—Ab) and/or the person's subjective norm concerning his or her performance of the behavior (i.e., the person's perception that his or her important others think that he or she should or should not perform the behavior in question—SN). Algebraically, this can be expressed as: $B \sim I = w_1 Ab + w_2 SN$, where w_1 and w_2 are weights indicating the relative importance of attitudes and subjective norms as determinants of intention. It is important to recognize that the relative importance of these two psychosocial variables as determinants of intention will depend upon both the behavior and the population being considered. Thus, for example, one behavior may be primarily determined by attitudinal considerations, while another may be primarily influenced by perceived norms. Similarly, a behavior that is attitudinally driven in one population or culture may be normatively driven in another. While some behaviors may be entirely under attitudinal control (i.e., w_2 may be zero), others may be entirely under normative control (i.e., w_1 may be zero).

The theory also considers the determinants of attitudes and subjective norms. Based on Fishbein's earlier (1963) expectancy-value model, attitudes are viewed as a function of behavioral beliefs and their evaluative aspects. Algebraically, $Ab = f(3b_i e_i)$, where Ab = the attitude toward performing the behavior, b_i = belief that performing the behavior will lead to outcome "I," and e_i = the evaluation of outcome "i."

Somewhat similar to this, subjective norms are viewed as a function of normative beliefs and motivations to comply. Algebraically, $SN = f(Nb_i Mc_i)$, where SN = the subjective norm, Nb_i = the normative belief that referent "i" thinks one should (or should not) perform the behavior, and Mc_i = the motivation to comply, in general, with referent "i."

Generally speaking, the more one believes that performing a given behavior will lead to positive outcomes and/or will prevent negative outcomes, the more favorable will be one's attitude toward performing that behavior. Similarly, the more one believes that specific referents (i.e., individuals or groups) think that one should (or should not) perform the behavior and the more one is motivated to comply with those referents, the stronger will be the perceived pressure (i.e., the subjective norm) to perform (or to not perform) that behavior.

It is at this level of behavioral and normative beliefs that the substantive uniqueness of each behavior comes into play. Clearly, the outcomes (or consequences) of performing one's behavior may be very different from those associated with performing some other behavior, even if the two behaviors appear quite similar. For example, the outcomes (or consequences) of always using a condom for vaginal sex with one's main partner may be very different from those associated with always using a condom for anal sex with one's main partner or for always using a condom for vaginal sex with an occasional partner. According to the theory, these behavioral and normative beliefs about the behavior in question must be identified in order to fully understand the determinants of that behavior. Although an investigator can sit in her or his office and develop measures of attitudes and subjective norms, she or he cannot tell you what a given population (or a given person) believes about performing a given behavior. Thus, one must go to members of that population to identify salient behavioral and normative beliefs. To put this somewhat differently, one must understand the behavior from the perspective of the population one is considering.

Finally, the TRA also considers the role played by more traditional demographic, economic, personality, attitudinal, and other individual difference variables (such as perceived risk or sensation seeking). According to the model, these types of variables play primarily an indirect role in influencing behavior. That is, these "background" or "distal" factors are expected to influence behavior only to the extent that they influence the behavioral or normative beliefs underlying attitudes and norms. Thus, for example, men and women may hold different beliefs about performing some behaviors but very similar beliefs with respect to others. Gender may therefore be related to some behaviors but not to others. According to the theory, although there is no necessary relation between "distal" or "background" variables and any given behavior, distal variables such as cultural and personality differences and differences in a wide range of values should be reflected in the underlying belief structure.

APPLYING THE MODEL

The first step in using the theory of reasoned action involves identifying the behavior (or behaviors) that one wishes to understand, predict, and/or change. Unfortunately, this is not as simple or straightforward as is often assumed. As indicated above, it is important to distinguish between behaviors, behavioral categories, and goals. Equally important, from the perspective of TRA, the definition of a behavior involves several elements: the action (enlisting, using, buying), the target (the army, condoms), and the context (after graduating high school, for vaginal sex with an occasional partner). Clearly, a change in any one of the elements changes the behavior under consideration. Thus, for example, enlisting in the army is a different behavior than enlisting in the navy (a change in target). Similarly, enlisting in the army after graduating high school is a different behavior than enlisting in the army after completing college (a change in context). Moreover, in considering behavior, it is also important to include an additional element—time. For example, assessing whether one enlisted in the army in the past 3 months is different from assessing whether one enlisted in the Army in the past 2 years. Consistent with this, the intention to enlist in the army in the next 3 months is very different from the intention to enlist in the army in the next 2 years. Changing any one element in the behavioral definition will usually lead to very different beliefs about the consequences of performing that behavior and about the expectations of relevant others, and thus to very different attitudes, subjective norms, and intentions. Although all four elements should be considered in arriving at one's behavioral criterion, the level of specificity or generality used to define each element should be determined by the substantive questions being asked. Thus, for example, behavior may be assessed at a fairly general level (i.e., people could be asked whether they have ever [time] purchased [action] cigarettes [targets]—[context unspecified]) or at a more specific level (i.e., they could be asked whether they had purchased [action] Marlboro Light 100's [target] from their local supermarket [context] in the past 2 weeks [time]).

The second step in applying the theory of reasoned action is to identify the specific population to be considered. As indicated above, for any given behavior, both the relative importance of attitudes and norms as determinants of intention (and/or behavior) and the substantive content of the behavioral and normative beliefs underlying these determinants may vary as a function of the population under consideration. Thus, it is imperative to define the population (or populations) to be considered.

Once one or more behaviors and populations have been identified, the theory of reasoned action can be used to understand why some members of a target population are performing the behavior and others are not. As indicated above, it is necessary to go to a representative sample of the target population to identify salient outcomes and referents for the behavior in question. This formative research provides input necessary for the development of belief measures. Central to the theory of reasoned action is the concept of correspondence or compatibility. That is, for accurate prediction and full understanding of a given behavior, measures of beliefs, attitudes, norms, and intention must all correspond exactly to the behavior to be predicted. For example, if one is interested in predicting whether one will or will not always use condoms for vaginal sex with one's main partner during the next 6 months, beliefs, attitudes, norms, and intentions must all be assessed with respect to "My always using a condom for vaginal sex with my main partner for the next 6 months." By obtaining correspondent measures of all of these variables, one can determine, for example, whether a given health behavior (e.g., getting a colonoscopy) is not being performed because people have not formed intentions to get a colonoscopy or because they are unable to act on their intentions. Similarly, one can determine, for the population under consideration, whether intention is influenced primarily by attitudes or norms. Finally, one can identify the specific behavioral or normative beliefs that discriminate between those who do or do not (intend to) perform the behavior.

This type of information is essential for developing interventions to reinforce or change behavior. Clearly, different interventions are necessary if one is unable to act on one's intentions than if appropriate intentions have been formed. If appropriate intentions have not been formed, different interventions will be necessary to change behaviors under attitudinal control than behaviors under normative control. Finally, if one is going to change attitudes or subjective norms, the more information one has about underlying beliefs, the more likely is one to develop a successful intervention.

The theory has been used successfully to predict and explain a wide variety of behaviors, including such things as wearing safety helmets, smoking marijuana, voting, eating at fast-food restaurants, smoking cigarettes, drinking alcohol, entering an alcohol treatment program, using birth control pills, breast feeding, donating blood, wearing seat belts, condom use, recycling, church attendance, and engaging in premarital sexual behavior. It has also served as the theoretical basis for the development of a number of successful health-related interventions, particularly in the area of HIV/AIDS prevention.

Extensions of reasoned action theory include Ajzen's (1991) theory of planned behavior and Fishbein's (2000) integrative model of behavioral prediction.

—*Martin Fishbein*

See also THEORY OF PLANNED BEHAVIOR; THEORY OF TRIADIC INFLUENCE; TRANSTHEORETICAL MODEL OF BEHAVIOR CHANGE

Further Reading

Ajzen, I. (1991). The theory of planned behaviour. *Organizational Behavior & Human Decision Processes, 50*, 179-211.

Ajzen, I., & Fishbein, M. (1980). *Understanding attitudes and predicting social behavior.* Englewood Cliffs, NJ: Prentice Hall.

Fishbein, M. (1963). An investigation of the relationships between beliefs about an object and the attitude toward that object. *Human Relations, 16*, 233-240.

Fishbein, M. (2000). The role of theory in HIV prevention. *AIDS Care, 12*, 273-278.

Fishbein, M., & Ajzen, I. (1975). *Belief, attitude, intention and behavior: An introduction to theory and research.* Boston: Addison-Wesley.

Terry, D. J., Gallois, C., & McCamish, M. (1993). *The theory of reasoned action: Its application to AIDS-preventive behavior.* Oxford, UK: Pergamon.

THEORY OF TRIADIC INFLUENCE

The theory of triadic influence (TTI) is one of the most integrative theories of health behavior (see Figure 1). It explains behavior as being the result of three streams of causes of behavior (*intrapersonal, interpersonal,* and *sociocultural-environmental*) that flow through several levels of causation (ultimate → distal → proximal). Factors in each of the three streams interact with factors in each of the other streams. All three streams converge on decisions/intentions as the final predictor of behavior. Finally, engaging in a behavior may have effects that feed back and alter the original causes of the behavior.

The TTI provides a single, unifying framework that organizes the constructs from many other theories, including theories of social control and social bonding, social development, peer clustering, personality, cognitive-affective predictors, social/cognitive learning, biological vulnerability, and other integrative theories (see Petraitis, Flay, & Miller, 1995, for a review). TTI also provides dozens of testable hypotheses about causal processes, including mediation, moderation, and reciprocal effects. The TTI is useful not only for explaining behavior but also for designing interventions for the treatment or prevention of health-compromising or other risky behaviors, the promotion of health-enhancing and other positive behaviors, and positive youth development.

THE CAUSES OF BEHAVIOR

In order to understand the mass of findings in the vast theoretical and empirical literature on the causes of health behavior, reviewers have proposed various groupings of causes. Three generally agreed-upon categories consist of (1) *individual/intrapersonal* (biological, personality, character traits), (2) *social contextual* (neighborhood, family, school, peers), and (3) *broader sociocultural-environmental* (economic, political, religious). These three categories underlie the three streams of the TTI.

Levels/Tiers of Influence

The common causes of behavior listed above are causally distant from behavior, and have their actions through intervening/mediating variables. That is, they influence other variables closer (i.e., more proximal) to behavior that, in turn, cause changes in behavior. For example, families' effects on youth smoking may occur through several other variables, such as how parents interact with their children (an ultimate factor), the parents' own smoking-related attitudes

THE THEORY OF TRIADIC INFLUENCE

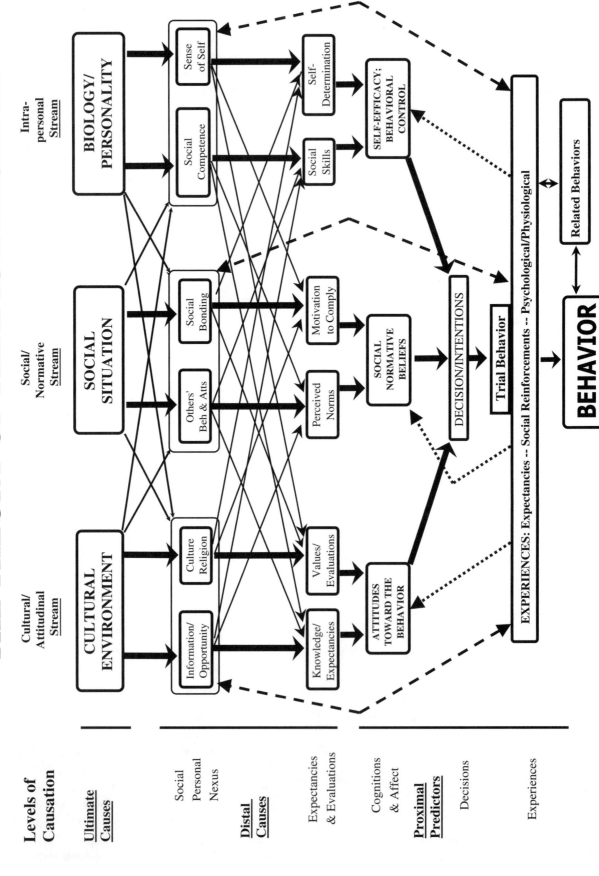

Figure 1   The Theory of Triadic Influence

800

and behaviors, and the children's perceptions of these (distal influences), and the children's general social normative beliefs about smoking, which in turn determine the children's decisions/intentions regarding smoking (the most proximal determinant). This is an example of a mediated causal chain and of the tiers/levels of causation in the TTI.

Ultimate influences are the furthest removed from behavior (e.g., neighborhood unemployment rate, rigid parenting style, biological susceptibility). As such, their effects are the most general, the most mediated, and often the most difficult for any one person or program to change. The well-known debate over the relative effects of genes and environment on behavior usually focuses on ultimate causes.

One step closer to behavior are the *distal causes*. The first level of distal causes are at the *social-personal nexus* (e.g., religious participation, bonding to parents or deviant role models, rebelliousness). Second-order distal causes, another step closer to behavior, are a set of cognitive/affective influences, called *expectancies and evaluations*. Compared to ultimate-level influences, distal-level influences are less far removed from behavior, have effects on behavior that are more specific and less mediated, and are usually less difficult to change.

Near the bottom of Figure 1 are the most *proximal causes* of behavior. Attitudes, social normative beliefs, and self-efficacy about the specific behavior (derived directly from the immediately preceding tier) have direct effects on decisions/intentions to engage in that behavior. The more proximal the cause to a behavior, the more likely it is to be specific to that behavior. For example, attitudes toward violence will be predictive of violence but less predictive of substance use or mental health. Proximal causes of behavior might be the easiest to alter in the short run.

Streams of Influence

The three streams of causes of behavior in the TTI are similar to the rings of influence in Bronfenbrenner's social ecology model; however, the social ecology model does not consider the levels/tiers of causation within its rings. The TTI is also broader and specifies more detailed causal links than other biopsychosocial models.

Sociocultural causes of behavior include societal, ethnic/cultural, religious, political/legal, and economic factors. They explain broad variations in behavior according to the society into which one is born and raised and one's ethnicity, culture, religion, education, and socioeconomic status. Religions, governmental regulations, educational institutions, economic systems, and opportunities place major constraints on the behavior of citizens. Witness the different behavioral patterns of people raised in different countries, political systems, or religions. They also influence the type of information and values systems available in a society (social-personal nexus). Mass media, education, religions, and other information/values systems carry many different kinds of information and values: news, that may be biased by the government of the country or locality; advertising, that may be regulated as to content or claims; and entertainment, that may help shape, as well as reflect, societal values, attitudes, and norms. Thus, the informational/values systems of society (ultimate) affect the knowledge that people learn and the values that they adopt (distal) that, in turn, influence people's decision making about their behavior (proximal).

Interpersonal or social causes of behavior include all of the social contexts or situations in which individuals interact with each other. These include communities or neighborhoods (ultimate), families, schools, peer groups, and friendships (distal). Communities and neighborhoods shape the general behavioral patterns of the people living in them. Families shape the behavior of their children's lives through their parenting styles and their own behavioral patterns, and by influencing selection of schools and how much time their children spend with peers versus family. These distal factors, in turn, determine individuals' perceptions of what others expect of them (perceived norms), and individuals' beliefs about how they think they should behave (motivation to comply or desire to please). These distal factors, in turn, determine social normative beliefs that, in turn, help determine decisions/intentions about how to behave (proximal).

Interstream Influences

It is clear from the above descriptions that *mediation* within streams lies at the core of TTI. In addition, some mediating processes flow between streams. For instance, weak bonds to school could foster strong bonds with deviant peers (distal social-personal nexus) that would then contribute to positive expectations for substance use (distal cultural/attitudinal). Another example is that poor behavioral control (distal intrapersonal), which might be the result of parenting, genetic predisposition, or some combination thereof, might contribute to risk-taking behavior through its contribution to involvement with risk-taking peers (distal social). Similarly, social influences might be mediated by attitudinal influences. For instance, weak bonds to school (distal social) help determine positive expectations for substance use (second-level distal attitudinal).

In addition to mediating influences between streams, there are *moderating processes* (statistical interactions) between streams (not shown in Figure 1). For example, exposure to a program (ultimate social-environmental) that teaches refusal skills might have no effect on adolescents who already have strong social skills (distal intrapersonal), but it might have its strongest effects on adolescents who have the weakest social skills. This is only one of numerous possible moderating processes within the TTI.

FEEDBACK

The TTI further posits that each instance of a behavior has a feedback influence on its predictors; that is, effects are bidirectional. Thus, adolescents' experimentation with smoking might change their relationships with peers and family, their own perceptions of the physiological effects of smoking, and their "knowledge" or expectancies about the personal and social effects of use. As this example makes clear, these changes might occur toward the top of the streams of influence and then filter down just as original causes did, or they might (also) occur at the proximal level.

The Role of Related Behaviors

Related behaviors influence or relate to each other in at least two ways. First, they have many of the same ultimate and distal causes. For example, youth raised in disadvantaged communities, raised by unconventional parents, or who are high on risk-taking propensity are more likely to engage in multiple problem behaviors. Second, engaging in one problem behavior alters, through the feedback mechanism described above, the causes of that behavior and closely related behaviors. For example, engaging in smoking cigarettes may change one's attitudes toward trying other substances.

Development

The multiple causes of behavior comprise a *dynamic system* that changes as people develop and have new experiences and as they experience particular behaviors. It is clear that biological and social development also play an important role in determining behavior. As children develop, the relative importance of attitudinal, normative, and self-efficacy variables changes, with attitudinal influences being most important for younger children, social and normative processes being more important during adolescence, and self-efficacy becoming more important as youth gain more experiences.

DESIGNING PREVENTION AND TREATMENT INTERVENTIONS

Many theories provide guidance for the design of prevention and treatment programs. The TTI is particularly useful because it is so comprehensive, addressing all of the causes of a particular behavior or class of behaviors, providing suggestions of how causal processes operate (mediating and moderating processes), and providing suggestions about how to achieve lasting effects.

First, the TTI can suggest which factors are modifiable with available resources and which are not. Clearly, interventions need to focus on those factors that are modifiable, rather than those that are not.

Second, the TTI makes it clear *why* a program's effectiveness is likely to be related to how well it addresses more rather than fewer risk and protective factors. However, the TTI, a "content" theory, does not inform us on *how* to achieve this—for this a "process" theory of change like Lawrence Green's PRECEDE-PROCEED model is also needed.

Third, the TTI suggests that it is better, in the long term, to address ultimate or distal factors rather than lower-level distal or proximal factors. If a program does not also address some of the determinants of these lower-level distal and proximal influences, they will soon be altered again, possibly changed back to their prior levels, by other influences in the students' homes, and broader social environments. Thus, to be long lasting, health promotion programs must also change the social ecologies in which people live.

Fourth, the TTI can suggest appropriate target audiences for interventions. Not all people have the same level of risk or the same reaction to a program.

For instance, a program that emphasizes the dangers of drug use might reduce the drug use of low risk takers but might promote drug use among high risk takers. Thus, the TTI, because it articulates moderating or interaction effects, can suggest populations for which programs are more appropriate, and whether prevention efforts should be universal, selective, or indicated.

Fifth, judging the potential impact of a program against the TTI might help planners anticipate the size of their program's impact. Many well-intended programs have been conducted under the assumption that simply teaching kids about the dangers of drugs will, by itself, have a meaningful impact. However, if program providers realized that information about drugs is only one variable in a more complex web of variables, they would come to expect more modest effects from their programs.

Sixth, the TTI can help locate the various effects of a particular intervention. Programs are designed to have an immediate effect on some variables that are expected to have subsequent effects on the targeted behavior. By spelling out the intervening (mediating) variables, theories allow us to measure the appropriate variables and help us locate the immediate, intermediate, and long-term effects of a program.

Finally, the TTI suggests that for program effects to be long lasting, programs must also be long lasting. After all, the influences in peoples' social environments to engage in unhealthy behavior do not go away, so programs must continue to influence or counteract them.

—*Brian R. Flay*

See also ADOPTION OF HEALTH BEHAVIOR; CULTURAL FACTORS AND HEALTH; THEORY OF PLANNED BEHAVIOR; THEORY OF REASONED ACTION; TRANSTHEORETICAL MODEL OF BEHAVIOR CHANGE

Further Reading

Flay, B. R. (1999). Understanding environmental, situational and intrapersonal risk and protective factors for youth tobacco use: The theory of triadic influence. *Discussant Comments. Nicotine & Tobacco Research, 1*, S111-S114.

Flay, B. (2002). Positive youth development requires comprehensive health promotion programs. *American Journal of Health Behavior, 26*, 407-424.

Flay, B. R., & Petraitis, J. (1994). The theory of triadic influence: A new theory of health behavior with implications for preventive interventions. In G. S. Albrecht (Ed.), *Advances in medical sociology: Vol. 4. A reconsideration of models of health behavior change* (pp. 19-44). Greenwich, CT: JAI.

Flay, B. R., Petraitis, J., & Hu, F. (1995). The theory of triadic influence: Preliminary evidence related to alcohol and tobacco use. In J. B. Fertig & J. P. Allen (Eds.), *NIAAA research monograph: Alcohol and tobacco: From basic science to clinical practice* (pp. 37-57). Bethesda, MD: Government Printing Office.

Flay, B. R., Petraitis, J., & Hu, F. B. (1999). Psychosocial risk and protective factors for adolescent tobacco use. *Nicotine & Tobacco Research, 1*, S59-S65.

Petraitis, J., & Flay, B. R. (2003). Bridging the gap between substance use prevention theory and practice. In W. Bukoski & Z. Sloboda (Eds.), *Handbook for drug abuse prevention: Theory, science, and practice*. New York: Plenum.

Petraitis, J., Flay, B. R., & Miller, T. Q. (1995). Reviewing theories of adolescent substance abuse: Organizing pieces of the puzzle. *Psychological Bulletin, 117*, 67-86.

Petraitis, J., Flay, B. R., Miller, T. Q., Torpy, E. J., & Greiner, B. (1998). Illicit substance use among adolescents: A matrix of prospective predictors. *Substance Use and Misuse, 33*, 2561-2604.

TRANSTHEORETICAL MODEL OF BEHAVIOR CHANGE

The transtheoretical model (TTM) provides a framework for understanding how people change behavior to prevent disease or enhance health. The model views behavior change as occurring in a series of *stages of change*, each of which requires different strategies or *processes of change* to best help individuals make progress toward healthier lifestyles. The basic principles of the TTM, first described by James Prochaska and Carlo DiClemente around 1980, were initially intended as a framework for describing how individuals change in psychotherapy. The first health applications focused on the addictions, especially smoking cessation, alcohol abuse, and weight control. The model has since been applied extensively, providing the basis for effective "stage-tailored" interventions for many important health behaviors, including smoking, diet, sun exposure, exercise, screening mammography, alcohol abuse, weight management, stress management, and diabetes self-management.

In addition to the stages and processes of change, the TTM also incorporates a series of intervening or intermediate outcome variables, including *decisional balance* (the pros and cons of change) and *self-efficacy* (*confidence* in the ability to change and *temptations* to engage in the unhealthy behavior across challenging situations). Together with the processes of change, these constructs provide a multidimensional view of how people change, and represent a variety of theoretical orientations to the behavior change process. It is in this sense that the TTM is thought of as *trans*theoretical. Distinctive characteristics of the TTM include explicit recognition of *all* stages of readiness as important components of the change process and the emphasis placed on transitions between stages as functions of other important dimensions of behavior change. In particular, the TTM stresses the importance of the early stages of change, which are undifferentiated in most other theoretical models.

STAGES OF CHANGE

The central organizing construct of the TTM is the concept of stages of change. Five ordered categories of readiness to change behavior have been defined: *precontemplation, contemplation, preparation, action,* and *maintenance.* The term *motivational readiness to change* is sometimes used synonymously to mean stages of change. The stages provide a temporal or developmental dimension that represents when change occurs.

Precontemplation

Individuals in the precontemplation stage of change have no intention of changing their unhealthy behavior in the near future, usually defined as within the next 6 months. People in this stage may feel that they do not have a problem, or that their unhealthy behavior is not serious enough to warrant attention. They may be uninformed or underinformed about the seriousness of their behavior and the potential consequences of not changing. Individuals in the precontemplation stage may wish to change their behavior but have no serious intention of trying to do so. They may be demoralized about their chances due to repeated unsuccessful attempts to change. They tend to avoid thinking, reading, or talking about their behavior and are frequently characterized as resistant, defensive, and unmotivated. For those in

precontemplation, the costs of change clearly outweigh the benefits.

Contemplation

Individuals in the contemplation stage of change admit that they may have a problem and are seriously considering changing their behavior within the next 6 months. They understand the benefits of change but are also very much aware of the costs, resulting in considerable ambivalence. As a result, these individuals typically do not act on their intentions and frequently remain stuck in the contemplation stage for lengthy periods of time ("chronic contemplation"). Distinctive characteristics of the contemplation stage include the substitution of thinking for action, constant struggling with weighing the costs and benefits of change, indecision, and lack of commitment.

Preparation

Individuals in the preparation stage of change intend to act on their unhealthy behavior in the immediate future, usually defined as within the next 30 days. This stage of change is characterized by having a plan of action and by taking small steps toward action, such as reducing the number of cigarettes smoked per day, quitting smoking for 24 hours, buying a self-help book, joining a health club, or talking to health professionals. The preparation stage is also characterized by recent unsuccessful attempts at behavior change. It is this combination of intention to change with a behavioral pattern of recent attempts to change that distinguishes individuals in the preparation stage from those in contemplation.

Action

The action stage of change is a period of active engagement in changing unhealthy behavior. The period of action is usually described as lasting for 6 months, as this typically encompasses the period of greatest risk of relapse. Not all behavior change is sufficient for an individual to be considered in the action stage. To reach action, individuals must meet a strict standard of behavior change, such as quitting smoking (rather than simply reducing the number of cigarettes smoked) or eating five or more servings of fruits and vegetables per day (rather than simply increasing the number of servings per day). The action criterion is dependent on the specific behavior and should represent the established consensus of experts in the field as to how much change is sufficient to promote health or meaningfully reduce the chances of disease.

Maintenance

Individuals achieve maintenance after 6 months of continuous successful action. The goal for this stage is to continue to work on preventing relapse and consolidate the gains made during the action stage. Situational temptations to engage in the unhealthy behavior decline, and confidence in coping with challenging situations increases throughout this period. Maintenance is thus a continuation of the change process and not a static period. There is still a risk of relapse, and for some individuals and for some behaviors, maintenance may be a lifelong struggle.

Progression from precontemplation to maintenance is assumed to be invariant in that individuals need to complete the tasks and consolidate the gains of one stage before they are ready to successfully progress to the next. Unfortunately, most individuals do not progress linearly through the stages. A cyclical pattern is more common: individuals reaching the action or maintenance stage may relapse and recycle to an earlier stage of change. Relapse was once considered one of the stages of change but is now viewed as an event that stops movement through action or maintenance, initiating the process of recycling. Fortunately, most individuals who relapse do not regress all the way back to precontemplation. Some of the gains made before the relapse episode are preserved, so that subsequent action attempts are more likely to be successful. The TTM views relapse not as a failure but as an opportunity to learn from previous mistakes, weed out unsuccessful change strategies, and try new approaches.

PROCESSES OF CHANGE

The processes of change are covert and overt cognitive, affective, evaluative, and behavioral strategies and activities used by individuals to progress through the stages of change. A comparative analysis of more than 300 theories of psychotherapy identified 10 fundamental processes of change, such as consciousness raising (Freudian), contingency management (Skinnerian), and helping relationships (Rogerian). While additional processes of change have since been identified as important for specific health behaviors, 10 have been consistently supported across a wide range of behaviors. The processes are organized into two general higher-order processes. The experiential processes incorporate cognitive, affective, and evaluative aspects of change, whereas the behavioral processes include more specific, observable change strategies. The experiential processes include *consciousness raising* (efforts by the individual to increase awareness, seek new information, and gain understanding and feedback about their behavior), *dramatic relief* (experiencing and expressing feelings about their behavior and potential solutions, resulting in increased, often intense, emotional experiences), *environmental reevaluation* (affective and cognitive consideration of how their behavior affects their physical and social environment), *self-reevaluation* (emotional and cognitive reappraisal of personal values and reassessment of self-image with respect to behavior), and *social liberation* (awareness of social norms and the fact that alternative, healthy lifestyles are both available and acceptable). The behavioral processes include *contingency (reinforcement) management* (rewarding oneself or being rewarded by others for making appropriate changes, including punishment, but more typically using positive reinforcement), *counterconditioning* (substitution of alternative healthier behaviors as replacements for unhealthy behaviors), *helping relationships* (trusting, accepting, and utilizing the support of caring others during attempts to change behavior), *self-liberation* (choosing and committing to change as well as personal belief in the ability to change), and *stimulus control* (removal of cues for unhealthy behaviors, addition of cues for healthy alternatives, avoiding challenging social situations, and seeking alternative environments that provide support for healthier behaviors).

DECISIONAL BALANCE: PROS AND CONS OF CHANGE

Part of the decision to move from one stage to the next is based on the relative weight given to the pros and cons of changing behavior. The pros represent positive aspects or advantages of change, and the cons represent negative aspects or disadvantages of change. The comparative weighting of the pros and cons varies depending on the individual's stage of change. In the precontemplation stage, the cons of change outweigh the pros, whereas in the action and maintenance stages, the pros outweigh the cons. The positive and negative aspects of change are usually about equal in the contemplation stage. The resulting indecision and lack of commitment is largely responsible for individuals becoming stuck in the contemplation stage, substituting thinking for action while continually struggling with the costs and benefits of change. Decisional balance serves as an intermediate outcome variable in the TTM, the increase in the pros from precontemplation to contemplation being especially striking. Thus, the pros are an excellent indicator of the decision to move out of the precontemplation stage. The relationship between the stages of change and decisional balance has been shown to be very consistent across a wide range of health behaviors.

Self-Efficacy: Confidence and Temptation

The self-efficacy component of the TTM was adapted from cognitive-social learning theory. In the TTM, self-efficacy typically takes the form of asking individuals how *confident* they are that they will not engage in an unhealthy behavior and how tempted they would be to engage in an unhealthy behavior across a range of challenging or difficult situations. Both constructs are usually designed to be multidimensional in assessing situational determinants of relapse. Confidence and temptation typically show only modest relationships to stage of change from precontemplation to preparation, followed by strong and essentially linear increases and decreases from preparation to maintenance, respectively. Both constructs serve as indicators of relapse risk for individuals in the action and maintenance stages.

INTEGRATION OF TTM CONSTRUCTS

The stages and processes of change are integrally related. Transitions between stages are mediated by the use of distinct subsets of change processes and are associated with substantial changes in decision making and self-efficacy. Individuals in the earlier stages of change tend to rely on the experiential processes of change and report relatively little confidence in their ability to change and relatively high temptation to engage in unhealthy behaviors across difficult situations. The cons of change typically outweigh the pros. Individuals in the later stages tend to rely on the behavioral processes, report more confidence in the ability to change and relatively less temptation to engage in unhealthy behaviors, and evaluate the pros of change more highly than the cons. Consideration of

these relationships is important for the development of effective interventions. When treatment programs ignore or mismatch processes to stages, behavior change attempts are likely to fail. Interventions that deliver stage-specific interventions may accelerate progress through the stages. An important advantage of this approach is that stage-tailored interventions can be applicable not just to individuals who are ready to change behavior but to the majority of the population who are neither prepared nor motivated to change.

—*Joseph S. Rossi*

See also ADOPTION OF HEALTH BEHAVIOR; MOTIVATIONAL INTERVIEWING; SELF-EFFICACY; SMOKING AND NICOTINE DEPENDENCE: INTERVENTIONS; TAILORED COMMUNICATIONS; THEORY OF PLANNED BEHAVIOR; THEORY OF REASONED ACTION; THEORY OF TRIADIC INFLUENCE

Further Reading

Joseph, J., Breslin, C., & Skinner, H. (1999). Critical perspectives on the transtheoretical model and stages of change. In J. A. Tucker, D. M. Donovan, & G. A. Marlatt (Eds.), *Changing addictive behavior: Bridging clinical and public health strategies* (pp. 160-190). New York: Guilford.

Prochaska, J. O., Norcross, J. C., & DiClemente, C. C. (1994). *Changing for good.* New York: William Morrow.

Prochaska, J. O., Redding, C. A., & Evers, K. (2002). The transtheoretical model and stages of change. In K. Glanz, B. K. Rimer, & F. M. Lewis (Eds.), *Health behavior and health education: Theory, research, and practice* (3rd ed., pp. 99-120). San Francisco: Jossey-Bass.

Rossi, J. S., Rossi, S. R., Velicer, W. F., & Prochaska, J. O. (1995). Motivational readiness to control weight. In D. B. Allison (Ed.), *Handbook of assessment methods for eating behaviors and weight-related problems: Measures, theory, and research* (pp. 387-430). Thousand Oaks, CA: Sage.

Spencer, L., Pagell, F., Hallion, M. E., & Adams, T. B. (2002). Applying the transtheoretical model to tobacco cessation and prevention: A review of literature. *American Journal of Health Promotion, 17,* 7-71.

TYPE A BEHAVIOR. *See* HEART DISEASE AND TYPE A BEHAVIOR

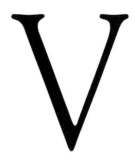

VIOLENCE PREVENTION

This entry provides a brief explanation of the three levels of preventive intervention, followed by an overview of the prevalence and prevention efforts for four major categories of violence in the United States: youth violence, suicide, child maltreatment, and intimate partner and sexual violence. Although space limits the breadth and depth of scope for this extensive topic, it is hoped that the reader will pursue more extensive readings on each of these and other violence-related topics as well as the many violence prevention efforts too numerous to mention. Before turning to the various manifestations of violence and their prevention, it is helpful to briefly explain the Institute of Medicine's report of summarizing the three levels of preventive intervention efforts. *Universal* violence prevention programs are designed to reach a wide audience of individuals who may or may not have experienced any aspect of violence. By exposing a large number of individuals to preventive information about violence, the goal is to decrease the prevalence of the behavior among a vast audience. *Selective* programs, however, are designed to target a specific audience with one or more risk factors associated with participating in violence behaviors such as exposure to interpersonal, community, or neighborhood violence. Selective interventions are typically designed to modify a malleable risk factor or to increase known protective factors in order to prevent violence behavior among individuals who have a higher likelihood of participating in violence.

Indicated programs are designed for individuals who are already participating in violence behaviors. The goal of indicated programs is to stop *future* participation in violence behaviors.

For all four violence areas, the vast majority of rigorously evaluated and funded interventions are selective and indicated programs.

YOUTH VIOLENCE

Homicide is the second leading cause of death among 15- to 24-year-olds overall. In 1999, 4,998 youths ages 15 to 24 were murdered—an average of 14 per day. Guns are a factor in most youth homicides. In 1999, 81% of homicide victims ages 15 to 24 were killed with firearms. Although typically overestimated, school-associated violent deaths represent less than 1% of all homicides and suicides that occur among school-aged children.

Historically, violence prevention and intervention efforts have been the purview of the criminal and juvenile justice system and as such have been mired by the fact that the justice system largely interacts with youth who have already committed a violent crime. Indicated intervention efforts aimed at rehabilitating youth to prevent recidivism have been somewhat successful; however, the juvenile justice system has had little to no impact in terms of preventing youth from becoming involved with violence.

Over the past decade, there have been efforts to develop and evaluate universal school-based violence prevention efforts. Four universal programs have emerged as effective: Promoting Alternative THinking

Strategies (PATHS), Bullying Prevention Program (BPP), Life Skills Training (LST), and the Midwestern Prevention Project (MPP). Interestingly, the latter two programs focus on drug prevention but appear to have more generalized effects for reducing youth violence. Community-based violence prevention efforts are selective programs that target areas particularly plagued with neighborhood or community violence. Because these community-based programs (e.g., Detroit's Save Our Sons and Daughters Program) are recent undertakings, they do not yet have reported results.

SUICIDE

Overall, suicide is the 11th leading cause of death for all Americans and is the third leading cause of death for young people aged 15 to 24. Males are four times more likely to die from suicide than are females. However, females are more likely to attempt suicide than are males. Nearly three of every five suicides in 1999 (57%) were committed with a firearm. Suicide rates tend to increase with age and are highest among Americans aged 65 years and older. This trend is marked by the fact that 1980-1990 was the first decade since the 1940s that the suicide rate for older individuals rose instead of declined.

Because of the high association of mental disorder, suicide prevention programs have tended to focus on identifying and treating clinical levels of depression or other mental illness. Suicide prevention programs can generally be classified into one of five types: (1) increasing training for community and institutional gatekeepers to identify and refer those at-risk for suicidal behavior, (2) treating the underlying risk factors associated with suicide such as depression or alcohol and drug abuse, (3) providing general education about suicide vulnerabilities, (4) reducing access to lethal means such as guns, and prescription drugs, and (5) developing self-referral sources such as hotlines. While each of the above programs has the potential to avert suicide, there are many and varied risk factors associated with suicidal behavior. The effectiveness of these five approaches has yet to be demonstrated, thus potentially hindering prevention program implementers, community/institutional gatekeepers, and policymakers in their efforts to educate their constituencies about the array of suicide prevention tools currently available.

CHILD MALTREATMENT

Child maltreatment includes physical abuse, neglect (physical, educational, emotional, and/or medical), sexual abuse, emotional abuse (psychological/verbal abuse/mental injury), and other types of maltreatment such as abandonment, exploitation, and/or threats to harm the child. Every year, an estimated 826,000 children experience nonfatal child maltreatment. Though the risk factors are varied, an ecological approach takes into account the parent's background, the child's temperament, and societal aspects related to child maltreatment. This framework underscores the need for prevention programs to go beyond simplistic parent education programs to better effectively target the complex interaction between parents, children, and the society in which they live.

Universal programs to prevent child maltreatment are typically public awareness messages where parents are informed about child maltreatment along with ways to get help when they feel out of control. There has been, however, no systematic evaluation of the value of these messages. Selective interventions are aimed at families where the risk factors for child maltreatment are high. An example is the Home Visitation Program by David Olds and associates. This program targeted young, single, low-income mothers using a comprehensive approach where mothers were visited in their homes with parent education and informal support, as well as being connected to available social and health services, including adequate health care. Evaluations of this program have demonstrated a reduction in child maltreatment along with a host of other positive benefits for the child and the mother. Indicated interventions are typically run by social and/or human service agencies, since these families have had one or more children who have been maltreated. While there is no data on the effectiveness of these state-run indicated programs, program officials have long advocated for comprehensive programs that deal with the wide spectrum of problems that these families face.

INTIMATE PARTNER AND SEXUAL VIOLENCE

Available data suggest that violence against women is a substantial public health problem in the United States. Every year, an estimated 4,000 females die as the result of homicide. Thirty percent of these women were known to have been murdered by a spouse or ex-spouse. Data on nonfatal cases of assault are less easily accessible, but recent survey data suggest that approximately 1.3 million women have been physically assaulted annually, and approximately 200,000 women have been raped annually by a current or former intimate partner.

Universally targeted public awareness messages about intimate partner and sexual violence prevention have not been systematically evaluated for their effectiveness. Examples of selective programs are those delivered on college campuses focusing on correcting intimate partner violence myths, understanding consequences for such violence, increasing assertiveness and self-defense skills, as well as helping students learn to avoid high-risk situations. Results of these programs have been mixed, partially due to the fact that these interventions have tended to be one-time, short duration programs, thus inhibiting their potential effectiveness. Indicated programs for offenders have also tended to focus on dispelling intimate partner violence myths, effective anger management, and engaging empathy for the victims. Indicated program results have relied on recommission of a crime (recidivism) as an index of program success and as such is a limited indicator of intimate partner violence prevention.

—*Paula Smith*

See also CHILD ABUSE, CHILD NEGLECT, AND HEALTH

Further Reading

Center for the Study and Prevention of Violence at the University of Colorado. (2003). Retrieved from http://www.colorado.edu/cspv/blueprints/index.html

Centers for Disease Control and Prevention. (1992). *Youth suicide prevention program: A resource guide*. Atlanta, GA: Department of Health and Human Services.

Harrington, D., & Dubowitz, H. (1999). Preventing child maltreatment. In R. Hampton (Ed.), *Family violence* (pp. 122-147). Thousand Oaks, CA: Sage.

Institute of Medicine. (1994). *Reducing the risk for mental disorders: Frontiers for preventive intervention research*. Washington, DC: National Academy Press.

Schewe, P. A. (2002). Guidelines for developing rape prevention and risk reduction interventions. In P. A. Schewe (Ed.), *Preventing violence in relationships: Interventions across the lifespan* (pp. 107-121). Washington, DC: American Psychological Association.

Spivak, H., Prothrow-Stith, D., & Hausman, A. (1988). Dying is no accident: Adolescents, violence and intentional injury. *Paediatric Clinics of North America, 35,* 1339-1347.

VITAL EXHAUSTION

Vital exhaustion is a psychosocial risk indicator for adverse cardiovascular health outcomes, including myocardial infarction and recurrent cardiac events following percutaneous coronary interventions. Exhaustion has three characteristic components: lack of energy, increased irritability, and demoralization. The duration of an episode of exhaustion can vary from 2 weeks to 2 years. Individuals should not be classified as exhausted if the condition lasts longer than 2 years without showing an increase within that period. Reliable questionnaire and interview-derived assessment instruments have been developed. In patients with cardiovascular disease, prevalence estimates of exhaustion range from 30% to 50%, compared to 5% in the general adult population. Exhaustion is purportedly the end stage of prolonged uncontrollable psychological distress and has biological correlates relevant to the pathophysiology of cardiovascular disease progression. Psychosocial intervention techniques have been proven feasible in patients with coronary artery disease.

The construct *vital exhaustion* was developed using empirical techniques aimed to identify premonitory symptoms of myocardial infarction. Pivotal research has been conducted by Dr. Ad Appels and his colleagues in the Netherlands. The prefix *vital* was included to reflect the far-reaching consequences of this condition on daily life function (similar to vital depression) and is not used in the remainder of this text.

ASSESSMENT

Exhaustion can be assessed with the 21-item Maastricht Questionnaire (MQ) or, preferably, with the Maastricht Interview for Vital Exhaustion.

The Maastricht Questionnaire has been used in a variety of clinical and epidemiological settings in over 15 countries. Factor analysis has confirmed that exhaustion has three main components (lack of energy, increased irritability, and demoralization), and possibly a separate factor indicating sleep problems. Items are scored from 0 (symptom absent) to 2 (symptom present), and question marks are coded as 1, resulting in a possible score range from 0 to 42. Two additional items have been added to the questionnaire to better assess the irritability component (the MQ-23). Validation for these additional 2 items is limited, and the 21-item version is most commonly used. The mean and standard deviation of the questionnaire is 8.8 ± 8.7 for healthy adults. Hospitalized patients without cardiovascular disease have MQ scores of 11.7 ± 9.8, and patients with documented cardiovascular disease have scores of 18.5 ± 9.5. The questionnaire's reliability is satisfactory (Cronbach's alpha = 0.80). Consistent with most psychological self-report measures, women tend to score 0.5 standard deviation higher then men. For clinical and research selection purposes, several cutoffs have been used to identify "exhausted" individuals, ranging from 14 to 18, depending on the importance of false positives or false negatives.

The Maastricht Interview for Vital Exhaustion has 23 items derived from the questionnaire and inquires about the presence and duration of exhaustion symptoms. The interview has adequate internal consistency (Cronbach's alpha = 0.86) and interrater reliability (kappa = 0.91). The correlation between questionnaire and interview scores is 0.74. Interviews are diagnostic for exhaustion if (a) seven or more of the items are scored positive and (b) at least one of the three exhaustion components shows an increase in severity in the past 2 years. The major advantage of the interview over the questionnaire is its superiority in preventing diagnosis of false positives.

PREVALENCE

Exhaustion is common in patients with established coronary artery disease, with prevalence estimates ranging from 30% to 50% (mean MQ scores 18.5 ± 9.5; see above). In healthy adults, the prevalence is substantially lower, and selection strategies for psychophysiological studies should target a prevalence of 5%.

Because fatigue and lack of energy are common symptoms of a variety of general medical conditions, exhaustion scores are often elevated in individuals attending health care clinics and those hospitalized for noncardiac medical conditions. There is also overlap between symptoms of depressive mood disorders and exhaustion. Research on the convergent and divergent validity of these two constructs is still in progress; preliminary data suggest that 57% of exhausted individuals do not meet criteria for major or minor depression. Most individuals (> 90%) meeting criteria for major depression also meet criteria for exhaustion. Important differences exist in the biological concomitants of exhaustion and depression, including circadian variation of cortisol and hemostatic measures. Exhaustion is also more common than major depression in cardiac patients, and may therefore be an additional psychosocial risk indicator for adverse disease progression.

ETIOLOGY AND THEORETICAL BACKGROUND

Exhaustion reflects the end stage of prolonged and uncontrollable psychological distress. The etiological theory for exhaustion builds on Selye's general adaptation syndrome, which postulates that prolonged physical or emotional challenges result in a state of exhaustion associated with elevated risk of morbidity and mortality. The psychosocial precursors as well as biological correlates of exhaustion support this etiological theory.

Exhaustion is more prevalent among individuals who experience prolonged psychological distress. For example, cross-sectional studies indicate that the prevalence of exhaustion is higher among individuals of low socioeconomic status and Type A behavior pattern and/or hostility. No studies have examined race and ethnicity as predictors of exhaustion.

Because exhaustion is commonly observed in patients with cardiovascular diseases, research has examined to what extent exhaustion reflects underlying disease severity. No associations have been found between exhaustion and the anatomical severity of coronary disease, cardiac pump function at rest, or inducible ischemia in response to exercise or mental arousal. In selected cases, however, complaints of exhaustion may reflect severe cardiac pathology. As described below, exhaustion has biological correlates, including elevated markers of inflammation and proinflammatory cytokines. These inflammatory factors could be secondary to underlying cardiovascular disease, and the role of immune system parameters in the etiology of exhaustion requires further investigation. Furthermore, there may be a circular influence between exhaustion and adverse health behaviors, including low exercise, smoking, and coffee consumption.

BIOLOGICAL CORRELATES

Research has indicated the following biological correlates of exhaustion: flattened diurnal cortisol profile; increased coagulation factors; impaired fibrinolysis upon awakening; and increased markers of low-grade inflammation (e.g., C-reactive protein), and possibly increased pathogen burden (e.g., cytomegalovirus). No consistent evidence has been found for altered cardiovascular reactivity or hypercortisolemia, or adverse lipid profile. Finally, exhaustion is characterized by reduced duration of deep sleep stages, altered autonomic nervous system function (reduced parasympathetic activity), and possibly impaired exercise tolerance (see Table 1).

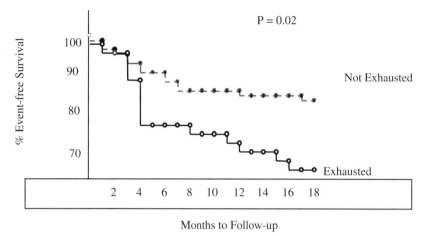

Figure 1 Predictive Value of Exhaustion for New Cardiac Events During 1.5-Year Follow-Up

Table 1 Biological Correlates of Exhaustion

Cardiovascular Factor	Measures
Hemostasis	
Low-grade Inflammation	C-reactive protein, white blood cell count
	Pro-inflammatory cytokines, lower albumin
Coagulation	Fibrinogen, Factor$_{1+2}$
Fibrinolysis (morning)	Plasminogen activator inhibitor-1 activity, t-PA antigen
Neuroendocrine	
Autonomic Nervous System	Heart rate variability reduced
Cortisol	Diurnal variation flattened
Sleep	Slow wave sleep reduced

HEALTH RISKS

The primary health risks associated with exhaustion include incident and recurrent cardiac events. Prospective studies in healthy individuals indicate that exhaustion is associated with an excess risk of first myocardial infarction (RR = 2.3, $p < .001$) and unstable angina during 4-year follow-up. In patients undergoing successful coronary angioplasty, exhaustion is associated with a greater than twofold risk of recurrent

cardiac events within 1.5 years (OR = 2.7; 95% CI = 1.1-6.3). As shown in Figure 1, cardiac events (cardiac death, myocardial infarction, bypass surgery, documented coronary disease progression) occurred more often in exhausted than nonexhausted patients during follow-up. Most research suggests that the predictive value of exhaustion is primarily observed within 2 years after assessment. Case-control studies indicate that exhaustion is also associated with elevated risk of sudden cardiac death, and that cardiovascular risks are similar for men and women.

The theoretical framework of the etiology of exhaustion, as well as its biological correlates, does not preclude exhaustion as a risk factor for adverse health outcomes other than cardiovascular disease. However, empirical evidence has as yet not supported such associations.

TREATMENT STRATEGIES

Interventions specifically targeting exhaustion have focused on stress-management strategies, including relaxation, management of hostile attitudes and behaviors, and breathing techniques. Preliminary analyses indicate that exhaustion can be successfully treated by psychosocial interventions. The most efficient setting for such interventions appears to be in small groups (approximately eight participants). Pharmacological trials using SSRIs and related compounds in different contexts (e.g., posttraumatic stress disorder) have resulted in significant reductions of exhaustion scores. A large randomized trial currently investigates the efficacy of psychological interventions in over 700 exhausted postangioplasty patients.

CONCLUSION

Exhaustion consists of three components: lack of energy, increased irritability, and demoralization. The duration of an episode of exhaustion can vary from 2 weeks to 2 years. The risk ratios of exhaustion for cardiovascular disease are similar to traditional risk factors such as hypertension and hypercholesterolemia. Exhaustion is hypothesized to result from prolonged uncontrollable psychological distress and has biological correlates relevant to the pathophysiology of cardiovascular disease progression. The role of inflammatory processes in the etiology of exhaustion requires further investigation. Understanding the mechanisms accounting for the relationship between exhaustion and cardiovascular disease may help to direct the timing and nature of psychosocial interventions in patients at risk for clinical coronary artery disease.

—*Willem J. Kop*

Further Reading

Appels, A. (1997). Depression and coronary heart disease: Observations and questions. *Journal of Psychosomatic Research, 43,* 443-452.

Kop, W. J. (1999). Chronic and acute psychological risk factors for clinical manifestations of coronary artery disease. *Psychosomatic Medicine, 61,* 476-487.

Kop, W. J., Appels, A. P., Mendes de Leon, C. F., de Swart, H. B., & Bar, F. W. (1994). Vital exhaustion predicts new cardiac events after successful coronary angioplasty. *Psychosomatic Medicine, 56,* 281-287.

Kop, W. J., & Cohen, N. (2001). Psychological risk factors and immune system involvement in cardiovascular disease. In R. Ader, D. L. Felten, & N. Cohen (Eds.), *Psychoneuroimmunology* (3rd ed., pp. 525-544). San Diego, CA: Academic Press.

Meesters, C. M., & Appels, A. (1996). An interview to measure vital exhaustion, I and II. *Psychological Health, 11,* 557-581.

van Diest, R., & Appels, A. (1991). Vital exhaustion and depression: A conceptual study. *Journal of Psychosomatic Research, 35,* 535-544.

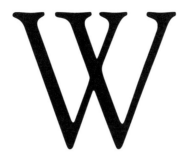

WOMEN'S HEALTH ISSUES

Women's health issues have traditionally been defined in terms of reproductive health such as menstrual cycles, infertility, pregnancy, and menopause. However, women's health is now considered to encompass a much wider range of topics, including diseases that are more common in women (such as osteoporosis, lupus, depression, and diabetes) as well as the leading causes of death among women (coronary heart disease, AIDS, and lung cancer). Women's health issues also include gender differences in health risks (such as substance abuse and physical inactivity); how societal influences such as social norms, poverty, and caregiving impact women's health; and violence against women. Sex differences in physiology and anatomy related to health consequences are also a growing area of interest. A 2001 report from the Institute of Medicine concludes that differences in the prevalence and severity of a broad range of diseases and conditions exist between the sexes and that the distinct anatomy and physiology of being male or female has a broader influence on health than previously thought. Differences in health are influenced by individual genetic and physiologic conditions as well as by one's experiences and interactions with environmental factors.

This entry is organized around a paradigm developed by Chesney and Ozer, which provides a model of ways to view women's health issues. First, there are key content areas such as the leading causes of death among women, diseases more common in women, reproductive health, and gender and societal influences

on health risk. Underlying this content layer are processes that span content areas that include the diversity of participants and use of gender-appropriate methods and measures in health research studies. Women's health issues encompass an extremely broad area, and this entry can only briefly mention some of these key areas.

CONTENT AREAS

Demographics and Leading Causes of Death Among Women

Demographic Patterns

Currently, the life expectancy of a non-Hispanic White woman in the United States is 80 years, and it is approximately 75 years for an African American woman. In the next 50 years, it is projected that the United States will experience a shift toward an increasingly older U.S. female population. The aging of the female population is likely to result in larger numbers of elderly women living with chronic illnesses and/or functional disabilities. The racial and ethnic mix of the U.S. female population will also change dramatically during that time. The Hispanic female population is expected to increase from the current 11% to approximately 20% of U.S. females by 2050. The Asian American female population is also projected to rise from 4% of the current total population to 9% of U.S. females in 2050. Non-Hispanic White women, who comprise approximately 70% of the female population, are anticipated to account for only 60% of the population in 2030 and only 35% in 2050. This diversity in the U.S. female population has implications for future health care delivery systems and the need for health care workers to be knowledgeable of health conditions affecting women of diverse ethnic backgrounds.

Leading Causes of Death

The leading causes of death in women across all age groups are (a) diseases of the heart, (b) cancer, (c) cerebrovascular diseases, (d) chronic obstructive pulmonary diseases, and (e) pneumonia and influenza. This rank order of causes of mortality is also the same for White and African American women. Hispanic women share the top three causes of death, but diabetes mellitus is the fourth leading cause of death for women of this ethnicity, followed by pneumonia and influenza and then chronic obstructive pulmonary disease as the sixth leading cause of death. Differences in this rank ordering are attributed largely to the lower rates of smoking among older Hispanic females. Causes of mortality also vary by age group, as well as ethnicity, with deaths in younger women occurring more from accidental, violent, or infectious causes rather than chronic conditions.

Cardiovascular disease. Although heart disease and stroke are still perceived by some as affecting men primarily, more than half of the deaths from cardiovascular disease occur among women. Cardiovascular disease is the leading cause of death among women, and mortality rates are higher for African American than White or Hispanic women. Cardiovascular disease kills more women each year than all forms of cancer combined, and stroke kills more than twice as many American women as breast cancer. Heart disease in women often goes undetected and untreated until the disease has progressed. As a result, approximately 40% of women who have heart attacks die within 1 year, compared to roughly 25% of men. African American women with heart disease have 3 to 4 times greater risk of death from heart disease than either White or Hispanic women and 2.5 times the mortality rate from cerebrovascular diseases. Similarly, women account for about 40% of new strokes each year, but approximately 60% of stroke deaths.

Cancer. Since 1987, lung cancer has been the primary cause of cancer mortality in U.S. women, followed by deaths from breast and colorectal cancers respectively.

The lung cancer mortality rate has been attributed to the increases in rates of women's cigarette smoking during the 1950s and subsequent decades. Breast cancer incidence rates declined during the early 1990s, primarily in younger women, due to improved treatments and early detection. Although rates of breast cancer are higher for Whites, African American women are more likely to die from breast cancer. Incident rates of endometrial and uterine cancer have remained relatively constant. Rates for cervical cancer have declined markedly over the past 30 years, due to widespread use of Pap tests to detect cancerous and precancerous lesions. For both endometrial and cervical cancers, mortality is highest for African American women than for Whites, Hispanics, and Asian Americans. Ovarian cancer accounts for approximately 4% of all cancer deaths, and although it is a rare cancer, the lack of techniques for the early detection of this condition have resulted in its being responsible for more deaths than any other cancer of the female reproductive system.

DISORDERS MORE COMMON IN WOMEN THAN MEN

Eating Disorders

Eating disorders, including anorexia nervosa and bulimia, are more prevalent and are on the increase among women in the United States. Eating disorders affect an estimated 5 million Americans annually, 90% of whom are young females. Approximately 1% of young women will develop anorexia nervosa, and bulimia affects approximately 1% to 3%. Both of these disorders are initiated primarily in mid to late adolescence. Only about half of those who develop both conditions will recover fully. The remainder will have some lifetime struggles with the illness, as well as some debilitation secondary to their eating disorders.

Mental Health

In any given year, approximately 13% of women will have a diagnosable depressive disorder. About one in five women will experience an episode of major depression during her lifetime, twice the rate seen in men. Anxiety disorders are also more common in women than in men. Although they often receive less attention than depressive disorders, anxiety disorders are the most common psychiatric disorders in the

United States. Slightly more than one third of women will experience an anxiety disorder in their lifetime; in any given year, almost a quarter of American women will be affected with an anxiety disorder. Anxiety disorders include such diagnoses as specific phobia, social phobia, agoraphobia, panic orders, and generalized anxiety disorder. Psychiatric disorders often go undetected and treated in women, and it is estimated that only 30% of patients with anxiety disorders actually receive treatment for their conditions.

Autoimmune Diseases

Autoimmune diseases, conditions where the body's immune system becomes defective and produces antibodies against normal parts of the body, comprise a list of approximately 80 serious, chronic conditions that are a major source of disability in women, including multiple sclerosis, fibromyalgia, scleroderma, and systemic lupus erythematosus. About three quarters of these autoimmune diseases occur in women, primarily during the childbearing years. Multiple sclerosis, one of the most common, is most often diagnosed in women in their 20s and 30s, at almost double the rate of men. Eighty percent of fibromyalgia occurs in women. Scleroderma affects women, particularly African American women, three times more often than men overall, and this rate increases drastically during the childbearing years. In addition, approximately 90% of all cases of systemic lupus erythematosus occur in women, and it is three times more common in African American than White women.

Diabetes

Diabetes mellitus is a common chronic illness characterized by defects in the body's ability to produce or use insulin. Approximately 8 million women in the United States have diabetes compared to 7.5 million cases in men. About a third of men and women do not know they have the disease. The prevalence of diabetes is higher in Native American, African American, and Hispanic women than White women. Diabetes increases the risk of cardiovascular disease, the primary cause of death among women, and is also a major cause of disability and dependency in older women. Diabetes also increases the risk of developing cerebrovascular disease, blindness, end stage renal disease, and nontraumatic lower extremity amputation due to peripheral vascular disease. In addition, epidemiological studies have established an association between diabetes and dementia secondary to Alzheimer's disease and cerebrovascular disease.

Arthritis

Approximately 30 million women are affected by some type of arthritis, which accounts for nearly two thirds of all persons living with these diseases. Arthritis causes an inflammation of a joint(s), usually accompanied by pain and swelling. Arthritis can limit an individual's use of the affected joints, such as the fingers, knees, or shoulder, making the performance of usual daily activities more challenging and painful. Osteoarthritis in women accounts for approximately 75% of all cases, and rheumatoid arthritis in women accounts for about 70%. Girls represent approximately 86% of all cases of juvenile rheumatoid arthritis.

Urinary Incontinence

Urinary incontinence, characterized by the involuntary loss of urine that is socially and hygienically undesirable, is a major health problem among women in the United States. One in four women ages 30 to 59 years has experienced an episode of urinary incontinence, and it is estimated that 30% of elderly American women have some form of urge incontinence. Health care costs related to incontinence are greater than $16 billion each year, with more than $1 billion alone being spent on disposable sanitary products. Urinary incontinence can result in reductions in one's life quality and roles, and is a major predictor of women's ability to live independently as they age.

Osteoporosis

Eighty percent of osteoporosis—a disease characterized by low bone mass and structural deterioration of bone tissue leading to bone fragility—occurs in women. Another significant portion of adult women have osteopenia (low bone mass), which puts them at increased risk for developing osteoporosis and/or fractures. About one out of two women and one out of eight men over the age of 50 years will have an osteoporotic-related fracture of the vertebrae or hip. Women lose up to 20% of their bone mass in the first 5 to 7 years following menopause, and intervention efforts have recently targeted this group of women to prevent the occurrence of fracture-related injuries or disabilities. About 15% to 20% of those who have a hip fracture will not survive the 6 months after the fracture. At least half of those who do survive will require assistance in performing their daily activities, and 15% to 20% enter a long-term care facility. Thus, the prevention of osteoporosis is a major focus in women's health currently.

Dementia

Dementia is a pathological age-related condition manifested by declines in cognitive, behavioral, and emotional functioning leading to dependency on others. Alzheimer's disease (AD) is the most common form of dementia, followed by vascular disease and degenerative diseases of the brain such as Parkinson's disease and other more obscure disorders. Dementia is a major health problem of older adults. Approximately 14 million Americans will develop AD alone by 2050 unless a cure or prevention is found. The rate of dementia is two to three times higher in women than men. Diseases most common to women that may also increase risk of dementia (Alzheimer's type and vascular) include heart disease, hypertension, and diabetes.

REPRODUCTIVE AND POSTREPRODUCTIVE HEALTH

Gynecological Health

Gynecological issues during childbearing years (ages 15-44) largely focus on problems related to menstruation (irregular periods, bleeding problems, painful menses and premenstrual-related symptoms, amenorrhea); contraception, sexual functioning, and sexually transmitted diseases; and pregnancy-related concerns. The term *premenstrual syndrome* is used to describe a range of symptoms, such as bloating, breast tenderness, abdominal cramps, and mood changes, that occur in 70% to 80% of women immediately prior to, during, or immediately following the monthly menstrual cycle. A more severe version of this syndrome, premenstrual dysphoric disorder, occurs in approximately 4% to 7% of all women, and can lead to major disruptions in a woman's daily activities. Endometriosis—dislocation of the endometrial lining of the uterus to other locations in the pelvis is more likely to occur in women between 25 and 40 years of age, and causes dysmenorrhea, pelvic

pain, heavy or irregular periods, and sometimes infertility. Uterine fibroids, which are more common in African American women, occur in 20% of women of reproductive age, and cause unusual or heavy menstrual bleeding, anemia, dysmenorrhea, pelvic pain, and infertility.

Hysterectomy is the second most frequently performed surgical procedure among women in the United States. Hysterectomy is performed most often between the ages of 35 and 54 years, peaking in the 40- to 44-year-old age group. The majority of hysterectomies do not occur for cancerous conditions, but in fact are performed due to complications related to uterine fibroids. In general, hysterectomy does not lead to serious complications, but the removal of the uterus and possibly the ovaries may have adverse effects on a woman's physical and emotional health. Alternatives to hysterectomy include endometrial ablation, used to control excessive uterine bleeding, myomectomy (the surgical removal of the fibroids without removing the uterus), and hormone-related therapies. Vaginal hysterectomy is also being performed more commonly to reduce the morbidity surrounding surgery as well as to reduce health care costs.

Pregnancy, Infertility, and Contraception

Teenage pregnancies have declined over the past decade, with the largest declines among African American and young Hispanic women. However, births to teenagers remain a continuing concern. Many young women lack access to adequate prenatal care, and face increased risks for premature and low birth weight infants.

Sexually transmitted diseases (STDs) are an ongoing concern in this age group and can also lead to infertility and other chronic health risks. Endometriosis and pelvic inflammatory diseases also place women at increased risk for infertility, as do smoking and high doses of caffeine. Methods such as oral contraceptives are highly effective when used properly to prevent pregnancy but offer no protection in the prevention of STDs, including HIV.

Success of contraception is largely dependent on behavior. Some women lack the ability to use contraceptive methods appropriately, and in some relationships, male partners refuse to use contraception. For these reasons, forms of contraception that are not directly linked to the sexual act are needed (e.g., injections, implants). However, as noted above, these do not protect against STDs.

Childbirth

Although maternal mortality related to pregnancy has declined steadily over the past 60 years, conditions such as pregnancy-induced hypertension and ectopic pregnancy have been increasing, and if left undetected or untreated, can cause maternal death. Deliveries by Cesarean section have also increased markedly since 1970, from 6% of all deliveries to 21% in 1998. The use of obstetric intervention during delivery, such as the use of medications to induce labor, fetal monitors, and forceps, is also on the rise. In addition, although systematic reviews of randomized research studies have concluded that there is no evidence of benefit to performing routine episiotomies, this procedure is still performed on approximately 50% of all women giving birth in hospitals—which is still the setting where 99% of births to women in the United States occur.

Menopause

At the other end of the reproductive cycle is the cessation of menses or menopause. Menopause is receiving increasing attention as baby boomers reach their 50s, as epidemiological data suggest that the decline in ovarian function may contribute to other conditions, and as the controversy over the use of hormone replacement therapy increases. Although the median age of menopause is between 51 and 52 years, the age at which women reach menopause varies considerably. The vast majority of women experience menopause between the ages of 45 and 55. Though many factors have been thought to influence a woman's age of menopause, the most consistent factor is smoking. Women who smoke experience menopause from 1 to 2 years earlier than nonsmokers. Although women have often been thought to experience a wide range of symptoms such as dizzy spells, irritability, depression, anxiety, trouble sleeping, and sexual dysfunction during the menopausal transition, only vasomotor symptoms (hot flashes and night sweats) have been clearly associated with menopause status, distinct from chronological aging. There is great variation among women in the frequency and severity to which these symptoms are experienced, but for some women they can be quite severe and are the primary reason that women seek hormonal therapy (HT). While HT has been shown to be the most effective treatment option for relieving vasomotor symptoms, many women are concerned about troubling side effects and potential risks associated with HT such as irregular bleeding, increased breast tenderness, increased risk of breast cancer and endometrial cancer, and thromboembolitic events. For these reasons, many women seek alternative therapies for relief, for example, herbal products. However, at this point in time, there is no scientific evidence of the effectiveness of these alternatives. This continues to be an active area of investigation.

GENDER INFLUENCES ON HEALTH RISKS

Another area of women's health includes gender differences in behaviors such as substance abuse and physical inactivity. Substance abuse is a preventable and treatable condition that imposes huge costs to society. These costs are measured by disease and death, lost productivity, violence, unwanted or unplanned sex, foster child care, and homeless shelters. A number of issues related to substance abuse differ by gender. Females are more likely than males to initiate substance use to manage depression and anxiety and escalate to abuse in response to these mood disturbances. Depression is also a more common sequelae of chronic substance abuse in women. Women begin using illicit substances at a slightly later age than men and are strongly influenced by spouses and boyfriends who use. Although males are more likely to report initial exposure to illicit drugs, data suggest that women may be as likely to make a transition to drug use after initial exposure.

A similar pattern is seen in exposure to cigarette smoking as more women are taking up the habit and fewer are quitting. Nicotine in cigarettes induces euphoric or relaxing sensations, which relieve symptoms of emotional stress and reinforce repeated use. Trying to quit smoking produces a withdrawal syndrome characterized by irritability, lack of concentration, and weight gain. There is consistent evidence that nicotine replacement via gum and/or patch is less successful for women than men. Yet, most smoking abstinence programs rely heavily on nicotine therapy. Other treatment strategies, such as behavioral interventions, counseling, and treatment with medications, may be more appropriate for women.

Age and gender interact to create special needs for treatment of younger and older women. Girls and young women are using drugs and alcohol at earlier ages, and larger numbers are becoming addicted. Traditional treatment programs, which are based on biological and behavioral aspects of men, do not necessarily work well for females. There is new evidence that, for physiological reasons, women may become addicted more easily than men.

Older women also need special consideration. Substance abuse among older women—particularly of alcohol and prescription drugs—is becoming one of the fastest growing health problems in the United States. Sometimes called the "invisible epidemic," the trend disproportionably affects older women, as evidenced by a 43% increase in admission to treatment centers by women age 55 and older, compared to a 25% increase by men. Insufficient data and awareness of health providers, peer disapproval, and individual shame have kept the issue invisible and created barriers to treatment.

Physical activity is an important factor in women's health that has only recently received the attention of clinicians and researchers. Integrating physical activity in early childhood is an important step in building a healthy lifestyle, and maintaining regular physical activity into midlife and beyond reduces the risk of age-related diseases such as heart disease, hypertension, colon cancer, and diabetes. Despite the benefits of physical activity, only about 27% of women participate in recommended levels of physical activity, and 70% exercise irregularly or not at all.

Findings on physical activity over the life span indicate erosion of regular vigorous physical activity from adolescence through young adulthood, with the sharpest decline between ages 15 and 18 years. Erosion continues through the 20s before stabilizing during midlife. At age 65 and beyond, there is a stable-to-slight increase in physical activity until late life. Most important, at all points during the life span, females report much lower rates of regular sustained activity as compared to males. The differences in vigorous physical activity are especially large between adolescent boys and girls in vigorous activity.

SOCIETAL INFLUENCES ON WOMEN'S HEALTH

Societal and cultural norms and socialization to gender roles are inextricably linked to women's health. Traditionally, these norms and roles suggest a way of life in which females are more responsible for care of the home and other people than providing for their own economic security. This makes women dependent on someone else who is in control of the income and has the power that accompanies this. Education and economic realities of recent times have done much to empower women with respect to role flexibility and a place in the workforce. However, traditional gender roles are deeply ingrained, and although most women work outside the home, they still bear primary responsibility for work inside the home and care of dependent others—including their children, the ill, and the elderly. Despite the expansion of "women's work," women—and their children—are still the most impoverished members of our society. It is not surprising, then, that the traditional focus on care of others rather than self-care, devotion to unpaid work, and poverty—each and collectively—takes a toll on women's health.

Attention to preventive health practices and self-care of health problems suffer because of role responsibilities. Women are more likely than men to report reduced control over daily decisions to practice healthy behaviors, such as regular exercise. Even women with chronic illness have difficulty attending to their own self-care needs because of their response to the needs of others. Women not only provide more care for others, they also report more burden from the caregiving experience. Burdensome outcomes of caregiving in women include declines in physical and emotional health, social isolation, and loss of income due to reduction in work hours or giving up paid work in order to provide care.

Finally, poor and minority women experience the most extreme threats to healthy living. Poor women, and their children, are at increased risk for inadequate nutrition and preventive health care as well as untreated and undertreated chronic disease. They are disproportionately exposed to substance abuse and the risk of injury due to crime and violence. Also, chronic stress associated with poor housing, dangerous neighborhoods, and financial insecurity are potent stressors that predict emotional and physical health problems. The highest number of depressive symptoms are found in unemployed poor women who are raising children without adequate social support.

VIOLENCE AGAINST WOMEN

While violence is a problem throughout our society, it affects men and women differently. Men are more likely to be victims of violent crime, but women are more likely to be assaulted, raped, or murdered by a current or former intimate partner. Violence can include physical or sexual assault, verbal abuse, threats, and social isolation. Violence against women has a number of repercussions for the woman, her children, and her family. In addition to the physical consequences of violence, victims of sexual assault are more likely to receive a psychiatric diagnosis of major depression, obsessive-compulsive disorder, or posttraumatic stress disorder and to suffer from alcohol and other substance abuse. Children are also affected by violence. Studies have shown that children who have witnessed violence show long-term behavioral effects and may show signs of posttraumatic stress disorder. Health care providers are increasingly being encouraged to conduct routine screenings for signs of violence.

PROCESSES

Research Participants and Health Care Policy

Who gets included in research is an important issue because research findings influence treatment and health care policy. It has been well documented that for many years women were underrepresented in research. Consequently, research was based on male subjects and then simply "applied" to women. However, we are now learning that because of differences in physiology and biology, women do not necessarily respond to diseases and treatments in the same way as men. For example, women with myocardial infarction present with different symptoms than men, and women respond differently to drugs such as potassium channel blockers as well as to chemotherapy.

As we begin to understand the importance of including women in research, we need to keep in mind that women cannot be considered a homogeneous group. In particular, as described throughout this entry, there are numerous differences in the health concerns of minority and majority women. African American women have a lower life expectancy than White women and have higher mortality rates for a number of diseases and conditions. For example, for women ages 25 to 44 years, HIV is the third leading cause of death among African American women, the fourth leading cause among Hispanic women, but is the tenth cause of death among White women. Although mortality rates due to HIV declined during the 1990s, chiefly due to improved therapies, this decline has been greater in men than in women.

Recognizing the importance of women's health issues, in 1990 the National Institutes of Health (NIH) established the Office of Research on Women's Health (ORWH). The ORWH has a broad mandate that includes enhancing research related to diseases, disorders, and conditions that affect women, ensuring that research conducted by the NIH adequately address issues regarding women's health, and ensuring that women are appropriately represented in NIH-funded research. The NIH is now making a concerted effort to ensure that women and minorities are included in research. However, recruitment can still be a problem, particularly with respect to minorities and rural populations. Often these women are not reached through traditional recruitment methods, do not have access to clinical trial sites, or have logistical issues that make participation difficult.

VARIABLES AND MEASURES

Another important issue concerns how we measure important concepts. In the behavioral and social sciences, many of our measures are based on self-report. We often use measures and concepts such as physical activity, social support, stress, depression, coping, quality of life, and Type A behavior. We need to ensure that these measures are appropriate for both men and women and people across ethnic groups. Often, measures developed for one population may not be valid for another. For example, when asking about physical activity, we need to ensure that specific items and activities are ones that both men and women engage in.

CONCLUSIONS

Women's health issues have clearly extended beyond reproductive-related concerns. We are increasingly learning how sex and gender influence health and behavior. It is critical that we understand and appreciate these differences as we continue to conduct research, provide treatment, and formulate policy.

—*Nancy E. Avis, Laura Coker,*
and Michelle Naughton

See also AFRICAN AMERICAN HEALTH AND BEHAVIOR; AIDS AND HIV: PREVENTION OF HIV INFECTION; AUTOIMMUNE

DISEASES: PSYCHOSOCIAL ASPECTS; EATING DISORDERS; GENDER DIFFERENCES IN HEALTH; LOW BIRTH WEIGHT: PSYCHOSOCIAL ASPECTS; PREGNANCY OUTCOMES: PSYCHOSOCIAL ASPECTS; PREGNANCY PREVENTION IN ADOLESCENTS; VIOLENCE PREVENTION

Further Reading

American Cancer Society. (2000). *Cancer facts and figures, 2000*. Atlanta, GA: Author.

Belle, D. (1990). Poverty and women's mental health. *American Psychologist, 45*, 385-389.

Caspersen, C. J., Pereira, M. A., & Curran, K. M. (2000). Changes in physical activity patterns in the United States by sex and cross-sectional age. *Medicine and Science in Sports and Exercise, 32*, 1601-1609.

Chesney, M. A., & Ozer, E. M. (1995). Women and health: In search of a paradigm. *Women's Health: Research on Gender, Behavior, and Policy, 1*, 3-26.

Institute of Medicine. (2001). *Exploring the biological contributions to human health: Does sex matter?* Washington, DC: National Academy Press.

Kumanyika, S. K., Morssink, C. B., & Nestle, M. (2001). Minority women and advocacy for women's health. *American Journal of Public Health, 91*, 1383-1388.

Misra, D. (Ed.). (2001). *The women's health data book: A profile of women's health in the United States* (3rd ed., pp. 14-45). Washington, DC: Jacobs Institute of Women's Health.

Murphy, S. L. (2000). Deaths: Final data for 1998. *National Vital Statistics Report, 48*, 1-105.

National Center for Health Statistics. (1999). *National vital statistics report, 47*(19). U.S. Department of Health and Human Services.

Ness, R. B., & Kuller, L. H. (Eds.). (1999). *Health and disease among women*. New York: Oxford University Press.

Pharmaceutical Research and Manufacturers of America. (1999). Facts about diseases/conditions affecting women. *New Medicines in Development for Women*, 29-34.

WORK-RELATED STRESS AND HEALTH

SHIFT WORK

In this entry, shift work, including night shifts, means a rotating schedule that includes work at night and during daytime. In modern shift work schedules, the most common solution is to change working hours over successive working days so rapidly that a long-term shift to a biological night schedule is never achieved. Such a rotation requires considerable biological adaptation. If the body has not adapted to work at night, it tries to keep the brain awake by increasing activity in the sympathoadrenomedullary system and other similar energy-mobilizing systems. On the other hand, it is also difficult to fall asleep during day hours when the biological clock promotes a high level of energy. This means reduced sleep, which results in fatigue the next day. To compensate for this fatigue, the body has to increase the energy level that day, for example, by increasing the excretion of adrenaline and noradrenaline. A constant sleep deficit may result. It is important to organize shift schedules in a way that corresponds as closely as possible to the body's needs. Possibilities for recuperation must be provided after periods of excessive night work.

A difficult problem in research on health effects of shift work is that there are strong selection effects. This means that workers who easily adapt themselves to shift work, including night shifts, will tend to stay in such work, whereas those who have difficulties will tend to "select themselves out." Particularly after many years, this may result in an attenuation of the observed effect of such work on the risk of developing myocardial infarction. One of the first prospective studies in the field (Knutsson, Akerstedt, Jonsson, & Orth-Gomer, 1986) may have suffered from this problem. A group of industry workers were followed for more than 20 years with regard to morbidity and mortality. The findings indicated that there was a significant association between exposure to such shift work up to 20 years. After a longer period of exposure, no association was found. Quite to the contrary, an inverse relationship was observed. The most obvious explanation may be that workers who have stayed in this kind of work for over 20 years stand shift work unusually well. After such long periods, it may therefore be impossible to measure the true effect of shift work, including night shifts, on health risks.

There is increasing convergence in opinion among epidemiological researchers that shift work is associated with increased risk of developing myocardial infarction. A number of recently published epidemiological studies have shown effects in the order of 1.4 (which means 40% excess risk associated with exposure) even when adjustment has been made for possible confounders (factors that are associated both with shift work and with cardiovascular illness risk—such factors may create spurious associations) such as serum lipids, blood pressure, smoking habits, overweight, social class, and educational level. One reason for this association could be that shift workers have a more unfavorable psychosocial job situation with regard to "job strain" (the combination of high psychological demands and low decision latitude; see Job Strain and Health in this volume) or imbalance between effort and reward at work (see Effort-Reward Imbalance in this volume). Adjustment for job strain did not change the association between shift work (including night shifts) and myocardial infarction risk, whereas adjustment for effort-reward imbalance did. Hence, it is not likely that the association is mediated by job strain but it could be partly mediated by effort-reward imbalance.

Two different possible pathways for the association between shift work, including night shifts, and cardiovascular disease have been discussed:

1. *Effects of shift work on personal habits of significance to cardiovascular illness risk.* Such effects may include effects on tobacco consumption, physical exercise, and eating habits. Shift workers have been observed in many studies to smoke more than other workers. It has been speculated that this may be due to the fact that shift workers have difficulties in staying awake and use tobacco as a stimulant. Shift work, which is prevalent among drivers, may prevent regular physical activity. Access to healthy food may also be limited in shift work. While all these factors may contribute to excess risk, they do not seem to explain all of it, since adjustment for them does not eliminate all of the risk associated with shift work, including night work.

2. *Direct effects of disturbed regulation of endocrine systems.* As mentioned above, the body tries to compensate for lack of sleep by increasing the activity in the sympathoadrenomedullary system, mainly the excretion of adrenaline and noradrenaline. This may have effects by itself, including increased coagulation, which may accelerate the atherosclerosis process. Lack of sleep is known to increase the risk of developing diabetes, which may also accelerate atherosclerosis. The body's ability to metabolize lipids and carbohydrates is weakened at night, and hence there is a possibility that food with a high content of fat and carbohydrates may have more adverse effects on cardiovascular illness risk in shift workers than in others.

LONG WORKING HOURS

In early epidemiological studies performed in the 1950s and 1960s, a relationship between long working hours (mostly above 70 hours per week) and risk of developing myocardial infarction early in life was shown. One of these was the cohort study of the U.S. Bell Telephone Company by Hinkle et al., which showed that men working full time and at the same time going to night college had an elevated risk of dying a coronary death. A Swedish study from this period showed that owners of small shops who had very long working weeks had an excess risk of developing myocardial infarctions. Kornitzer et al. showed that bank employees working in a state-owned bank system had a lower risk of developing myocardial infarction than bank employees in private banks. During later years, very few studies have been published on the relationship between long working hours and myocardial infarction risk. The small number of publications could be due either to lack of interest among researchers (which is unlikely) or to lack of positive findings in studies exploring this relationship. It could be that it has become increasingly difficult for participants in questionnaire studies to respond to questions about number of working hours. Leisure-time activities are more and more often mixed with paid work, for example, due to increased homework facilitated by small computers. A Japanese study of male office workers in 1998 showed that men both with low (equal to or less than 7 hours of work per day) and high (more than 11 hours of work per day) numbers of working hours had elevated risks of developing myocardial infarction. It could be suspected that men with a low number of working hours have reduced their working hours due to illness, but the authors argued that the design of their study made this explanation unlikely. Instead, they point at the fact that working a low number of working hours could be caused by financial crisis and could cause loss of self-esteem and anxiety, which could per se cause increased risk.

It could be argued that in future studies, the number of working hours should not be studied as a single factor. Being forced by someone else to work long hours and to work long hours in boring work that requires a high level of vigilance all the time (for example, taxi or truck driving) is much more dangerous to health than working long hours in joyful work that one does voluntarily. One also has to combine the information regarding number of working hours with information about unpaid work, for example, in household work. A study by our group published in 1985 pointed in this direction. It was based on all male and female employees in four counties in Sweden. For each person, there was information regarding job title (three-digit international code, Nordic version). For each one of these occupation titles, there was information from national surveys regarding the distribution of responses to questions about working conditions. This made it possible to impute information regarding the "typical working conditions" for the individual's occupation. It was, for example, possible to identify individuals who were working in occupations in which at least 10 hours of overwork per week were common. Such individuals were compared with others with regard to risk of hospitalization during a 1-year follow-up.

Men working in "typical overtime work occupations" had a lower incidence and women working in such occupations a higher incidence of hospitalization for myocardial infarction than others. The reason for this discrepancy in findings between men and women could be either women's double role (paid and unpaid work) or differences in women's and men's labor market. The double role means that even moderate overtime could create an unbearable total workload. The difference in men's and women's labor market is of relevance, because women more frequently than men work in jobs with low decision latitude. Accordingly, overtime work may often be involuntary. The combination of long working hours and low decision latitude may be particularly hazardous to health. The effect of the double workload in women was studied in 199 Canadian women whose blood pressure was monitored by means of fully automated equipment during work hours, leisure hours, and sleep. This study, which was published in 1999, indicated that women who reported both job strain and strenuous family conditions had higher blood pressure at work, during leisure, and during sleep than other women.

PROFESSIONAL DRIVING

In some studies, professional drivers have been shown to have a higher myocardial infarction incidence than other occupational groups. After adjustment for possible confounders, the findings have only been consistent for inner-city bus drivers, however. Unhealthy diet, lack of physical exercise, Type A behavior, and adverse psychosocial conditions have been discussed as possible underlying etiological factors. Among psychosocial factors, job strain (high demands and lack of decision latitude; see Job Strain and Health in this volume) and imbalance between effort and reward (see Effort/Reward Imbalance in this volume) have been discussed. One important factor in professional driving is that there is constant vigilance and more or less conscious avoidance of threats. This is particularly common in inner-city traffic, where there are many unexpected and uncontrollable events around the bus, with pedestrians, bicyclists, and car drivers doing unexpected and potentially dangerous things. The driver has to have a high level of attention in order to be able to act adequately in all these situations. Studies have shown that such long-lasting hyperaroused states have adverse effects on the central nervous (electroencephalogram and evoked potentials) and cardiovascular systems (blood pressure and heart rate).

An additional possibly relevant factor that has been insufficiently studied in relation to the bus driver work is the relationship with passengers who may sometimes pose threats.

Other kinds of professional driving have also been studied in relation to the risk of developing cardiovascular disease. In some studies, taxi drivers as well as truck drivers have been found to have excess risk of developing cardiovascular disease, but these findings have been less consistent.

—*Töres Theorell*

See also Effort-Reward Imbalance; Job Strain and Health

Further Reading

Belkic, K., Savic, C., Theorell, T., Rakic, L., Ercegovac, D., & Djordjevic, M. (1994, April). Mechanisms of cardiac risk among professional drivers. *Scandinavian Journal of Work, Environment and Health,* pp. 73-86.

Brisson, C., Laflamme, N., Moisan, J., Milot, A., Masse, B., & Vezina, M. (1999). Effect of family responsibilities and job strain on ambulatory blood pressure among white-collar women. *Psychosomatic Medicine, 61,* 205-213.

Hinkle, L. F., Jr., Whitney, L. H., Lehman, E. Q., Dunn, J., Benjamin, B., King, R., et al. (1968). Occupation, education and coronary heart disease. *Science 161,* 238-246.

Knutsson, A., & Boggild, H. (2000). Shiftwork and cardiovascular disease: Review of disease mechanisms. *Review of Environmental Health, 15,* 359-372.

Knutsson, A., Akerstedt, T., Jonsson, B. G., & Orth-Gomer, K. (1986). Increased risk of ischaemic heart disease in shift workers. *Lancet, 12,* 89-92.

Kornitzer, J., Kittel, F., Dramaix, M., & deBacker, G. (1982). Job stress and coronary heart disease. *Advances in Cardiology, 19,* 56-61.

Sokejima, S., & Kagamimori, S. (1998). Working hours as a risk factor for acute myocardial infarction in Japan: Case-control study. *British Medical Journal, 19,* 775-780.

Steenland, K., Fine, L., Belkic, K., Landsbergis, P., Schnall, P., Baker, D., et al. (2000). Research findings linking workplace factors to CVD outcomes. *Occupational Health, 15,* 7-68.

WORKSITE HEALTH PROMOTION

Worksite health promotion includes programs, policies, and other initiatives based in worksites aimed at the promotion of workers' health. As such, worksite health promotion may include efforts to (a) reduce risk-related behaviors, such as tobacco use, unhealthy dietary patterns, physical inactivity, or sun exposure; (b) reduce risk-related exposures at work, such as to environmental tobacco smoke, occupational hazards, or job stressors; and (c) increase utilization of screening for early detection of disease, including, for example, screening for high blood pressure or high cholesterol, or mammography or Pap screening.

Worksites are an important channel for influencing the health of a large proportion of the adult population. Since the 1980s, the number of organizations offering worksite health promotion programs has grown rapidly. In 1999, approximately 90% of companies employing at least 50 workers reported offering at least one health promotion program for their employees in the last 12 months.

Worksite health promotion may focus on all workers and/or seek to identify and intervene with high-risk employees. There is some evidence pointing to the cost-effectiveness of programs targeting high-risk employees. From a public health perspective, the *impact* of an intervention is a product of both its *efficacy* in changing behavior and its *reach,* meaning the proportion of the population reached either through their direct participation or indirectly through diffusion of intervention messages throughout the worksite. Worksite-wide programs designed to reach a broad audience within the worksite are likely to create an overall climate supportive of worker health. Individualized risk reduction counseling of high-risk employees is likely to be most effective when conducted in the overall context of a worksite health promotion effort for all employees.

The evolution of worksite health promotion programs has progressed through several generations. Early efforts often were conducted in response to safety regulations, or for similar reasons, and commonly were delivered in a lecture format with minimal employee input. Programs then progressed to a stage where they were focused on a single risk factor or behavior and were designed to reach one population. Later programs offered an array of interventions aimed at a variety of risk factors or behaviors for all employees. Recent efforts focus on comprehensive approaches that incorporate all activities, policies, and decisions related to the health of employees, their families, and the communities in which they reside. Several reviews of worksite health promotion have suggested that the most efficacious programs are those that are comprehensive, which means they provide multiple and coordinated interventions, offered in a coherent, ongoing program, focus on both workers and management, and address multiple levels of influence on worker and workplace health.

Effective comprehensive programs generally are based on strong theoretical foundations. A range of theoretical frameworks has suggested that worker health is the result of a complex interplay of factors involving individual workers and their immediate work environments, as well as characteristics of the larger contexts in which both the individual worker and the worksite are embedded. The social ecological model provides a structure for understanding and intervening on these multiple levels of influence. Accordingly, worksite health promotion programs aim to promote healthful change among individual workers, build social support and social norms that support healthful behavior, engage management in ensuring a healthful work environment, involve workers' families in health-promoting activities, and provide links to community and public policy initiatives that support health-promoting behaviors and organizations. This model provides a framework for moving beyond the individual as the locus of intervention and responsibility for health, recognizing the central roles of management, unions, coworkers, families, and public policy initiatives in engaging in healthful behaviors that lead to reduced chronic disease risk. Thus, comprehensive worksite health promotion programs require coordinated efforts at the individual, interpersonal, and organizational levels.

INTERVENING AT THE INDIVIDUAL LEVEL

For maximum reach, interventions for individuals must be designed for workers at varying stages of readiness to change their health behavior. A comprehensive program needs to provide a full spectrum of activities, ranging from minimal interventions for workers not yet ready to make significant investments in health behavior change, to incentives and competitions, to group programs that build skills for change, provide counseling for high-risk workers, and are a source of social support for change. Increasingly, health promotion programs are moving away from a one-size-fits-all approach to interventions for individuals, to utilize "tailored" approaches. Tailoring provides a method for addressing the unique needs, interests, and concerns of participants, thus providing health education that is salient to the individual and more likely to lead to health behavior change. In the tailoring process, participants complete an assessment that elicits information such as sociodemographic characteristics, stage of readiness for behavior change, current health behavior status, and personal facilitators and barriers of health behavior change. These factors are fashioned into health messages, which are compiled into tailored feedback reports that are conveyed to individual participants in print or electronic media. Because it is possible to automate the tailoring process, it is now feasible to reach large numbers of people with personalized risk reduction messages. Interventions must also address structural barriers influencing worker participation. For example, blue-collar workers are less likely than white-collar workers to participate in health promotion programs. To increase participation, it may be necessary to garner supervisor support or incorporate interventions with management to reduce exposures to occupational hazards.

INTERVENING AT THE INTERPERSONAL LEVEL

Interventions at the interpersonal level include promoting coworker, supervisor, and family social support and worksite social norms supportive of employee health. For example, buddy systems and peer support groups have been shown to enhance the effectiveness of worksite wellness programs. Similarly, peer-led programs may provide a strategy for dissemination of health information, a source of role models for behavior change, and a means of fostering positive social norms. Programs that build family support for health behavior change have been shown to be effective in promoting the adoption of healthy eating patterns. Social norms and social support, from both coworkers and supervisors, are also important in workers' compliance with protective recommendations. The social contexts in which workers live and work also influence their health behaviors and the effectiveness of interventions. For example, it is important to understand and incorporate into program planning ways in which time on the job is structured, the meaning attached to health behaviors within one's work group, and work stressors.

INTERVENING AT THE ENVIRONMENTAL/ORGANIZATIONAL LEVEL

Policies supporting worker health include those influencing the work environment and the organization of work. The work environment directly influences worker health through the presence of health-compromising exposures, such as exposures to occupational hazards or environmental tobacco smoke, and by the access to health-promoting environments, such as cafeterias that serve healthful foods or fitness facilities. Also, work environments may shape social norms associated with worker health. Job characteristics and the organization of work are also important correlates of worker health. For example, there is strong evidence that job strain is a risk factor for heart disease and is associated with smoking, sedentary behavior, and other deleterious health outcomes. Assessment of job content and job design may lead to necessary changes in the organization of work, and are important elements of a range of worksite interventions.

Interventions at the organizational level must involve key stakeholders, including management, workers, and unions. Management sets the direction for worker health, either through clear statements of priorities or through tacit understandings transmitted through administrative hierarchies. Management support may be reflected in corporate mission statements, worker participation in health and safety committees, and the extent to which employees are afforded the flexibility necessary to participate in worksite health promotion programs. All of these factors have been associated with positive health behavior. Management support also serves to sustain and institutionalize programs over the long term. To observe change in health outcomes, programs must be of sufficient duration to provide ongoing, persistent messages supporting health.

In unionized worksites, unions provide a voice for workers. Labor-management relationships, however, are likely to influence workers' response to health promotion programs, and need to be addressed by program planners. If labor-management relationships are strained and programs are perceived by workers to be closely aligned with management, union members may view them with skepticism. Historically, unions have espoused a philosophy that members' private lives are not the prerogative of management. This belief may have an impact on the way union members respond to workplace programs that address personal health behaviors. In addition, unions have expressed concern that health promotion programs may draw attention away from the competing needs to address workplace risks. Another concern expressed by some union members is that health promotion efforts may enter into areas that traditionally have been reserved for collective bargaining, thus taking power and control away from the union. There are effective approaches to overcoming these potential barriers. Researchers have found that in worksites that offer health programs addressing occupational health as well as health promotion, blue-collar workers are more likely to participate in program activities and have higher rates of smoking cessation than programs that address only health promotion. When unions are represented at the table along with management to plan and implement programs and policies and their voices are heard, unions are likely to support programs that benefit the health of their members. For example, a recent study of organized labor's positions on worksite tobacco control policies found that nearly 50% of the local unions surveyed supported worksite smoking bans or restrictions and only 8% actively opposed them. When unions have grieved worksite smoking policies, the most common reason has been that policies were unilaterally imposed by management without involvement of the union.

Worker participation in planning can ensure that interventions respond to worker needs and priorities.

Programs are likely to be more effective when they are based on an understanding of workers' concerns about health risks on the job. Also, participatory methods are important as a basis for educational strategies. Use of learner-centered models can build a sense of worker control, which goes beyond transmission of information and skills, and may facilitate joint problem solving. These methods may be health enhancing in and of themselves.

In summary, the current evidence points to the feasibility and potential efficacy of worksite health promotion programs. Much research to date has tested intervention "packages," making it difficult to disentangle the effects of specific intervention components. Future research can help to identify those program elements that hold particular promise within a range of work settings and with differing types of workers. Programs to date have been less successful with low-income, less-educated workers than with middle and upper income, well-educated workers. Future research needs to attend to social disparities in health; to recognize demographic changes in the U.S. workforce, such as the increasing diversity by race/ethnicity and aging; and to understand the changing nature of work within the United States. Future worksite health promotion programs need to be designed to respond to these changes.

—*Glorian Sorensen and Mary Kay Hunt*

See also HEALTH COMMUNICATION; HEALTH PROMOTION AND DISEASE PREVENTION; OBESITY: PREVENTION AND TREATMENT; PHYSICAL ACTIVITY INTERVENTIONS; TAILORED COMMUNICATIONS

Further Reading

Baker, E., Israel, B., & Schurman, S. (1996). The integrated model: Implications for worksite health promotion and occupational health and safety practice. *Health Education Quarterly, 23*, 175-188.

Buller, D. B., Morrill, C., Taren, D., Aickin, M., Sennott-Miller, L., Buller, M. K., et al. (1999). Randomized trial testing: The effect of peer education at increasing fruit and vegetable intake. *Journal of the National Cancer Institute, 91*, 1491-1500.

DeJoy, D., & Southern, D. (1993). An integrative perspective on worksite health promotion. *Journal of Medicine, 35*, 1221-1230.

Eakin, J. M. (1997). Work-related determinants of health behavior. In D. S. Gochman (Ed.), *Handbook of health* behavior research, I: Personal and social determinants (pp. 337-357). New York: Plenum.

Erfurt, J. C., Foote, A., & Heirich, M. A. (1991). Worksite wellness programs: Incremental comparison of screening and referral alone, health education, follow-up counseling, and plant organization. *American Journal of Health Promotion, 5*, 438-449.

Glasgow, R. E., Vogt, T. M., & Boles, S. M. (1999). Evaluating the public health impact of health promotion interventions: The RE-AIM framework. *American Journal of Public Health, 89*, 1322-1327.

Heaney, C. A., & Goetzel, R. Z. (1997). A review of health-related outcomes of multicomponent worksite health promotion programs. *American Journal of Public Health, 11*, 290-308.

Kreuter, M., Farrell, D., Olevitch, L., & Brennan, L. (2000). *Tailoring health messages: Customizing communication with computer technology.* Mahwah, NJ: Lawrence Erlbaum.

Landsbergis, P. A., Schnall, P. L., Deitz, D. K., Pickering, W. K., & Schwartz, J. E. (1998). Job strain and health behaviors: Results of a prospective study. *American Journal of Health Promotion, 12*, 237-245.

Pelletier, K. R. (2001). A review and analysis of the clinical- and cost-effectiveness studies of comprehensive health promotion and disease management programs at the worksite: 1998-2000 update. *American Journal of Health Promotion, 16*, 107-116.

Ringen, K. (2001). Working with labor-management health and welfare funds to provide coverage for smoking cessation treatment. In E. Barbeau, K. Yous, D. McLellan, C. Levenstein, R. Youngstrom, C. E. Siqueira, et al. (Eds.), *Organized labor, public health, and tobacco control policy: A dialogue toward action* [Conference report]. *New Solutions, 11*, 121-126.

Sorensen, G. (2001). Worksite tobacco control programs: The role of occupational health. *Respiration Physiology, 189*, 89-102.

Sorensen, G., Emmons, K., Hunt, M. K., & Johnston, D. (1998). Implications of the results of community intervention trials. *Annual Review of Public Health, 19,* 379-416.

Sorensen, G., Stoddard, A., Peterson, K., Cohen, N., Hunt, M. K., Stein, E., et al. (1999). Increasing fruit and vegetable consumption through worksites and families in the Treatwell 5-A-Day Study. *American Journal of Public Health, 89*, 54-60.

Stokols, D., Pelletier, K., & Fielding, J. (1996). The ecology of work and health: Research and policy directions for the promotion of employee health. *Health Education Quarterly, 23*, 137-158.

Wallerstein, N. (1992). Health and safety education for workers with low-literacy or limited English skills. *American Journal of Industrial Medicine, 22*, 751-765.

Willemsen, M., de Vries, H., van Breukelen, G., & Genders, R. (1998). Long-term effectiveness of two Dutch work site smoking cessation programs. *Health Education and Behavior, 25*, 418-435.

WOUND HEALING AND STRESS

Damage to any soft or hard tissue is followed by an ordered set of events aimed at restoring tissue function and integrity. Injured tissues heal by partial or complete regeneration or by repair. Regeneration implies complete reestablishment of the original tissue structure. Repair results in replacement with scar tissue that is structurally and functionally inferior to the original tissue. Although there can be substantial diversity in the type and severity of wounds, healing is typically divided into three general phases that overlap considerably. These are the inflammatory, proliferative (new tissue generation), and remodeling phases.

The first phase or inflammatory phase begins immediately after injury. This inflammatory phase is the localized response elicited by injury and destruction of tissues, and serves to remove or wall off both the injurious agent and the injured tissues. This inflammatory phase begins almost immediately upon wounding with the accumulation of platelets to establish a clot to limit blood loss and limit further tissue injury. Also within the first minutes after wounding, neutrophils are recruited to the wound to control infection. The inflammatory environment stimulates the release of toxic reactive oxygen intermediates from neutrophils. These reactive oxygen intermediates include substances such as hydrogen peroxide and are toxic to invading bacteria and fungi. Once bacterial contamination has been controlled, neutrophils become entrapped within the clot or are ingested and thus removed by macrophages that follow into the wound to begin the reparative process. Wound macrophages continue to eliminate deleterious materials, generate substances called chemotactic factors that recruit additional inflammatory cells to the injury site, and release collagenases, which are degrading enzymes that digest and remove dead or nonviable material. Wound macrophages also synthesize growth factors that stimulate new tissue formation.

These growth factors include platelet-derived growth factor, transforming growth factor-beta, fibroblast growth factors, and interleukin-1. Once the macrophage begins to produce these growth factors, the next phase of wound healing begins.

The second phase of wound healing is the proliferative phase. In cutaneous wounds, it is characterized by reepithelialization and granulation tissue formation. Reepithelialization is the reconstitution of the cells of the epidermis in order to cover the injured site and restore barrier function. Granulation tissue formation consists of fibroplasia and angiogenesis and occurs in the healing of all wounded tissues. Fibroplasia is the process of fibroblast recruitment into the wound site and the ensuing synthesis and secretion of a temporary extracellular matrix of structural collagens and space-filling sugars (i.e., glycosaminoglycans and proteoglycans). The extracellular matrix and the cells within it give a tissue its physical structure and provide for its function. The provisional and immature matrix produced during the proliferative phase provides for temporary scaffolding upon which the wound heals. It will be gradually replaced with a mature and organized extracellular matrix. Angiogenesis is the process of new blood vessel formation, and it occurs simultaneously with fibroplasia, commencing within days of injury. The assembly of a dense network of capillaries in the healing scar helps provide the energy and nutrients necessary for the proliferation of fibroblasts, the production of large quantities of provisional matrix, and the secretion of growth factors by macrophages. As this new tissue is forming, contraction begins to lessen the size of the wound. Wound contraction is the reduction in the defect by centripetal movement (i.e., movement toward the center) of the surrounding undamaged skin.

The third and final phase of wound healing, the remodeling phase, begins soon after the first molecules of connective tissue are produced during the previous phases. The provisional matrix or granulation tissue that is produced during the proliferative phase is immature and poorly organized. In an attempt to regenerate the characteristics of the original tissue, provisional matrix molecules are progressively replaced by mature forms of collagens and proteoglycans. Remodeling is normally considered the final phase of wound healing because it continues for months to years after granulation tissue has been resolved. Through remodeling, the highly cellular and highly vascular granulation tissue is gradually replaced, forming scar tissue, which is less cellular and less vascular than the temporary granulation tissue. Although repaired tissues will not be identical to the original, the resultant remodeled matrix should resemble it in both strength and function, whether it is bone, skin, liver, or any other type of tissue.

When these three stages proceed normally, wounds heal without serious consequences to the host. However, the timing of each event during the phases of healing is important, as each component is dependent on the one that came before. Therefore, influences at any of these stages could impact the healing process and delay wound closure. Behavioral stress is one of those influences that alter healing. Studies in both animals and humans have shown that psychological stress (e.g., emotional distress, depression, anxiety, helplessness) can delay the closure of small cutaneous wounds by several days. Psychological and behavioral stressors reduce the onset and magnitude of the inflammatory phase of healing as the production of proinflammatory factors is diminished in stressed subjects. Thus, the recruitment of neutrophils and macrophages is diminished as well as their ability to kill and remove microorganisms. This results in impaired bacterial elimination and delayed wound debridement (i.e., removal of dead, devitalized, or contaminated tissue). Not only is the inflammatory phase affected, but every step along the way to scar maturation can be altered by stress. For example, reepithelialization is impaired as keratinocyte proliferation is delayed. In addition, fibroblast proliferation, the production of the provisional matrix, and angiogenesis are all diminished in the wounds of stressed subjects. Consequences due to this delay include a prolonged chance for bacterial contamination of the open wound.

How does stress slow wound healing? Psychological stressors activate a bodywide set of physiologic adaptations mediated primarily by the hypothalamic-pituitary-adrenal axis through the production of glucocorticoids (e.g., cortisol and corticosterone) and by the sympathetic nervous system via the production of catecholamines (e.g., epinephrine and norepinephrine). These neuroendocrine systems regulate many components of the healing cascade. For example, the use of exogenous glucocorticoids in the clinic has been associated with increased risk of wound contamination and delayed healing of open wounds. Glucocorticoids produce these effects by interfering with inflammation, fibroblast proliferation, collagen synthesis and degradation, angiogenesis, wound contraction, reepithelialization, and remodeling. Glucocorticoids, whether exogenously administered by a physician or endogenously elevated due to psychological stress, regulate the expression of various genes at the wound site that encode key players in each of these wound repair processes. For example, proinflammatory cytokines (interleukin-1 and tumor necrosis factor alpha), growth factors (keratinocyte growth factor, transforming growth factor beta, and platelet-derived growth factor), and remodeling enzymes (macrophage- and fibroblast-derived matrix metalloproteinases) are targets of glucocorticoid action in wounded skin.

—*David A. Padgett*

See also ALLOSTATIS, ALLOSTATIC LOAD, AND STRESS; CAREGIVING AND STRESS; IMMUNE RESPONSES TO STRESS; PSYCHONEUROIMMUNOLOGY; STRESS: BIOLOGICAL ASPECTS

Further Reading

Hom, D. B., Thatcher, G., & Tibesar, R. (2002). Growth factor therapy to improve soft tissue healing. *Facial Plastic Surgery, 18*, 41-52.

Marucha, P. T., Sheridan, J. F., & Padgett, D. A. (2001). Stress and wound healing. In R. Ader, D. L. Felten, & N. Cohen (Eds.), *Psychoneuroimmunology: Vol. 2* (3rd ed., pp. 613-626). San Diego, CA: Academic Press.

Singer, A. J., & Clark, R. A. (1999). Cutaneous wound healing. *New England Journal of Medicine, 341*, 738-746.

Appendix A

Online Resources and Health and Behavior Organizations

Agency for Healthcare Research and Quality
2101 E. Jefferson Street, Suite 501
Rockville, MD 20852
Telephone: 301-594-1364
http://www.ahcpr.gov/

According to its Web site, the "mission of the Agency for Health Care Policy and Research is to support, conduct, and disseminate research that improves access to care and the outcomes, quality, cost, and utilization of health care services. The research sponsored and conducted by the Agency provides better information that enables better decisions about health care" (in 1999, the Agency for Health Care Policy and Research changed its name to the Agency for Healthcare Research and Quality, AHRQ).

Alan Guttmacher Institute
120 Wall Street, 21st Floor
New York, NY 10005
Telephone: 212-248-1111
www.agi-usa.org/

The Alan Guttmacher Institute is a nonprofit organization focused on sexual and reproductive health research, policy analysis, and public education. The institute's mission is to protect the reproductive choices of all women and men in the United States and throughout the world. It is to support their ability to obtain the information and services needed to achieve their full human rights, safeguard their health, and exercise their individual responsibilities in regard to sexual behavior and relationships, reproduction, and family formation.

Alzheimer's Association
225 North Michigan Avenue, Suite 1700
Chicago, IL 60601-7633
Telephone: 312-335-8700
http://www.alz.org/

The Alzheimer's Association, a national network of chapters, is the largest national voluntary health organization dedicated to advancing Alzheimer's research and helping those affected by the disease. Having awarded $136 million in research grants, the association ranks as the top private funder of research into the causes, treatments, and prevention of Alzheimer's disease. The association also provides education and support for people diagnosed with the condition, their families, and caregivers.

American Academy of Child and Adolescent Psychiatry
3615 Wisconsin Avenue N.W.
Washington, DC 20016-3007
Telephone: 202-966-7300
http://www.aacap.org

The American Academy of Child and Adolescent Psychiatry (AACAP) is a membership-based organization, composed of more than 6,500 child and adolescent psychiatrists and other interested physicians. Its members actively research, evaluate, diagnose, and treat psychiatric disorders and pride themselves on giving direction to and responding quickly to new developments in addressing the health care needs of children and their families.

American Academy of Nursing
600 Maryland Avenue, S.W., Suite 100 West
Washington, DC 20024-2571
Telephone: 202-651-7238
www.nursingworld.org/aan/

The American Academy of Nursing is constituted to potentiate the contributions of nursing leaders in transforming the health care system to optimize public well-being. This leadership is grounded in a global perspective, enriched by diversity, and actualized through partnerships with other health care and consumer groups.

American Academy of Pediatrics
141 Northwest Point Boulevard
Elk Grove Village, IL 60007-1098
Telephone: 847-434-4000
http://www.aap.org/

The American Academy of Pediatrics (AAP) and its member pediatricians dedicate their efforts and resources to the health, safety, and well-being of all infants, children, adolescents, and young adults. The AAP has 57,000 members in the United States, Canada, and Latin America. Members include pediatricians, pediatric medical subspecialists, and pediatric surgical specialists. More than 41,000 members are board certified and are called Fellows of the American Academy of Pediatrics (FAAP).

American Association of Colleges of Nursing
One Dupont Circle, N.W., Suite 530
Washington, DC 20036
Telephone: 202-463-6930
http://www.aacn.nche.edu/

The American Association of Colleges of Nursing (AACN) is the national voice for America's baccalaureate- and higher-degree nursing education programs. AACN's educational, research, government advocacy, data collection, publications, and other programs work to establish quality standards for bachelor's- and graduate-degree nursing education, assist deans and directors to implement those standards, influence the nursing profession to improve health care, and promote public support of baccalaureate and graduate education, research, and practice in nursing.

American Association of Spinal Cord Injury Psychologists
   and Social Workers
75–20 Astoria Boulevard.
Jackson Heights, NY 11370

Telephone: 718-803-3782
http://www.aascipsw.org/

The American Association of Spinal Cord Injury Psychologists and Social Workers (AASCIPSW) is an organization of psychologists and social workers who provide for the emotional, behavioral, and psychosocial care of persons affected by spinal cord impairment (SCI). AASCIPSW, incorporated in 1986, operates exclusively for scientific, charitable, and educational purposes. AASCIPSW provides members the opportunity to develop and refine leadership skills through active participation in the association.

American Association of Suicidology
4201 Connecticut Avenue, N.W., Suite 408
Washington, DC 20008
Telephone: 202-237-2280
www.suicidology.org/

The goal of the American Association of Suicidology (AAS) is to understand and prevent suicide. AAS promotes research, public awareness programs, public education, and training for professionals and volunteers. In addition, AAS serves as a national clearinghouse for information on suicide. The membership of AAS includes mental health and public health professionals, researchers, suicide prevention and crisis intervention centers, school districts, crisis center volunteers, survivors of suicide, and a variety of laypersons who have an interest in suicide prevention.

American Cancer Society
http://www.cancer.org
Telephone: 1-800-ACS-2345

The American Cancer Society (ACS) is a nationwide, community-based voluntary health organization. With chartered divisions throughout the country and more than 3,400 local offices, the ACS is committed to fighting cancer through balanced programs of research, education, patient service, advocacy, and rehabilitation.

American College of Preventive Medicine
1307 New York Avenue, N.W., Suite 200
Washington, DC 20005
Telephone: 202-466-2044
www.acpm.org

The American College of Preventive Medicine (ACPM) is the national professional society for physicians committed to disease prevention and health promotion.

American Counseling Association
5999 Stevenson Avenue
Alexandria, VA 22304
Telephone: 1-800-347-6647
www.counseling.org

The American Counseling Association (ACA) is a not-for-profit, professional and educational organization dedicated to the growth and enhancement of the counseling profession. Founded in 1952, ACA is the world's largest association exclusively representing professional counselors in various practice settings. ACA has been instrumental in setting professional and ethical standards for the counseling profession.

American Diabetes Association
National Center
1701 North Beauregard Street
Alexandria, VA 22311
Telephone: 1-800-DIABETES (1-800-342-2383)
www.diabetes.org

The American Diabetes Association is the nation's leading nonprofit health organization providing diabetes research, information, and advocacy. The mission of the organization is to prevent and cure diabetes and to improve the lives of all people affected by diabetes.

American Heart Association
National Center
7272 Greenville Avenue
Dallas, TX 75231
Telephone: 1-800-AHA-USA-1 or 1-800-242-8721
www.americanheart.org

The American Heart Association is a national voluntary health agency whose mission is to reduce disability and death from cardiovascular diseases and stroke.

American Institute of Stress
124 Park Avenue
Yonkers, NY 10703
Telephone: 914-963-1200
http://www.stress.org/

The American Institute of Stress is committed to developing a better understanding of how to tap into the vast innate potential that resides in each of us for preventing disease and promoting health.

American Psychiatric Association
1000 Wilson Boulevard, Suite 1825

Arlington, VA 22209-3901
Telephone: 703-907-7300
www.psych.org

The American Psychiatric Association is a medical specialty society recognized worldwide. Its 37,000 U.S. and international member physicians work together to ensure humane care and effective treatment for all persons with mental disorders, including mental retardation and substance-related disorders. It is the voice and conscience of modern psychiatry. Its vision is a society that has available accessible quality psychiatric diagnosis and treatment.

American Psychological Association
750 First Street, N.E.
Washington, DC 20002-4242
Telephone: 1-800-374-2721 or 202-336-5500
www.apa.org

The American Psychological Association (APA) is a scientific and professional organization that represents psychology in the United States. With more than 155,000 members, APA is the largest association of psychologists worldwide. APA's initiatives include supporting psychology as a science, profession, and means to improve health and human welfare; educating the public and the media on the value of psychology; advocating in legislatures, educational settings, and major social institutions on behalf of the discipline and psychologists; and working to advance education and training in psychology from preschool to postdoctorate levels.

American Psychological Society
1010 Vermont Avenue N.W., Suite 1100
Washington, DC 20005-4907
Telephone: 202-783-2077
http://www.psychologicalscience.org/

The mission of the American Psychological Society (APS) is to promote, protect, and advance the interests of scientifically oriented psychology in research, application, teaching, and the improvement of human welfare. The APS is a nonprofit membership organization founded in 1988 to advance scientific psychology and its representation as a science on the national level. APS grew quickly, surpassing 5,000 members in its first 6 months. In 2003, APS membership exceeded 13,500 and includes the leading psychological scientists and academics, clinicians, researchers, teachers, and administrators.

American Psychosocial Oncology Society
2365 Hunters Way
Charlottesville, VA 22911
Telephone: 434-293-5350
www.apos-society.org/

The mission of American Psychosocial Oncology Society is to promote the psychological, social, and physical well-being of patients with cancer and their families at all stages of disease and survivorship through clinical care, education, research, and advocacy.

American Psychosomatic Society
6728 Old McLean Village Drive
McLean, VA 22101-3906
Telephone: 703-556-9222
www.psychosomatic.org

The mission of the American Psychosomatic Society is to promote and advance the scientific understanding of the interrelationships among biological, psychological, social, and behavioral factors in human health and disease, and the integration of the fields of science that separately examine each, and to foster the application of this understanding in education and improved health care.

American Public Health Association
800 I Street, N.W.
Washington, DC 20001
Telephone: 202-777-2742
http://www.apha.org/

The American Public Health Association (APHA) is the oldest and largest organization of public health professionals in the world, representing more than 50,000 members from over 50 occupations of public health. APHA brings together researchers, health service providers, administrators, teachers, and other health workers in a unique, multidisciplinary environment of professional exchange, study, and action. APHA is concerned with a broad set of issues affecting personal and environmental health, including federal and state funding for health programs, pollution control, programs and policies related to chronic and infectious diseases, a smoke-free society, and professional education in public health.

American Social Health Association
P.O. Box 13827
Research Triangle Park, NC 27709
Telephone: 919-361-8400
http://www.ashastd.org/

The American Social Health Association is recognized by the public, patients, providers, and policymakers for developing and delivering accurate, medically reliable information about sexually transmitted diseases.

American Society for Clinical Nutrition
9650 Rockville Pike
Bethesda, MD 20814-3998
Telephone: 301-530-7110
www.faseb.org/ascn/

The American Society for Clinical Nutrition (ASCN) is the clinical division of the American Society for Nutritional Sciences. The goals and objectives of the ASCN are to encourage and implement undergraduate and graduate education in basic and clinical nutrition, particularly in medical schools; expand research and clinical training opportunities in nutrition science for health professionals; and provide opportunities for investigators to present and discuss current research in human nutrition.

American Society for Nutritional Sciences
9650 Rockville Pike, Suite 4500
Bethesda, MD 20814
Telephone: 301-530-7050
www.asns.org/

The American Society for Nutritional Sciences is the premier research society dedicated to improving the quality of life through the science of nutrition.

American Sociological Association
1307 New York Avenue, N.W., Suite 700
Washington, DC 20005
Telephone: 202-383-9005
http://www.asanet.org/

The American Sociological Association (ASA) is a membership association dedicated to advancing sociology as a scientific discipline and profession serving the public good. With approximately 13,000 members, ASA encompasses sociologists who are faculty members at colleges and universities, researchers, practitioners, and students.

Association for Applied Psychophysiology and
    Biofeedback
10200 W. 44th Avenue, Suite 304
Wheat Ridge, CO 80033-2840, USA
Telephone: 303-422-8436
www.aapb.org

The mission of the Association for Applied Psychophysiology and Biofeedback (AAPB) is to advance the development, dissemination, and utilization of knowledge about applied psychophysiology and biofeedback to improve health and the quality of life through research, education, and practice. The goals of the association are to promote a new understanding of biofeedback and advance the methods used in this practice.

Association for the Advancement of Behavior Therapy
305 7th Avenue, 16th Floor
New York, NY 10001
Telephone: 212-647-1890
www.aabt.org

The Association for the Advancement of Behavior Therapy (AABT) is a professional, interdisciplinary organization that is concerned with the application of behavioral and cognitive sciences to the understanding of human behavior, developing interventions to enhance the human condition, and promoting the appropriate utilization of these interventions. AABT is a not-for-profit membership organization of more than 4,500 mental health professionals and students who are interested in behavior therapy and cognitive behavior therapy in order to gain a better understanding of human behavior; develop, assess, and apply interventions to assist in behavior change; help people deal with personal and social problems and issues; and further the empirical study, theory, and practice of these therapies.

Association of Behavior Analysis
1219 South Park Street
Kalamazoo, MI 49001
Telephone: 269-492-9310
http://www.abainternational.org/

The mission of the Association of Behavior Analysis is to develop, enhance, and support the growth and vitality of behavioral analysis through research, education, and practice.

Association of State and Territorial Directors of
  Health Promotion and Public Health Education
1101 15th Street, N.W., Suite 601
Washington, DC 20005
Telephone: 202-659-2230
www.astdhpphe.org

The Association of State and Territorial Directors of Health Promotion and Public Health Education

(ASTDHPPHE) was founded in 1946 (as the Conference of State Directors of Public Health Education) as a joint effort between directors of health education in state health departments and deans of health education in schools of public health. In 1994, the association changed its name to the Association of State and Territorial Directors of Health Promotion and Public Health Education to better reflect the mission and roles of the membership in promoting health and preventing disease in states and communities.

Association of Teachers of Preventive Medicine
1660 L Street, N.W., Suite 208
Washington, DC 20036
Telephone: 202-463-0550
http://www.atpm.org/

The Association of Teachers of Preventive Medicine (ATPM) is the national association supporting health promotion and disease prevention educators and researchers. Since 1942, ATPM and its members have been in the forefront of advancing, promoting, and supporting health promotion and disease prevention in the education of physicians and other health professionals.

Behavior OnLine
www.behavior.net/about.html

Behavior OnLine aspires to be the premier World Wide Web gathering place for mental health professionals and applied behavioral scientists—a place where professionals of every discipline can feel at home.

Center for Behavioral Neuroscience
www.cbn-atl.org

The Center for Behavioral Neuroscience examines the neural mechanisms underlying the social behaviors that are essential for species survival, such as fear, affiliation, aggression, and reproductive behaviors.

Center for Communication Programs
Johns Hopkins Bloomberg School of Public Health
111 Market Place, Suite 310
Baltimore, MD 21202
Telephone: 410-659-6300
www.jhuccp.org/

The Center for Communication Programs (CCP) works with international agencies, foundations, governments, and nongovernmental organizations in the United States and overseas to promote healthy behavior.

The CCP's work focuses on the field of strategic, research-based communication for behavior change and health promotion that has helped transform the theory and practice of public health.

Center for the Advancement of Health
2000 Florida Avenue, N.W., Suite 210
Washington, DC 20009–1231
Telephone: 202-387-2829
www.cfah.org/

The Center for the Advancement of Health promotes a view of health that recognizes that where we live, how we are educated, and what we eat, drink, breathe, and do affect health as much as, if not more than, access to health care. Its mission is to translate research on this expanded view of health into effective policy and practice.

Centers for Disease Control and Prevention
1600 Clifton Road
Atlanta, GA 30333
Telephone: 404-639-3311
www.cdc.gov

The Centers for Disease Control and Prevention (CDC) is recognized as the lead federal agency for protecting the health and safety of people, at home and abroad, providing credible information to enhance health decisions and promoting health through strong partnerships. The CDC serves as the national focus for developing and applying disease prevention and control, environmental health, and health promotion and education activities designed to improve the health of the people of the United States. The CDC's mission is to promote health and quality of life by preventing and controlling disease, injury, and disability.

College on Problems of Drug Dependence
3420 N. Broad Street
Philadelphia, PA 19140
Telephone: 215-707-3242
http://www.cpdd.vcu.edu/

The College on Problems of Drug Dependence (CPDD), formerly the Committee on Problems of Drug Dependence, has been in existence since 1929 and is the longest-standing group in the United States addressing problems of drug dependence and abuse. CPDD serves as an interface among government, industrial, and academic communities maintaining liaisons with regulatory and research agencies as well as educational, treatment, and prevention facilities in the drug abuse field. It also functions as a collaborating center of the World Health Organization.

Commission on Accreditation of Rehabilitation Facilities
4891 E. Grant Road
Tucson, AZ 85712
Telephone: 520-325-1044
www.carf.org

The Commission on Accreditation of Rehabilitation Facilities (CARF) is an independent, not-for-profit accrediting body promoting quality, value, and optimal outcomes of services through a consultative accreditation process that centers on enhancing the lives of the persons receiving services. Founded in 1966 as the Commission on Accreditation of Rehabilitation Facilities, the accrediting body is now known as CARF. The mission of CARF is to promote the quality, value, and optimal outcomes of services through a consultative accreditation process that centers on enhancing the lives of the persons served.

Consortium of Social Science Associations
1522 K Street, N.W., Suite 836
Washington, DC 20005
Telephone: 202-842-3525
http://www.cossa.org/

The Consortium of Social Science Associations (COSSA) is an advocacy organization supported by more than 100 professional associations, scientific societies, universities, and research institutions. COSSA stands alone in representing the full range of social scientists. COSSA represents the needs and interests of social and behavioral scientists; educates federal officials about social and behavioral science; informs the science community about relevant federal policies; and cooperates with other science and education groups in pursuit of common goals. COSSA lobbies Congress and the Executive Branch on issues affecting the social science portfolios of the National Science Foundation, the National Institutes of Health, the Departments of Agriculture, Commerce, Education, Justice, and Labor, and many other federal agencies.

Council of Graduate Departments of Psychology
http://psych.wfu.edu/cogdop/

The Council of Graduate Departments of Psychology (COGDOP) is a society constituted of chairs and heads of departments of psychology or other equivalent administrative units, which are authorized to offer graduate degrees in psychology in institutions accredited by their regional accrediting association. Membership is held by the department, not by the individual.

Decade of Behavior
750 First Street, N.E.
Washington, DC 20002-4242
Telephone: 202-336-6166
www.decadeofbehavior.org

The Decade of Behavior, launched in September 2000, is a multidisciplinary initiative to focus the talents, energy, and creativity of the behavioral and social sciences on meeting many of society's most significant challenges. These include improving education and health care; enhancing safety in homes and communities; actively addressing the needs of an aging population; and helping to curb drug abuse, crime, high-risk behaviors, poverty, racism, and cynicism toward government.

Federation of Behavioral, Psychological and Cognitive
  Sciences
750 First Street, N.E.
Washington, DC 20002
Telephone: 202-336-5920
http://www.thefederationonline.org/

The Federation of Behavioral, Psychological and Cognitive Sciences is a dues-supported coalition of member organizations, university departments of psychology, schools of education, research centers, regional psychological associations, and science divisions of the American Psychological Association. The federation represents the interests of scientists who do research in the areas of behavioral, psychological, and cognitive sciences. The efforts of the federation are focused on legislative and regulatory advocacy, education, and the communication of information to scientists.

Gerontological Society of America
1030 15th Street, N.W., Suite 250
Washington, DC 20005
Telephone: 202-842-1275
http://www.geron.org/

The Gerontological Society of America (GSA) is a nonprofit professional organization with more than 5,000 members in the field of aging. GSA provides researchers, educators, practitioners, and policymakers with opportunities to understand, advance, integrate, and use basic and applied research on aging to improve the quality of life as one ages.

Healthfinder
P.O. Box 1133
Washington, DC 20013-1133
www.healthfinder.gov/

Healthfinder is a guide to reliable health information from the Department of Health and Human Services. The guide includes a health library of hand-picked health information from A to Z—prevention and wellness, diseases and conditions, and alternative medicine—plus medical dictionaries, an encyclopedia, journals, and more.

Health Psychology, Division 38 of the American
  Psychological Association
750 First Street, N.E.
Washington, DC 20002-4242
Telephone: 202-336-6013
www.apa.org/about/division/div38.html

Division 38 seeks to advance contributions of psychology to the understanding of health and illness through basic and clinical research, education, and service activities and encourages the integration of biomedical information about health and illness with current psychological knowledge. The division has a nursing and health group and special interest groups in aging, women, and minority health issues. The division publishes the bimonthly journal *Health Psychology* and the quarterly newsletter *Health Psychologist*. Division 38 offers a listing of training programs in health psychology and presents an annual student paper award.

Human Factors and Ergonomics Society
P.O. Box 1369
Santa Monica, CA 90406-1369
Telephone: 310-394-2410
http://www.hfes.org/

The mission of the Human Factors and Ergonomics Society is to promote the discovery and exchange of knowledge concerning the characteristics of human beings that are applicable to the design of systems and devices of all kinds. The society was founded in 1957 as the Human Factors Society of America. Later, the name was changed to the Human Factors Society, Inc., to reflect its international influence and membership. In 1992, the name was changed to the Human Factors and Ergonomics Society.

Institute for the Advancement of Human Behavior
4370 Alpine Road, Suite 209

Portola Valley, CA 94028
Telephone: 1-800-258-8411
www.iahb.org

The Institute for the Advancement of Human Behavior (IAHB) is a fully accredited sponsor of continuing education and continuing medical education for mental health, chemical dependency, and substance abuse treatment providers in the United States and Canada. IAHB's mission is to provide high-quality clinical training to health care professionals as well as to companies and individuals with health care-related interests.

Institute for the Advancement of Social Work Research
750 First Street, N.E., Suite 700
Washington, DC 20002-4241
Telephone: 202-336-8385
http://www.iaswresearch.org/

The Institute for the Advancement of Social Work Research (IASWR) is a Washington, D.C.-based nonprofit organization. IASWR works to improve the lives of vulnerable populations by advocating for the importance of research to strengthen the social work profession's capacity to address complex social needs, and to contribute to improved prevention and treatment interventions, services, and policies. The overarching, single mission of IASWR is to promote and strengthen research in the social work profession.

Institute of Medicine
The National Academies
500 Fifth Street, N.W.
Washington, DC 20001
Telephone: 202-334-2138
www.iom.edu/

The mission of the Institute of Medicine (IOM) is to advance and disseminate scientific knowledge to improve human health. The institute provides objective, timely, authoritative information and advice concerning health and science policy to government, the corporate sector, the professions, and the public. IOM is part of the National Academy of Sciences organizations and does not receive direct federal appropriations for its work. The National Academy of Sciences was created by the federal government to be an adviser on scientific and technological matters.

Intercultural Cancer Council
6655 Travis, Suite 322
Houston, TX 77030-1312

Telephone: 713-798-4617
http://iccnetwork.org

The Intercultural Cancer Council (ICC) promotes policies, programs, partnerships, and research to eliminate the unequal burden of cancer among racial and ethnic minorities and medically underserved populations in the United States and its associated territories.

International Psycho-Oncology Society
2365 Hunters Way
Charlottesville, VA 22911
Telephone: 434-971-4788
http://www.ipos-society.org

The International Psycho-Oncology Society (IPOS) was created to foster international multidisciplinary communication about clinical, educational, and research issues that relate to the subspecialty of psycho-oncology. The society seeks to provide leadership and development of standards for educational training and research in the two psychosocial dimensions of cancer: the response of patients, families, and staff to cancer and its treatment at all stages, and the psychological, social, and behavioral factors that influence tumor progression and survival. It has boundaries with all clinical oncologic specialties, epidemiology and cancer control, basic sciences, bioethics, palliative care, rehabilitation, clinical trials, and decision making.

International Social Science Council
UNESCO House
1, rue Miollis
75732 Paris Cedex 15, France
http://www.unesco.org/ngo/issc/sommaire.htm

The International Social Science Council (ISSC) is an international nonprofit scientific organization with its headquarters in UNESCO House in Paris. The ISSC has as its aims and objectives the promotion of the understanding of human society in its environment by fostering the social and behavioral sciences throughout the world and their application to major contemporary problems and by enhancing cooperation by means of a global international organization of social and behavioral scientists and social and behavioral science organizations, encouraging multidisciplinary and interdisciplinary cooperation among the members of the ISSC.

International Society for Developmental Psychobiology
http://www.oswego.edu/isdp/

The purposes of the International Society for Developmental Psychobiology are to (a) promote and encourage research on the development of behavior in all organisms including humans, with special attention to the effects of biological factors operating at any level of organization; (b) facilitate communication of research results and theory in the area of developmental psychobiology through the use of both professional and popular printed media and through the presentation of papers at meetings of the society; and (c) foster application of the valid findings of research to human affairs in a way beneficial to humankind.

International Society of Behavioral Medicine
www.isbm.miami.edu

The International Society of Behavioral Medicine (ISBM) is a federation of national societies whose goal is to serve the needs of all health-related disciplines concerned with issues relevant to behavioral medicine. Each national society includes both biomedical and behavioral scientists.

MEDLINEplus
http://medlineplus.gov/

MEDLINEplus is a Web site with authoritative consumer health information from the National Institutes of Health and others.

MEDLINE/PubMed
www.ncbi.nih.gov/entrez/query.fcgi

MEDLINE/PubMed is a database with references, primarily from MEDLINE, to journal articles in life sciences with a concentration on articles in the biomedical field.

The Metanexus Institute
3624 Market Street, Suite 301
Philadelphia, PA 19104
Telephone: 215-789-2200
www.metanexus.net

The Metanexus Institute advances research, education, and outreach on the constructive engagement of science and religion. It seeks to create an enduring intellectual and social movement by collaborating with persons and communities from diverse religious traditions and scientific disciplines.

National Academy of Neuropsychology
2121 South Oneida Street, Suite 550
Denver, CO 80224–2594

Telephone: 303-691–3694
http://www.nanonline.org/

The National Academy of Neuropsychology is a professional society that includes clinicians, scientist practitioners, and researchers interested in neuropsychology.

National Academy of Sciences
500 Fifth Street, N.W.
Washington, DC 20001
Telephone: 202-334-2000
http://www4.nationalacademies.org/nas/nashome.nsf

The National Academy of Sciences (NAS) is a private, nonprofit, self-perpetuating society of distinguished scholars engaged in scientific and engineering research, dedicated to the furtherance of science and technology and to their use for the general welfare. The academy is governed by a council composed of 12 members (councilors) and five officers, elected from among the academy membership. The council is responsible to the membership for the activities undertaken by the organization and for the corporate management of the National Academy of Sciences, a corporation created by act of Congress that also includes the National Academy of Engineering (NAE), the Institute of Medicine (IOM), and the National Research Council (NRC). Collectively, these organizations are called the National Academies.

National Cancer Institute
6116 Executive Boulevard, MSC 8322
Bethesda, MD 20892-8322
Telephone: 1-800-422-6237
www.nci.nih.gov/

The National Cancer Institute (NCI) leads a national effort to reduce the burden of cancer morbidity and mortality. Its goal is to stimulate and support scientific discovery and its application to achieve a future when all cancers are uncommon and easily treated. Through basic and clinical biomedical research and training, NCI conducts and supports programs to understand the causes of cancer; prevent, detect, diagnose, treat, and control cancer; and disseminate information to the practitioner, patient, and public.

National Center for Complementary and Alternative Medicine
Bethesda, MD 20892
Telephone: 1-888-644-6226
www.nccam.nih.gov/

The National Center for Complementary and Alternative Medicine (NCCAM) is dedicated to exploring complementary and alternative medical (CAM) practices in the context of rigorous science, training CAM researchers, and disseminating authoritative information.

National Center for Research Resources
One Democracy Plaza, Room 984
6701 Democracy Boulevard, MSC 4874
Bethesda, MD 20892-4874
Telephone: 301-435-0888
www.ncrr.nih.gov/

The National Center for Research Resources (NCRR) advances biomedical research and improves human health through research projects and shared resources that create, develop, and provide a comprehensive range of human, animal, technological, and other resources. NCRR's support is concentrated in four areas: biomedical technology, clinical research, comparative medicine, and research infrastructure.

National Center on Minority Health and Health Disparities
6707 Democracy Boulevard, Suite 800, MSC 5465
Bethesda, MD 20892-5465
Telephone: 301-402-1366
www.ncmhd.nih.gov/

The mission of the National Center on Minority Health and Health Disparities (NCMHD) is to promote minority health and to lead, coordinate, support, and assess the National Institutes of Health effort to reduce and ultimately eliminate health disparities. In this effort, NCMHD will conduct and support basic, clinical, social, and behavioral research; promote research infrastructure and training; foster emerging programs; disseminate information; and reach out to minority and other health disparity communities.

National Heart, Lung, and Blood Institute
Bethesda, MD 20892
Telephone: 301-592-8573
www.nhlbi.nih.gov/

The National Heart, Lung, and Blood Institute (NHLBI) provides leadership for a national program in diseases of the heart, blood vessels, lung, and blood; blood resources; and sleep disorders. NHLBI plans, conducts, fosters, and supports an integrated and coordinated program of basic research, clinical investigations and trials, observational studies, and demonstration and education projects.

National Human Genome Research Institute
www.nhgri.nih.gov/

The National Human Genome Research Institute (NHGRI) supports the National Institutes of Health component of the Human Genome Project, a worldwide research effort designed to analyze the structure of human DNA and determine the location of the estimated 30,000 to 40,000 human genes.

National League for Nursing
61 Broadway
New York, NY 10006
Telephone: 1-800-669-1656 or 212-363-5555
http://www.nln.org/

The National League for Nursing advances quality nursing education that prepares the nursing workforce to meet the needs of diverse populations in an ever-changing health care environment.

National Institute of Allergy and Infectious Diseases
Building 31, Room 7A-50, MSC 2520
31 Center Drive
Bethesda, MD 20892-2520
www.niaid.nih.gov/

National Institute of Allergy and Infectious Diseases (NIAID) research strives to understand, treat, and ultimately prevent the myriad infectious, immunologic, and allergic diseases that threaten millions of human lives.

National Institute of Arthritis and
    Musculoskeletal and Skin Diseases
1 AMS Circle
Bethesda, MD 20892-3675
Telephone: 301-495-4484
www.niams.nih.gov/

The National Institute of Arthritis and Musculoskeletal and Skin Diseases (NIAMS) supports research into the causes, treatment, and prevention of arthritis and musculoskeletal and skin diseases, the training of basic and clinical scientists to carry out this research, and the dissemination of information on research progress in these diseases.

National Institute of Child Health and Human
    Development
Building 31, Room 2A32, MSC 2425
31 Center Drive
Bethesda, MD 20892-2425
www.nichd.nih.gov/

National Institute of Child Health and Human Development (NICHD) research on fertility, pregnancy, growth, development, and medical rehabilitation strives to ensure that every child is born healthy and wanted and grows up free from disease and disability.

National Institute of Dental and Craniofacial Research
Bethesda, MD 20892-2190
Telephone: 301-496-4261
www.nidcr.nih.gov/

The National Institute of Dental and Craniofacial Research (NIDCR) provides leadership for a national research program designed to understand, treat, and ultimately prevent the infectious and inherited craniofacial-oral-dental diseases and disorders that compromise millions of human lives.

National Institute of Diabetes and Digestive and Kidney Diseases
Building 31, Room 9A04, MSC 2560
Center Drive
Bethesda, MD 20892
www.niddk.nih.gov/

The National Institute of Diabetes and Digestive and Kidney Diseases (NIDDK) conducts and supports basic and applied research and provides leadership for a national program in diabetes, endocrinology, and metabolic diseases; digestive diseases and nutrition; and kidney, urologic, and hematologic diseases. Several of these diseases are among the leading causes of disability and death; all seriously affect the quality of life of those who have them.

National Institutes of Health
9000 Rockville Pike
Bethesda, MD 20892
www.nih.gov/

The National Institutes of Health (NIH) is the steward of medical and behavioral research for the United States. Its mission is science in pursuit of fundamental knowledge about the nature and behavior of living systems and the application of that knowledge to extend healthy life and reduce the burdens of illness and disability. The goals of the agency are as follows: (1) foster fundamental creative discoveries, innovative research strategies, and their applications as a basis to advance significantly the nation's capacity to protect and improve health; (2) develop, maintain, and renew scientific human and physical resources that will assure the nation's capability to prevent disease;

(3) expand the knowledge base in medical and associated sciences in order to enhance the nation's economic well-being and ensure a continued high return on the public investment in research; and (4) exemplify and promote the highest level of scientific integrity, public accountability, and social responsibility in the conduct of science.

National Institute of Mental Health
6001 Executive Boulevard, Room 8184, MSC 9663
Bethesda, MD 20892
Telephone: 301-443-4513
www.nimh.nih.gov/

The National Institute of Mental Health (NIMH) provides national leadership dedicated to understanding, treating, and preventing mental illnesses through basic research on the brain and behavior, and through clinical, epidemiological, and services research.

National Institute of Neurological Disorders and Stroke
P.O. Box 5801
Bethesda, MD 20824
Telephone: 1-800-352-9424
www.ninds.nih.gov/

The mission of the National Institute of Neurological Disorders and Stroke (NINDS) is to reduce the burden of neurological diseases—a burden borne by every age group, every segment of society, and people all over the world. To accomplish this goal, the NINDS supports and conducts research, both basic and clinical, on the normal and diseased nervous system, fosters the training of investigators in the basic and clinical neurosciences, and seeks better understanding, diagnosis, treatment, and prevention of neurological disorders.

National Institute of Nursing Research
www.ninr.nih.gov/

The National Institute of Nursing Research (NINR) supports clinical and basic research to establish a scientific basis for the care of individuals across the life span—from the management of patients during illness and recovery to the reduction of risks for disease and disability; the promotion of healthy lifestyles; the promotion of quality of life in those with chronic illness; and the care for individuals at the end of life. This research may also include families within a community context, and it also focuses on the special needs of at-risk and underserved populations, with an emphasis on health disparities.

National Institute on Aging
Building 31, Room 5C27, MSC 2292
31 Center Drive
Bethesda, MD 20892
Telephone: 301-496-1752
www.nia.nih.gov/

The National Institute on Aging (NIA) leads a national program of research on the biomedical, social, and behavioral aspects of the aging process; the prevention of age-related diseases and disabilities; and the promotion of a better quality of life for all older Americans.

National Institute on Alcohol Abuse and Alcoholism
6000 Executive Boulevard, Willco Building
Bethesda, MD 20892-7003
www.niaaa.nih.gov/

The National Institute on Alcohol Abuse and Alcoholism (NIAAA) conducts research focused on improving the treatment and prevention of alcoholism and alcohol-related problems to reduce the enormous health, social, and economic consequences of this disease.

National Institute on Deafness and
    Other Communication Disorders
MSC 2320
31 Center Drive
Bethesda, MD 20892-2320
www.nidcd.nih.gov/

The National Institute on Deafness and Other Communication Disorders (NIDCD) conducts and supports biomedical research and research training on normal mechanisms as well as diseases and disorders of hearing, balance, smell, taste, voice, speech, and language that affect 46 million Americans.

National Institute on Drug Abuse
www.nida.nih.gov/

The National Institute on Drug Abuse (NIDA) leads the nation in bringing the power of science to bear on drug abuse and addiction through support and conduct of research across a broad range of disciplines and rapid and effective dissemination of results of that research to improve drug abuse and addiction prevention, treatment, and policy.

National Library of Medicine
8600 Rockville Pike
Bethesda, MD 20894
www.nlm.nih.gov/

The National Library of Medicine (NLM) collects, organizes, and makes available biomedical science information to investigators, educators, and practitioners and carries out programs designed to strengthen medical library services in the United States. Both health professionals and the public use its electronic databases, including MEDLINE and MEDLINEplus, extensively throughout the world.

National Science Foundation
4201 Wilson Boulevard
Arlington, VA 22230
Telephone: 703-292-5111
www.nsf.gov

The National Science Foundation (NSF) is an independent agency of the U.S. government. The NSF's mission is to promote the progress of science; to advance the national health, prosperity, and welfare; and to secure the national defense.

Neurobehavioral Teratology Society
http://www.nbts.org/

The purpose of the Neurobehavioral Teratology Society (NBTS) is to understand the behavioral and developmental alterations that result from genetic and environmental perturbations of the nervous system during the pre- and perinatal period. NBTS is also focused on communicating such findings to physicians, scientists, public health officials, and the general public to promote awareness and lessen the risks for teratologic occurrences in the population at large. NBTS also has a special focus of educating scientists in the appropriate methodology for conducting teratologic research.

Office of Behavioral and Social Sciences Research
http://obssr.od.nih.gov/

The Office of Behavioral and Social Sciences Research (OBSSR) mission is to stimulate behavioral and social sciences research throughout the National Institutes of Health (NIH) and to integrate these areas of research more fully into others of the NIH health research enterprise, thereby improving our understanding, treatment, and prevention of disease.

Office of Disease Prevention and Health Promotion
200 Independence Avenue S.W., Room 738G
Washington, DC 20201
Telephone: 202-205-8611
www.odphp.osophs.dhhs.gov/

Created by Congress in 1976, the Office of Disease Prevention and Health Promotion (ODPHP) plays a vital role in developing and coordinating a wide range of national disease prevention and health promotion strategies.

Psychology.info
http://psychology.info/

Psychology.info is the easiest starting point for psychology and mental health information on the Internet. The links are handpicked psychology destinations with reliable information and include recent headlines in the field of psychology.

PsychoNeuroImmunology Research Society
6619 Palma Lane
Morton Grove, IL 60053
www.pnirs.org

The PsychoNeuroImmunology Research Society (PNIRS) is an international organization for researchers in a number of scientific and medical disciplines, including psychology, neurosciences, immunology, pharmacology, psychiatry, behavioral medicine, infectious diseases, and rheumatology, who are interested in interactions between the nervous system and the immune system, and the relationship between behavior and health.

Psychonomic Society
1710 Fortview Road
Austin, TX 78704
Telephone: 512-462-2442
http://www.psychonomic.org/

The Psychonomic Society promotes the communication of scientific research in psychology and allied sciences. Its members are qualified to conduct and supervise scientific research, must hold a PhD degree or equivalent, and must have published significant research other than the doctoral dissertation.

Psych web
www.psywww.com/

Psych web is a Web site containing lots of psychology-related information for students and teachers of psychology.

Public Health Institute
2001 Addison Street, Second Floor
Berkeley, CA 94704-1103
Telephone: 510-644-8200
http://www.phi.org/

The Public Health Institute (PHI) is an independent, nonprofit organization dedicated to promoting health, well-being, and quality of life for people throughout California, across the nation, and around the world. As one of the largest and most comprehensive public health organizations in the nation, the PHI focuses its efforts in two distinct but complementary ways. PHI promotes and sustains independent, innovative research, training, and demonstration programs—many in collaboration with the private health care system and community-based organizations. PHI also serves as a partner with government to support its role in assessment, policy development, and assurance.

Research Society on Alcoholism
4314 Medical Parkway, Suite 12
Austin, TX 78756-3332
Telephone: 512-454-0022
http://www.rsoa.org/

The Research Society on Alcoholism (RSA) serves as a meeting ground for scientists in the broad areas of alcoholism and alcohol-related problems. The society promotes research and the acquisition and dissemination of scientific knowledge.

Robert Wood Johnson Foundation
P.O. Box 2316
Princeton, NJ 08543
Telephone: 1-888-631-9989
www.rwjf.org

The Robert Wood Johnson Foundation is the largest philanthropy devoted exclusively to health and health care in the United States. The Robert Wood Johnson Foundation seeks to improve the health and health care of all Americans. To achieve the most impact with its funds, it prioritizes grants into four goal areas: to ensure that all Americans have access to quality health care at reasonable cost; to improve the quality of care and support for people with chronic health conditions; to promote healthy communities and lifestyles; and to reduce the personal, social, and economic harm caused by substance abuse—tobacco, alcohol, and illicit drugs.

Science.gov
www.science.gov

Science.gov is a gateway to authoritative selected science information provided by U.S. government agencies, including research and development results. It contains reliable information resources selected by the respective agencies as their best science information. Two major types of information are included—selected authoritative science Web sites and databases of technical reports, journal articles, conference proceedings, and other published materials. The selected Web sites can be explored from the science.gov homepage. The Web pages and the databases can be searched individually or simultaneously from the search page.

Social Sciences Institute
North Carolina AT&T University
Charles H. Moore Building, A-35
Greensboro, NC 27411
www.ssi.nrcs.usda.gov/ssi/

The Social Sciences Institute (SSI) integrates customer opinion and fieldwork with science-based analysis to discover how social and economic aspects of human behavior can be applied to natural resource conservation programs, policies, and activities.

Society of Behavioral Medicine
7600 Terrace Avenue, Suite 203
Middleton, WI 53562
Telephone: 608-827-7267
www.sbm.org

The Society of Behavioral Medicine (SBM) is the nation's largest multidisciplinary organization dedicated to advancing the science and practice of behavioral medicine. Behavioral medicine is defined as an interdisciplinary field dedicated to improving individual and population health through the integration of scientific knowledge from the behavioral, biomedical, social, and public health disciplines and through the application of this evidence-based knowledge to improve prevention, treatment, rehabilitation, chronic illness management, quality of life, and coping during all phases of the life cycle.

Society for Behavioral Neuroendocrinology
4327 Ridge Road
Palmyra, VA 22963
www.sbn.org

The Society for Behavioral Neuroendocrinology (SBN) is a scientific society committed to understanding interactions between behavior and neuroendocrine function to advance understanding of behavioral neuroendocrinology. The society promotes exchanges between investigators approaching this problem from diverse perspectives. Researchers working in

laboratory, field, or clinical settings and on invertebrates, vertebrates, or cell lines both in vitro and in vivo are encouraged to join the society. Scientists interested in behavioral ecology, animal behavior, biological timing, neurosciences, endocrinology, development, cell biology, and genetics are all welcome. One's research need not explicitly employ behavioral techniques as long as the research is relevant to behavior. Similarly, behavioral research need not employ neuroendocrine techniques, but only be related to neuroendocrine function. Integrating cellular and molecular concepts into a functional framework is crucial to understanding how neuroendocrine function affects behavior and is, in turn, affected by behavior.

Society for Medical Decision Making
1211 Locust Street
Philadelphia, PA 19107
Telephone: 215-545-7697
http://www.smdm.org/

The Society for Medical Decision Making's mission is to improve health outcomes through the advancement of proactive systematic approaches to clinical decision making and policy formation in health care by providing a scholarly forum that connects and educates researchers, providers, policymakers, and the public.

Society for Neuroscience
11 Dupont Circle, N.W., Suite 500
Washington, DC 20036
Telephone: 202-462-6688
www.sfn.org

The Society for Neuroscience (SfN) is a nonprofit membership organization of basic scientists and physicians who study the brain and nervous system. Neuroscience includes the study of brain development, sensation and perception, learning and memory, movement, sleep, stress, aging, and neurological and psychiatric disorders. It also includes the molecules, cells, and genes responsible for nervous system functioning.

Society of Pediatric Psychology
P.O. Box 170231
Atlanta, GA 30317
www.apa.org/divisions/div54/

The Society of Pediatric Psychology (SPP) provides a forum for scientists and professionals interested in the health care of children, adolescents, and their families. The field of pediatric psychology is defined by the concerns of psychologists and allied professionals who work in interdisciplinary settings such as children's hospitals, developmental clinics, and pediatric or medical group practices, as well as traditional clinical child or academic arenas. It focuses on the rapidly expanding role of behavioral medicine and health psychology in the care of children, adolescents, and their families. As Division 54 of the American Psychological Association (APA), it provides an annual forum for research and practice presentations at the annual APA convention.

Society for Prevention Research
1300 I Street, N.W., Suite 250 West
Washington, DC 20005
Telephone: 202-216-9670
http://info@preventionresearch.org

One of the primary goals of the Society for Prevention Research (SPR) is to create a scientific, multidisciplinary forum for prevention science, and a concerted effort is being made to invite investigators whose research specialties are not represented in the current membership to join SPR.

Society for Psychophysiological Research
1010 Vermont Avenue, N.W., Suite 1100
Washington, DC 20005-4907
Telephone: 202-393-4810
www.wlu.edu/~spr/

The Society for Psychophysiological Research is an international scientific society with worldwide membership. The purpose of the society is to foster research on the interrelationships between the physiological and psychological aspects of behavior.

Society for Public Health Education
750 First Street N.E., Suite 910
Washington, DC 20002-4242
Telephone: 202-408-9804
http://www.sophe.org/

The Society for Public Health Education (SOPHE) is an independent, international professional association made up of a diverse membership of health education professionals and students. The society promotes healthy behaviors, healthy communities, and healthy environments through its membership, its network of local chapters, and its numerous partnerships with other organizations. With its primary focus on public health education, SOPHE provides leadership

through a code of ethics; standards for professional preparation, research, and practice; professional development; and public outreach.

Society for Research in Child Development
University of Michigan
3131 South State Street, Suite 302
Ann Arbor, MI 48108-1623
http://www.srcd.org/

The purposes of the Society for Research in Child Development are to promote multidisciplinary research in the field of human development, to foster the exchange of information among scientists and other professionals of various disciplines, and to encourage applications of research findings. The society is a multidisciplinary, not-for-profit, professional association with a membership of approximately 5,500 researchers, practitioners, and human development professionals from more than 50 countries.

Society for Research on Nicotine and Tobacco
7600 Terrace Avenue, Suite 203
Middleton, WI 53562, USA
Telephone: 608-836-3787
www.srnt.org/

The mission of the Society for Research on Nicotine and Tobacco (SRNT) is to stimulate the generation of new knowledge concerning nicotine in all its manifestations—from molecular to societal.

Society for Stimulus Properties of Drugs
http://www.sspd.org.uk/

The Society for Stimulus Properties of Drugs (SSPD) supports the use of drug discrimination methods and some related approaches in teaching and research on psychoactive drugs. Many of these drugs have medical uses in psychiatry and neurology, whereas others have no recognized medical uses but may be under development for such use, or are subject to abuse. Both licit and illicit substances are included. Membership of SSPD is open to individuals with bachelor or higher degrees in relevant subjects and with a genuine interest in the field.

Substance Abuse and Mental Health Services Agency
5600 Fishers Lane
Rockville, MD 20857
www.samhsa.gov/

The Substance Abuse and Mental Health Services Agency (SAMHSA) is the federal agency charged with improving the quality and availability of prevention, treatment, and rehabilitative services in order to reduce illness, death, disability, and cost to society resulting from substance abuse and mental illnesses.

U.S. National Committee of the International Union of Psychological Science
http://www.iupsys.org/

The International Union of Psychological Science serves as an umbrella international voice supporting "the development of psychological science, whether biological or social, normal or abnormal, pure or applied." It has national members from close to 70 countries, and works to represent the full breadth of psychology as a profession and as a science.

Women's Health Initiative
www.nhlbi.nih.gov/whi/
www.whi.org/

The Women's Health Initiative (WHI) is one of the largest preventive studies of its kind in the United States. The WHI is a 15-year research program that is composed of three major components: a randomized controlled clinical trial of promising but unproven approaches to prevention, an observational study to identify predictors of disease, and a study of community approaches to developing healthful behaviors.

World Health Organization
Avenue Appia 20
1211 Geneva 27, Switzerland
Telephone: (+ 41 22) 791 21 11
http://www.who.int

The World Health Organization (WHO), the United Nations specialized agency for health, was established in 1948. WHO's mission is the attainment by all peoples of the highest possible level of health. Health is defined in WHO's constitution as a state of complete physical, mental, and social well-being and not merely the absence of disease or infirmity.

Appendix B
Bibliography

Abraído-Lanza, A. F., Dohrenwend, B. P., Ng-Mak, D. S., & Turner, J. B. (1999). The Latino mortality paradox: A test of the "salmon bias" and healthy migrant hypotheses. *American Journal of Public Health, 89,* 1543-1548.

Abramson, L. Y., Seligman, M. E. P., & Teasdale, J. D. (1978). Learned helplessness in humans: Critique and reformulation. *Journal of Abnormal Psychology, 87,* 49-74.

ACCP/AACVPR Pulmonary Rehabilitation Guidelines Panel. (1997). Pulmonary rehabilitation: Evidence-based guidelines. *Chest, 112,* 1363-1396.

Ackerman, M. D., & Carey, M. P. (1995). Psychology's role in the assessment of erectile disorder: Historical precedents, current knowledge, and methods. *Journal of Consulting and Clinical Psychology, 63,* 862-876.

Adams, J. S. (1963). Towards an understanding on inequity. *Journal of Abnormal and Social Psychology, 67,* 422-436.

Adams, L. A., & Rickert, V. I. (1989). Reducing bedtime tantrums: Comparison between positive routines and graduated extinction. *Pediatrics, 84,* 756-761.

Aday, L. A. (2001). *At risk in America: The health and health care needs of vulnerable populations in the United States.* San Francisco: Jossey-Bass.

Adelman, R. D., Greene, M. G., & Ory, M. (2000). Communication between older patients and their doctors. *Clinics in Geriatric Medicine, 16,* 1-24.

Ader, R. (2000). On the development of psychoneuroimmunology. *European Journal of Pharmacology, 405* (1-3), 167-176.

Ader, R., Felten, D. L., & Cohen, N. (2001). *Psychoneuroimmunology.* San Diego, CA: Academic Press.

Ades, P. A. (2001). Cardiac rehabilitation and secondary prevention of coronary heart disease. *New England Journal of Medicine, 345,* 892-902.

Adler, N. E., Boyce, T., Chesney, M., Cohen, S., Folkman, S., Kahn, R., & Syme, L. (1994). Socioeconomic status and health: The challenge of the gradient. *American Psychologist, 49,* 15-24.

Adler, N. E., Marmot, M., McEwen, B. S., & Stewart, J. E. (1999). *Socioeconomic status and health in industrial nations: Social, psychological, and biological pathways.* New York: New York Academy of Sciences.

Adler, N. E., & Newman, K. (2002). Socioeconomic disparities in health: Pathways and policies. *Health Affairs, 21*(2), 60-76.

Adler, N. E., & Ostrove, J. M. (1999). SES and health: What we know and what we don't. *Annals of the New York Academy of Sciences, 896,* 3-15.

Affleck, G., & Tennen, H. (1996). Construing benefits from adversity. *Journal of Personality, 64,* 900-922.

Affleck, G., Tennen, H., & Rowe, J. (1991). *Infants in crisis: How parents cope with newborn intensive care and its aftermath.* New York: Springer-Verlag.

Agargun, M. Y. (2002). Serum cholesterol concentration, depression, and anxiety. *Acta Psychiatrica Scandinavica, 105,* 81-83.

Agency for Healthcare Research and Quality. (2003). *Practice guideline databases.* Retrieved from www.ahrq.gov

Agras, W. S. (2001). The consequences and costs of eating disorders. *Psychiatric Clinics of North America, 24,* 371-379.

Aguirre-Molina, M., Molina, C., & Zambrana, R. E. (Eds.). (2001). *Health issues in the Latino community.* San Francisco: Jossey-Bass.

Airhihenbuwa, C. O. (1995). *Health and culture: Beyond the Western paradigm.* Thousand Oaks, CA: Sage.

Aitkin, M., Anderson, D., & Hinde, J. (1981). Statistical modelling of data on teaching styles (with discussion). *Journal of the Royal Statistical Society A, 144,* 148-161.

Ajzen, I. (1988). *Attitudes, personality, and behavior.* Chicago: Dorsey.

Ajzen, I. (1991). The theory of planned behavior. *Organizational Behavior and Human Decision Processes, 50,* 179-211.

Ajzen, I., & Fishbein, M. (1980). *Understanding attitudes and predicting social behavior.* Englewood Cliffs, NJ: Prentice Hall.

Akerlind, I., & Hornquist, J. O. (1992). Loneliness and alcohol abuse: A review of evidences of an interplay. *Social Science and Medicine, 34,* 405-413.

al'Absi, M., Bongard, S., Buchanan, T., Pincomb, G. A., Licinio, J., & Lovallo, W. R. (1997). Cardiovascular and neuroendocrine adjustment to public-speaking and mental arithmetic stressors. *Psychophysiology, 34,* 266-275.

al'Absi, M., Everson, S. A., & Lovallo, W. R. (1995). Hypertension risk factors and cardiovascular reactivity to mental stress in young men. *International Journal of Psychophysiology, 20,* 155-160.

Aldwin, C. M. (1990). The elders life stress inventory: Egocentric and nonegocentric stress. In M. A. P. Stevens, J. H. Crowther, S. E. Hobfoll, & D. L. Tennenbaum, *Stress and coping in later life families* (pp. 49-69). New York: Hemisphere.

Aldwin, C. M., & Gilmer, D. F. (2003). *Health, illness, and optimal aging: Biological and psychosocial perspectives.* Thousand Oaks, CA: Sage.

Allen, M. T., Matthews, K. A., & Sherman, F. S. (1997). Cardiovascular reactivity to stress and left ventricular mass in youth. *Hypertension, 30,* 782-787.

Allensworth, D., Lawson, E., Nicholson, L., & Wyche, J. (Eds.). (1997). *Schools and health: Our nation's investment.* Washington, DC: National Academy Press.

Allison, D. B. (Ed.). (1995). *Handbook of assessment methods for eating behaviors and weight related problems: Measures, theory, and research.* Thousand Oaks, CA: Sage.

Allison, T. G., Williams, D. E., Miller, T. D., Patten, C. A., Bailey, K. R., Squires, R. W., et al. (1995). Medical and economic costs of psychologic distress in patients with coronary artery disease. *Mayo Clinic Proceedings, 70,* 734-742.

Altman, D. G., Schulz, K. F., Moher, D., Egger, M., Davidoff, F., Elbourne, D., et al. (2001). The revised CONSORT Statement for reporting randomized trials: Explanation and elaboration. *Annals of Internal Medicine, 134,* 663-694.

Altman, I. (1975). *The environment and social behavior.* Monterey, CA: Brooks-Cole.

Amaro, H., Whitaker, R., Coffman, G., & Heeren, T. (1990). Acculturation and marijuana and cocaine use: Findings from HHANES 1982-84. *American Journal of Public Health, 80*(Suppl.), 54-60.

American Academy of Pediatrics, Committee on Public Education. (2001). Children, Adolescents, and Television. *Pediatrics, 2,* 423-426.

American Cancer Society. (2000). *Cancer facts and figures, 2000.* Atlanta, GA: Author.

American College of Occupational and Environmental Medicine. (2003). Retrieved from http://www.acoem. org

American Diabetes Association. (2002). Nutritional recommendations and principles for people with diabetes mellitus. *Diabetes Care.* Retrieved from www.diabetes.org

American Geriatrics Society. (1998). The management of chronic pain in older persons: AGS Panel on Chronic Pain in Older Persons. [Published erratum appears in *Journal of the American Geriatrics Society, 46*(7), 913, 1998, July] [See comments]. *Journal of the American Geriatrics Society, 46*(5), 635-651.

American Psychiatric Association. (1987). *Diagnostic and statistical manual of mental disorders* (3rd ed., rev.). Washington, DC: Author.

American Psychiatric Association. (1994). *Diagnostic and statistical manual of mental disorders* (4th ed.). Washington, DC: Author.

American Psychiatric Association. (2000a). *Diagnostic and statistical manual of mental disorders* (4th ed.). Washington, DC: Author.

American Psychiatric Association. (2000b). Practice guidelines for the treatment of patients with eating disorders (Rev. ed.). *American Journal of Psychiatry, 157*(Suppl. 1), 1-39.

American Psychiatric Association. (2003). *Practice guidelines.* Retrieved from www.psych.org/clin_res/prac_guide.cfm

American Psychological Association. (2003). *Recommendations for psychotherapy treatment.* Retrieved from http://www.apa.org/divisions/div12/journals.html

American Sleep Disorders Association. (1997). *International Classification of Sleep Disorders, revised: Diagnostic and coding manual.* Rochester, MN: Author.

Amick, B. C., III, Kawachi, I., Coakley, E. H., Lerner, D. J., Levine, S., & Colditz, G. A. (1998). Relationship of job strain and iso-strain to health status in a cohort of women in the U.S. *Scandinavian Journal of Work, Environment & Health, 24,* 54-61.

Amick, B. C., III, McDonough, P., Chang, H., Rogers, W. H., Duncan, G., & Pieper, C. (2002). The relationship between all-cause mortality and cumulative working life course psychosocial and physical exposures in the United States labor market from 1968-1992. *Psychosomatic Medicine, 64:* 370-381.

Amir, N., & Kozak, M. J. (1998). Anxiety. In H. S. Friedman (Ed.), *Encyclopedia of mental health* (Vol. 1, pp. 129-135). Boston: Academic Press.

Anda, R. F., Williamson, D. F., Escobedo, L. G., Remington, P. L., Mast, E. E., & Madans, J. H. (1992). Self-perceived stress and the risk of peptic ulcer disease: A longitudinal study of U.S. adults. *Archives of Internal Medicine, 152*, 829-833.

Andersen, B. L., Anderson, B., & deProsse, C. (1989). Controlled prospective longitudinal study of women with cancer, II: Psychological outcomes. *Journal of Consulting and Clinical Psychology, 57*, 692-697.

Andersen, B. J., Auslander, W. F., Jung, K. C., Miller, J. P., & Santiago, J. V. (1990). Assessing family sharing of diabetes responsibilities. *Journal of Pediatric Psychology, 15*, 477-492.

Anderson, I. M. (2000). Selective serotonin reuptake inhibitors versus tricyclic antidepressants: A meta-analysis of efficacy and tolerability. *Journal of Affective Disorders, 58*, 19-36.

Anderson, J., Moeschberger, M., Chen, M. S., Jr., Kunn, P., Wewers, M. E., & Guthrie, R. (1993). An acculturation scale for Southeast Asians. *Social Psychiatry & Psychiatric Epidemiology, 28*, 134-141.

Anderson, L. M., Wood, D. L., & Sherbourne, C. D. (1997). Maternal acculturation and childhood immunization levels among children in Latino families in Los Angeles. *American Journal of Public Health, 87*, 2018-2021.

Andreasen, A. R. (1995). *Marketing social change: Changing behavior to promote health, social development, and the environment.* San Francisco: Jossey-Bass.

Andrews, L., & Friedland, G. (2000). Progress in HIV therapeutics and the challenges of adherence to antiretroviral therapy. *Infectious Disease Clinics of North America, 14*(4), 901-928.

Angel, J. L., & Angel, R. J. (1992). Age at migration, social connections, and well-being among elderly Hispanics. *Journal of Aging and Health, 4*, 480-499.

Angeleri, F., Angeleri, V. A., Foschi, N., Giaquinto, S., & Nolfe, G. (1993). The influence of depression, social activity, and family stress on functional outcome after stroke. *Stroke, 24*, 1478-1483.

ANON. (2001). Executive summary of the Third Report of the National Cholesterol Education Program (NCEP) Expert Panel on Detection, Evaluation, and Treatment of High Blood Cholesterol in Adults (Adult Treatment Panel III). *Journal of the American Medical Association, 285*, 2486-2497.

Antonovsky, A. (1967). Social class, life expectancy, and overall mortality. *Milbank Quarterly, 45*, 31-73.

Antonuccio, D. O. (1998). The coping with depression course: A behavioral treatment for depression. *Clinical Psychologist, 51*(5), 3-5.

Appels, A. (1997). Depression and coronary heart disease: Observations and questions. *Journal of Psychosomatic Research, 43*, 443-452.

Aranda, M. P., & Knight, B. G. (1997). The influence of ethnicity and culture of the caregiver on the caregiver stress and coping process: A sociocultural review and analysis. *Gerontologist, 37*, 342-354.

Arcia, E., Skinner, M., Bailey, D., & Correa, V. (2001). Models of acculturation and health behaviors among Latino immigrants to the U.S. *Social Science & Medicine, 53*, 41-53.

Argyle, M. (2001). *The psychology of happiness.* London: Routledge.

Armeli, S., Gunthert, K. C., & Cohen, L. H. (2001). Stressor appraisals, coping, and post-event outcomes: The dimensionality and antecedents of stress-related growth. *Journal of Social and Clinical Psychology, 20*, 366-395.

Armitage, C. J., & Conner, M. (2001). Efficacy of the theory of planned behavior: A meta-analytic review. *British Journal of Social Psychology, 40*, 471-499.

Arno, P. S., Levine, C., & Memmott, M. M. (1999). The economic value of informal caregiving. *Health Affairs, 18*, 182-188.

Ascher, J., Cole, J., Colin, J.-N., Feighner, J., Ferris, R., Fibiger, H., Golden, R., Martin, P., Potter, W., Richelson, E., et al. (1995). Bupropion: A review of its mechanism of antidepressant activity. *Journal of Clinical Psychiatry, 56*, 395-401.

Ascherio, A., Katan, M. B., Zock, P. L., Stampfer, M. J., & Willett, W.C. (1999). Trans fatty acids and coronary heart disease. *New England Journal of Medicine, 340*, 1994-1998.

Ashby, F. G., Isen, A. M., & Turken, A. U. (1999). A neurophysiological theory of positive affect and its influence on cognition. *Psychological Review, 106*, 529-550.

Aspinwall, L. G., & Taylor, S. E. (1997). A stitch in time: Self-regulation and proactive coping. *Psychological Bulletin, 121*, 417-436.

Astin, J. A. (1998). Why patients use alternative medicine: Results of a national study. *Journal of the American Medical Association, 279*, 1548-1553.

Astin, J. A., Beckner, W., Soeken, K., Hochberg, M. C., & Berman, B. (2002). Psychological interventions for rheumatoid arthritis: A meta-analysis of randomized controlled trials. *Arthritis & Rheumatism (Arthritis Care & Research), 47*, 291-302.

Atienza, A. A., Henderson, P. C., Wilcox, S., & King, A. C. (2001). Gender differences in cardiovascular response to dementia caregiving. *Gerontologist, 41,* 490-498.

Atienza, A. A., & King, A. C. (2002). Community-based health intervention trials: An overview of methodological issues. *Epidemiologic Reviews, 24*(1), 72-79.

Ayman, D. A., & Goldshine, A. D. (1938). Cold as a standard stimulus of blood pressure: A study of normal and hypertensive subjects. *New England Journal of Medicine, 219,* 650-655.

Babyak, M., Blumenthal, J. A., Herman, S., Khatri, P., Doraiswamy, M., Moore, K., Craighead, W. E., Baldewicz, T. T., & Krishnan, K. R. (2000). Exercise treatment for major depression: maintenance of therapeutic benefit at 10 months. *Psychosomatic Medicine, 62,* 633-638.

Bagley, S. P., Angel, R., Dilworth-Anderson, P., Liu, W., & Schinke, S. (1995). Panel V: Adaptive health behaviors among ethnic minorities. *Health Psychology, 14,* 632-640.

Baker, E., Israel, B., & Schurman, S. (1996). The integrated model: Implications for worksite health promotion and occupational health and safety practice. *Health Education Quarterly, 23,* 175-188.

Balady, G. J., Ades, P. A., Comoss, P., Limacher, M., Pina, I. L, Southard, D., et al. (2000). Core components of cardiac rehabilitation/secondary prevention programs: A statement for healthcare professionals from the American Heart Association and the American Association of Cardiovascular and Pulmonary Rehabilitation Writing Group. *Circulation, 102,* 1069-1073.

Baltes, M. M., & Carstensen, L. L. (1996). The process of successful aging. *Ageing and Society, 16,* 397-422.

Bandura, A. (1977a). Self-efficacy: Toward a unifying theory of behavior change. *Psychological Bulletin, 84,* 191-215.

Bandura, A. (1977b). *Social learning theory.* Englewood Cliffs, NJ: Prentice Hall.

Bandura, A. (1986). *Social foundations of thought and action: A social cognitive theory.* Englewood Cliffs, NJ: Prentice Hall.

Bandura, A. (1994). Social cognitive theory and exercise of control over HIV infection. In R. J. DiClemente & J. L. Peterson (Eds.), *Preventing AIDS: Theories and methods of behavioral interventions.* New York: Plenum.

Bandura, A. (1997). *Self-efficacy: The exercise of control.* New York: W. H. Freeman.

Bandura, A. (2002). Environmental sustainability by sociocognitive deceleration of population growth. In P. Schmuch & W. Schultz (Eds.), *The psychology of*

sustainable development (pp. 209-238). Dordrecht, the Netherlands: Kluwer.

Barbarin, O. (1999). Do parental coping, involvement, religiosity and racial identity mediate children's psychological adjustment to sickle cell disease? *Journal of Black Psychology, 25,* 391-426.

Barbarin, O., Whitten, C., & Bonds, S. (1994). Estimating rates of psychosocial problems in urban and poor children with sickle cell anemia. *Health and Social Work, 19,* 112-119.

Barefoot, J. C. (1992). Developments in the measurement of hostility. In H. Friedman (Ed.), *Hostility, coping, and health* (pp. 13-31). Washington, DC: American Psychological Association.

Barefoot, J. C., Dodge, K. A., Peterson, B. L., Dahlstrom, W. G., & Williams, R. B., Jr. (1989). The Cook-Medley Hostility Scale: Item content and ability to predict survival. *Psychosomatic Medicine, 51,* 46-57.

Barker, D. J. P. (1998). *Mothers, babies and health in later life.* Edinburgh: Churchill Livingstone.

Barlow, D. H. (1986). Causes of sexual dysfunction: The role of anxiety and cognitive interference. *Journal of Consulting and Clinical Psychology, 54,* 140-148.

Barlow, D. H. (1988). *Anxiety and its disorders.* New York: Guilford.

Barlow, J., Wright, C., Sheasby, J., Turner, A., & Hainsworth, J. (2002). Self-management approaches for people with chronic conditions: A review. *Patient Education & Counseling, 1603,* 1-11.

Baron-Epel, O., & Kaplan, G. (2001). General subjective health status or age-related health status: Does it make a difference? *Social Science & Medicine, 53,* 1373-1381.

Barrera, M., Jr., Sandler, I. N., & Ramsay, T. B. (1981). Preliminary development of a scale of social support: Studies on college students. *American Journal of Community Psychology, 9,* 435-447.

Barrett, D., Wisotzek, I. E., Abel, G. G., Rouleau, J. L., Plat, A. F., Pollard, W. E., & Eckman, J. R. (1988). Assessment of psychosocial functioning of patients with sickle cell disease. *Southern Medical Journal, 81,* 745-750.

Bartlett, J. A. (2002). Addressing the challenges of adherence. *JAIDS, 29,* S2-S10.

Baskin, M. L. (2001). Conducting health interventions in Black churches: A model for building effective partnerships. *Ethnicity and Disease, 11,* 823-833.

Basmajian, J. V. (1962). *Muscles alive.* Baltimore: Williams and Wilkins.

Bass, D. M., McClendon, M. J., Deimling, G. T., & Mukherjee, S. (1994). The influence of a diagnosed mental impairment on family caregiver strain. *Journal of Gerontology, 49,* S146-S155.

Bassuk, S., Glass, T., & Berkman, L. (1999). Social disengagement and incident cognitive decline in community-dwelling elderly persons. *Annals of Internal Medicine, 131,* 165-173.

Bastani, R., Berman, B. A., Belin, T. R., Crane, L. A., Marcus, A. C., Nasseri, K., et al. (2002). Increasing cervical cancer screening among underserved women in a large county health system: Can it be done? What does it take? *Medical Care, 40,* 891-907.

Baum, A. (1987). Toxins, technology, and natural disasters. In G. R. VandenBos & B. K. Bryant (Eds.), *Cataclysms, crises, and catastrophes: Psychology in action. The master lectures* (pp. 9-53). Washington, DC: American Psychological Association.

Baum, A., & Andersen, B. L. (Eds.). (2001). *Psychosocial interventions for cancer.* Washington, DC: American Psychological Association.

Baum, A., Gatchel, R. J., Aiello, J. R., & Thompson, D. (1981). Cognitive mediation of environmental stress. In J. H. Harvey (Ed.), *Cognition, social behavior and the environment* (pp. 513-533). Hillsdale, NJ: Lawrence Erlbaum.

Baum, A., & Paulus, P. B. (1987). Crowding. In D. Stokols & I. Altman (Eds.), *Handbook of environmental psychology* (pp. 533-570). New York: John Wiley.

Baumstark, K. E., & Buckelew, S. P. (1992). Fibromyalgia: Clinical signs, research findings, treatment implications, and future directions. *Annals of Behavioral Medicine, 14,* 282-291.

Bausell, R. B., & Berman, B. M. (2002). Commentary: Alternative medicine: Is it a reflection of the continued emergence of the biopsychosocial paradigm? *American Journal of Medical Quality, 17*(1), 28-32.

Beaglehole, R. (1990). International trends in coronary heart disease mortality, morbidity, and risk factors. *Epidemiological Reviews, 12,* 1-16.

Beck, A. T. (1967). *Depression: Causes and treatment.* Philadelphia: University of Pennsylvania Press.

Beck, A. T., Rush, A. J., Shaw, B. F., & Emery, G. (1979). *Cognitive therapy of depression.* New York: Guilford.

Beck, A. T., & Steer, R. A. (1989). Clinical predictors of eventual suicide: A five- to ten-year study of suicide attempters. *Journal of Addictive Disorders, 17,* 203-209.

Beck, A. T., & Steer, R. A. (1993). *Manual for the Beck Depression Inventory.* San Antonio, TX: Psychological Corporation.

Beck, A. T., Steer, R. A., & Brown, G. K. (1996). *Manual for Beck Depression Inventory-II.* San Antonio, TX: Psychological Corporation.

Beck, A. T., Steer, R. A., & Brown, G. K. (2000). *Manual for Beck Depression Inventory FastScreen for Medical Settings.* San Antonio, TX: Psychological Corporation.

Beck, A. T., Ward, C. H., Mendelson, M., Mock, J., & Erbaugh, J. (1961). An inventory for measuring depression. *Archives of General Psychiatry, 4,* 561-571.

Beck, J. S., Beck, A. T., & Jolly, J. (2001). *Manual for the Beck Youth Inventories of Emotional and Social Impairment.* San Antonio, TX: Psychological Corporation.

Becker, M. H. (1974). The health belief model and personal health behavior. *Health Education Monographs, 2,* 324-473.

Beckham, E. E., & Leber, W. R. (Eds.). (1995). *Handbook of depression* (2nd ed.). New York: Guilford.

Bedi, M., Varshney, V. P., & Babbar, R. (2000). Role of cardiovascular reactivity to mental stress in predicting future hypertension. *Clinical and Experimental Hypertension, 22,* 1-22.

Belgrave, F., & Molock, S. (1991). The role of depression in hospital admissions and emergency treatment of patients with sickle cell disease. *Journal of the National Medical Association, 83,* 777-781.

Belkic, K., Savic, C., Theorell, T., Rakic, L., Ercegovac, D., & Djordjevic, M. (1994, April). Mechanisms of cardiac risk among professional drivers. *Scandinavian Journal of Work, Environment and Health,* pp. 73-86.

Bellamy, N., Buchanan, W. W., Goldsmith, C. H., Campbell, J., & Stitt, L. W. (1988). Validation study of WOMAC. *Journal of Rheumatology 15,* 1833-1840.

Belle, D. (1990). Poverty and women's mental health. *American Psychologist, 45,* 385-389.

Bendtsen, L., Norregaard, J., Jensen, R., & Olesen, J. (1997). Evidence of qualitatively altered nociception in patients with FM. *Arthritis Rheumatology, 40,* 98-102.

Benfari, R. C. (1981). The Multiple Risk Factor Intervention (MRFIT): The model for intervention. *Preventive Medicine, 10,* 426-442.

Bennett, G. G., Merritt, M. M., Edwards, C. L., Sollers, J., & Williams, R. B. (n.d.). *High effort coping, job demands, and the cortisol response to awakening.* Unpublished manuscript.

Bennett, N. (1976). *Teaching styles and pupil progress.* London: Open Books.

Bennett, R. (1998). Fibromyalgia, chronic fatigue syndrome, and myofascial pain. *Current Opinions in Rheumatology, 10,* 95-103.

Bennett, R. M. (1995). Fibromyalgia: The commonest cause of widespread pain. *Comprehensive Therapy, 21,* 269-275.

Bennett, R. M. (1996). Multidisciplinary group programs to treat fibromyalgia patients. *Rheumatic Diseases Clinics of North America, 22*, 351-367.

Bergner, M., Bobbitt, R. A., Kressel, S., Pollard, W., Gilson, B., & Morris, J. (1976). The Sickness Impact Profile: Conceptual formulation and methodology for the development of health status measure. *International Journal of Health Services 6*, 393-415.

Berkman, L. F., & Glass, T. (2000). Social integration, social networks, social support and health. In L. F. Berkman & I. Kawachi (Eds.), *Social epidemiology* (pp. 137-173). New York: Oxford University Press.

Berkman, L. F., & Syme, S. L. (1979). Social networks, host resistance, and mortality: A nine-year follow-up study of Alameda County residents. *American Journal of Epidemiology, 109*, 186-204.

Berlin, J. A., & Colditz, G. A. (1990). A meta-analysis of physical activity in the prevention of coronary heart disease. *American Journal of Epidemiology, 1332*, 612-628.

Bernard, H. R. (2000). *Social research methods: Qualitative and quantitative approaches.* Thousand Oaks, CA: Sage.

Bernard-Bonnin, A., Stachenko, S., Bonnin, D., Charette, C., & Rousseau, E. (1995). Self-management teaching programs and morbidity of pediatric asthma: A meta-analysis. *Journal of Allergy and Clinical Immunology, 90*, 135-138.

Berne, R. M., & Levy, M. N. (1997). *Cardiovascular physiology.* St. Louis, MO: C. V. Mosby.

Berntson, G. G., Bigger, J. T., Eckberg, D. L., Grossman, P., Kaufmann, P. G., Malik, M., et al. (1997). Heart rate variability: Origins, methods, and interpretive caveats. *Psychophysiology, 34*, 623-648.

Beutler, L. E. (2000). David and Goliath: When empirical and clinical standards of practice meet. *American Psychologist, 55*, 997-1007.

Biddle, S. J. H., & Mutrie, N. (2001). *Psychology of physical activity.* London: Routledge.

Bien, T., & Burge, R. (1990). Smoking and drinking: A review of the literature. *International Journal of Addictions, 25*, 1429-1454.

Births: Final data for 2000. (2002). *National Vital Statistics Reports, 50*(5). Public Health Service Report No. 2002-1120. Retrieved from http://www.cdc.gov/nchs/data/nvsr/nvsr50/nvsr50_05.pdf

Black, D., Morris, J. N., Smith, C., et al. (1982). *Inequalities in health: The Black report.* Middlesex: Penguin.

Blackburn, H., Luepker, R. V., Kline, F. G., Bracht, N., Carlaw, R. W., Jacobs, D. R., et al. (1984). The Minnesota Heart Health Program: A research and demonstration project in cardiovascular disease prevention. In J. D. Matarazzo, N. E. Miller, & S. M. Weiss (Eds.), *Behavioral health: A handbook of health enhancement and disease prevention* (pp. 1171-1178). New York: John Wiley.

Blair, S. N., Kohl, H. W., III, Barlow, C. E., Paffenbarger, R. S., Jr., Gibbons, L. W., & Marera, C. A. (1995). Changes in physical fitness and all-cause mortality. *Journal of the American Medical Association, 273*, 1093-1098.

Blair, S. N., & Morrow, J. R. (Eds.). (1998). Theme issue: Physical activity interventions [Special issue]. *American Journal of Preventive Medicine, 15*(4).

Blanchard, E. B. (2001). *Irritable bowel syndrome: Psychosocial assessment and treatment.* Washington, DC: American Psychological Association.

Blanchard, E. B., Schwarz, S. P., Suls, J. M., Gerardi, M. A., Scharff, L., Greene, B., et al. (1992). Two controlled evaluations of multicomponent psychological treatment of irritable bowel syndrome. *Behaviour Research and Therapy, 30*, 175-189.

Blascovich, J., & Katkin, E. S. (1993). *Cardiovascular reactivity to psychological stress and disease.* Washington, DC: American Psychological Association.

Blazer, D. (2000). Psychiatry and the oldest old. *American Journal of Psychiatry, 157*, 1915-1924.

Blazer, D., Hybels, C., & Pieper, C. (2001). The association of depression and mortality in elderly persons: A case for multiple independent pathways. *Journal of Gerontology: Medical Science, 56A*, M505-M509.

Block, J., & Kremen, A. M. (1996). IQ and ego-resiliency: Conceptual and empirical connections and separateness. *Journal of Personality and Social Psychology, 70*, 349-361.

Block, L., Morwitz, V. G., Putsis, W. P., & Sen, S. K. (2002). Assessing the impact of anti-drug advertising on adolescent drug consumption: Results from a behavioral model. *American Journal of Public Health, 92*, 1346-1351.

Blumenthal, J. A., Sherwood, A., Gullette, E. C. D., Georgiades, A., & Tweedy, D. (2002). Biobehavioral approaches to the treatment of essential hypertension. *Journal of Consulting and Clinical Psychology, 70*(3), 569-589.

Bobo, J. (1989). Nicotine dependence and alcoholism epidemiology and treatment. *Journal of Psychoactive Drugs, 21*(3), 323-329.

Bogden, J. F. (2000). *Fit, healthy, and ready to learn: A school health policy guide, Part I: Physical activity, healthy eating, and tobacco-use prevention.* Alexandria, VA: National Association of State Boards of Education.

Bolger, N., Zuckerman, A., & Kessler, R. C. (2000). Invisible support and adjustment to stress. *Journal of Personality and Social Psychology, 79,* 953-961.

Booth-Kewley, S., & Friedman, H. S. (1987). Psychological predictors of heart disease: A quantitative review. *Psychological Bulletin, 101,* 343-362.

Borkum, J. (in press). *Chronic headaches: Biology, psychology and behavioral treatment.* Hillsdale, NJ: Laurence Erlbaum.

Botvin, G. J., Baker, E., Dusenbury, L., Botvin, E. M., & Diaz, T. (1995). Long-term follow-up results of a randomized drug abuse prevention trial in a White middle-class population. *Journal of the American Medical Association, 273,* 1106-1112.

Bowlby, J. (1969). *Attachment and loss* (Vol. 1). London: Hogarth.

Bowling, A. (1995). *Measuring disease.* Buckingham, UK: Open University Press.

Bradley, C., Riazi, A., Barendse, S., Pierce, M., & Hendrieck, C. (2001). Diabetes mellitus. In D. W. Johnston (Ed.), *Health psychology* (pp. 277-304). Amsterdam: Elsevier Science.

Bradley, L. A., & McKendree-Smith, N. L. (2002). Central nervous system mechanisms of pain in fibromyalgia and other musculoskeletal disorders: Behavioral and psychologic treatment approaches. *Current Opinion in Rheumatology, 14,* 45-51.

Brady, J. V., Porter, R. W., Conrad, D. G., & Mason, J. W. (1958). Avoidance behavior and the development of gastroduodenal ulcers. *Journal of the Experimental Analysis of Behavior, 1,* 69-71.

Brassington, J. C., & Marsh, N. V. (1998). Neuropsychological aspects of multiple sclerosis. *Neuropsychological Review, 8,* 43-77.

Brickman, P., Coates, D., & Janoff-Bulman, R. (1978). Lottery winners and accident victims: Is happiness relative? *Journal of Personality and Social Psychology, 36,* 917-927.

Brisson, C., Laflamme, N., Moisan, J., Milot, A., Masse, B., & Vezina, M. (1999). Effect of family responsibilities and job strain on ambulatory blood pressure among white-collar women. *Psychosomatic Medicine, 61,* 205-213.

Broadhead, W., Blazer, D., George, L., & Tse, C. (1990). Depression, disability days and days lost from work: A prospective epidemiologic survey. *Journal of the American Medical Association, 264,* 2524-2528.

Brody, H., with Brody, D. (2000). *The placebo response: How to release the body's inner pharmacy for better health.* New York: Harper Collins.

Bross, I. D. J. (1967). Pertinency of an extraneous variable. *Journal of Chronic Diseases, 20,* 487-495.

Brown, P. C., & Smith, T. W. (1992). Social influence, marriage, and the heart: cardiovascular consequences of interpersonal control in husbands and wives. *Health Psychology, 11*(2), 88-96.

Brown, P. C., Smith, T. W., & Benjamin, L. S. (1998). Perceptions of spouse dominance predict blood pressure reactivity during marital interactions. *Annals of Behavioral Medicine, 20*(4), 286-293.

Brown, R. T., Armstrong, F. D., & Eckman, J. R. (1993). Neurocognitive aspects of paediatric sickle cell disease. *Journal of Learning Disabilities, 26,* 33-45.

Browne, A., Miller, B., & Maguin, E. (1999). Prevalence and severity of lifetime physical and sexual victimization among incarcerated women. *International Journal of Law and Psychiatry, 22,* 301-322.

Brownell, K. D. (2000). *The LEARN program for weight management.* Dallas, TX: American Health.

Brownley, K. A., Hurwitz, B. E., & Schneiderman, N. (2000). Cardiovascular psychophysiology. In J. T. Cacioppo, L. G. Tassinary, & G. G. Berntson (Eds.), *Handbook of psychophysiology* (2nd ed.). Cambridge, UK: Cambridge University Press.

Brownson, R. C., Housemann, R. A., Brown, D. R., Jackson-Thompson, J., King, A. C., Malone, B. R., & Sallis, J. F. (2000). Promoting physical activity in rural communities: Walking trail access, use, and effects. *American Journal of Preventive Medicine, 18,* 235-241.

Bruehl, S., McCubbin, J. A., & Harden, R. N. (1999). Theoretical review: Altered pain regulatory systems in chronic pain. *Neuroscience and Biobehavioral Reviews, 23,* 877-890.

Brunner, E. J. (1997). Stress and the biology of inequality. *British Medical Journal, 314,* 1472-1476.

Brunner, E. J. (2000). Toward a new social biology. In L. F. Berkman & I. Kawachi (Eds.), *Social epidemiology.* New York: Oxford University Press.

Brunner, E. J., Hemingway, H., Walker, B. R., Page, M., Clarke, P., Juneja, M., Shipley, M. J., Kumari, M., Andrew, R., Seckl, J. R., Papadopoulos, A., Checkley, S., Rumley, A., Lowe, G. D. O., Stansfeld, S. A., & Marmot, M. G. (2002), Adrenocortical, autonomic and inflammatory causes of the metabolic syndrome: Case-control study. *Circulation, 106,* 2659-2665.

Brunner, E. J., Marmot, M. G., Nanchahal, K., Shipley, M. J., Stansfeld, S. A., Juneja, M., & Alberti, K. G. M. M. (1997). Social inequality in coronary risk: Central obesity and the metabolic syndrome. Evidence from the WII Study. *Diabetologia, 40,* 1341-1349.

Buchholz, W. M. (1988). The medical uses of hope. *Western Journal of Medicine, 148,* 69.

Budney, A. J., & Higgins, S. T. (1998). *The community reinforcement plus vouchers approach: Manual 2: National Institute on Drug Abuse therapy manuals for drug addiction.* (NIH Pub. No. 98-4308). Rockville, MD: National Institute on Drug Abuse.

Buller, D. B., Morrill, C., Taren, D., Aickin, M., Sennott-Miller, L., Buller, M. K., et al. (1999). Randomized trial testing: The effect of peer education at increasing fruit and vegetable intake. *Journal of the National Cancer Institute, 91,* 1491-1500.

Burg, M. M., & Seeman, T. E. (1994). Families and health: The negative side of social ties. *Annals of Behavioral Medicine, 16*(2), 109-115.

Burke, L. E., & Ockene, I. S. (Eds.). (2001). *Compliance in healthcare and research.* Armonk, NY: Futura.

Burt, R. S. (1982). *Toward a structural theory of action.* New York: Academic Press.

Buss, A. H., & Durkee, A. (1957). An inventory for assessing different kinds of hostility. *Journal of Consulting Psychology, 21,* 343-349.

Buss, A. H., & Perry, M. (1992). The aggression questionnaire. *Journal of Personality and Social Psychology, 63,* 452-459.

Byrd, W. M., & Clayton, L. A. (2000). *An American health dilemma: The medical history of African Americans and the problem of race.* New York: Routledge.

Byrne, D. (1964). Repression-sensitization as a dimension of personality. In B. A. Maher (Ed.), *Progress in experimental personality research* (Vol. 1, pp. 169-220). New York: Academic Press.

Cabana, M. D., Ebel, B. E., Cooper-Patrick, L., Powe, N. R., Rubin, H. R., & Rand, C. S. (2000). Barriers pediatricians face when using asthma practice guidelines. *Archives of Pediatric & Adolescent Medicine, 154,* 685-693.

Cacioppo, J. T., Ernst, J. M., Burleson, M. H., McClintock, M. K., Malarkey, W. B., Hawkley, L. C., Kowalewski, R. B., Paulsen, A., Hobson, J. A., Hugdahl, K., Spiegel, D., & Berntson, G. G. (2000). Lonely traits and concomitant physiological processes: The MacArthur social neuroscience studies. *International Journal of Psychophysiology, 35,* 143-154.

Cacioppo, J. T., Tassinary, L. G., & Berntson, G. G. (Eds.). (2000). *Handbook of psychophysiology.* New York: Cambridge University Press.

Caetano, R., & Mora, M. E. (1988). Acculturation and drinking among people of Mexican descent in Mexico and the United States. *Journal of Studies on Alcohol. 49,* 462-471.

Calfas, K. J., Sallis, J. F., Nichols, J. F., Sarkin, J. A., Johnson, M. F., & Caparosa, S. (1999). Project GRAD: Two-year outcomes of a randomized controlled physical activity intervention among young adults. *American Journal of Preventive Medicine, 18,* 28-37.

Cameron, N. (1947). *The psychology of behavior disorders: A bio-social interpretation.* Boston: Houghton Mifflin.

Campbell, J. K., Penzien, D. B., & Wall, E. M. (2000). *Evidence-based guidelines for migraine headache: Behavioral and physical treatments.* U.S. Headache Consortium. Retrieved May 15, 2001, from http://www.aan.com/public/practiceguidelines/headache_gl.htm

Campbell, M. K. (2000). The North Carolina Black Churches United for Better Health Project: Intervention and process evaluation. *Health Education and Behavior, 27,* 241-253.

Campbell, R. S., & Pennebaker, J. W. (in press). The secret life of pronouns: Flexibility in writing style and physical health. *Psychological Science.*

Cannon, W. B. (1929). *Bodily changes in pain, hunger, fear, and rage.* New York: Appleton.

Cannuscio, C. C., Jones, C., Kawachi, I., Colditz, G. A., Berkman, L., & Rimm, E. (2002). Reverberations of family illness: A longitudinal assessment of informal caregiving and mental health status in the Nurses' Health Study. *American Journal of Public Health, 92,* 1305-1312.

Caplin, D. L., & Creer, T. L. (2001). A self-management program for adult asthma, III: Maintenance and relapse of skills. *Journal of Asthma, 38,* 343-356.

Cappelli, P., Bassi, L., Katz, H., Knoke, D., Osterman, P., & Useem, M. (1997). *Change at work.* New York: Oxford University Press.

Carels, R. A., Sherwood, A., Szczepanski, R., & Blumenthal, J. A. (2000). Ambulatory blood pressure and marital distress in employed women. *Behavioral Medicine, 26*(2), 80-85.

Carey, K. B., & Carey, M. P. (1993). Changes in self-efficacy resulting from unaided attempts to quit smoking. *Psychology of Addictive Behaviors, 7,* 219-224.

Carey, M. P., & Vanable, P. A. (2003). HIV/AIDS. In A. M. Nezu, C. M. Nezu, & P. A. Geller (Eds.), *Comprehensive handbook of psychology: Vol. 9. Health psychology.* New York: John Wiley.

Carleton, R. A., Lasater, T. M., Assaf, A. R., Feldman, H. A., & McKinlay, S. (1995). The Pawtucket Heart Health Program: Community changes in cardiovascular risk factors and projected disease risk. *American Journal of Public Health, 85,* 777-785.

Carleton, R. A., Lasater, T. M., Assaf, A. R., Lefebvre, R. C., & McKinlay, S. M. (1987). The Pawtucket Heart Health Program: An experiment in population-based disease prevention. *Rhode Island Medical Journal, 70,* 533-538.

Carrasquillo, O., Carrasquillo, A. I., & Shea, S. (2000). Health insurance coverage of immigrants living in the United States: Differences by citizenship status and country of origin. *American Journal of Public Health, 90,* 917-923.

Carroll, D. (1992). *Health psychology: Stress, behaviour and disease.* London: Falmer.

Carroll-Ghosh, T., Victor, B., & Bourgeois, J. (2002). Suicide. In R. Hales & S. Yudofsky (Eds.), *Textbook of clinical psychiatry* (pp. 1457-1483). Washington, DC: American Psychiatric Press.

Carter-Pokras, O., & Zambrana, R. E. (2001). Latino health status. In M. Aguirre-Molina, C. Molina, & R. E. Zambrana (Eds.), *Health issues in the Latino community* (pp. 23-54). San Francisco: Jossey-Bass.

Carver, C. S. (1998). Resilience and thriving: Issues, models and linkages. *Journal of Social Issues, 54,* 245-266.

Carver, C. S. (2001). Depression, hopelessness, optimism, and health. In N. J. Smelser & P. T. Baltes (Eds.), *International encyclopedia of the social and behavioral sciences* (Vol. 5, pp. 3516-3522). Oxford, UK: Elsevier.

Carver, C. S., & Scheier, M. F. (1998). *On the self-regulation of behavior.* New York: Cambridge University Press.

Carver, C. S., & Scheier, M. F. (2002). Optimism. In C. R. Snyder & S. J. Lopez (Eds.), *Handbook of positive psychology* (pp. 231-243). New York: Oxford University Press.

Carver, C. S., Scheier, M. F., & Weintraub, J. K. (1989). Assessing coping strategies: A theoretically based approach. *Journal of Personality and Social Psychology, 56,* 267-283.

Case, A., & Paxson, C. (2002). Parental behavior and child health. *Health Affairs, 21*(2), 164-178.

Caspersen, C. J., Merritt, R. K., & Stephens, T. (1994). International activity patterns: A methodological perspective. In R. K. Dishman (Ed.), *Advances in exercise adherence* (pp. 73-110). Champaign, IL: Human Kinetics.

Caspersen, C. J., Pereira, M. A., & Curran, K. M. (2000). Changes in physical activity patterns in the United States by sex and cross-sectional age. *Medicine and Science in Sports and Exercise, 32,* 1601-1609.

Cassel, J. (1976). The contribution of the social environment to host resistance. *American Journal of Epidemiology, 104,* 107-123.

Cassel, J. C., Patrick, R., & Jenkins, C. D. (1960). Epidemiological analysis of the health implications of culture change. *Annals of the New York Academy of Sciences, 84,* 938-949.

Catanzaro, S. J., & Greenwood, G. (1994). Expectancies for negative mood regulation, coping, and dysphoria among college students. *Journal of Counseling Psychology, 41,* 34-44.

Cattell, R. B. (1957). *Handbook for the I.P.A.T. Anxiety Scale.* Chicago: University of Chicago Press.

Cattell, R. B. (1966). Patterns of change: Measurement in relation to state-dimension, trait change, lability, and process concepts. In *Handbook of multivariate experimental psychology.* Chicago: Rand McNally.

Cattell, R. B., & Scheier, I. H. (1958). The nature of anxiety: A review of thirteen multivariate analyses comprising 814 variables. *Psychological Reports, 4,* 351.

Cattell, R. B., & Scheier, I. H. (1963). *Handbook for the IPAT Anxiety Scale* (2nd ed.). Champaign, IL: Institute for Personality and Ability Testing.

Catz, S. L., Kelly, J. A., Bogurt, L. M., Benotsch, E. G., & McAuliffe, T. L. (2000). Patterns, correlates, and barriers to medication adherence among persons prescribed new treatments for HIV disease. *Health Psychology, 19*(2), 124-133.

Caudill, M. (2001). *Managing pain before it manages you* [Patient workbook] (Rev. ed.). New York: Guilford.

Center for the Study and Prevention of Violence at the University of Colorado. (2003). Retrieved from http://www.colorado.edu/cspv/blueprints/index.html

Centers for Disease Control and Prevention. (1988). Guidelines for effective school health education to prevent the spread of AIDS. *Morbidity and Mortality Weekly Report, 37,* 1-14.

Centers for Disease Control and Prevention. (1992). *Youth suicide prevention program: A resource guide.* Atlanta, GA: Department of Health and Human Services.

Centers for Disease Control and Prevention. (1993a). Mandatory bicycle helmet use: Victoria, Australia. *Morbidity and Mortality Weekly Report, 42,* 359-363.

Centers for Disease Control and Prevention. (1993b). Sexually transmitted diseases treatment guideline. *Morbidity and Mortality Weekly Report, 42* (No. RR-14), 56-66.

Centers for Disease Control and Prevention. (1993c). Use of race and ethnicity in public health surveillance. Summary of the CDC/ATSDR Workshop. *Morbidity and Mortality Weekly Report, 42,* 1-28.

Centers for Disease Control and Prevention. (1994a). Current trends: Prevalence of disabilities and associated health conditions—United States, 1991-1992. *Morbidity and Mortality Weekly Report, 43*(40), 737-739.

Centers for Disease Control and Prevention. (1994b). Guidelines for school health programs to prevent tobacco use and addiction. *Morbidity and Mortality Weekly Report, 43,* 1-18.

Centers for Disease Control and Prevention. (1996a). Guidelines for school health programs to promote life-long healthy eating. *Morbidity and Mortality Weekly Report, 45,* 1-41.

Centers for Disease Control and Prevention. (1996b). Ten leading nationally notifiable infectious diseases—United States, 1995. *Morbidity and Mortality Weekly Report, 45,* 883-884.

Centers for Disease Control and Prevention. (1997). Guidelines for school and community programs to promote lifelong physical activity among young people. *Morbidity and Mortality Weekly Report, 46,* 1-36.

Centers for Disease Control and Prevention. (1999a, March). *Best practices for comprehensive tobacco control programs.* Atlanta, GA: U.S. Department of Health and Human Services, Centers for Disease Control and Prevention, National Center for Chronic Disease Prevention and Health Promotion, Office on Smoking and Health.

Centers for Disease Control and Prevention. (1999b). Cigarette smoking among adults—United States, 1997. *Morbidity and Mortality Weekly Report, 48,* 993-996.

Centers for Disease Control and Prevention. (2001). Births to teenagers in the United States, 1940-2000. *National Vital Statistics Reports, 49*(10), 1-24.

Centers for Disease Control and Prevention. (2002). *A glance at the HIV epidemic.* Retrieved December 31, 2002, from http://www.cdc.gov/hiv/pubs/facts.htm

Centers for Disease Control and Prevention. (2003). Revised birth and fertility rates for the United States in 2000-2001. *National Vital Statistics Reports, 51*(4), 1-24.

Chambless, D. L., & Ollendick, T. H. (2001). Empirically supported psychological interventions: Controversies and evidence. *Annual Review of Psychology, 52,* 685-716.

Chaney, E. F., O'Leary, M. R., & Marlatt, G. A. (1978). Skill training in alcoholics. *Journal of Consulting and Clinical Psychology, 46,* 1092-1104.

Chang, E. C. (Ed.). (2001). *Optimism and pessimism: Implications for theory, research, and practice.* Washington, DC: American Psychological Association.

Chang, E. C., D'Zurilla, T. J., & Maydeu-Olivares, A. (1997). Optimism and pessimism as partially independent constructs: Relations to positive and negative affectivity

and psychological well-being. *Personality and Individual Differences, 23,* 433-440.

Chapman, C. R., & Okifuji, A. (in press). Pain: Basic mechanisms and conscious experience. In R. H. Dworkin & W. S. Breibart (Eds.), *Psychosocial and psychiatric aspects of pain: A handbook for health care providers.*

Chen, X., Unger, J. B., & Johnson, C. A. (1999). Is acculturation a risk factor for early smoking initiation among Chinese American minors? A comparative perspective. *Tobacco Control, 8,* 402-410.

Chesney, M. A., Morin, M., & Sherr, L. (2000). Adherence to combination therapy. *Social Science & Medicine, 50,* 1599-1605.

Chesney, M. A., & Ozer, E. M. (1995). Women and health: In search of a paradigm. *Women's Health: Research on Gender, Behavior, and Policy, 1,* 3-26.

Cheung, F. K., & Snowden, L. R. (1990). Community mental health and ethnic minority populations. *Community Mental Health Journal, 26,* 277-291.

Child Trends, Inc. (2001). *Facts at a glance, 12/99 overview.* Retrieved from http://www.childtrends.org/.8

Chobanian, A. V., and the National High Blood Pressure Education Program Coordinating Committee. (2003). The seventh report of the Joint National Committee on Prevention, Detection, Evaluation, and Treatment of High Blood Pressure: The JNC 7 report. *Journal of the American Medical Association, 289,* 2560-2572.

Chrousos, G. P. (1998). Stressors, stress, and neuroendocrine integration of the adaptive response: The 1997 Hans Selye Memorial Lecture. *Annals of the New York Academy of Sciences, 851,* 311-335.

Chun, K. M., Balls Organista, P., & Marín, G. (Eds.). (2003). *Acculturation: Advances in theory, measurement and applied research.* Washington, DC: American Psychological Association.

Clark, L. A., & Watson, D. (1991). A tripartite model of anxiety and depression: Psychometric evaluation and taxonomic implications. *Journal of Abnormal Psychology, 100,* 316-336.

Clark, N. M. (1998). Management of asthma by parents and children. In H. Kotses & A. Harver (Eds.), *Self-management of asthma* (pp. 271-291). New York: Marcel Dekker.

Clark, N. M. (2002, March). *Evaluation and results of 3 NHLBI-funded studies of school-based asthma education.* Presentation at American Academy of Allergy Asthma & Immunology Annual Meeting, New York.

Clark, N. M., Feldman, C. H., Evans, D., Duzey, O., Levison, M. J., Wasilewski, Y., et al. (1986). Managing better: Children, parents, and asthma. *Patient Education & Counseling, 8,* 27-38.

Clark, N. M., Gong, M., & Kaciroti, N. (2001). A model of self-regulation for control of chronic disease. *Health Education & Behavior, 28,* 769-782.

Clark, N. M., Gong, M., Schork, M. A., Kaciroti, N., Evans, D., Roloff, D., et al. (2000). Long-term effects of asthma education for physicians on patient satisfaction and use of health services. *European Respiratory Journal, 16,* 15-21.

Clark, N. M., Nothwehr, F., Gong, M., Evans, D., Maiman, L. A., Hurwitz, M. E., et al. (1995). Physician-patient partnership in managing chronic illness. *Academic Medicine, 70,* 957-959.

Clark, R., Anderson, N. B., Clark, V. R., & Williams, D. R. (1999). Racism as a stressor for African Americans: A biopsychosocial model. *American Psychologist, 54,* 805-816.

Clarke, A. (Ed.). (1998). *The genetic testing of children.* Oxford, UK: Bios Scientific Publishers.

Clauw, D. J. (1995). The pathogenesis of chronic pain and fatigue syndromes, with special reference to fibromyalgia. *Medical Hypotheses, 44,* 369-378.

Clauw, D. J., & Chrousos, G. P. (1997). Chronic pain and fatigue syndromes: Overlapping clinical and neuroendocrine features and potential pathogenic mechanisms. *Neuroimmunomodulation, 4,* 134-153.

Clayton, D., & Hills, M. (1993). *Statistical models in epidemiology.* New York: Oxford University Press.

Cleary, P. D., Van Devanter, N., Steilen, M., Stuart, A., Shipton-Levy, R., McMullen, W., Rogers, T. F., Singer, E., Avorn, J., & Pindyck, J. (1995). A randomized trial of an education and support program for HIV-infected individuals. *AIDS, 9,* 1271-1278.

Clifford, J. (1988). *Predicament of culture: Twentieth-century ethnography, literature and art.* Cambridge, MA: Harvard University Press.

Coates, T. J., McKusick, L., Kuno, R., & Stites, D. P. (1989). Stress reduction training changed number of sexual partners but not immune function in men with HIV. *American Journal of Public Health, 79,* 885-887.

Cobas, J. A., Balcazar, H., Benin, M. B., Keith, V. M., & Chong, Y. (1996). Acculturation and low-birthweight infants among Latino women: A reanalysis of HHANES data with structural equation models [See comments]. *American Journal of Public Health, 86,* 394-396.

Cobb, S. (1976). Social support as a moderator of life stress. *Psychosomatic Medicine, 38,* 300-314.

Cochran Collaboration. (2003). *Recent reviews of treatments.* Retrieved from www.cochrane.org

Coe, C. L., & Lubach, G. R. (2003). Critical periods of special health relevance for psychoneuroimmunology. *Brain, Behavior, and Immunity, 17*(1), 3-12.

Cohen, S. (1988). Psychosocial models of the role of social support in the etiology of physical disease. *Health Psychology, 7,* 269-297.

Cohen, S., Gottlieb, B. H., & Underwood, L. G. (2000). Social relationships and health. In S. Cohen, L. G. Underwood, & B. H. Gottlieb (Eds.), *Social support measurement and intervention: A guide for health and social scientists* (pp. 1-25). New York: Oxford University Press.

Cohen, S., & Herbert, T. B. (1996). Health psychology: Psychological factors and physical disease from the perspective of human psychoneuroimmunology. *Annual Review of Psychology, 47,* 113-142.

Cohen, S., Kessler, R. C., & Underwood, L. G. (1995). *Measuring stress: A guide for health and social scientists.* New York: Oxford University Press.

Cohen, S., & McKay, G. (1984). Social support, stress and the buffering hypothesis: A theoretical analysis. In A. Baum, S. E. Taylor, & J. E. Singer (Eds.), *Handbook of psychology and health* (pp. 253-267). Hillsdale, NJ: Lawrence Erlbaum.

Cohen, S., Mermelstein, R., Kamarck, T., & Hoberman, H. M. (1985). Measuring the functional components of social support. In I. G. Sarason & B. R. Sarason (Eds.), *Social support: Theory research and applications.* Dordrecht, the Netherlands: Martinus Nijhoff.

Cohen, S., Underwood, S., & Gottlieb, B. (2000). *Social support measures and intervention.* New York: Oxford University Press.

Cohen, S., & Wills, T. A. (1985). Stress, social support, and the buffering hypothesis. *Psychological Bulletin, 98,* 310-357.

Cole, S. W., & Kemeny, M. E. (2000). Psychosocial influences on the progression of HIV infection. In R. Ader, D. L. Felten, & N. Cohen (Eds.), *Psychoneuroimmunology* (3rd ed., pp. 583-612). New York: Academic Press.

Coleman, J. S. (1990). *Foundations of social theory.* Cambridge, MA: Harvard University Press.

Collins, J. W., Jr., David, R. J., Symons, R., Handler, A., Wall, S. N., & Dwyer, L. (2000). Low-income African-American mothers' perception of exposure to racial discrimination and infant birth weight. *Epidemiology, 11,* 337-339.

Collins, J., & David, R. (1990). The differential effect of traditional risk factors on infant birth weight among Blacks and Whites in Chicago. *American Journal of Public Health, 80,* 679-681.

Committee on the Consequences of Uninsurance, Board on Health Care Services. (2002). *Care without courage: Too little, too late.* IOM report. Washington, DC: National Academy Press.

Committee on Diet and Health; National Research Council. (1989). *Diet and health: Implications for reducing chronic disease risk.* Washington, DC: National Academy Press.

Conklin, C. A., & Tiffany, S. T. (2002). Applying extinction research and theory to cue-exposure addiction treatments. *Addiction, 97,* 155-167.

Conner Christensen, T., Feldman Barrett, L., Bliss-Moreau, E., Lebo, K., & Kaschub, C. (2003). A practical guide to experience sampling procedures. *Journal of Happiness Studies, 4,* 53-78.

Connolly, K. J., Edelmann, R. J., Bartlett, H., Cooke, I. D., Lenton, E., & Pike, S. (1993). An evaluation of counselling for couples undergoing treatment for in-vitro fertilization. *Human Reproduction, 8,* 1332-1338.

CONSORT Statement. (2003). Retrieved from www.consort-statement.org

Cook, W. W., & Medley, D. M. (1954). Proposed hostility and pharisaic-virtue scales for the MMPI. *Journal of Applied Psychology, 38,* 414-418.

Cooper, J. O., Heron, T. E., & Heward, W. L. (1987). *Applied behavior analysis.* Upper Saddle River, NJ: Merril.

Cooper-Patrick, L., et al. (1999). Race, gender, and partnership in the patient-physician relationship. *Journal of the American Medical Association, 282,* 583-589.

Corcoran, J., Franklin, C., & Bennett, P. (2000). Ecological factors associated with adolescent pregnancy and parenting. *Social Work Research, 24,* 29-39.

Cornelius, L. J. (2000). Limited choices for medical care among minority populations. In C. J. R. Hogue, M. A. Hargraves, & K. S. Collins (Eds.), *Minority health in America: Findings and policy implications from the Commonwealth Fund minority survey* (pp. 176-193). Baltimore: Johns Hopkins University Press.

Cousins, N. (1979). *Anatomy of an illness.* New York: Bantam Books.

Covey, L., Glassman, A., & Stetner, F. (1998). Cigarette smoking and major depression. In M. Gold & B. Stimmel (Eds.), *Smoking and illicit drug use* (pp. 35-46). Binghamton, NY: Haworth Medical Press.

Cox, V. C., Paulus, P. B., McCain, G., & Karlovac, M. (1982). The relationship between crowding and health. In A. Baum & J. E. Singer (Eds.), *Advances in environmental psychology* (Vol. 4, pp. 271-294). Hillsdale, NJ: Lawrence Erlbaum.

Cram, J. R. (Ed.). (1990). *Clinical EMG for surface recordings* (Vol. 2). Nevada City, CA: Clinical Resources.

Cram, J. R., & Kasman, G. (1998). *Introduction to surface electromyography.* Gaithersburg, MD: Aspen.

Creed, F. (1999). The relationship between psychosocial parameters and outcome in irritable bowel syndrome. *American Journal of Medicine, 107,* 74S-80S.

Creer, T. L., Levstek, D. A., & Reynolds, R. C. V. (1998). History and evaluation. In H. Kotses & A. Harver (Eds.), *Self-management of asthma* (pp. 379-405). New York: Marcel Dekker.

Crellin, J. K., Andersen, R. R., & Connor, J. T. H. (Eds.). (1997). *Alternative health care in Canada: Nineteenth and twentieth century perspectives.* Toronto, Ontario, Canada: Canadian Scholars' Press.

Crespo, C. J., Smit, E., Troiano, R. P., Bartlett, S. J., Macera, C. A., & Andersen, R. E. (2001). Television watching, energy intake, and obesity in U.S. children: Results from the third National Health and Nutrition Examination Survey, 1988-1994. *Archives of Pediatric and Adolescent Medicine, 155,* 360-365.

Cromley, E. K. (2002). *GIS and Public Health.* New York: Guilford.

Cronin-Stubbs, D., Mendes de Leon, C. F., Beckett, L. A., Field, T. S., Glynn, R. J., & Evans, D. A. (2000). Six-year effect of depressive symptoms on the course of physical disability in community-living older adults. *Archives of Internal Medicine, 160,* 3074-3080.

Cruess, D. G., Leserman, J., Petitto, J. M., Golden, R. N., Szuba, M. P., Morrison, M. F., & Evans, D. L. (2001). Psychosocial-immune relationships in HIV disease. *Seminars in Clinical Neuropsychiatry, 6,* 241-251.

Cutrona, C. E., & Russell, D. W. (1990). Type of social support and specific stress: Toward a theory of optimal matching. In B. R. Sarason, I. G. Sarason, & G. R. Pierce (Eds.), *Social support: An interactional view.* New York: John Wiley.

Dabelea, D., Pettitt, D. J., Jones, K. L., & Arsianian, S. A. (1999). Type 2 diabetes mellitus in minority children and adolescents: An emerging problem. *Endocrinology and Metabolism Clinics of North America, 28,* 709-729.

da Costa, I. G., Rapoff, M. A., Lemanek, K., & Goldstein, G. L. (1997). Improving adherence to medication regimens for children with asthma and its effects on clinical outcome. *Journal of Applied Behavior Analysis, 30,* 687-691.

Dannenberg, A. L., Gielen, A. C., Beilenson, P. L., Wilson, M. H., & Joffe, A. (1993). Bicycle helmet laws and educational campaigns: An evaluation of strategies to increase children's helmet use. *American Journal of Public Health, 83,* 667-674.

Danner, D. D., Snowden, D. A., & Friesen, W. V. (2001). Positive emotions in early life and longevity: Findings from the Nun Study. *Journal of Personality and Social Psychology, 80,* 801-813.

Dantzer, R. (2001). Cytokine-induced sickness behavior: Mechanisms and implications. *Annals of the New York Academy of Sciences, 933,* 222-234.

The Dartmouth atlas of health care. (2002). Center for the Evaluative Clinical Sciences, Dartmouth Medical School. Chicago: American Hospital Publishing.

Darwin, C. (1965). *The expression of emotions in man and animals.* Chicago: University of Chicago Press. (Original work published 1872)

D'Atri, D. A., Fitzgerald, E. F., Kasl, S. K., & Ostfeld, A. M. (1981). Crowding in prison: The relationship between changes in housing mode and blood pressure. *Psychosomatic Medicine, 43,* 95-105.

Dautzenberg, M. G., Diederiks, J. P., Philipsen, H., & Tan, F. E. (1999). Multigenerational caregiving and well-being: Distress of middle-aged daughters providing assistance to elderly parents. *Women and Health, 29,* 57-74.

Davidson, K. W., Goldstein, M., Kaplan, R. M., Kaufmann, P. G., Knatterud, G. L., Orleans, C. T., et al. (in press). Evidence-based behavioral medicine: What is it, and how do we achieve it? *Annals of Behavioral Medicine.*

Davidson, L. L., Durkin, M. S., Kuhn, L., O'Connor, P., Barlow, B., & Heagarty, M. C. (1994). The impact of the Safe Kids/Healthy Neighborhoods Injury Prevention Program in Harlem, 1988 through 1991. *American Journal of Public Health, 84,* 580-586.

Davidson, R. J. (2000). Affective style, psychopathology, and resilience: Brain mechanisms and plasticity. *American Psychologist, 55,* 1196-1214.

Davison, G. C. (1998). Being bolder with the Boulder model: The challenge of education and training in empirically supported treatments. *Journal of Consulting and Clinical Psychology, 66*(1), 163-167.

Davis, C. G., Nolen-Hoeksema, S., & Larson, J. (1998). Making sense of loss and benefiting from experience: Two construals of meaning. *Journal of Personality and Social Psychology, 75,* 561-574.

Davison, K. P., Pennebaker, J. W., & Dickerson, K. P. (2000). Who talks? The social psychology of illness support groups. *American Psychologist, 55*(2), 205-217.

DeBusk, R. F., Miller, N. H., Superko, H. R., Dennis, C. A., Thomas, R. J., Lew, H. T., Berger, W. E., III, Heller, R. S., Rompf, J., Gee, D., Kraemer, H. C., Bandura, A., Ghandour, G., Clark, M., Shah, R. V., Fisher, L., & Taylor, C. B. (1994). A case-management system for coronary risk factor modification after acute myocardial infarction. *Annals of Internal Medicine, 120,* 721-729.

de Groot, M., Anderson, R., Freedland, K. E., Clouse, R. E., & Lustman, P. J. (2001). Association of depression and diabetes complications: A meta-analysis. *Psychosomatic Medicine, 63,* 619-630.

DeJong, W., & Hingson, R. (1998). Strategies to reduce driving under the influence of alcohol. *Annual Review of Public Health, 19,* 359-378.

DeJoy, D., & Southern, D. (1993). An integrative perspective on worksite health promotion. *Journal of Medicine, 35,* 1221-1230.

deKoning, K., & Martin, M. (Eds.). (1996). *Participatory research in health: Issues and experiences.* London: Zed Books.

dela Cruz, F. A., Padilla, G. V., & Butts, E. (1998). Validating a short acculturation scale for Filipino-Americans. *Journal of the American Academy of Nurse Practitioners, 10,* 453-460.

Delahanty, D. L., Dougall, A. L., & Baum, A. (2000). Neuroendocrine and immune alterations following natural disasters and traumatic stress. In R. Ader, D. L. Felten, & N. Cohen (Eds.), *Psychoneuroimmunology: Vol. 2* (3rd ed., pp. 335-345). San Diego, CA: Academic Press.

Delamater, A. M., Jacobson, A. M., Anderson, B., Cox, D., Fisher, L., Lustman, P., et al. (2001). Psychosocial therapies in diabetes: Report of the Psychosocial Therapies Working Group. *Diabetes Care, 24,* 1286-1292.

Dember, W. N., Martin, S., Hummer, M. K., Howe, S., & Melton, R. (1989). The measurement of optimism and pessimism. *Current Psychology: Research and Reviews, 8,* 102-119.

Dembroski, T. M., MacDougall, J. M., Williams, R. B., Haney, T. L., & Blumenthal, J. (1985). Components of Type A, hostility, and anger-in: Relationship to angiographic findings. *Psychosomatic Medicine, 47,* 219-233.

De Meyer, G. R. Y., & Herman, A. G. (1997). Vascular endothelial dysfunction. *Progress in Cardiovascular Disease, 34,* 325-342.

Demitrack, M. (1998). Chronic fatigue syndrome and fibromyalgia: Dilemmas in diagnosis and clinical management. *Psychiatric Clinics of North America, 21,* 671-692.

Demitrack, M. A., & Crofford, L. J. (1998). Evidence for and pathophysiologic implications of hypothalamic-pituitary-adrenal axis dysregulation in fibromyalgia and chronic fatigue syndrome. *Annals of the New York Academy of Sciences, 840,* 684-697.

Dennis, M., O'Rourke, S., Slattery, J., Staniforth, T., & Warlow, C. (1997). Evaluation of a stroke family care worker: Results of a randomised controlled trial. *British Medical Journal, 314,* 1071-1076.

Derogatis, L. R. (1983). *SCL-90-R administration, scoring, and procedures manual-II.* Towson, MD: Clinical Psychometric Research.

Derr, J., Forst, L., Yun Chen, H., & Conroy, L. (2002). Fatal falls in the construction industry, 1990-1999. *Journal of Occupational and Environmental Medicine, 43,* 853-860.

DeRubeis, R. J., Gelfand, L. A., Tang, T. Z., & Simons, A. D. (1999). Medication versus cognitive behavioral therapy for severely depressed outpatients: Mega-analysis of four randomized comparisons. *American Journal of Psychiatry, 156,* 1007-1013.

Desbiens, N. A., Mueller-Rizner, N., Virnig, B., & Lynn, J. (2001). Stress in caregivers of hospitalized oldest-old patients. *Journal of Gerontology, 56,* M231-M235.

DeWalt, K., & DeWalt, B. (2002). *Participant observation: A guide for fieldworkers.* Walnut Creek, CA: AltaMira.

DiClemente, C., Prochaska, J., Fairhurst, S., Velicer, W., Velasquez, M., & Rossi, J. (1991). The process of smoking cessation: An analysis of precontemplation, contemplation, and preparation stages of change. *Journal of Consulting and Clinical Psychology, 59*(2), 295-304.

Diener, E., & Seligman, M. E. P. (2002). Very happy people. *Psychological Science, 13,* 81-84.

Dietz, W. H., & Gortmaker, S. L. (2001). Preventing obesity in children and adolescents. *Annual Review of Public Health, 22,* 237-253.

Diez Roux, A. V. (2001). Investigating neighborhood and area effects on health. *American Journal of Public Health, 91,* 1783-1789.

Diez Roux, A. V., Merkin, S. S., Arnett, D., Chambless, L., Massing, M., Nieto, F. J., et al. (2001). Neighborhood of residence and incidence of coronary heart disease. *New England Journal of Medicine, 345,* 99-106.

DiGuiseppi, C., & Roberts, I. G. (2000) Individual-level injury prevention strategies in the clinical setting. *Future of Children, 10*(1), 53-82.

DiGuiseppi, C. G., Rivara, F. P., Koepsell, T. D., & Polissar, L. (1989). Bicycle helmet use by children: Evaluation of a community-wide helmet campaign. *Journal of the American Medical Association, 262,* 2256-2261.

Dijkstra, A., & De Vries, H. (1999). The development of computer-generated tailored interventions. *Patient Education and Counseling, 36,* 193-203.

Dilworth-Anderson, P., & Anderson, N. B. (1994). Dementia caregiving in Blacks: A contextual approach to research. In B. Lebowitz, E. Light, & G. Neiderehe (Eds.), *Mental and physical health of Alzheimer's caregivers* (pp. 385-409). New York: Springer.

Dilworth-Anderson, P., Williams, I. C., & Gibson, B. E. (2002). Issues of race, ethnicity, and culture in caregiving research: A 20-year review (1980-2000). *Gerontologist, 42,* 237-272.

DiMatteo, M. R. (1998). The role of the doctor in the emerging health care environment. *Western Journal of Medicine, 168,* 328-333.

DiMatteo, M. R., & Martin, L. R. (2002). *Health psychology.* Boston: Allyn & Bacon.

DiMatteo, M. R., Reiter, R. C., & Gambone, J. C. (1994). Enhancing medication adherence through communication and informed collaborative choice. *Health Communication, 6,* 253-265.

Dion, K. L. (2001). The social psychology of perceived prejudice and discrimination. *Canadian Psychology, 43*(1), 1-10.

Dishion, T. J., & Andrews, D. W. (1995). Preventing escalation in problem behaviors with high risk young adolescents: Immediate and 1-year outcomes. *Journal of Consulting & Clinical Psychology, 63,* 538-548.

Djeddah, C., Facchin, P., Ranzato, C., & Romer, C. (2000). Child abuse: Current problems and key public health challenges. *Social Science & Medicine, 51,* 905-915.

Dobkin, P. L., Da Costa, D., Lawrence, J., Fortin, P. R., Edworthy, S., Barr, S., Ensworth, S., Esfaile, J. M., Beaulieu, A., Zummer, M., Senecal, J. L., Goulet, J. R., Choquette, D., Rich, E., Smith, D., Cividino, A., Gladman, D., St. Pierre, Y., & Clarke, A. W. (2002). Counterbalancing patient demands with evidence: Results from a Pan-Canadian randomized clinical trial of brief supportive-expressive group psychotherapy for women with systemic lupus erythematosus. *Annals of Behavioral Medicine, 24,* 88-99.

Dobson, K. S. (1989). A meta-analysis of the efficacy of cognitive therapy for depression. *Journal of Consulting and Clinical Psychology, 57,* 414-419.

Doka, K. J. (1989). *Disenfranchised grief: Recognizing hidden sorrow.* New York and Toronto: Lexington Books.

Doll, R., & Peto, R. (1981). The causes of cancer: Quantitative estimates of avoidable risks of cancer in the United States today. *Journal of the National Cancer Institute, 66,* 1191-1308.

Doll, R., Peto, R., Wheatley, K., Gray, R., & Sutherland, I. (1994). Mortality in relation to smoking: 40 years observations on male British doctors. *BMJ, 309,* 901-911.

Domar, A. D., Clapp, D., Slawsby, E., Kessel, B., Orav, J., & Freizinger, M. (2000). The impact of group psychological interventions on distress in infertile women. *Health Psychology, 19,* 568-575.

Donald, A. (2002). Evidence-based medicine: Key concepts. *Medscape Psychiatry & Mental Health eJournal, 7*(2), 1-6.

Donatelle, R., Prows, S. L., Champeau, D., & Hudson, L. D. (2000). Randomized controlled trial using social support and financial incentives for high-risk pregnant smokers: The Significant-Other Supporter (SOS) program. *Tobacco Control, 9*(Suppl. 3), III67-III69.

Donohew, L., Sypher, H. E., & Bukowski, W. J. (1991). *Persuasive communication and drug abuse prevention.* Hillsdale, NJ: Lawrence Erlbaum.

Douglas, J. C., and the Hypertension in African Americans Working Group. (2003). Management of high blood pressure in African Americans: Consensus statement of the Hypertension in African Americans Working Group of the International Society on Hypertension in Blacks. *Archives of Internal Medicine, 163,* 525-541.

Dressler, W. W. (1991). Social support, lifestyle incongruity, and arterial blood pressure in a southern Black community. *Psychosomatic Medicine, 53,* 608-620.

Dressler, W. W. (1993). Social and cultural dimensions of hypertension in Blacks: Underlying mechanisms. In J. G. Douglas & J. C. S. Fray (Eds.), *Pathophysiology of hypertension in Blacks* (pp. 69-89). New York: Oxford University Press.

Dressler, W. W. (1999). Modernization, stress and blood pressure: New directions in research. *Human Biology, 71,* 583-605.

Dressler, W. W., & Bindon, J. R. (2000). The health consequences of cultural consonance: Cultural dimensions of lifestyle, social support and arterial blood pressure in an African American community. *American Anthropologist, 102,* 244-260.

Drolet, G., Dumont, E. C., Gosselin, I., Kinkead, R., Laforest, S., & Trottier, J. F. (2001). Role of endogenous opioid system in the regulation of the stress response. *Progress in Neuropsychopharmacology and Biological Psychiatry, 4,* 729-741.

Drossman, D. A. (1999). Do psychosocial factors define symptom severity and patient status in irritable bowel syndrome? *American Journal of Medicine, 107,* 41S-50S.

Drossman, D. A., Creed, F. H., Olden, K. W., Svedund, J., Toner, B. B., & Whitehead, W. E (1999). Psychosocial aspects of the functional gastrointestinal disorders. *Gut, 45*(Suppl. 2), II25-II30.

Drummond, D. C., Tiffany, S. T., Glautier, S., & Remington, B. (Eds.). (1995). *Addictive behaviour: Cue exposure theory and practice.* Chichester, UK: Wiley.

Druss, B. G., & Rosenheck, R. A. (1999). Association between use of unconventional therapies and conventional medical services. *Journal of the American Medical Association, 282,* 651-656.

Dunbar-Jacob, J., Erlen, J. A., Schlenk, E., Ryan, C., Sereika, S., & Doswell, E. (2000). Adherence in chronic disease. In J. Fitzpatrick & J. Goeppinger (Eds.), *Annual review of nursing research* (Vol. 18, pp. 48-90). New York: Springer.

Dunbar-Jacob, J., Sereika, S., Rohay, J., & Burke, L. (1998). Electronic methods in assessing adherence to medical regimens. In D. Krantz & A. Baum (Eds.), *Technology and methods in behavioral medicine* (pp. 95-113). Mahwah, NJ: Lawrence Erlbaum.

Dunham, J. (Ed.). (2001). *Stress in the workplace: Past, present and future.* London: Whurr.

Dunkel Schetter, C., Gurung, R. A., Lobel, M., & Wadhwa, P. (2000). Stress processes in pregnancy and birth: Psychological, biological, and sociocultural influences. In A. Baum, T. Revenson, & J. Singer (Eds.), *Handbook of health psychology.* Hillsdale, NJ: Lawrence Erlbaum.

Dunkel-Schetter, C. (1998). Maternal stress and preterm delivery. *Prenatal and Neonatal Medicine, 3,* 39-42.

Dusenbury, L., & Falco, M. (1995). Eleven components of effective drug abuse prevention curricula. *Journal of School Health, 65,* 420-425.

Dusseldorp, E., Van Elderen, T., Maes, S., Meulman, J., & Kraaij, V. (1999). A meta-analysis of psychoeducational programs for coronary heart disease. *Health Psychology, 18,* 506-519.

Dzewaltowski, D. A., Estabrooks, P. A., & Johnston, J. A. (2002). Healthy Youth Places promoting nutrition and physical activity. *Health Education Research: Theory and Practice, 17,* 541-551.

Eakin, J. M. (1997). Work-related determinants of health behavior. In D. S. Gochman (Ed.), *Handbook of health behavior research, I: Personal and social determinants* (pp. 337-357). New York: Plenum.

Ebbeling, C. B., Pawlak, D. B., & Ludwig, D. S. (2002). Childhood obesity: Public health crisis, common sense cure. *Lancet, 360,* 473-482.

Ebrahim, S., & Smith, G. D. (1998). Lowering blood pressure: A systematic review of sustained effects of non-pharmacological interventions. *Journal of Public Health Medicine, 20*(4), 441-448.

Eckenrode, J. E., & Wethington, E. (1990). The process and outcome of mobilizing social support. In S. Duck (Ed.), *Personal relationships and social support* (pp. 83-103). Newbury Park, CA: Sage.

EDK Associates. (1994). *Women and sexually transmitted diseases: The danger of denial.* New York: Author.

EDK Associates. (1995). *The ABCs of STDs.* New York: Author.

Edwards, C. L., Fillingim, R. B., & Keefe, F. (2001). Race, ethnicity and pain. *Pain, 94,* 133-137.

Edwards, R. R., Doley, D. M., Fillingim, R. B., & Lowery, D. (2001). Ethnic differences in pain tolerance: Clinical implications in a chronic pain population. *Psychosomatic Medicine, 63*(2), 316-323.

Eisenberg, D. M., Davis, R. B., Ettner, S. L., Appel, S., Wilkey, S., Rompay, M. V., et al. (1998). Trends in alternative medicine use in the United States, 1990-1997: Results of a follow-up national survey. *Journal of the American Medical Association, 280*, 1569-1575.

Eisenberg, D. M., Kessler, R. C., Foster, C., Norlock, F. E., Calkins, D. R., & Delbanco, T. L. (1993). Unconventional medicine in the United States: Prevalence, costs, and patterns of use. *New England Journal of Medicine, 328,* 246-252.

Elkin, I., Shea, M. T., Watkins, J. T., Imber, S. D., Sotsky, S. M., Collins, J. F., et al. (1989). National Institute of Mental Health treatment of collaborative research program: General effectiveness of treatments. *Archives of General Psychiatry, 46*, 971-982.

Elliott, A. M., Smith, B. H., Penny, K. I., Smith, W. C., & Chambers, W. A. (1999). The epidemiology of chronic pain in the community. *Lancet, 354*(9186), 1248-1252.

Elliott, D. S. (Ed.). (1997). *Blueprints for violence prevention.* Boulder: Center for the Study and Prevention of Violence, University of Colorado.

Ellison, C. G., & Levin, J. S. (1998). The religion-health connection: Evidence, theory, and future directions. *Health Education and Behavior, 25*, 700-720.

Elo, I. T., & Preston, S. H. (1996). Educational differentials in mortality: United States, 1979-85. *Social Science and Medicine, 42*(1), 47-57.

Emery, C. F., Schein, R. L., Hauck, E. R., & MacIntyre, N. R. (1998). Psychological and cognitive outcomes of a randomized trial of exercise among patients with chronic obstructive pulmonary disease. *Health Psychology, 17*, 232-240.

Emmons, K. M., & Rollnick, S. (2001). Motivational interviewing in health care settings: Opportunities and limitations. *American Journal of Preventive Medicine, 20*, 68-74.

Engel, G. L. (1977). The need for a new medical model: A challenge for biomedicine. *Science, 196*, 129-136.

Enzlin, P., Mathieu, C., & Demyttenaere, K. (2002). Gender differences in the psychological adjustment to Type 1 diabetes mellitus: An explorative study. *Patient Education & Counseling, 48*, 139-145.

Epstein, J. A., Botvin, G. J., & Diaz, T. (1998). Linguistic acculturation and gender effects on smoking among Hispanic youth. *Preventive Medicine, 27*, 583-589.

Epstein, L. H., Myers, M. D., Raynor, H. A., & Saelens, B. E. (1998). Treatment of pediatric obesity. *Pediatrics, 101*(3, Pt. 2), 554-570.

Erfurt, J. C., Foote, A., & Heirich, M. A. (1991). Worksite wellness programs: Incremental comparison of screening and referral alone, health education, follow-up counseling, and plant organization. *American Journal of Health Promotion, 5*, 438-449.

Eriksson, J., Taimela, S., & Koivisto, V. A. (1997). Exercise and the metabolic syndrome. *Diabetologia, 40*, 125-135.

Erlen, J. A., & Mellors, M. P. (1999). Adherence to combination therapy in persons living with HIV: Balancing the hardships and the blessings. *Journal of the Association of Nurses in AIDS Care, 10*(4), 75-84.

Ernst, J. M., & Cacioppo, J. T. (1999). Lonely hearts: Psychological perspectives on loneliness. *Applied and Preventive Psychology, 8*, 1-22.

Estrada, C. A., Isen, A. M., & Young, M. J. (1997). Positive affect facilitates integration of information and decreases anchoring in reasoning among physicians. *Organizational Behavioral and Human Decision Processes, 77*, 117-136.

EuroQol Group. (1990). EuroQol: A new facility for the measurement of health-related quality of life. *Health Policy 16,* 199-208.

Evans, G. W. (2001). Environmental stress and health. In A. Baum, T. Revenson, & J. E. Singer (Eds.), *Handbook of health psychology* (pp. 365-385). Mahwah, NJ: Lawrence Erlbaum.

Evans, G. W., & Cohen, S. (1987). Environmental stress. In D. Stokols & I. Altman (Eds.), *Handbook of environmental psychology* (pp. 571-610). New York: John Wiley.

Evans, G. W., & Kantrowitz, E. (2002). Socioeconomic status and health: The potential role of environmental risk exposure. *Annual Review of Public Health, 23*, 303-331.

Evans, R. L., Connis, R. T., Bishop, D. S., Hendricks, R. D., & Haselkorn, J. K. (1994). Stroke: A family dilemma. *Disability and Rehabilitation, 16*, 110-118.

Everson, S., Goldberg, D., Kaplan, G., Julkunen, J., & Salanen, J. (1998). Anger expression and incident hypertension. *Psychosomatic Medicine, 60,* 730-735.

Everson, S. A., Goldberg, D. E., Kaplan, G. A., Cohen, R. D., Pukkala, E., Tuomilehto, J., & Salonen, J. T. (1996). Hopelessness and risk of mortality and incidence of myocardial infarction and cancer. *Psychosomatic Medicine, 58,* 113-121.

Everson, S. A., Kaplan, G. A., Goldberg, D. E., & Salonen, J. T. (1996). Anticipatory blood pressure response to exercise predicts future high blood pressure in middle-aged men. *Hypertension, 27,* 1059-1064.

Everson, S. A., McKey, B. S., & Lovallo, W. R. (1995). Effect of trait hostility on cardiovascular responses to harassment in young men. *International Journal of Behavioral Medicine, 2,* 172-191.

Ewart, C. K. (1991). Social action theory for a public health psychology. *American Psychologist, 46,* 931-946.

Ewart, C. K. (2003). How integrative theory building can improve health promotion and disease prevention. In R. G. Frank, J. Wallander, & A. Baum (Eds.), *Models and perspectives in health psychology.* Washington, DC: American Psychological Association.

Ewart, C. K., & Suchday, S. (2002). Discovering how urban poverty and violence affect health: Development and validation of a neighborhood stress index. *Health Psychology, 21*(3), 254-262.

Fagerstrom, K. (1991). Towards better diagnoses and more individual treatment of tobacco dependence. Special issue: Future directions in tobacco research. *Brit J Addiction, 86*(5), 543-547.

Fairburn, C. G., & Brownell, K. D. (Eds.). (2002). *Eating disorders and obesity: A comprehensive handbook* (2nd ed.). New York: Guilford.

Fairey, A. S., Courneya, K. S., Field, C. J., & Mackey, J. R. (2002). Physical exercise and immune system function in cancer survivors: A comprehensive review and future directions. *Cancer, 94,* 539-551.

Fardy, P. S., White, R. E., Haltiwanger-Schmitz, K., Magel, J. R., McDermott, K. J., Clark, L. T., et al. (1996). Coronary disease risk factor reduction and behavior modification in minority adolescents: The PATH program. *Journal of Adolescent Health, 18,* 247-253.

Farquhar, J. W., Fortmann, S. P., Flora, J. A., Taylor, C. B., Haskell, W. L., Williams, P. T., et al. (1990). Effects of communitywide education on cardiovascular disease risk factors: The Stanford Five-City Project. *Journal of the American Medical Association, 264,* 359-365.

Farquhar, J. W., Fortmann, S. P., Maccoby, N., Haskell, W. L., Williams, P. T., Flora, J., et al. (1985). The Stanford Five-City Project: Design and methods. *American Journal of Epidemiology, 122,* 323-334.

Farran, C. J., Miller, B. H., Kaufman, J. E., & Davis, L. (1997). Race, finding meaning, and caregiver distress. *Journal of Aging and Health, 9,* 316-333.

Fawzy, F. I., Cousins, N., Fawzy, N. W., Kemeny, M. E., Elashoff, R., & Morton, D. (1990). A structured psychiatric intervention for cancer patients: I. Changes over time in methods of coping and affective disturbance. *Archives of General Psychiatry, 47,* 720-725.

Fazio, R. H. (1990). Multiple processes by which attitudes guide behavior: The MODE model as an integrative framework. In M. P. Zanna (Ed.), *Advances in experimental social psychology* (Vol. 23, pp. 75-109). San Diego, CA: Academic Press.

Feldman Barrett, L., & Barrett, D. J. (2001). An introduction to computerized experience sampling in psychology. *Social Science Computer Review, 19,* 175-185.

Feldman, L. (2001). Gender roles, role quality and health in Venezuelan working women. In S. P. Wamala & Lynch (Eds.), *Gender and social inequities in health: A public health issue.* Lund, Sweden: Studentlitteratur.

Ferber, R. (1985). *Solve your children's sleep problems.* New York: Simon & Schuster.

Ferguson, S. A., Leaf, W. A., Williams, A. F., & Preusser, D. F. (1996). Differences in young driver crash involvement in states with varying licensure practices. *Accident Analysis and Prevention, 28,* 171-180.

Fernandez, E., & Turk, D. C. (1989). The utility of cognitive coping strategies for altering pain perception: A meta-analysis. *Pain, 38*(2), 123-135.

Feuerstein, M., Labbe, E. E., & Kuczmierczyk, A. R. (1986). *Health psychology: A psychobiological perspective.* New York: Plenum.

Fields, H. L., & Basbaum, A. I. (1999). Central nervous system mechanisms of pain modulation. In P. D. Wall & R. Melzack (Eds.), *Textbook of pain* (pp. 309-329). Edinburgh: Churchill Livingstone.

Finch, B., Kolody, B., & Vega, W. (2000). Perceived discrimination and depression among Mexican-origin adults in California. *Journal of Health & Social Behavior, 41,* 295-313.

Fiore, M., Bailey, W., Cohen, S., Dorfman, S., Goldstein, M., Gritz, E., Heyman, R., Holbrook, J., Jaen, C., Kottke, T., Lando, H., Mecklenburg, R., Mullen, P., Nett, L., Robinson, L., Stitzer, M., Tommasello, A., Villejo, L., & Wewers, M. (2000, June). *Treating tobacco use and dependence* [Clinical practice guideline]. Rockville, MD: U.S. Department of Health and Human Services, Public Health Service, Agency for Healthcare Research and Quality.

First, M. B., Spitzer, R. L., Gibbon, M., & Williams, J. B. W. (1996). *User's guide for structured clinical interview for DSM-IV Axis I disorders: SCID-I clinician version.* Washington, DC: American Psychiatric Press.

Fischer, C. S., Jackson, R. M., Steuve, C. A., Gerson, K., Jones, L. M., & Baldassare, M. (1977). *Networks and places.* New York: Free Press.

Fishbein, M. (1963). An investigation of the relationships between beliefs about an object and the attitude toward that object. *Human Relations, 16,* 233-240.

Fishbein, M. (1997). *Theoretical models of HIV prevention. NIH Consensus Development Conference: Interventions to prevent HIV risk behaviors* [Program and Abstracts]. Bethesda, MD: National Institutes of Health.

Fishbein, M. (2000). The role of theory in HIV prevention. *AIDS Care, 12,* 273-278.

Fishbein, M., & Ajzen, I. (1975). *Belief, attitude, intention, and behavior: An introduction to theory and research.* Reading, MA: Addison-Wesley.

Fishbein, M., Bandura, A., Triandis, H. C., Kanfer, F. H., Becker, M. H., Middlestadt, S. E., & Eichler, A. (1992). *Factors influencing behavior and behavior change: Final report—Theorist's workshop.* Rockville, MD: National Institute of Mental Health.

Fishbein, M., Middlestadt, S. E., & Hitchcock, P. J. (1991). Using information to change sexually transmitted diseases-related behaviors: An analysis based on the theory of reasoned action. In N. J. Wasserheti, S. O. Aral, & K. K. Holmes (Eds.), *Research issues in human behavior and sexually transmitted diseases in the AIDS era.* Washington, DC: American Society for Microbiology.

Fisher, J. D., Nadler, A., & Whitcher-Alagna, S. (1982). Recipient reactions to aid. *Psychological Bulletin, 91,* 27-54.

Fisher, R. A. (1935). *The design of experiments.* Edinburgh: Oliver & Boyd.

Fitzpatrick, R., Davey, C., Buxton, M., & Jones, D. (1998). Evaluating patient-based outcome measures for use in clinical trials. *Health Technology Assessment 2,* 1-74.

Fitzpatrick, T. R. (1998). Bereavement events among elderly men: The effects of stress and health. *Journal of Applied Gerontology, 17,* 204-228.

Fitzpatrick, T. R., Spiro, A., III, Kressin, N. R., Greene, E., & Bossé, R. (2001). Leisure activities, stress, and well-being among bereaved and non-bereaved elderly men: The normative aging study. *OMEGA, 43,* 217-245.

Fix, M., & Struyk, R. J. (1993). *Clear and convincing evidence: Measurement of discrimination in America.* Washington, DC: Urban Institute Press.

Flay, B. (2002). Positive youth development requires comprehensive health promotion programs. *American Journal of Health Behavior, 26,* 407-424.

Flay, B. R. (1999). Understanding environmental, situational and intrapersonal risk and protective factors for youth tobacco use: The theory of triadic influence. *Discussant Comments. Nicotine & Tobacco Research, 1,* S111-S114.

Flay, B. R., & Petraitis, J. (1994). The theory of triadic influence: A new theory of health behavior with implications for preventive interventions. In G. S. Albrecht (Ed.), *Advances in medical sociology: Vol. 4. A reconsideration of models of health behavior change* (pp. 19-44). Greenwich, CT: JAI.

Flay, B. R., Petraitis, J., & Hu, F. (1995). The theory of triadic influence: Preliminary evidence related to alcohol and tobacco use. In J. B. Fertig & J. P. Allen (Eds.), *NIAAA research monograph: Alcohol and tobacco: From basic science to clinical practice* (pp. 37-57). Bethesda, MD: Government Printing Office.

Flay, B. R., Petraitis, J., & Hu, F. B. (1999). Psychosocial risk and protective factors for adolescent tobacco use. *Nicotine & Tobacco Research, 1,* S59-S65.

Fletcher, G. F., Balady, G. J., Amsterdam, E. A., Chaitman, B., et al. (2001). Exercise standards for testing and training. A statement for healthcare professionals from the American Heart Association. *Circulation, 104,* 1694-1740.

Fletcher, G. F., Balady, G., Blair, S. N., Blumenthal, J., et al. (1996). Statement on exercise: benefits and recommendations for physical activity programs for all Americans. *Circulation, 94,* 857-862.

Flor, H., Turk, D. C., & Scholz, O. B. (1987). Impact of chronic pain on the spouse: Marital, emotional and physical consequences. *Journal of Psychosomatic Research, 31*(1), 63-71.

Foerster, S. B., Kizer, K. W., DiSogra, L. K., Bal, D. G., Krieg, B. F., & Bunch, K. L. (1995). California's 5 a Day—for Better Health! campaign: An innovative population-based effort to effect large-scale dietary change. *American Journal of Preventive Medicine, 11*(2), 124-131.

Folkman, S. (1997). Positive psychological states and coping with severe stress. *Social Science and Medicine, 45,* 1207-1221.

Folkman, S., & Lazarus, R. S. (1988). *The Ways of Coping.* Palo Alto, CA: Mind Garden.

Folkman, S., & Moskowitz, J. T. (2000). Positive affect and the other side of coping. *American Psychologist, 55,* 647-654.

Foner, N. (2000). Anthropology and the study of immigration. In N. Foner, R. G. Rumbaut, & S. G. Gold (Eds.), *Immigration research for a new century: Multidisciplinary perspectives* (pp. 49-53). New York: Russell Sage Foundation.

Fontana, A., & Frey, J. H. (1994). Interviewing: The art of science. In N. Denzin & Y. Lincoln (Eds.), *The handbook of qualitative research* (pp. 361-376). Thousand Oaks, CA: Sage.

Ford, D. E. (2000). Managing patients with depression: Is primary care up to the challenge? *Journal of General Internal Medicine, 15,* 344-345.

Ford, D. E., Mead, L. A., Chang, P. P., Cooper-Patrick, L., Wang, N. Y., & Klag, M. J. (1998). Depression is a risk factor for coronary artery disease in men. *Archives of Internal Medicine, 158,* 1422-1426.

Ford, E. S., Giles, W. H., & Dietz, W. H. (2002). Prevalence of the metabolic syndrome among U.S. adults: Findings from the Third National Health and Nutrition Examination Survey. *Journal of the American Medical Association, 287,* 356-359.

Forster, J. L., Murray, D., Wolfson, M., Blaine, T., Wagenaar, A., & Hennrikus, D. (1998). The effects of community policies to reduce youth access to tobacco. *American Journal of Public Health, 88,* 1193-1198.

Fos, P. J., & Fine, D. J. (1998). *Designing health care for populations: Applied epidemiology in health care administration.* San Francisco: Jossey-Bass.

Foxx, R., & Brown, R. (1979). Nicotine fading and self-monitoring for cigarette abstinence or controlled smoking. *Journal of Applied Behavior Analysis, 12,* 111-125.

France, K. G., & Hudson, S. M. (1990). Behavior management of infant sleep disturbance. *Journal of Applied Behavior Analysis, 23,* 91-98.

Frank, E., & Thase, M. E. (1999). Natural history and preventive treatment of recurrent mood disorders. *Annual Review of Medicine, 50,* 453-468.

Frankenhaeuser, M., Lundberg, U., Fredrikson, M., Melin, B., Toumisto, M., Myrsten, A. L., Hedman, M., Bergman-Losman, B., & Wallin, L. (1989). Stress on and off the job as related to sex and occupational status in white-collar workers. *Journal of Organizational Behavior, 10,* 321-346.

Franklin, C., & Corcoran, J. (1999). Preventing adolescent pregnancy: A review of programs and practices. *Social Work, 45*(1), 40-52.

Franklin, C., Corcoran, J., & Harris, M. B. (in press). Risk, protective factors, and effective interventions for adolescent pregnancy. In M. W. Fraser (Ed.), *Risk and resilience in childhood and adolescents* (2nd ed.). Washington, DC: NASW Press.

Franklin, C., Grant, D., Corcoran, J., O'Dell, P., & Bultman, L. (1997). Effectiveness of prevention programs for adolescent pregnancy: A meta-analysis. *Journal of Marriage and the Family, 59*(3), 551-567.

Franklin, S. S., Khan, S. A., Wong, N. D., Larson, M. G., & Levy, D. (1999). Is pulse pressure useful in predicting risk for coronary heart disease? The Framingham Heart Study. *Circulation, 100,* 354-360.

Franzini, L., Ribble, J. C., & Keddie, A. M. (2001). Understanding the Hispanic paradox. *Ethnicity & Disease, 11,* 496-518.

Frasure-Smith, N., Lesperance, F., & Talajic, M. (1995). Depression and 18-month prognosis after myocardial infarction. *Circulation, 91,* 999-1005.

Fredman, L., & Daly, M. P. (1997). Weight change. *Journal of Aging & Health, 9,* 43-70.

Fredrickson, B. L. (1998). What good are positive emotions? *Review of General Psychology: New Directions in Research on Emotion, 2* [Special Issue], 300-319.

Fredrickson, B. L. (2000). Cultivating positive emotions to optimize health and well-being. *Prevention and Treatment, 3.* Retrieved from http://journals.apa.org/prevention

Fredrickson, B. L. (2001). The role of positive emotions in positive psychology: The broaden-and-build theory of positive emotions. *American Psychologist, 56* [Special Issue], 218-226.

Fredrickson, B. L., & Branigan, C. A. (2002). *Positive emotions broaden the scope of attention and thought-action repertoires: Evidence for the broaden-and-build theory.* Manuscript submitted for publication.

Fredrickson, B. L., & Joiner, T. (2002). Positive emotions trigger upward spirals toward emotional well-being. *Psychological Science, 13,* 172-175.

Fredrickson, B. L., & Levenson, R. W. (1998). Positive emotions speed recovery from the cardiovascular sequelae of negative emotions. *Cognition and Emotion, 12,* 191-220.

Fredrickson, B. L., Mancuso, R. A., Branigan, C., & Tugade, M. M. (2000). The undoing effect of positive emotions. *Motivation and Emotion, 24,* 237-258.

Fredrickson, B. L., Maynard, K. E., Helms, M. J., Haney, T. L., Siegler, I. C., & Barefoot, J. C. (2000). Hostility predicts magnitude and duration of blood pressure response to anger. *Journal of Behavioral Medicine, 23,* 229-243.

Fredrickson, B. L., Tugade, M. M., Waugh, C. E., & Larkin, G. (2002). *What good are positive emotions in crises? A prospective study of resilience and emotions following the terrorist attacks on the United States on September 11th, 2001.* Manuscript submitted for publication.

Freedman, R. R. (1991). Physiological mechanisms of temperature biofeedback. *Biofeedback and Self-Regulation, 16,* 95-115.

Freud, S. (1917). *Mourning and melancholia* (Standard ed., Vol. 14). New York: W. W. Norton.

Freud, S. (1924). *Collected papers* (Vol. 1). London: Hogarth.

Freud, S. (1936). *The problem of anxiety.* New York: W. W. Norton.

Freud, S. (1959). Why war? In J. Strachey (Ed.), *Collected papers* (Vol. 5). London: Hogarth. (Original work published 1933)

Fried, L., & Walston, J. (1999). Frailty and failure to thrive. In W. Hazzard, J. Blass, W. Ettinger, J. Halter, & J. Ouslander (Eds.), *Principles of geriatric medicine and gerontology* (pp. 1387-1402). New York: McGraw-Hill.

Friedberg, F., & Jason, L. A. (1998). *Understanding chronic fatigue syndrome: An empirical guide to assessment and treatment.* Washington, DC: American Psychological Association.

Friedman, M., & Ghandour, G. (1993). Medical diagnosis of Type A behavior. *American Heart Journal, 126,* 607-618.

Friedman, M., & Rosenman, R. H. (1971). Type A behavior pattern: Its association with coronary heart disease. *Annals of Clinical Research, 3,* 300-312.

Friedman, M., & Rosenman, R. (1974). *Type A behavior and your heart.* New York: Random House. (Original work published 1959)

Friedman, M., Thoresen, C. E., & Gill, J. J. (1986). Alteration of Type A behavior and its effect on cardiac recurrences in post-myocardial infarction patients: Summary results of the Recurrent Coronary Prevention Project. *American Heart Journal, 112,* 653-662.

Friedman, R., Schwartz, J., Schnall, P., Landsbergis, P., Pieper, C., Gerin, W., & Pickering, T. (2001). Psychological variables in hypertension: Relationship to casual or ambulatory blood pressure in men. *Psychosomatic Medicine, 63,* 19-31.

Fries, J. F. (1995). *Arthritis: A take care of yourself health guide for understanding your arthritis* (4th ed.). Reading, MA: Perseus.

Frijda, N. H. (1986). *The emotions.* Cambridge, UK: Cambridge University Press.

Froom, P., Melamed, S., & Benbasal, J. (1998). Smoking cessation and weight gain. *Journal of Family Practice, 46*(6), 460-464.

Frumkin, L. R., & Leonard, J. M. (1997). *Questions and answers on AIDS* (3rd ed.). Los Angeles: Health Information Press.

Fukuda, K., Straus, S. E., Hickie, I., Sharpe, M. C., Dobbins, J. G., & Komaroff, A. (1994). The chronic fatigue syndrome: A comprehensive approach to its definition and study. *Annals of Internal Medicine, 121,* 953-959.

Fuller-Jonap, F., & Haley, W. (1995). Mental and physical health of male caregivers of a spouse with Alzheimer's disease. *Journal of Aging and Health, 7,* 99-118.

Furnham, A. (1994). Why people choose complementary medicine. In W. Andritzky (Ed.), *Yearbook of cross-cultural medicine and psychotherapy 1992* (pp. 165-198). Berlin, Germany: VWB—Verlag für Wissenschaft und Bildung.

Gallagher, D., Wrabetz, A., Lovett, S., Del Maestro, S., & Rose, J. (1989). Depression and other negative affects in family caregivers. In E. Light & B. Lebowitz (Eds.), *Alzheimer's disease treatment and family stress: Future directions of research* (pp. 218-244). Washington, DC: Government Printing Office.

Gallinelli, A., Roncaglia, R., Matteo, M. L., Ciaccio, I., Volpe, A., & Facchinetti, F. (2001). Immunological changes and stress are associated with different implantation rates in patients undergoing in vitro fertilization embryo transfer. *Fertility & Sterility, 76,* 85-91.

Gallo, L. C., & Matthews, K. A. (2003). Understanding the association between socioeconomic status and physical health: Do negative emotions play a role? *Psychological Bulletin, 129*(1), 10-51.

Gasper, K., & Clore, G. L. (2002). Attending to the big picture: Mood and global versus local processing of visual information. *Psychological Science, 13,* 34-40.

Gass-Sternas, K. A. (1995). Single parent widows: Stressors, appraisal, coping, grieving responses and health. *Marriage and Family Review, 20,* 411-445.

Gatchel, R., & Turk, D. C. (Eds.). (1999). *Psychological factors in pain.* New York: Guilford.

Gaudry, E., Spielberger, C. D., & Vagg, P. R. (1975). Validation of the state-trait distinction in anxiety research. *Multivariate Behavior Research, 10,* 331-341.

Gaugler, J. E., Kane, R. A., & Langlois, J. (2000). Assessment of family caregivers of older adults. In R. L. Kane & R. A. Kane (Eds.), *Assessing older persons: Measures, meaning, and practical applications* (pp. 320-359). New York: Oxford University Press.

Geleziunas, R., & Greene, W. C. (1999). Molecular insights into HIV-1 infection and pathogenesis. In M. A. Sande & P. A. Volberding (Eds.), *The medical management of AIDS* (6th ed., pp. 23-39). Philadelphia: W. B. Saunders.

George, L. K., & Gwyther, L. (1986). Caregiver well-being: A multidimensional examination of family caregivers of demented adults. *Gerontologist, 26,* 253-259.

Gerin, W., Pickering, T. G., Glynn, L., Christenfeld, N., Schwartz, A., Carroll, D., & Davidson, K. (2000). An historical context for behavioral models of hypertension. *Journal of Psychosomatic Research, 48,* 369-377.

Getzen, T. E. (1997). *Health economics: Fundamentals and flow of funds.* New York: John Wiley.

Ghione, S. (1996). Hypertension-associated hypalgesia: Evidence in experimental animals and humans, pathophysiological mechanisms and potential clinical consequences. *Hypertension, 28,* 494-504.

Gibrar, O. (1996). The connection between the psychological condition of breast cancer patients and survival: A follow-up after eight years. *General Hospital Psychiatry, 18*(4), 266-270.

Gilchrist, V. (1992). Key informant interviews. In B. F. Crabtree & W. Miller (Eds.), *Doing qualitative research* (pp. 70-92). Newbury Park, CA: Sage.

Gillham, J. E., Reivich, K. J., Jaycox, L. H., & Seligman, M. E. P. (1995). Prevention of depressive symptoms in schoolchildren: Two-year follow-up. *Psychological Science, 6*, 343-351.

Gilligan, I., Fung, L., Piper, D. W., & Tennant, C. (1987). Life event stress and chronic difficulties in duodenal ulcer: A case control study. *Journal of Psychosomatic Research, 31*(1), 117-123.

Giovengo, S. L., Russell, I. J., & Larson, A. A. (1996). Increases in nerve growth factor concentrations in cerebrospinal fluid (CSF) of fibromyalgia patients [Abstract]. *Pain, 66* (Suppl.), 225.

Glantz, S. A., Slade, J., Bero, L. A., Hanauer, P., & Barnes, D. E. (1996). *The cigarette papers*. Berkeley: University of California Press.

Glanz, K., Lewis, F. M., & Rimer, B. K. (Eds.). (1997). *Health behavior and health education*. San Francisco: Jossey-Bass.

Glanz, K., Rimer, L., & Lewis, F. M. (2002). *Health behavior and health education*. San Francisco: Jossey-Bass.

Glaser, R., & Kiecolt-Glaser, J. K. (Eds.). (1994). *Handbook of human stress and immunity*. San Diego, CA: Academic Press.

Glaser, R., Kiecolt-Glaser, J. K., Malarkey, W. B., & Sheridan, J. F. (1998). The influence of psychological stress on the immune response to vaccines. *Annals of the New York Academy of Sciences, 840*, 649-655.

Glasgow, M. S., Gaarder, K. R., & Engel, B. T. (1982). Behavioral treatment of high blood pressure: II. Acute and sustained effects of relaxation and systolic blood pressure biofeedback. *Psychosomatic Medicine, 44*(2), 155-170.

Glasgow, R. E., & Eakin, E. G. (1998). *Issues in diabetes self-management* (2nd ed.). New York: Springer.

Glasgow, R. E., Fisher, E. F., Anderson, B. J., La Greca, A., Marrero, D., Johnson, S. B., et al. (1999). Behavioral science in diabetes: Contributions and opportunities. *Diabetes Care, 22*, 832-843.

Glasgow, R. E., Vogt, T. M., & Boles, S. M. (1999). Evaluating the public health impact of health promotion interventions: The RE-AIM Framework. *American Journal of Public Health, 89*, 1322-1327.

Glass, J. M., & Park, D. C. (2001). Cognitive dysfunction in fibromyalgia. *Current Rheumatology Reports, 3*, 123-127.

Glass, T., Mendes de Leon, C., Marottoli, R., & Berkman, L. (1999). Population based study of social and productive activities as predictors of survival among elderly Americans. *BMJ, 319*, 478-483.

Glass, T. A., & Maddox, G. L. (1992). The quality and quantity of social support: Stroke recovery as psycho-social transition. *Social Science & Medicine, 34*, 1249-1261.

Glassman, A. (1993). Cigarette smoking: Implications for psychiatric illness. *American Journal of Psychiatry 150*, 546-553.

Glassman, A. H., & Shapiro, P. A. (1998). Depression and the course of coronary artery disease. *American Journal of Psychiatry, 155*, 4-11.

Glavin, G. B., Murison, R., Overmier, J. B., Paré, W. P., Bakke, H. K., Henke, P. G., & Hernandez, D. E. (1991). The neurobiology of stress ulcers. *Brain Research Reviews, 16*, 301-343.

Glynn, R. J., Chae, C. U., Guralnik, J. M., Taylor, J. O., & Hennekens, C. H. (2000). Pulse pressure and mortality in older people. *Archives of Internal Medicine, 160*, 2765-2772.

Goadsby, P. J., Lipton, R. B., & Ferrari, M. D. (2002). Migraine-current understanding and treatment. *New England Journal of Medicine, 346*, 257-270.

Gold, M. R. (1996). *Cost-effectiveness in health and medicine*. New York: Oxford University Press.

Goldberg, A. D., Becker, L. C., Bonsall, R., Cohen, J. D., Ketterer, M. W., Kaufman, P. G., Krantz, D. S., Light, K. C., McMahon, R. P., Noreuil, T., Pepine, C. J., Raczynski, J., Stone, P. H., Strother, D., Taylor, H., & Sheps, D. S. (1996). Ischemic, hemodynamic, and neurohormonal responses to mental and exercise stress: Experience from the Psychophysiological Investigations of Myocardial Ischemia Study (PIMI). *Circulation, 94*, 2402-2409.

Goldman, D. P., & Smith, J. P. (2002). Can patient self-management help explain the SES health gradient? *Proceedings of the National Academy of Sciences of the United States of America, 99*(16), 10929-10934.

Goldman, M. S., Boyd, G. M., & Faden, V. (Eds.). (2002). College drinking, what it is, and what to do about it: A review of the state of the science. *Journal of Studies on Alcohol, S14*.

Goldman, S. L., Kraemer, D. T., & Salovey, P. (1996). Beliefs about mood moderate the relationship of stress to illness and symptom reporting. *Journal of Psychosomatic Research, 41*, 115-128.

Goldstein, H. (1995). *Multilevel statistical models* (2nd ed.). London: Arnold.

Gollwitzer, P. M. (1999). Implementation intentions: Strong effects of simple plans. *American Psychologist, 54*, 493-503.

Gonder-Frederick, L. A., Cox, D. J., & Ritterband, L. M. (2002). Diabetes and behavioral medicine: The second decade. *Journal of Consulting and Clinical Psychology, 70*, 611-625.

Goodenough, W. H. (1963). *Cooperation in change.* New York: Russell Sage.

Goodkin, K., Feaster, D. J., Asthana, D., Blaney, N. T., Kumar, M., Baldewicz, T., Tuttle, R. S, Maher, K. J., Baum, M. K., Shapshak, P., & Fletcher, M. A. (1998). Bereavement support group intervention is longitudinally associated with salutary effects on the CD4 cell count and number of physician visits. *Clinical & Diagnostic Laboratory Immunology, 5,* 382-391.

Gordon, M. (1964). *Assimilation in American life: The role of race, religion, and national origins.* New York: Oxford University Press.

Gore, S. (1981). Stress-buffering functions of social supports: An appraisal and clarification of research models. In B. S. Dohrenwend & B. P. Dohrenwend (Eds.), *Stressful life events and their contexts* (pp. 202-222). New York: Prodist.

Gortmaker, S. L., Peterson, K., Wiecha, J., Sobol, A. M., Dixit, S., Fox, M. K., et al. (1999). Reducing obesity via a school-based interdisciplinary intervention among youth: Planet Health. *Archives of Pediatric and Adolescent Medicine, 153,* 409-418.

Gove, W. R., & Hughes, M. (1983). *Overcrowding in the household.* New York: Academic Press.

Gowers, S. G., & Shore, A. (2001). Development of weight and shape concerns in the aetiology of eating disorders. *British Journal of Psychiatry, 179,* 236-242.

Grace, G. M., Nielson, W. R., Hopkins, M., & Berg, M. A. (1999). Concentration and memory deficits in patient with fibromyalgia syndrome. *Journal of Clinical and Experimental Neuropsychology, 21,* 477-487.

Grahl, C. (1994). Improving compliance: Solving a $100 billion problem. *Managed Health Care,* pp. S11-S13.

Granovetter, M. (1973). The strength of weak ties. *American Journal of Sociology, 78,* 1360-1380.

Green, C. R., Baker, T. A., Smith, E. M., & Sato, T. (2003). The effect of race in older adults presenting for chronic pain management: A comparative study of African and Caucasian Americans. *Journal of Pain, 4*(2), 82-90.

Green, C. R., Flowe-Valencia, H., Rosenblum, L., & Tait, A. R. (2001). The role of childhood and adulthood abuse among women presenting for chronic pain management. *Clinical Journal of Pain, 17,* 359-364.

Green, C. R., Wheeler, J., Laporte, F., Marchant, B., & Guerrero, E. (2002). How well is chronic pain managed? Who does it well? *Pain Medicine, 3*(1), 56-65.

Green, L. W., George, M. A., Daniel, M., Frankish, C. J., Herbert, C. J., Bowie, W. R., et al. (1995). *Study of participatory research in health promotion.* Vancouver, BC, Canada: University of British Columbia, Royal Society of Canada.

Green, L. W., & Kreuter, M. W. (1999). *Health promotion planning: An educational and ecological approach.* Mountain View, CA: Mayfield.

Green, L. W., & Mercer, S. L. (2001). Participatory research: Can public health researchers and agencies reconcile the push from funding bodies and the pull from communities? *American Journal of Public Health, 91,* 1926-1929.

Greenland, S. (1993). Basic problems in interaction assessment. *Environmental Health Perspectives, 101*(Suppl. 4), 59-66.

Greenland, S., & Brumback, B. A. (2002). An overview of relations among causal modelling methods. *International Journal of Epidemiology, 31,* 1030-1037.

Greenland, S., & Morgenstern, H. (2001). Confounding in health research. *Annual Reviews of Public Health, 22,* 189-212.

Greenland, S., & Poole, C. (1988). Invariants and noninvariants in the concept of interdependent effects. *Scandinavian Journal of Work, Environment, and Health, 14,* 125-129.

Greenland, S., & Robins, J. M. (1986). Identifiability, exchangeability, and epidemiological confounding. *International Journal of Epidemiology, 15,* 413-419.

Greenland, S., Robins, J. M., & Pearl, J. (1999). Confounding and collapsibility in causal inference. *Statistical Science, 14,* 29-46.

Greenland, S., & Rothman, K. J. (1998). Measures of effect and measures of association. In K. J. Rothman & S. Greenland (Eds.), *Modern Epidemiology* (2nd ed., Chap. 4). Philadelphia: Lippincott.

Gross, J. J., Fredrickson, B. L., & Levenson, R. W. (1994). The psychophysiology of crying. *Psychophysiology, 31,* 460-468.

Grossman, D. C. (2000). The history of injury control and the epidemiology of child and adolescent injuries. *Future of Children, 10*(1), 23-52.

Groves, E. R., & Ogburn, W. F. (1928). *American marriage and family relationships.* New York: Henry Holt.

Gudino, A., Jr. (1997). Biopsychosocial correlates of HIV/AIDS infected African-American males. *Dissertation Abstracts International: Section B: The Sciences and Engineering, 57*(10-B), 6572.

Guidelines for the Diagnosis and Management of Asthma. (1997). *National asthma education and prevention program: Expert panel report II.* Bethesda, MD: National Asthma Education Program, Office of Prevention, Education, and Control: National Heart, Lung, and Blood Institute.

Gumnick, J. F., & Nemeroff, C. B. (2000). Problems with currently available antidepressants. *Journal of Clinical Psychiatry, 61*(Suppl. 10), 5-15.

Guthrie, E., Creed, F., Dawson, D., & Tomenson, B. (1991). A controlled trial of psychological treatment for the irritable bowel syndrome. *Gastroenterology, 100*, 450-457

Gutin, B., & Barbeau, P. (2000). Physical activity and body composition in children and adolescents. In C. Bouchard (Ed.), *Physical activity and obesity* (pp. 213-245). Champaign, IL: Human Kinetics.

Gutmann, M. C. (1999). Ethnicity, alcohol, and acculturation. *Social Science & Medicine, 48*, 173-184.

Guy, W. (1976). *ECDEU assessment manual of psychopathology—Revised* (DHEW Pub. No. ADM 76-338). Rockville, MD: U.S. Department of Health, Education and Welfare.

Gybels, J. M., & Tasker, R. R. (1999). Central neurosurgery. In P. D. Wall & R. Melzack (Eds.), *Textbook of pain* (4th ed., pp. 1307-1339). Edinburgh: Churchill Livingston.

Haan, M. N., Shemanski, L., Jagust, W. J., Manolio, T. A., & Kuller, L. (1999). The role of APOE E4 in modulating effects of other risk factors for cognitive decline in elderly persons. *Journal of the American Medical Association, 282*, 40-46.

Haddon, W., Jr. (1970). On the escape of tigers: An ecologic note. *American Journal of Public Health, 60*, 2229-2234.

Haddon, W., Jr. (1972). A logical framework for categorizing highway safety phenomena and activity. *Journal of Trauma, 12*, 193-207.

Hahn, B. A. (1993). Marital status and women's health: The effect of economic marital acquisitions. *Journal of Marriage and the Family, 55*, 495-504.

Haines, A. P., Imeson, J. D., & Meade, T. W. (1987). Phobic anxiety and ischaemic heart disease. *British Medical Journal Clinical Research Ed., 295*(6593), 297-299.

Hajat, A., Lucas, J., & Kington, R. (2000). *Health outcomes among Hispanic subgroups: United States, 1992-95.* Advance data from Vital and Health Statistics, No. 310. Hyattsville, MD: National Center for Health Statistics.

Haley, W. E., Roth, D. L., Coleton, M. I., Ford, G. R., West, C. A., Collins, R. P., & Isobe, T. L. (1996). Appraisal, coping, and social support as mediators of well-being in Black and White family caregivers of patients with Alzheimer's disease. *Journal of Consulting and Clinical Psychology, 64*, 121-129.

Hall, A., & Wellman, B. (1985). Social networks and social support. In S. Cohen & S. L. Syme (Eds.), *Social support and health* (pp. 23-41). Orlando, FL: Academic Press.

Halley, F. M. (1991). Self-regulation of the immune system through biobehavioral strategies. *Biofeedback & Self Regulation, 16*, 55-74.

Hallqvist, J., Diderichsen, F., Theorell, T., Reuterwall, C., & Ahlbom, A. (1998). Is the effect of job strain due to interaction between high psychological demand and low decision latitude? *Social Science and Medicine, 46*, 1405-1411.

Hamazaki, T., Sawazaki, S., Itomura, M., Asaoka, E., Nagao, Y., Nishimura, N., Yazawa, K., Kuwamori, T., & Kobayashi, M. (1996). The effect of docosahexaenoic acid on aggression in young adults: A placebo-controlled double-blind study. *Journal of Clinical Investigation, 97*, 1129-1133.

Hamburg, D. A., & Adams, J. E. (1967). A perspective on coping behavior: Seeking and utilizing information in major transitions. *Archives of General Psychiatry, 17*, 277-284.

Hamilton, M. (1960). A rating scale for depression. *Journal of Neurology and Neurosurgical Psychiatry, 23*, 56-62.

Hammer Burns, L., & Covington, S. N. (1998). *Infertility counselling: A comprehensive handbook for clinicians.* New York: Parthenon.

Hampson, S. E., Skinner, T. C., Hart, J., Storey, L., Gage, H., Foxcroft, D., et al. (2000). Behavioral interventions for adolescents with Type 1 diabetes: How effective are they? *Diabetes Care, 23*, 1416-1422.

Handy, S. L., Boarnet, M. G., Ewing, R., & Killingsworth, R. E. (2002). How the built environment affects physical activity. *American Journal of Preventive Medicine, 23*(Suppl. 2), 64-73.

Haney, T. L., Maynard, K. E., Houseworth, S. J., Scherwitz, L. W., Williams, R. B., & Barefoot, J. C. (1996). Interpersonal hostility assessment technique: Description and validation against the criterion of coronary artery disease. *Journal of Personality Assessment, 66*, 386-401.

Hansen, W. B., & Dusenbury, L. (2001). Building capacity for prevention's next generation. *Prevention Science, 2*, 207-208.

Harburg, E., Erfurt, J. C., Hauenstein, L. S., et al. (1973). Socio-ecological stressor areas and Black-White blood pressure: Detroit. *Psychosomatic Medicine, 35*, 276-296.

Harpham, T., Grant, E., & Thomas, E. (2002). Measuring social capital within health surveys: Key issues. *Health Policy and Planning, 17*(1), 106-111.

Harrell, J., Hall, S., & Taliaferro, J. (2003). Physiological responses to racism and discrimination: An assessment of the evidence. *American Journal of Public Health, 93*, 243-248.

Harrell, J. S., McMurray, R. G., Gansky, S. A., Bangdiwala, S. I., & Bradley, C. B. (1999). A public health vs. a risk-based intervention to improve cardiovascular health in elementary school children: The Cardiovascular Health in Children Study. *American Journal of Public Health, 89,* 1529-1535.

Harrington, D., & Dubowitz, H. (1999). Preventing child maltreatment. In R. Hampton (Ed.), *Family violence* (pp. 122-147). Thousand Oaks, CA: Sage.

Harris, K. M. (1999). The health status and risk behaviors of adolescents in immigrant families. In D. J. Hernandez (Ed.), *Children of immigrants: Health, adjustment and public assistance* (pp. 286-315). Washington, DC: National Academy Press.

Harris, M. B., & Franklin, C. (in press). Effects of a cognitive-behavioral, school-based, group intervention with Mexican-American pregnant and parenting mothers. *Social Work Research.*

Harvard Center for Cancer Prevention. (1996). Harvard report on cancer prevention: Vol. 1. Causes of human cancer. *Cancer Causes & Control, 7*(Suppl. 1), 53-59.

Haskell, W. L., Alderman, E. L., Fair, J. M., Maron, D. J., Mackey, S. F., Superko, H. R., Williams, P. T., Johnstone, I. M., Champagne, M. A., Krauss, R. M., & Farquhar, J. W. (1994). Effects of intensive multiple risk factor reduction on coronary atherosclerosis and clinical cardiac events in men and women with coronary artery disease. *Circulation, 89,* 975-990.

Hatch, J. (1992). Empowering Black churches for health promotion. *Health Values, 16,* 3-9.

Hathaway, S. R., & McKinley, J. C. (1942). A multiphasic personality schedule (Minnesota): I. Construction of the schedule. *Journal of Psychology, 10,* 249-254.

Hathaway, S. R., & McKinley, J. C. (1951). *The Minnesota Multiphasic Personality Inventory manual* (Rev.). New York: Psychological Corporation.

Hathaway, S. R., & McKinley, J. C. (1989). *Minnesota Multiphasic Personality Inventory-2 manual for administration and scoring.* Minneapolis: University of Minnesota Press.

Haugaard, J. J. (2000). The challenge of defining child sexual abuse. *American Psychologist, 55,* 1036-1039.

Havenaar, J. M., Cwikel, J. G., & Bromet, E. J. (2002). *Toxic turmoil: Psychological and societal consequences of ecological disasters. Plenum series on stress and coping.* New York: Kluwer Academic/Plenum.

Hawkins, J. D., Catalano, R. F., Kosterman, R., Abbott, R., & Hill, K. G. (1999). Preventing adolescent health-risk behaviors by strengthening protection during childhood. *Archives of Pediatrics & Adolescent Medicine, 153,* 226-234.

Haynes, J., Manci, E., & Voelkel, N. (1994). Pulmonary complications. In S. H. Embury, R. P. Hebbel, N. Mohandas, & M. Steinberg (Eds.), *Sickle cell disease: Basic principles and clinical practice* (pp. 623-631). New York: Raven.

Haynes, R. B., McDonald, H., Garg, A. X., & Montague, P. (2002). *Interventions for helping patients to follow prescriptions for medications* [Systematic review]. Cochrane Database of Systematic Reviews. Victoria, Australia: La Trobe University, Cochrane Consumers and Communication Group.

Haynes, R. B., McKibbon, K. A., & Kanani, R. (1996). Systematic review of randomised trials of interventions to assist patients to follow prescriptions for medications. *Lancet, 348,* 383-386.

Haynes, S. G., Feinleib, M., & Kannel, W. B. (1980). The relationship of psychosocial factors to coronary heart disease in the Framingham Study: Eight-year incidence of coronary heart disease. *American Journal of Epidemiology, 111,* 37-58.

Hays, R. D., Wells, K. B., Sherbourne, C. D., Rogers, W., & Spritzer, K. (1995). Functioning and well-being outcomes of patients with depression compared with chronic general medical illnesses. *Archives of General Psychiatry, 52,* 11-19.

Hazuda, H. P., Stern, M. P., & Haffner, S. M. (1988). Acculturation and assimilation among Mexican Americans: Scales and population-based data. *Social Science Quarterly, 69,* 687-705.

Health Canada. (2001). *Perspectives on complementary and alternative health care: A collection of papers prepared for Health Canada* (Cat. No. H39-572/2001E). Ottawa, Ontario, Canada: Author.

Heaney, C. A., & Goetzel, R. Z. (1997). A review of health-related outcomes of multicomponent worksite health promotion programs. *American Journal of Public Health, 11,* 290-308.

Heather, N., Peters, T. J., & Stockwell, T. (Eds.). (2001). *International handbook of alcohol dependence and problems.* Chichester, UK: Wiley.

Hecht, S. S. (1999). Tobacco smoke carcinogens and lung cancer. *Journal of the National Cancer Institute, 91*(14), 1194-1210.

Heck, K., Wagener, D., Schatzkin, A., et al. (1997). Socioeconomic status and breast cancer mortality, 1989 through 1993: An analysis of education data from death certificates. *American Journal of Public Health, 87,* 1218-1222.

Heckman, T. G., Kockman, A., Sikkema, K. J., Kalichman, S. C., Masten, J., & Goodkin, K. (2000). Late middle-aged and older men living with HIV/AIDS: Race differences in coping, social support and psychological distress. *Journal of the National Medical Association, 92*(9), 436-444.

Heiman, J. R., & Meston, C. M. (1997). Empirically validated treatment for sexual dysfunction. *Annual Review of Sex Research, 8,* 148-195.

Heimendinger, J., Van Duyn, M. A., Chapelsky, D., Foerster, S., & Stables, G. (1996). The National 5 a Day for Better Health Program: A large-scale nutrition intervention. *Journal of Public Health Management Practice, 2,* 27-35.

Heisler, M., Bouknight, R. R., Hayward, R. A., Smith, D. M., & Kerr, E. A. (2002). The relative importance of physician communication, participatory decision making, and patient understanding in diabetes self-management. *Journal of General Internal Medicine, 17,* 243-252.

Helgeson, V., & Cohen, S. (1996). Social support and adjustment to cancer: Reconciling descriptive, correlational, and intervention research. *Health Psychology, 15,* 135-148.

Helman, C. G. (2000). *Culture, health and illness* (4th ed.). Woburn, MA: Reed.

Henderson, S., Duncan-Jones, P., Byrne, D. G., & Scott, R. (1980). Measuring social relationships. The Interview Schedule for Social Interaction. *Psychological Medicine, 10*(4), 723-734.

Henkel, G., & Pincus, T. (2000). *The Arthritis Foundation's guide to good living with rheumatoid arthritis.* Atlanta, GA: Arthritis Foundation

Hermens, H., Freriks, B., Merletti, R., Stegeman, D., Joleen, B., Gner, R., Disselhorst-Klug, C., & Hagg, G. (1999). *SENIAM: European recommendations for surface electromyography.* Enschede, the Netherlands: Roessingh Research and Development.

Hester, R. K., & Miller, W. R. (1989). *Handbook of alcoholism treatment approaches: Effective alternatives.* New York: Pergamon.

Hester, R. K., & Miller, W. R. (1995). *Handbook of alcoholism treatment approaches: Effective alternatives* (2nd ed.). Boston: Allyn & Bacon.

Hiatt, R. A., & Rimer, B. K. (1999). A new strategy for cancer control research. *Cancer Epidemiology, Biomarkers, and Prevention, 8,* 957-964.

Higgins, S. T., & Silverman, K. (1999). *Motivating behavior change among illicit-drug abusers: Research on contingency management interventions.* Washington, DC: American Psychological Association.

Higgins, S. T., Wong, C. J., Badger G. J., Haug Ogden, D., & Dantona, R. L. (2000). Contingent reinforcement increases cocaine abstinence during outpatient treatment and one year of follow-up. *Journal of Consulting and Clinical Psychology, 68,* 64-72.

Hill, J. O., & Peters, J. C. (1998). Environmental contributions to the obesity epidemic. *Science, 280,* 1371-1377.

Hilton, J. L., & von Hippel, W. (1996). Stereotypes. *Annual Review of Psychology, 47,* 237-271.

Hines, E. A., & Brown, G. E. (1936). The cold pressor test for measuring the reactibility of the blood pressure: Data concerning 571 normal and hypertensive subjects. *American Heart Journal, 11,* 1-9.

Hingson, R., Heeren, T., Zakocs, R. C., Kopstein, A., & Wechsler, H. (2002). Magnitude of alcohol related mortality and morbidity among U.S. college students ages 18-24. *Journal of Studies on Alcohol, 63,* 136-144.

Hinkle, L. F., Jr., Whitney, L. H., Lehman, E. Q., Dunn, J., Benjamin, B., King, R., et al. (1968). Occupation, education and coronary heart disease. *Science, 161,* 238-246.

Hinrichsen, G. A., & Ramirez, M. (1992). Black and White dementia caregivers: A comparison of their adaptation, adjustment, and service utilization. *Gerontologist, 32,* 375-381.

Hobel, C. J., Dunkel-Schetter, C., & Roesch, S. (1999). Maternal stress as a signal to the fetus. *Prenatal and Neonatal Medicine, 3,* 116-120.

Hochbaum, G. M. (1958). *Public participation in medical screening program: A sociopsychological study.* Public Health Service Publication No. 572. Washington, DC: Government Printing Office.

Hodgkin, J., Connors, G., & Celli, B. (Eds.). (2000). *Pulmonary rehabilitation* (4th ed.). Philadelphia: Lippincott, Williams, & Wilkins.

Hogue, C. J., Hoffman, S., & Hatch, M. C. (2001). Stress and preterm delivery: A conceptual framework. *Paediatric and Perinatal Epidemiology, 15*(Suppl. 2), 30-40.

Holland, J. C. (Ed.). (1998). *Psycho-oncology.* New York: Oxford University Press.

Holmes, G. P., Kaplan, J. E., Gantz, N. M., Komaroff, A. L., Schonberger, L. B., Strauss, S. S., et al. (1988). Chronic fatigue syndrome: A working case definition. *Annals of Internal Medicine, 108,* 387-389.

Holmes, T. H., & Rahe, R. H. (1967). The social readjustment rating scale. *Journal of Psychosomatic Research, 11,* 213-218.

Holroyd, K. A. (2002). Assessment and psychological treatment of recurrent headache disorders. *Journal of Consulting and Clinical Psychology, 70,* 656-677.

Holroyd, K. A., O'Donnell, F. J., Stensland, M., Lipchik, G. L., Cordingley, G. E., & Carlson, B. (2001). Management of chronic tension-type headache with tricyclic antidepressant medication, stress-management therapy, and their combination: a randomized controlled trial. *Journal of the American Medical Association, 285,* 2208-2215.

Holtmann, G., Armstrong, D., Pöppel, E., Bauerfeind, A., Goebell, H., Arnold, R., Classen, M., Witzel, L., Fischer, M., Heinisch, M., Blum, A. L., & Members of the RUDER Study Group. (1992). Influence of stress on the healing and relapse of duodenal ulcers. *Scandinavian Journal of Gastroenterology, 27,* 917-923.

Hom, D. B., Thatcher, G., & Tibesar, R. (2002). Growth factor therapy to improve soft tissue healing. *Facial Plastic Surgery, 18,* 41-52.

Hooker, K., Monahan, D. J., Bowman, S. R., Frazier, L. D., & Shifren, K. (1998). Personality counts for a lot: Predictors of mental and physical health of spouse caregivers in two disease groups. *Journal of Gerontology, 53,* P73-P85.

Hopper, J. (2000). The symbolic origins of conflict in divorce. *Journal of Marriage and the Family, 63,* 430-445.

Horsten, M., Mittleman, A. M., Wamala, S. P., Schenck-Gustafsson, K., & Orth-Gomér, K. (2000). Depression and social isolation in relation to prognosis of coronary heart disease in women. *European Heart Journal, 21*(13), 1072-1080.

Horwitz, A. V., Raskin White, H., & Howell-White, S. (1996). Becoming married and mental health: A longitudinal study of a cohort of young adults. *Journal of Marriage and the Family, 58,* 895-907.

House, J., Robbins, C., & Metzner, H. (1982). The association of social relationships and activities with mortality: Prospective evidence from the Tecumseh Community Health Study. *American Journal of Epidemiology, 116,* 123-140.

House, J. S. (1981). *Work stress and social support.* Reading, MA: Addison-Wesley.

House, J. S., Kessler, R. C., Herzog, A. R., et al. (1990). Age, socioeconomic status, and health. *Milbank Quarterly, 68,* 383-411.

House, J. S., & Williams, D. R. (2000). Understanding and reducing socioeconomic and racial/ethnic disparities in health. In B. D. Smedley & S. L. Syme (Eds.), *Promoting health: Intervention strategies from social and behavioral research* (pp. 81-124). Washington, DC: National Academy Press.

Houston, B. K. (1988). Cardiovascular and neuroendocrine reactivity, global Type A, and components of Type A behavior. In B. K. Houston & C. R. Snyder (Eds.), *Type A behavior pattern: Research, theory, and intervention* (pp. 212-253). New York: John Wiley.

Houston, B. K. (1994). Anger, hostility, and psychophysiological reactivity. In A. W. Siegman & T. W. Smith (Eds.), *Anger, hostility, and the heart* (pp. 97-115). Hillsdale, NJ: Lawrence Erlbaum.

Houts, A. C., Liebert, R. M., & Padawer, W. (1983). A delivery system for the treatment of primary enuresis. *Journal of Abnormal Child Psychology, 11,* 513-519.

Hox, J. (2002). *Multilevel analysis: Techniques and applications.* Mahwah, NJ: Lawrence Erlbaum.

Hu, F. B., Manson, J. E., & Willett, W. C. (2001). Types of dietary fat and risk of coronary heart disease: A critical review. *Journal of the American College of Nutrition, 20,* 5-19.

Hu, F. B., Rimm, E., Smith-Warner, S. A., Feskanich, D., Stampfer, M. J., Ascherio, A., Sampson, L., & Willett, W. C. (1999). Reproducibility and validity of dietary patterns assessed by a food frequency questionnaire. *American Journal of Clinical Nutrition, 69,* 243-249.

Hu, F. B., Stampfer, M. J., Manson, J. E., Rimm, E., Colditz, G. A., Rosner, B. A., Hennekens, C. H., & Willett, W. C. (1997). Dietary fat intake and risk of coronary heart disease in women. *New England Journal of Medicine, 337,* 1491-1499.

Hu, F. B., Stampfer, M. J., Rimm, E. B., Manson, J. E., Ascherio, A., Colditz, G. A., Rosner, B. A., Spiegelman, D., Speizer, F. E., Sacks, F. M., Hennekens, C. H., & Willett, W. C. (1999). A prospective study of egg consumption and risk of cardiovascular disease in men and women. *Journal of the American Medical Association, 281,* 1387-1394.

Hu, F. B., & Willett, W. C. (2002). Diet and coronary heart disease in women. In P. S. Douglas (Ed.), *Cardiovascular health and disease in women* (2nd ed.). Philadelphia: W. B. Saunders.

Hughes, E. C. (1944). Dilemmas and contradictions of status. *American Journal of Sociology, 50,* 353-359.

Hughes, J., Fiester, S., Goldstein, M., Resnick, M., Rock, N., & Ziedonis, D. (1996). American Psychiatric Association practice guideline for the treatment of patients with nicotine dependence. *American Journal of Psychiatry, 153*(Suppl. 10), S1-S31.

Hughes, J., Goldstein, M., Hurt, R., & Shiffman, S. (1999). Recent advances in the pharmacotherapy of smoking. *Journal of the American Medical Association, 281,* 72-76.

Hughes, J., & Hatsukami, D. (1992). The nicotine withdrawal syndrome: A brief review and update. *International Journal of Smoking Cessation, 1,* 21-26.

Humpel, N., Owen, N., & Leslie, E. (2002). Environmental factors associated with adults' participation in physical activity: A review. *American Journal of Preventive Medicine, 22,* 188-199.

Hunt, L. M. (1999). *The concept of acculturation in health research: Assumptions about rationality and progress.* East Lansing: Julian Samora Research Institute, Michigan State University.

Hunt, S., McEwen, J., & McKenna, S. (1986). *Measuring health status.* London: Croom Helm.

Huyser, B. A., & Parker, J. C. (1998). Stress and rheumatoid arthritis: An integrative review. *Arthritis Care and Research, 11,* 135-145.

Ickovics, J., & Park, C. L. (1998). Thriving: Broadening the paradigm beyond illness to health [Special issue]. *Journal of Social Issues, 54.*

Idler, E. L., & Benyamini, Y. (1997). Self-rated health and mortality: A review of twenty-seven community studies. *Journal of Health and Social Behavior, 38,* 21-37.

Illsley, R., & Mullen, K. (1985). The health needs of disadvantaged client groups. In W. W. Holland, R. Detels, & G. Know (Eds.), *Oxford textbook of public health* (pp. 389-402). Oxford, UK: Oxford University Press.

Institute of Health Promotion Research, University of British Columbia. (1996). *Study of participatory research in health promotion: Review and recommendations for the development of participatory research in health promotion in Canada.* Ottawa: Royal Society of Canada. Available from http://www.rsc.ca/english/publications.html

Institute of Medicine. (1994a). *Growing up tobacco free: Preventing nicotine addiction in children and youth.* Washington, DC: National Academy Press.

Institute of Medicine. (1994b). *Reducing the risk for mental disorders: Frontiers for preventive intervention research.* Washington, DC: National Academy Press.

Institute of Medicine. (2001a). *Exploring the biological contributions to human health: Does sex matter?* Washington, DC: National Academy Press.

Institute of Medicine. (2001b). *Health and behavior: The interplay of biological, behavioral, and societal influences.* Washington, DC: National Academy Press.

Institute of Medicine. (2002). Assessing potential sources of racial and ethnic disparities in care: The clinical encounter. In *Unequal treatment: Confronting racial and ethnic disparities in health care.* Washington, DC: National Academy Press.

International Agency for Research on Cancer. (2002a). *IARC Handbooks of cancer prevention: Vol. 6. Weight control and physical activity.* Lyon, France: Author.

International Agency for Research on Cancer. (2002b). Tobacco smoke and involuntary smoking. *IARC monographs on the evaluation of carcinogenic risks to humans* (Vol. 82). Lyon, France: Author.

International Association for the Study of Pain. (1986). Classification of chronic pain: Descriptions of chronic pain syndromes and definitions of pain terms. *Pain, 3,* S1-S226.

Iribarren, C., Sidney, S., Liu, K., Markovitz, J. H., Bild, D. E., Roseman, J. M., & Mathews, K. (2000). Association of hostility with coronary artery calcification in young adults: The CARDIA Study. *Journal of the American Medical Association, 283,* 2546-2551.

Irving, L. M., Snyder, C. R., & Crowson, J. J., Jr. (1998). Hope and the negotiation of cancer facts by college women. *Journal of Personality, 66,* 195-214.

Irwin, M. (2002). Psychoneuroimmunology of depression: Clinical implications. *Brain, Behavior, and Immunity, 16*(1), 1-16.

Isen, A. M., & Daubman, K. A. (1984). The influence of affect on categorization. *Journal of Personality and Social Psychology, 47,* 1206-1217.

Isen, A. M., Daubman, K. A., & Nowicki, G. P. (1987). Positive affect facilitates creative problem solving. *Journal of Personality and Social Psychology, 52,* 1122-1131.

Isen, A. M., Johnson, M. M. S., Mertz, E., & Robinson, G. F. (1985). The influence of positive affect on the unusualness of word associations. *Journal of Personality and Social Psychology, 48,* 1413-1426.

Isen, A. M., & Means, B. (1983). The influence of positive affect on decision-making strategy. *Social Cognition, 2,* 118-131.

Isen, A. M., Rosenzweig, A. S., & Young, M. J. (1991). The influence of positive affect on clinical problem solving. *Medical Decision Making, 11,* 221-227.

Ismail, A. I., & Szpunar, S. M. (1990). Oral health status of Mexican-Americans with low and high acculturation status: Findings from southwestern HHANES, 1982-84. *Journal of Public Health Dentistry, 50,* 24-31.

Israel, A. C., Guile, C. A., Baker, J. E., & Silverman, W. K. (1994). An evaluation of enhanced self-regulation training in the treatment of childhood obesity. *Journal of Pediatric Psychology, 19,* 737-749.

Israel, B. A., Lichtenstein, R., Lantz, P., McGranaghan, R., Allen, A., Guzman, J. R., et al. (2001). The Detroit Community-Academic Urban Research Center: Development, implementation and evaluation. *Journal of Public Health Management and Practice, 7*(5), 1-19.

Israel, B. A., Schulz, A. J., Parker, E. A., & Becker, A. B. (1998). Review of community-based research: Assessing partnership approaches to improve public health. *Annual Review of Public Health, 19,* 173-202.

Israel, B. A., Schulz, A. J., Parker, E. A., Becker, A. B., Allen, A. J., & Guzman, J. R. (2002). Critical issues in developing and following community-based participatory research principles. In M. Minkler & N. Wallerstein (Eds.), *Community-based participatory research for health* (pp. 56-73). San Francisco: Jossey-Bass.

Istvan, J., & Matarazzo, J. (1984). Tobacco, alcohol and caffeine use: A review of their interrelationships. *Psychological Bulletin, 95,* 301-326.

Jackson, L. A., & Adams-Campbell, L. L. (1994). John Henryism and blood pressure in Black college students. *Journal of Behavioral Medicine, 17,* 69-79.

Jacob, R. G., Thayer, J. F., Manuck, S., Muldoon, M., Tamres, L., Williams, D., Ding, Y., & Gatsonis, C. (1999). Ambulatory blood pressure responses and the circumplex model of mood: A four-day study. *Psychosomatic Medicine, 61,* 319-333.

Jacobson, A. M. (1996). The psychological care of patients with insulin-dependent diabetes mellitus. *New England Journal of Medicine, 334,* 1249-1253.

Jahoda, M. (1958). *Current conceptions of positive mental health.* New York: Basic Books.

James, S. A. (1994). John Henryism and the health of African Americans. *Culture, Medicine and Psychiatry, 18,* 163-182.

James, S. A., Hartnett, S. A., & Kalsbeek, W. D. (1983). John Henryism and blood pressure differences among Black men. *Journal of Behavioral Medicine, 6*(3), 259-278.

James, S. A., Keenan, N. L., Strogatz, D. S., Browning, S. R., & Garrett, J. M. (1992). Socioeconomic status, John Henryism, and blood pressure in Black adults: The Pitt County Study. *American Journal of Epidemiology, 135,* 59-67.

James, S. A., Strogatz, D. S., Wing, S. B., & Ramsey, D. L. (1987). Socioeconomic status, John Henryism, and hypertension in Blacks and Whites. *American Journal of Epidemiology, 126*(4), 664-673.

Janz, N. K., & Becker, M. H. (1984). The health belief model: A decade later. *Health Education Quarterly, 11,* 1-47.

Jason, L. A., & Taylor, R. R. (2003). Chronic fatigue syndrome. In A. M. Nezu, C. M. Nezu, & P. A. Geller (Eds.), *Comprehensive handbook of psychology: Vol. 9. Health Psychology.* New York: John Wiley.

Jason, L. A., Richman, J. A., Friedberg, F., Wagner, L., Taylor, R., & Jordan, K. M. (1997). Politics, science,

and the emergence of a new disease: The case of chronic fatigue syndrome. *American Psychologist, 52,* 973-983.

Jason, L. A., Richman, J. A., Rademaker, A. W., Jordan, K. M., Plioplys, A. V., Taylor, R., et al. (1999). A community-based study of chronic fatigue syndrome. *Archives of Internal Medicine, 159,* 2129-2137.

Jemmott, J. B., Jemmott, L. S., & Fong, G. T. (1998). Abstinence and safer sex HIV risk-reduction interventions for African American adolescents: A randomized controlled trial. *Journal of the American Medical Association, 279,* 1529-1536.

Jenkins, D. J., Wolever, T. M., Taylor, R. H., Barker, H., Fielden, H., Baldwin, J. M., Bowling, A. C., Newman, H. C., Jenkins, A. L., & Goff, D. V. (1981). Glycemic index of foods: A physiological basis for carbohydrate exchange. *American Journal of Clinical Nutrition, 34,* 362-366.

Jennings, G. L. R. (1995). Mechanisms for reduction of cardiovascular risk by regular exercise. *Clinical and Experimental Pharmacology and Physiology, 22,* 209-211.

Jess, P., & Eldrup, J. (1994). The personality patterns in patients with duodenal ulcer and ulcer-like dyspepsia and their relationship to the course of the diseases. Hvidovre Ulcer Project Group. *Journal of Internal Medicine, 235*(6), 589-594.

Jessor, R. (1982). Problem behavior and developmental transition in adolescence. *Journal of School Health, 52,* 295-300.

Johnson, B. T., Carey, M. P., Marsh, K. L., Levin, K. D., & Scott-Sheldon, L. A. J. (2003). Interventions to reduce behavioral risk of HIV infection in adolescents (1985-2000): A meta-analysis. *Archives of Pediatrics and Adolescent Medicine.*

Johnson, D. W., & Johnson, F. P. (2003). *Joining together: Group theory and group skills* (7th ed.). Boston: Allyn & Bacon.

Johnson, J. V., & Stewart, W. F. (1993). Measuring work organization exposure over the life course with a job-exposure matrix. *Scandinavian Journal of Work, Environment, and Health, 19,* 21.

Johnson, K., Grossman, W., & Cassidy, A. (Eds.). (1996). *Collaborating to improve community health: Workbook and guide to best practices in creating healthier communities and populations.* San Francisco: Jossey-Bass.

Johnston, L. D., O'Malley, P. M., & Bachman, J. G. (2001). *Monitoring the future national survey results on drug use, 1975-2000: Volume 1, Secondary school students.* (NIH Publication No. 01-4924). Rockville, MD: U.S. Department of Health and Human Services.

Joint Committee on Health Education Terminology. (1991). Report of the Joint Committee on Health Education Terminology. *Journal of Health Education, 22*(2), 97-108.

Jonas, W. (2000). The social dynamics of medical pluralism. In M. Kelner, B. Wellman, B. Pescosolido, & M. Saks (Eds.), *Complementary and alternative medicine: Challenge and change* (pp. xi-xv). Amsterdam: Harwood Academic.

Jones, D. W., Appel, L. J., Sheps, S. G., Rocella, E. J., & Lenfant, C. (2003). Measuring blood pressure accurately: New and persistent challenges. *Journal of the American Medical Association, 289,* 1027-1030.

Jones, K., & Duncan, C. (1995). Individuals and their ecologies: Analysing the geography of chronic illness within a multilevel modelling framework. *Health Place, 1,* 27-40.

Jones, W. H., & Carver, M. D. (1991). Adjustment and coping implications of loneliness. In C. R. Snyder & D. R. Forsyth (Eds.), *Handbook of social and clinical psychology: The health perspective* (pp. 395-415). New York: Pergamon.

Jorgensen, R. S., Johnson, B. T., Kolodziej, M. E., & Schreer, G. E. (1996). Elevated blood pressure and personality: A meta-analytic review. *Psychological Bulletin, 120,* 293-320.

Joseph, J., Breslin, C., & Skinner, H. (1999). Critical perspectives on the transtheoretical model and stages of change. In J. A. Tucker, D. M. Donovan, & G. A. Marlatt (Eds.), *Changing addictive behavior: Bridging clinical and public health strategies* (pp. 160-190). New York: Guilford.

Julius, S. (1988). The blood pressure seeking properties of the central nervous system. *Journal of Hypertension, 6,* 177-185.

Kagawa-Singer, M., & Chung, R. C.-Y. (2002). Towards a new paradigm: A cultural systems approach. In K. S. Kurasaki, S. Okazaki, & S. Sue (Eds.), *Asian American mental health: Assessments, theories and methods* (pp. 47-66). New York: Kluwer Academic/Plenum.

Kahn, B. E., & Isen, A. M. (1993). The influence of positive affect on variety seeking among safe, enjoyable products. *Journal of Consumer Research, 20,* 257-270.

Kahn, E. B., Ramsay, L. T., Brownson, R. C., Heath, G. W., Howze, E. H., Powell, K. E., et al. (2002). The effectiveness of interventions to increase physical activity: A systematic review. *American Journal of Preventive Medicine, 22*(Suppl. 4), 73-107.

Kahneman, D., Diener, E., & Schwarz, N. (1999). *Wellbeing: Foundations of a hedonic psychology*. New York: Russell Sage Foundation.

Kalichman, S. C. (1998). *Preventing AIDS: A sourcebook for behavioral interventions*. Hillsdale, NJ: Lawrence Erlbaum.

Kalichman, S. C., Rompa, D., Cage, M., DiFonzo, K., Simpson, D., Austin, J., Luke, W., Buckles, J., Kyomugisha, F., Benotsch, E., Pinkerton, S., & Graham, J. (2001). Effectiveness of an intervention to reduce HIV transmission risks in HIV-positive people. *American Journal of Preventive Medicine, 21,* 84-92.

Kalish, R. (1987, Spring). Older people and grief. *Generations,* pp. 33-38.

Kalman, D. (1998). Smoking cessation treatment for substance misusers in early recovery: A review of the literature and recommendations for practice. *Substance Use and Misuse, 33,* 2021-2047.

Kamarck, T. W., & Lovallo, W. R. (2003). Progress and prospects in the conceptualization and measurement of cardiovascular reactivity. *Psychosomatic Medicine, 65,* 9-21.

Kamarck, T. W., Jennings, J. R., Debski, T. T., Glickman-Weiss, E., & Johnson, P. S. (1992). Reliable measures of behaviorally evoked cardiovascular reactivity from a PC-based test battery: Results from student and community samples. *Psychophysiology, 29,* 17-28.

Kamb, M. L., Fishbein, M., Douglas, J. M., Rhodes, F., Rogers, J., Bolan, G., Zenilman, J., Hoxworth, T., Malotte, K., Iatesta, M., Kent, C., Lentz, A., Graziano, S., Byers, R. H., Peterman, T. A., & Project RESPECT Study Group. (1998). Efficacy of risk-reduction counseling to prevent human immunodeficiency virus and sexually transmitted diseases—A randomized controlled trial. *Journal of the American Medical Association, 280,* 1161-1167.

Kaplan, G., & Baron-Epel, O. (2003). What lies behind the subjective evaluation of health status? *Social Science & Medicine, 56*(8), 1669-1676.

Kaplan, G., Salonen, J., Cohen, R., Brand, R., Syme, S., & Puska, P. (1988). Social connections and mortality from all causes and cardiovascular disease: Prospective evidence from eastern Finland. *American Journal of Epidemiology, 128,* 370-380.

Kaplan, G. A. (1996). People and places: Contrasting perspectives on the association between social class and health. *International Journal of Health Services 26,* 507-519.

Kaplan, R. M., & Bush, J. W. (1982). Health-related quality of life measurement for evaluation research and policy analysis. *Health Psychology, 1,* 61-80.

Kaplan, R. M., & Groessl, E. J. (2002). Applications of cost-effectiveness methodologies in behavioral medicine.

Journal of Clinical and Consulting Psychology, 70, 482-493.

Kaptein, A. A., & Creer, T. L. (Eds.). (2002). *Respiratory disorders and behavioral medicine.* London: Martin Dunitz.

Kar, S. B., Alcalay, R., & Alex, S. (Eds.). (2001). *Health communication: A multicultural perspective.* Thousand Oaks, CA: Sage.

Karasek, R., Baker, D., Marxer, F., Ahlbom, A., & Theorell, T. (1981). Job decision latitude, job demands, and cardiovascular diseases: A prospective study of Swedish men. *American Journal of Public Health, 71*(7), 694-705.

Karasek, R. A. (1979). Job demands, job decision latitude, and mental strain: Implications for job redesign. *American Society for Quality, 24,* 285-308.

Karasek, R. A., Brisson, C., Kawakami, N., Bongers, P., Houtman, I., & Amick, B. (1998). The job content questionnaire (JCQ): An instrument for internationally comparative assessments of psychosocial job characteristics. *Journal of Occupational Health and Psychology, 3,* 322-355.

Karasek, R. A., & Theorell, T. (1990). *Healthy work: Stress, productivity, and the reconstruction of working life.* New York: Basic Books.

Karlamangla, A. S., Singer, B. H., McEwen, B. S., Rowe, J. W., & Seeman, T. E. (2002). Allostatic load as a predictor of functional decline: MacArthur Studies of Successful Aging. *Journal of Clinical Epidemiology, 55,* 696-710.

Karoly, P., & Kanfer, F. H. (1982). *Self-management and behavior change.* New York: Pergamon.

Kasl, S. V. (1998). Measuring job stressors and studying the health impact of the work environment: An epidemiologic commentary. *Journal of Occupational Health and Psychology, 3,* 390-401.

Kasman, G., Cram, J. R., & Wolf, S. (1998). *Clinical applications in SEMG.* Gaithersburg, MD: Aspen.

Katz, L. F., King, J., & Liebman, J. B. (2001). Moving to opportunity in Boston: Early results of a randomized mobility experiment. *Quarterly Journal of Economics, 116,* 607-654.

Kaufman, J., Cooper, R., & McGee, D. (1997). Socioeconomic status and health in Backs and Whites: The problem of residual confounding and the resiliency of race. *Epidemiology, 8,* 621-628.

Kaufman, N. J., Castrucci, B. C., Mowery, P. D., Gerlach, K. K., Emont, S., & Orleans, T. (2002). Predictors of change on the smoking uptake continuum among adolescents. *Archives of Pediatrics and Adolescent Medicine, 156,* 581-587.

Kawachi, I., & Berkman, L. F. (2000). Social cohesion, social capital, and health. In L. F. Berkman & I. Kawachi (Eds.), *Social epidemiology* (pp. 174-190). New York: Oxford University Press.

Kawachi, I., Colditz, G. A., Ascherio, A., Rimm, E. B., Giovannucci, E., Stampfer, M. J., et al. (1996). A prospective study of social networks in relation to total mortality and cardiovascular disease in men in the U.S.A. *Journal of Epidemiology and Community Health, 50,* 245-251.

Kawachi, I., Colditz, G. A., Stampfer, M. J., Willett, W. C., Manson, J. E., Rosner, B., Speizer, F. E., & Hennekens, C. H. (1994). Smoking cessation and time course of decreased risk of coronary heart disease in women. *Archives of Internal Medicine, 154,* 169-175.

Kawachi, I., & Kennedy, B. P. (1999). Income inequality and health: Pathways and mechanisms. *Health Services Research, 34,* 215-227.

Kawachi, I., & Kennedy, B. P. (2002). *The health of nations.* New York: New Press.

Kawachi, I., Kennedy, B. P., & Glass, R. (1999). Social capital and self-rated health: A contextual analysis. *American Journal of Public Health, 89,* 1187-1193.

Kawachi, I., Kennedy, B. P., & Prothrow-Stith, D. (1997). Social capital, income inequality and mortality. *American Journal of Public Health, 87,* 1491-1498.

Kawachi, I., Kennedy, B. P., & Wilkinson, R. G. (Eds.). (1999). *Income inequality and health: A reader.* New York: New Press.

Kawachi, I., Sparrow, D., Spiro, A., III, Vokonas, P., & Weiss, S. T. (1996). A prospective study of anger and coronary heart disease: The Normative Aging Study. *Circulation, 94,* 2090-2095.

Kazarian, S. S., & Evans, D. R. (Eds.). (2001). *Handbook of cultural health psychology.* San Diego, CA: Academic Press.

Keefe, F., Lumley, M. A., Buffington, A., Carson, J., Studts, J., Edwards, C. L., Macklem, D. J., Aspnes, A., Fox, L., & Steffey, D. (2002). The changing face of pain: The evolution of pain research. *Psychosomatic Medicine, 64,* 921-938.

Keefe, F. J., Smith, S. J., Buffington, A. L. H., Gibson, J., Studts, J. L., & Caldwell, D. S. (2002). Recent advances and future directions in the biopsychosocial assessment and treatment of arthritis. *Journal of Consulting and Clinical Psychology, 70,* 640-655.

Kelley, M. L., Jarvie, G. J., Middlebrook, J. L., McNeer, M. F., & Drabman, R. S. (1984). Decreasing burned children's pain behavior: Impacting the trauma of hydrotherapy. *Journal of Applied Behavior Analysis, 1984,* 147-158.

Kelly, J. A. (1995). *Changing HIV risk behavior: Practical strategies.* New York: Guilford.

Kelly, J. A. (1999). Community-level interventions are needed to prevent new HIV infections. *American Journal of Public Health, 89,* 299-301.

Kelly, J. A., Murphy, D. A., Bahr, G. R., Koob, J. J., Morgan, M. G., Kalichman, S. C., Stevenson, L. Y., Brasfield, T. L., Bernstein, B. M., & St. Lawrence, J. S. (1993). Factors associated with severity of depression and high-risk sexual behavior among persons diagnosed with human immunodeficiency virus (HIV) infection. *Health Psychology, 12,* 215-219.

Kelly, J. A., St. Lawrence, J. S., Diaz, Y. E., Stevenson, L. Y., Hauth, A. C., & Brasfied, T. L. (1991). HIV risk behavior following intervention with key opinion leaders of a population: An experimental community level analysis. *American Journal of Public Health, 81,* 168-171.

Kemeny, M. E., Weiner, H., Taylor, S. E., Schneider, S., Visscher, B., & Fahey, J. L. (1994). Repeated bereavement, depressed mood, and immune parameters in HIV seropositive and seronegative gay men. *Health Psychology, 13,* 14-24.

Kempe, C. H., Silverman, F. N., Steele, B. F., Droegemueller, W., & Silver, H. K. (1962). The battered-child syndrome. *Journal of the American Medical Association, 181,* 17-24.

Kemper, T. D. (Ed.). (1990). *Social structure and testosterone: Explorations of the socio-bio-social chain.* Portland, OR: Book News.

Kennedy, S., Kiecolt-Glaser, J.-K., & Glaser, R. (1988). Immunological consequences of acute and chronic stressors: Mediating role of interpersonal relationships. *British Journal of Medical Psychology, 61,* 77-85.

Kerns, R. D., Turk, D. C., & Rudy, T. E. (1985). The West Haven-Yale Multidimensional Pain Inventory (WHYMPI). *Pain, 23,* 345-356.

Kessler, R. C. (1997). The effects of stressful life events on depression. In *Annual review of psychology* (pp. 191-214). Palo Alto, CA: Annual Reviews.

Kessler, R. C., McGonagle, K. A., Zhao, S., Nelson, C. B., Hughes, M., Eshelman, S., Wittchen, H. U., & Kendler, K. S. (1994). Lifetime and 12-month prevalence of *DSM-III-R:* Psychiatric disorders in the United States. Results from the National Comorbidity Survey. *Archives of General Psychiatry, 51,* 8-19.

Kessler, R. C., Zhao, S., Blazer, D. G., & Swartz, M. (1997). Prevalence, correlates, and course of minor depression and major depression in the national comorbidity survey. *Journal of Affective Disorders, 45,* 19-30.

Ketterer, M. W., Denollet, J., Goldberg, A. D., McCullough, P. A., Farha, A. J., Clark, V., et al. (2002). The big mush: Psychometric measures are confounded and nonindependent in their association with age at initial diagnosis of ICHD. *Journal of Cardiovascular Risk, 9,* 41-48.

Ketterer, M. W., Freedland, K. E., Krantz, D. S., Kaufman, P., Forman, S., Greene, A., et al. (2000). Psychological correlates of mental stress-induced ischemia in the laboratory: The psychophysiological investigations of myocardial ischemia (PIMI) study. *Journal of Health Psychology, 5,* 75-85.

Ketterer, M. W., Kenyon, L., Folet, B. A., Brymer, J., Rhoads, K., Kraft, P., et al. (1996). Denial of depression as an independent correlate of coronary artery disease. *Journal of Health Psychology, 1,* 93-105.

Ketterer, M. W., Mahr, G., & Goldberg, A. D. (2000). Psychological factors affecting a medical condition: Ischemic coronary heart disease. *Journal of Psychosomatic Research, 48,* 357-367.

Keys, A. (1980). *Seven countries: A multivariate analysis of death and coronary heart disease.* Cambridge, MA: Harvard University Press.

Khoshaba, D. M., & Maddi, S. R. (2001). *HardiTraining.* Newport Beach, CA: Hardiness Institute.

Kiecolt-Glaser, J. K., Dura, J. R., Speicher, C. E. Trask, O. J., & Glaser, R. (1991). Spousal caregivers of dementia victims: Longitudinal changes in immunity and health. *Psychosomatic Medicine, 53,* 345-362.

Kiecolt-Glaser, J. K., Fisher, L. D., Ogrocki, P., Stout, J. C., Speicher, C. E., & Glaser, R. (1987). Marital quality, marital disruption, and immune function. *Psychosomatic Medicine, 49,* 13-34.

Kiecolt-Glaser, J. K., & Glaser, R. (1999). Chronic stress and mortality among older adults. *Journal of the American Medical Association, 282,* 2259-2261.

Kiecolt-Glaser, J. K., McGuire, L., et al. (2002). Psychoneuroimmunology and psychosomatic medicine: Back to the future. *Psychosomatic Medicine, 64*(1), 15-28.

Kiecolt-Glaser, J. K., McGuire, L., Robles, T. F., & Glaser, R. (2002). Emotions, morbidity, and mortality: New perspectives from psychoneuroimmunology. *Annual Review of Psychology, 53,* 83-107.

Killen, J. D., Telch, M. J., Robinson, T. N., Maccoby, N., Taylor, C. B., & Farquhar, J. W. (1988). Cardiovascular disease risk reduction for tenth graders. *Journal of the American Medical Association, 260,* 1728-1733.

Killough, A. L., Webster, W., Brown, V., Houck, E., & Edwards, C. L. (2003). African American violence exposure: An emerging health issue. In C. C. Yeakey & R. D. Henderson (Eds.), *Surmounting all odds:*

Educational opportunities in the new millennium. Greenwich, CT: Information Age.

King, A. C. (2001). Interventions to promote physical activity by older adults. *Journal of Gerontology, 56A,* 36-46.

King, A. C., Stokols, D., Talen, E., Brassington, G. S., & Killingsworth, R. (2002). Theoretical approaches to the promotion of physical activity: Forging a transdisciplinary paradigm. *American Journal of Preventive Medicine, 23*(Suppl. 2), 15-25.

Kington, R. S., & Nickens, H. W. (2001). Racial and ethnic differences in health: Recent trends, current patterns, future directions. In N. J. Smelser, W. J. Wilson, & F. Mitchell (Eds.), *America becoming: Racial trends and their consequences* (Vol. 2, pp. 253-310). Washington, DC: National Academy Press.

Kirby, D. (2001). *Emerging answers: Research findings on programs to reduce teenage pregnancies.* Washington, DC: National Campaign to Prevent Teenage Pregnancy.

Kirsch, I. (1997). Specifying nonspecifics: Psychological mechanisms of placebo effects. In A. Harrington (Ed.), *The placebo effect: An interdisciplinary exploration* (pp. 166-186). Cambridge, MA: Harvard University Press.

Kirsch, I. S., Jungeblut, A., Jenkins, L., & Kolstad, A. (1993). *Adult literacy in America.* Washington, DC: Office of Educational Research and Improvement.

Kirscht, J. P. (1974). The health belief model and illness behavior. *Health Education Monographs, 2,* 387-408.

Kissner, S., & Pratt, S. (1997). Occupational fatalities among older workers in the United States. *Journal of Occupational and Environmental Medicine, 39,* 715-721.

Kitagawa, E. M. (1955). Components of a difference between two rates. *Journal of the American Statistical Association, 50,* 1168-1194.

Klassen, T. P., MacKay, J. M., Moher, D., Walker, A., & Jones, A. L. (2000). Community-based injury prevention interventions. *Future of Children, 10*(1), 83-110.

Klein, R. B., Penza-Clyve, S., McQuaid, E. L., & Fritz, G. K. (2000). Behavior modification as adjunctive therapy for asthma. *Clinical Practice Management, 7,* 326-330.

Klerman, G. L., Weissman, M. M., Rounsaville, B. J., & Chevron, E. S. (1984). *Interpersonal psychotherapy of depression.* New York: Basic Books.

Klippel, J. H., & Crofford, L. (Eds.). (2001). *Primer on the rheumatic diseases* (12th ed.). Atlanta, GA: Arthritis Foundation.

Klohnen, E. C. (1996). Conceptual analysis and measurement of the construct of ego-resiliency. *Journal of Personality and Social Psychology, 70,* 1067-1079.

Klonoff, E. A., & Landrine, H. (1999). Do Blacks believe that HIV/AIDS is a government conspiracy against them? *Preventive Medicine, 28,* 451-457.

Klump, K. L., Kaye, W. H., & Strober, M. (2001). The evolving genetic foundations of eating disorders. *Psychiatric Clinics of North America, 24,* 215-225.

Knight, B., Silverstein, M., McCallum, T. J., & Fox, L. (2000). A sociocultural stress and coping model for mental health outcomes among African American caregivers in Southern California. *Journal of Gerontology: Psychological Sciences, 55B,* P142-P150.

Knight, B. G., & McCallum, T. J. (1998). Heart rate reactivity and depression in African-American and White dementia caregivers: Reporting bias or positive coping. *Aging and Mental Health, 2,* 212-221.

Knutsson, A., & Boggild, H. (2000). Shiftwork and cardiovascular disease: Review of disease mechanisms. *Review of Environmental Health, 15,* 359-372.

Knutsson, A., Akerstedt, T., Jonsson, B. G., & Orth-Gomer, K. (1986). Increased risk of ischaemic heart disease in shift workers. *Lancet, 12,* 89-92.

Koenig, H. G., McCullough, M. E., & Larson, D. B. (2001). *Handbook of religion and health.* New York: Oxford University Press.

Koloski, N. A., Talley, N. J., & Boyce, P. M. (2001). Predictors of health care seeking for irritable bowel syndrome and nonulcer dyspepsia: A critical review of the literature on symptom and psychosocial factors. *American Journal of Gastroenterology, 96,* 1340-1349.

Koob, G. F., & LeMoal, M. (2001). Drug addiction, dysregulation of reward, and allostasis. *Neuropsychopharmacology, 24,* 97-129.

Kop, W. J. (1999). Chronic and acute psychological risk factors for clinical manifestations of coronary artery disease. *Psychosomatic Medicine, 61*(4), 476-487.

Kop, W. J., Appels, A. P., Mendes de Leon, C. F., de Swart, H. B., & Bar, F. W. (1994). Vital exhaustion predicts new cardiac events after successful coronary angioplasty. *Psychosomatic Medicine, 56,* 281-287.

Kop, W. J., & Cohen, N. (2001). Psychological risk factors and immune system involvement in cardiovascular disease. In R. Ader, D. L. Felten, & N. Cohen (Eds.), *Psychoneuroimmunology* (3rd ed., pp. 525-544). San Diego, CA: Academic Press.

Kornitzer, J., Kittel, F., Dramaix, M., & deBacker, G. (1982). Job stress and coronary heart disease. *Advances in Cardiology, 19,* 56-61.

Kotler, P., Roberto, N., & Lee, N. (2002). *Social marketing: Improving the quality of life* (2nd ed.). Thousand Oaks, CA: Sage.

Kotses, H., & Harver, A. (Eds.). (1998). *Self-management of asthma.* New York: Marcel Dekker.

Kovacs, M. (1992). *Children's Depression Inventory.* North Tonawanda, NY: Multi-Health Systems.

Kramer, B. J. (1997). Gain in the caregiving experience: Where are we? What next? *Gerontologist, 37,* 218-232.

Kramer, M. S., Goulet, L., Lydon, J., et al. (2001). Socio-economic disparities in preterm birth: Causal pathways and mechanisms. *Paediatric and Perinatal Epidemiology, 15*(Suppl. 2), 104-123.

Krantz, D. S., & Manuck, S. B. (1984). Acute psychophysiologic reactivity and risk for cardiovascular disease: A review and methodologic critique. *Psychological Bulletin, 96,* 435-464.

Kreuter, M. W., & Skinner, C. S. (2000). Tailoring: What's in a name? *Health Education Research, 15,* 1-4.

Kreuter, M. W., Strecher, V. J., & Glassman, B. (1999). One size does not fit all: The case for tailoring print materials. *Annals of Behavioral Medicine, 21,* 276-283.

Kreuter, M., Farrell, D., Olevitch, L., & Brennan, L. (2000). *Tailoring health messages: Customizing communication with computer technology.* Mahwah, NJ: Lawrence Erlbaum.

Krieger, N. (1994). Epidemiology and the web of causation: Has anyone seen the spider? *Social Science and Medicine, 39,* 887-903.

Krieger, N. (1999). Embodying inequality: A review of concepts, measures, and methods for studying health consequences of discrimination. *International Journal of Health Services, 29,* 295-352.

Krieger, N. (2000). Epidemiology and social sciences: Towards a critical reengagement in the 21st century. *Epidemiologic Reviews, 11,* 155-163.

Krieger, N. (2001a). A glossary for social epidemiology. *Journal of Epidemiology and Community Health, 55,* 693-700.

Krieger, N. (2001b). Theories for social epidemiology in the 21st century: An ecosocial perspective. *International Journal of Epidemiology, 30,* 668-677.

Krieger, N., & Sidney, S. (1996). Racial discrimination and blood pressure: The CARDIA study of young Black and White adults. *American Journal of Public Health, 86,* 1370-1378.

Krieger, N., Sidney, S., & Coakley, E. (1998). Racial discrimination and skin color in the CARDIA Study: Implications for public health research. *American Journal of Public Health, 88,* 1308-1313.

Kromhout, D., Bosschieter, E. B., & Coulander, C. (1985). The inverse relation between fish consumption and 20-year mortality from coronary heart disease. *New England Journal of Medicine, 312*(19), 1205-1209.

Kronfol, Z., & Remick, D. G. (2000). Cytokines and the brain: Implications for clinical psychiatry. *American Journal of Psychiatry, 157*(5), 683-694.

Kubzansky, L. D., & Kawachi, I. (2000). Going to the heart of the matter: Do negative emotions cause coronary heart disease? *Journal of Psychosomatic Research, 48,* 323-337.

Kubzansky, L. D., Kawachi, I., Weiss, S., & Sparrow, D. (1998). Anxiety and coronary heart disease: A synthesis of epidemiological, psychological, and experimental evidence. *Annals of Behavioral Medicine, 20*(2), 47-58.

Kubzansky, L. D., Sparrow, D., Vokonas, P., & Kawachi, I. (2001). Is the glass half empty or half full? A prospective study of optimism and coronary heart disease in the normative aging study. *Psychosomatic Medicine, 63,* 910-916.

Kuh, G. D. (1994). The influence of college environments on student drinking. In G. Gonzalez & V. Clement (Eds.), *Research and intervention: Preventing substance abuse in higher education* (pp. 45-71). Washington, DC: Office of Educational Research and Improvement.

Kulik, J. A., & Mahler, H. I. M. (1987). Effects of pre-operative roommate assignment on pre-operative anxiety and recovery from coronary bypass surgery. *Health Psychology, 6,* 525-543.

Kumanyika, S. K., Morssink, C. B., & Nestle, M. (2001). Minority women and advocacy for women's health. *American Journal of Public Health, 91,* 1383-1388.

Kumpfer, K. L. (1999). Factors and processes contributing to resilience: The resilience framework. In M. D. Glantz & J. L. Johnson (Eds.), *Resilience and development: Positive life adaptations* (pp. 179-224). New York: Kluwer Academic/Plenum.

Kunst, A. E., Feikje, G., Mackenbach, J. P., et al. (1998). Occupational class and cause-specific mortality in middle-age men in 11 European countries. *BMJ, 316,* 1636-1642.

Kuper, H., & Marmot, M. G. (2003). Job strain, job demands, decision latitude, and risk of coronary heart disease within the Whitehall II Study. *Journal of Epidemiology and Community Health, 57*(2), 147-153.

LaDou, J. (Ed.). (1997). *Occupational and environmental medicine* (2nd ed.). Stamford, CT: Appleton & Lange.

Lakey, B., & Cohen, S. (2000). Social support theory and measurement. In S. Cohen, L. G. Underwood, & B. H. Gottlieb (Eds.), *Social support measurement and intervention: A guide for health and social scientists* (pp. 29-52). New York: Oxford University Press.

Landro, N. I., Stiles, T. C., & Sletvold, H. (1997). Memory functioning in patients with primary fibromyalgia and major depression and healthy controls. *Journal of Psychosomatic Research, 42,* 297-306.

Landsbergis, P. A., Schnall, P. L., Deitz, D. K., Pickering, W. K., & Schwartz, J. E. (1998). Job strain and health behaviors: Results of a prospective study. *American Journal of Health Promotion, 12,* 237-245.

Langley, J. D., Wagenaar, A. C., & Begg, D. J. (1996). An evaluation of the New Zealand graduated driver licensing system. *Accident Analysis and Prevention, 28,* 139-146.

Lantz, P. M., House, J. S., Lepowski, J. M., et al. (1998). Socioeconomic factors, health behaviors, and mortality: Results from a nationally-representative prospective study of U.S. adults. *Journal of the American Medical Association, 279,* 1703-1708.

Lantz, P., Jacobson, P., Warner, J., Wasserman, J., Pollack, H., Berson, J., & Ahlstrom, A. (2000). Investing in youth tobacco control: A review of smoking prevention and control strategies. *Tobacco Control, 9,* 47-63.

Lantz, P., Viruell-Fuentes, E., Israel, B. A., Softley, D., & Guzman, J. R. (2001). Can communities and academia work together on public health research? Evaluation results from a community-based participatory research partnership in Detroit. *Journal of Urban Health, 78,* 495-507.

LaPiere, R. T. (1934). Attitudes vs. actions. *Social Forces, 13,* 230-237.

LaRosa, J. C., He, J., & Vupputuri, S. (1999). Effect of statins on risk of coronary disease: A meta-analysis of randomized controlled trials. *Journal of the American Medical Association, 282,* 2340-2346.

Lasater, T. M. (1997). Synthesis of findings and issues from religious-based cardiovascular disease prevention trials. *Annals of Epidemiology, 7,* S46-S53.

Last, J. M. (Ed.). (1983). *A dictionary of epidemiology.* New York: Oxford University Press.

Laumann, E. O., Paik, A., & Rosen, R. C. (1999). Sexual dysfunction in the United States. *Journal of the American Medical Association, 281,* 537-544.

Lavie, C. J., & Milani, R. V. (1999). Effects of cardiac rehabilitation and exercise training programs on coronary patients with high levels of hostility. *Mayo Clinic Proceedings, 74,* 959-966.

Lavoie, J. P. (1995). Support groups for informal caregivers don't work! Refocus the groups or the evaluations? *Canadian Journal on Aging, 14,* 580-595.

Lawlor, D. A., Ebrahim, S., & Davey-Smith, G. (2001). Sex matters: secular and geographical trends in sex differences in coronary heart disease mortality. *BMJ, 323*(7312), 541-545.

Lawton, M. P., Rajagopal, D., Brody, E., & Kleban, M. H. (1992). The dynamics of caregiving for a demented elder among Black and White families. *Journal of Gerontology, 47,* S156-S164.

Lazarus, R. S. (1993). From psychological stress to the emotions: A history of changing outlooks. *Annual Review of Psychology, 44,* 1-21.

Lazarus, R. S., & Folkman, S. (1984). *Stress, appraisal, and coping.* New York: Springer.

Lazarus, R. S., Kanner, A. D., & Folkman, S. (1980). Emotions: A cognitive-phenomenological analysis. In R. Plutchik & H. Kellerman (Eds.), *Theories of emotion* (pp. 189-217). New York: Academic Press.

Le Bars, D., Dickenson, A. H., & Besson, J. M. (1983). Opiate analgesia and descending control systems. In J. J. Bonica, U. Lindblom, & A. Iggo (Eds.), *Advances in pain research and therapy: Proceedings of the 3rd World Congress on Pain* (Vol. 5, pp. 341-372). New York: Raven.

LeCompte, M., & Schensul, J. (1999). Introduction to research methods. In J. Schensul & M. LeCompte (Eds.), *Ethnographer's toolkit: Vol. 1.* Walnut Creek, CA: AltaMira.

Lee, I-M. (1994). Physical activity, fitness, and cancer. In C. Bouchard, R. J. Shepard, & T. Stephens (Eds.), *Physical activity, fitness, and health: International proceedings and consensus statement* (pp. 814-831). Champaign, IL: Human Kinetics.

Lee, I-M., Hsieh, C.-c., & Paffenbarger, R. S., Jr. (1995). Exercise intensity and longevity in men: The Harvard Alumni Health Study. *Journal of the American Medical Association, 273,* 1179-1184.

Lee, I-M., Paffenbarger, R. S., Jr., & Hsieh, C.-c. (1991). Physical activity and risk of developing colorectal cancer among college alumni. *Journal of the National Cancer Institute, 83,* 1324-1329.

Lefcourt, H. M., Davidson-Katz, K., & Kueneman, K. (1990). Humor and immune-system functioning. *Humor: International Journal of Humor Research, 3,* 305-321.

Lefcourt, H. M., & Thomas, S. (1998). Humor and stress revisited. In W. Ruch (Ed.), *The sense of humor: Explorations of a personality characteristic* (pp. 179-202). Berlin, Germany: Walter de Gruyter.

Lefebvre, R. C., Doner, L., Johnston, C., Loughrey, K., Balch, G. I., & Sutton, S. M. (1995). Use of database marketing and consumer-based health communications in message design: An example from the 5 a Day for Better Health Program. In E. Maibach & R. I. Parrot (Eds.), *Designing health messages: Approaches from communications theory and public health practice* (pp. 217-246). Thousand Oaks, CA: Sage.

Lefebvre, R. C., & Flora, J. A. (1988). Social marketing and public health intervention. *Health Education Quarterly, 15,* 299-315.

Legler, J., Meissner, H. I., Coyne, C., Breen, N., Chollette, V., & Rimer, B. K. (2002). The effectiveness of interventions to promote mammography among women with historically lower rates of screening. *Cancer Epidemiology, Biomarkers & Prevention, 11,* 59-71.

Lehrer, P. M., Vaschillo, E., Vaschillo, B., Lu, S. E., Eckberg, D. L., Edelberg, R., Shih, W. J., Lin, Y., Kuusela, T. A., Tahvanainen, K. U. O., & Hamer, R. M. (in press). Heart rate variability biofeedback increases baroreflex gain and peak expiratory flow. *Psychosomatic Medicine.*

Leiblum, S. R. (1997). *Infertility: Psychological issues and counseling strategies.* New York: John Wiley.

Lemanek, K. L., Horwitz, W. L., & Ohene-Frempong, K. (1994). A multi-perspective investigation of social competence in children with sickle cell disease. *Journal of Pediatric Psychology, 19,* 443-456.

Lemanek, K. L., Moore, S. L., Gresham, F. M., Williamson, D. A., & Kelley, M. L. (1986). Psychological adjustment of children with sickle cell anemia. *Journal of Pediatric Psychology, 11,* 397-410.

Lepore, S. J., Evans, G. W., & Schneider, M. (1991). The dynamic role of social support in the link between chronic stress and psychological distress. *Journal of Personality and Social Psychology, 61,* 899-909.

Lepore, S. J., Silver, R. C., Wortman, C. B., & Wayment, H. A. (1996). Social constraints, intrusive thoughts, and depressive symptoms among bereaved mothers. *Journal of Personality and Social Psychology, 70,* 271-282.

Lepore, S. J., & Smyth, J. M. (2002). *The writing cure: How expressive writing promotes health and emotional well-being.* Washington, DC: American Psychological Association.

LeResche, L. (1999). *Gender considerations in the epidemiology of chronic pain.* In I. K. Crombie et al. (Eds.), *Epidemiology of pain.* Seattle, WA: International Association for the Study of Pain.

Leserman, J. (in press). HIV disease progression: Depression, stress and possible mechanisms. *Biological Psychiatry.*

Leserman, J., Petitto, J. M., Gu, H., Gaynes, B. N., Barroso, J., Golden, R. N., Perkins, D. O., Folds, J. D., & Evans, D. L. (2002). Progression to AIDS, a clinical AIDS condition, and mortality: Psychosocial and physiological predictors. *Psychological Medicine, 32,* 1-14.

Levenson, H. (1973). Multidimensional locus of control in psychiatric patients. *Journal of Consulting and Clinical Psychology, 41,* 397-404.

Levenson, R. W., Ekman, P., & Friesen, W. V. (1990). Voluntary facial action generates emotion-specific autonomic nervous system activity. *Psychophysiology, 27,* 363-384.

Levenstein, S. (2002a). Commentary: Peptic ulcer and its discontents. *International Journal of Epidemiology, 31*(1), 29-33.

Levenstein, S. (2002b). Psychosocial factors in peptic ulcer and inflammatory bowel disease. *Journal of Consulting and Clinical Psychology, 70,* 739-750. Retrieved from http://www.apa.org/journals/ccp/press_releases/june_2002/special_issue/ccp703739.pdf

Levenstein, S. (2000c). The very model of a modern etiology: A biopsychosocial view of peptic ulcer. *Psychosomatic Medicine, 62,* 176-185.

Levenstein, S., Prantera, C., Scribano, M. L., Varvo, V., Berto, E., & Spinella, S. (1996). Psychologic predictors of duodenal ulcer healing. *Journal of Clinical Gastroenterology, 22*(2), 84-89.

Leventhal, H., Nerenz, D. R., & Steele, D. J. (1984). Illness representations and coping with health threats. In A. Baum, S. E. Taylor, & J. E. Singer (Eds.), *Handbook of psychology and health* (pp. 219-252). Hillsdale, NJ: Lawrence Erlbaum.

Levy, D. (1999, January 19). [Data from the Framingham Heart Study]. *Washington Post,* Health Section, p. 5.

Lewin, B. (1997). The psychological and behavioral management of angina. *Journal of Psychosomatic Research, 43,* 453-462.

Lewinsohn, P. M., & Arconad, M. (1981). Behavioral treatment of depression: A social learning approach. In J. F. Clarkin & H. I. Glazer (Eds.), *Depression: Behavioral and directive interventional strategies.* New York: Garland STPM.

Lewinsohn, P. M., Youngren, M. A., & Grosscup, S. J. (1979). Reinforcement and depression. In R. A. DePue (Ed.), *The psychobiology of depressive disorders: Implications for the effects of stress.* New York: Academic Press.

Lewit, E., Schuurmann, B. L., Corman, H., & Shiono, P. (1995). The direct cost of low birth weight. *Future of Children, 5,* 35-56.

Leyland, A. H., & Goldstein, H. (Eds.). (2001). *Multilevel modelling of health statistics.* Wiley Series in Probability and Statistics. Chichester, UK: Wiley.

Lichtenstein, B., Laska, M. K., & Clair, J. M. (2002). Chronic sorrow in the HIV-positive patient: Issues of race, gender, and social support. *AIDS Patient Care & STDs, 16*(1), 27-38.

Lieberson, S. (1985). *Making it count: The improvement of social research and theory.* Berkeley: University of California Press.

Liebeskind, J. C., & Paul, L. A. (1977). Psychological and physiological mechanisms of pain. *Annual Review of Psychology, 28,* 41-60.

Light, K. C., Brownley, K. A., Turner, J. R., Hinderliter, A. L., Girdler, S. S., Sherwood, A., et al. (1995). Job status and high-effort coping influence work blood pressure in women and Blacks. *Hypertension, 25,* 554-559.

Light, K. C., Girdler, S. S., Sherwood, A., Bragdon, E. E., Brownley, K. A., West, S. G., & Hinderleiter, A. L. (1999). High stress responsivity predicts later blood pressure only in combination with positive family history and high life stress. *Hypertension, 33,* 1458-1464.

Lillard, L. A., & Panis, C. (1996). Marital status and mortality: The role of health. *Demography, 33,* 313-327.

Lillard, L. A., & Waite, L. J. (1995). Til death do us part: Marital disruption and mortality. *American Journal of Sociology, 100,* 1131-1156.

Lindemann, E. (1944). Symptomatology and management of acute grief. *American Journal of Psychiatry, 101.*

Linden, W., Lenz, J. W., & Con, A. (2001). Individualized stress management for primary hypertension: A controlled trial. *Archives of Internal Medicine, 161,* 1071-1080.

Lindsey, L. L. (Ed.). (1997). *Gender roles: A sociological perspective.* Upper Saddle River, NJ: Prentice Hall.

Link, B. G., Northridge, M., Phelan, J. C., et al. (1998). Social epidemiology and the fundamental cause concept: On the structuring of effective cancer screens by socioeconomic status. *Milbank Quarterly, 76,* 375-402.

Link, B. G., & Phelan, J. C. (1995). Social conditions as fundamental causes of disease. *Journal of Health and Social Behavior,* pp. 80-94 [Extra issue].

Lionberger, H. F. (1960). *Adoption of new ideas and practices.* Ames: Iowa State University Press.

Lipchik, G. L., Holroyd, K. A., & Nash, J. M. (2002). Cognitive-behavioral management of recurrent headache disorders: A minimal-therapist contact approach. In D. C. Turk & R. S. Gatchel (Eds.), *Psychological approaches to pain management* (2nd ed., pp. 356-389). New York: Guilford.

Lipton, R. B., Hamelsky, S. W., & Stewart, W. A. (2001). Epidemiology and impact of headache. In S. D. Silberstein, R. B. Lipton, & D. J. Dalessio (Eds.), *Wolff's headache and other head pain* (7th ed., pp. 85-107). New York: Oxford University Press.

Littlefield, C. H., & Rushton, J. P. (1986). When a child dies: The sociobiology of bereavement. *Journal of Personality and Social Psychology, 51*(4), 797-802.

Livingston, W. K. (1943). *Pain mechanisms.* New York: Macmillan.

Lochner, K., et al. (2003). Social capital and neighborhood mortality rates in Chicago. *Social Science and Medicine, 56,* 1797-1805.

Lochner, K., Kawachi, I., & Kennedy, B. P. (1999). Social capital: A guide to its measurement. *Health and Place, 5,* 259-270.

Logan, P. D. L. (1982). *Cancer mortality by occupation and social class 1951-1971.* London: HMSO.

Longford, N. (1993). *Random coefficient models.* Oxford, UK: Clarendon.

Loof, L., Adami, H., Fagerstrom, K., Gustavsson, S., Nyberg, A., Nyren, O., & Brodin, U. (1987). Psychological group counseling for the prevention of ulcer relapse. *Journal of Clinical Gastroenterology, 9*(4), 400-407.

Lorig, K., Chastain, R., Ung, E., Shoor, S., & Holman, H. (1989). Development and evaluation of a scale to measure the perceived self-efficacy of people with arthritis. *Arthritis and Rheumatism, 32,* 37-44.

Lorig, K., & Fries, J. F. (1990). *The arthritis helpbook.* New York: Addison-Wesley.

Lotufo-Neto, F., Trivedi, M., and Thase, M. E. (1999). Meta-analysis of the reversible inhibitors of monoamine oxidase type A moclobemide and brofaromine for the treatment of depression. *Neuropsychopharmacology, 20*(3), 226-247.

Loue, S. (Ed.). (1998). *Handbook of immigrant health.* New York: Plenum.

Loue, S., & Bunce, A. (1999). The assessment of immigration status in health research. *Vital Health Statistics, 2.*

Lovallo, W. R. (1997). *Stress and health: Biological and psychological interactions.* Thousand Oaks, CA: Sage.

Lowie, R. H. (1916). Plains Indians age societies, anthropological papers. *American Museum of Natural History, 11,* 877-1031.

Lox, C. L., Martin, K. A., & Petruzello, S. J. (2003). *The psychology of exercise: Integrating theory and practice.* Scottsdale, AZ: Holcomb Hathaway.

Luepker, R. V., Murray, D. M., Jacobs, D. R., Jr., Mittelmark, M. B., Bracht, N., Carlaw, R., et al. (1994). Community education for cardiovascular disease prevention: Risk factor changes in the Minnesota Heart Health Program. *American Journal of Public Health, 84,* 1383-1393.

Luepker, R. V., Perry, C. L., McKinlay, S. M., Nader, P. R., Parcel, G. S., Stone, E. J., Webber, L. S., Elder, J. P., Feldman, H. A., Johnson, C. C., Kelder, S. H., & Wu, M. (1996). Outcomes of a field trial to improve children's dietary patterns and physical activity: The Child and Adolescent Trial for Cardiovascular Health (CATCH). *Journal of the American Medical Association, 275,* 768-776.

Lundberg, U., & Frankenhaeuser, M. (1999). Stress and workload of men and women in high ranking positions. *Journal of Occupational Health Psychology, 4,* 142-151.

Lutgendorf, S. K., Garand, L., Buckwalter, K. C., Reimer, T. T., Hong, S. Y., & Lubaroff, D. M. (1999). Life stress, mood disturbance, and elevated interleukin-6 in healthy older women. *Journal of Gerontology, 54,* M434-M439.

Lyness, J. M., Caine, E. D., King, D. A., Cox, C., & Yoediono, Z. (1999). Psychiatric disorders in older primary care patients. *Journal of General Internal Medicine, 14,* 249-254.

Lyubomirsky, S., King, L. A., & Diener, E. (2003). *A review of the benefits of happiness.* Manuscript in preparation, University of California, Riverside.

Maccoby, E. E. (Ed.). (1998). *The two sexes: Growing up apart, coming together.* Cambridge, MA: Harvard University Press.

MacIntyre, S., & Hunt, K. (1997). Socioeconomic position, gender and health. How do they interact? *Journal of Health Psychology, 2*(3), 315-334.

MacIntyre, S., Ellaway, A., & Cummins, S. (2002). Place effects on health: How can we conceptualise, operationalise and measure them? *Social Science and Medicine, 55,* 125-139.

MacIntyre, S., Ellaway, A., Der, G., Ford, G., & Hunt, K. (1998). Do housing tenure and car access predict health because they are simply markers of income or self-esteem? A Scottish study. *Journal of Epidemiology and Community Health, 52,* 657-664.

MacIntyre, S., Maciver, S., & Sooman, A. (1993). Area, class, and health: Should we be focusing on places or people? *Journal of Social Policy, 22,* 213-234.

Mackay, J., & Eriksen, M. (2002). *The tobacco atlas.* Geneva: World Health Organization.

MacLean, D. R. (1994). Theoretical rationale of community intervention for the prevention and control of cardiovascular disease. *Health Reports, 6,* 174-180.

MacLennan, A. H., Wilson, D. H., & Taylor, A. W. (1996). Prevalence and cost of alternative medicine in Australia. *Lancet, 347,* 569-573.

Maddi, S. R. (1997). Personal Views Survey II: A measure of dispositional hardiness. In C. P. Zalaquett & R. J. Woods (Eds.), *Evaluating stress: A book of resources.* New York: University Press.

Maddi, S. R. (2002). The story of hardiness: Twenty years of theorizing, research, and practice. *Consulting Psychology Journal, 54,* 173-185.

Maddi, S. R., & Khoshaba, D. M. (2001a). *HardiSurvey III-R®: Test development and Internet instruction manual.* Newport Beach, CA: Hardiness Institute.

Maddi, S. R., & Khoshaba, D. M. (2001b). *Personal Views Survey III-R: Internet instruction manual.* Newport Beach, CA: Hardiness Institute.

Maddi, S. R., & Kobasa, S. C. (1984). *The hardy executive: Health under stress.* Homewood, IL: Dow Jones-Irwin.

Maes, M., Song, C., Lin, A., et al. (1998). The effects of psychological stress on humans: Increased production of pro-inflammatory cytokines and Th1-like response in stress-induced anxiety. *Cytokine, 10,* 313-318.

Maibach, E., Flora, J., & Nass, C. (1991). Changes in self-efficacy and health behavior in response to a minimal contact community health campaign. *Health Communication, 3,* 1-15.

Maibach, E., & Parrott, R. L. (1995). *Designing health messages: Approaches from communication theory and public health practice.* Thousand Oaks, CA: Sage.

Maier, S. F., & Watkins, L. R. (1998). Cytokines for psychologists: Implications of bidirectional immune-to-brain communication for understanding behavior, mood, and cognition. *Psychological Review, 105*(1), 83-107.

Mallin, K., & Anderson, K. (1988). Cancer mortality in Illinois Mexican and Puerto Rican immigrants, 1979-1984. *International Journal of Cancer, 41,* 670-676.

Mant, J., Carter, J., Wade, D. T., & Winner, S. (2000). Family support for stroke: A randomised controlled trial. *Lancet, 356,* 808-813.

Manuck, S. B. (1994). Cardiovascular reactivity in cardiovascular disease: "Once more unto the breach." *International Journal of Behavioral Medicine, 1,* 4-31.

Manuck, S. B., Kaplan, J. R., Adams, M. R., & Clarkson, T. B. (1988). Effects of stress and the sympathetic nervous system on coronary artery atherosclerosis in the cynomolgus macaque. *American Heart Journal, 116,* 328-333.

Marcus, G., & Fischer, M. (1986). *Anthropology as cultural critique: An experimental moment in the human sciences.* Chicago: University of Chicago Press.

Marín, G., & Marín, B. V. (1991). *Research with Hispanic populations.* Newbury Park, CA: Sage.

Marin, G., Perez-Stable, E. J., & Marin, B. V. (1989). Cigarette smoking among San Francisco Hispanics: The role of acculturation and gender. *American Journal of Public Health, 79,* 196-198.

Markides, K. S., Boldt, J. S., & Ray, L. A. (1986). Sources of helping and intergenerational solidarity: A three-generation study of Mexican Americans. *Journal of Gerontology, 41,* 506-511.

Markides, K. S., & Coreil, J. (1986). The health of Hispanics in the southwestern United States: An epidemiologic paradox. *Public Health Reports, 101,* 253-265.

Markovic, N., Bunker, C. H., Ukoli, F. A., & Kuller, L. H. (1998). John Henryism and blood pressure among Nigerian civil servants. *Journal of Epidemiology and Community Health, 52,* 186-190.

Markovitz, J., Matthews, K., Kannel, W., Cobb, J., & D'Agostino, R. (1993). Psychological predictors of hypertension in the Framingham Study: Is there tension in hypertension? *Journal of the American Medical Association, 270,* 2439-2443.

Markovitz, J. H., Matthews, K. A., Wing, R. R., Kuller, L. H., & Meilahn, E. N. (1991). Psychological, biological and health behavior predictors of blood pressure changes in middle-aged women. *Journal of Hypertension, 9*(5), 399-406.

Markowitz, J. C., Spielman, L. A., Sullivan, M., & Fishman, B. (2000). An exploratory study of ethnicity and psychotherapy outcome among HIV-positive patients with depressive symptoms. *Journal of Psychotherapy Practice and Research, 9,* 226-231.

Marks, N. F., & Lambert, J. A. (1998). Marital status continuity and change among young and midlife adults: Longitudinal effects on psychological well-being. *Journal of Family Issues, 19,* 652-686.

Marmot, M., Theorell, T., & Siegrist, J. (2002). Work and coronary heart disease. In S. A. Stansfeld & M. G. Marmot (Eds.), *Stress and the heart* (pp. 50-71). London: Oxford University Press.

Marmot, M. G., Davey Smith, G., Stansfeld, S., Patel, C., North, F., Head, J., White, I., Brunner, E., & Feeney, A. (1991). Health inequalities among British civil servants: The Whitehall II Study. *Lancet, 337,* 1387-1393.

Marmot, M. G., & Wilkinson, R. G. (1999). *Social determinants of health.* Oxford, UK: Oxford University Press.

Marris, P. (1978-1979). Conservatism, innovation and old age. *International Journal of Aging and Human Development, 9,* 127-135.

Marsella, A. J., Hirschfeld, R. M., & Katz, M. M. (Eds.). (1987). *The measurement of depression.* New York: Guilford.

Marshall, G. N., Wortman, C. B., Kusulas, J. W., Hervig, L. K., & Vickers, R. R., Jr. (1992). Distinguishing optimism from pessimism: Relations to fundamental dimensions of mood and personality. *Journal of Personality and Social Psychology, 62,* 1067-1074.

Marteau, T., & Richards, M. (Eds.). (1996). *The troubled helix: Social and psychological implications of the new genetics.* Cambridge, UK: Cambridge University Press.

Martin, R., Watson, D., & Wan, C. K. (2000). A three-factor model of trait anger: Dimensions of affect, behavior, and cognition. *Journal of Personality, 86,* 869-897.

Marucha, P. T., Sheridan, J. F., & Padgett, D. A. (2001). Stress and wound healing. In R. Ader, D. L. Felten, & N. Cohen (Eds.), *Psychoneuroimmunology: Vol. 2* (3rd ed., pp. 613-626). San Diego, CA: Academic Press.

Marx, E., Wooley, S. F., & Northrop, D. (Eds.). (1998). *Health is academic: A guide to coordinated school health programs.* New York: Teachers College Press.

Mason, F. (Ed.). (1954). *Balanchine's complete stories of the great ballets.* Garden City, NY: Doubleday.

Masten, A. S., Best, K. M., & Garmezy, N. (1990). Resilience and development: Contributions from the study of children who overcome adversity. *Development and Psychopathology, 2,* 425-444.

Masters, W. H., & Johnson, V. E. (1970). *Human sexual inadequacy.* Boston: Little, Brown.

Matarazzo, J. D. (1982). Behavioral health's challenge to academic, scientific, and professional psychology. *American Psychologist, 37,* 1-14.

Matsushima, Y., Aoyama, N., Fukuda, H., Kinoshita, Y., Todo, A., Himeno, S., Fujimoto, S., Kasuga, M., Nakase, H., & Chiba, T. (1999). Gastric ulcer formation after the Hanshin-Awaji earthquake: A case study of Helicobacter pylori infection and stress-induced gastric ulcers. *Helicobacter, 4*(2), 94-99.

Matthews, K. A., & Haynes, S. G. (1986). Type A behavior pattern and coronary disease risk: Update and critical evaluation. *American Journal of Epidemiology, 123,* 923-960.

May, R. (1977). *The meaning of anxiety.* New York: W. W. Norton. (Original work published 1950)

May, R. M., & Anderson, R. M. (1987). Transmission dynamics and HIV infection. *Nature, 326,* 137-142.

Mayne, T. J. (1999). Negative affect and health: The importance of being earnest. *Cognition and Emotion, 13,* 601-635.

Mays, V. M., & Cochran, S. D. (1998). *Racial discrimination and health outcomes in African Americans.* Proceedings of the Public Health Conference on Records and Statistics and Data User's Conference (PHCRS/DUC Proceedings CD-ROM No. 1). Washington, DC.

Mazur, A., & Michalek, J. (1998). Marriage, divorce and male testosterone. *Social Forces, 77,* 315-330.

McAdams, D. P. (1993). *The stories we live by: Personal myths and the making of the self.* New York: Morrow.

McAlister, A. L., Puska, P., Orlandi, M., Bye, L. L., & Zbylot, P. (1991). Behaviour modification: Principles and illustrations. In W. W. Holland, R. Detels, & E. G. Knox (Eds.), *Oxford textbook of public health: Vol. 3. Applications in public health* (2nd ed., pp. 3-16). Oxford, UK: Oxford University Press.

McCabe, M. P., & Cobain, M. J. (1998). The impact of individual and relationship factors on sexual dysfunction among males and females. *Sexual and Marital Therapy, 13,* 131-143.

McCrory, D., Penzien, D., Hasselblad, V., & Gray, R. (2001). *Behavioral and physical treatments for tension-type and cervicogenic headache (2085).* Des Moines, IA: Foundation for Chiropractic Education and Research.

McCubbin, J. (1993). Stress and endogenous opioids: Behavioral and circulatory interactions. *Biological Psychology, 35,* 91-122.

McCunney, R. J. (Ed.). (2003). *A practical approach to occupational and environmental medicine* (3rd ed.). Philadelphia: Lippincott, Williams & Wilkins.

McDonald, H. P., Garg, A. X., & Haynes, R. B. (2002). Interventions to enhance patient adherence to medication prescriptions. *Journal of the American Medical Association, 288*(22), 2868-2879.

McEwen, B. S. (1998). Protective and damaging effects of stress mediators. *New England Journal of Medicine, 338,* 171-179.

McEwen, B. S. (2000). The neurobiology of stress: from serendipity to clinical relevance. *Brain Research, 886,* 172-189.

McEwen, B. S. (2001). From molecules to mind: Stress, individual differences, and the social environment. *Annals of the New York Academy of Sciences, 925,* 42-49.

McEwen, B. S. (2002). Research to understand the mechanisms through which social and behavioral factors influence health. In L. F. Berkman (Ed.), *Through the kaleidoscope: Viewing the contributions of the behavioral and social sciences to health* (pp. 31-35). Washington, DC: National Academy Press.

McEwen, B. S., & Wingfield, J. C. (2003). The concept of allostasis in biology and biomedicine. *Hormones and Behavior, 43,* 2-15.

McGinnis, J. M., & Foege, W. H. (1993). Actual causes of death in the United States. *Journal of the American Medical Association 270,* 2207-2212.

McGinnis, J. M., Williams-Russo, P., & Knickman, J. R. (2002). The case for more active policy attention to health promotion. *Health Affairs, 21*(2), 78-93.

McGrady, A., & Bailey, B. (1995). Biofeedback-assisted relaxation and diabetes mellitus. In M. S. Schwartz (Ed.), *Biofeedback: A practitioner's guide* (2nd ed., pp. 471-492). New York: Guilford.

McKeigue, P. M., Ferrie, J. E., Pierpoint, T., & Marmot, M. G. (1993). Association of early-onset coronary heart disease in South Asian men with glucose intolerance and hyperinsulinemia. *Circulation, 87,* 153-161.

McKetney, E. C., & Ragland, D. R. (1996). John Henryism, education, and blood pressure in young adults: The CARDIA study. *American Journal of Epidemiology, 143,* 787-791.

McKhann, G., Drachman, D., Folstein, M., Katzman, R., Price, D., & Stadlan, E. M. (1984). Clinical diagnosis of Alzheimer's disease. Report of the NINCDS-ADRDA Work Group under the auspices of Department of Health and Human Services Task Force on Alzheimer's Disease. *Neurology, 34,* 939-944.

McNeilly, M. D., Anderson, N. B., Armstead, C. A., Clark, R., Corbett, M., Robinson, E. L., et al. (1996). The perceived racism scale: A multidimensional assessment of the experience of White racism among African Americans. *Ethnicity and Disease, 6,* 154-166.

McSweeny, A. J., & Grant, I. (Eds.). (1988). *Chronic obstructive pulmonary disease: A behavioral perspective.* New York: Marcel Dekker.

McTiernan, A., Ulrich, C., Slate, S., & Potter, J. (1998). Physical activity and cancer etiology: Associations and mechanisms. *Cancer Causes and Control, 9,* 487-509.

Meenan, R. F. (1982). The AIMS approach to health status measurement. *Journal of Rheumatology 9,* 785-788.

Meesters, C. M., & Appels, A. (1996). An interview to measure vital exhaustion, I and II. *Psychological Health, 11,* 557-581.

Melzack, R. (1975). The McGill Pain Questionnaire: Major properties and scoring methods. *Pain, 1,* 277-299.

Melzack, R. (1987). The short-form McGill Pain Questionnaire. *Pain, 30,* 191-197.

Melzack, R. (1989). Phantom limbs, the self and the brain (The D. O. Hebb Memorial Lecture). *Canadian Psychology, 30,* 1-14.

Melzack, R. (1990). Phantom limbs and the concept of a neuromatrix. *Trends in Neuroscience, 13,* 88-92.

Melzack, R. (1991). The gate control theory 25 years later: New perspectives on phantom limb pain. In M. R. Bond, J. E. Charlton, & C. J. Woolf (Eds.), *Pain research and* therapy: Proceedings of the 6th World Congress on Pain (pp. 9-21). Amsterdam: Elsevier.

Melzack, R. (1998). Pain and stress: Clues toward understanding chronic pain. In M. Sabourin, F. Craik, & M. Robert (Eds.), *Advances in psychological science: Vol. 2. Biological and cognitive aspects* (pp. 63-85). Hove, UK: Psychology Press.

Melzack, R. (1999). Pain and stress: A new perspective. In R. J. Gatchel & D. C. Turk (Eds.), *Psychological factors in pain*. New York: Guilford.

Melzack, R. (2001). Pain and the neuromatrix in the brain. *Journal of Dental Education, 65*, 1378-1382.

Melzack, R., & Casey, K. L. (1968). Sensory, motivational and central control determinants of pain: A new conceptual model. In D. Kenshalo (Ed.), *The skin senses* (pp. 423-443). Springfield, IL: Charles C Thomas.

Melzack, R., & Loeser, J. D. (1978). Phantom body pain in paraplegics: Evidence for a central "pattern generating mechanism" for pain. *Pain, 4*, 195-210.

Melzack, R., & Wall, P. D. (1965). Pain mechanisms: A new theory. *Science, 150*, 971-979.

Melzack, R., & Wall, P. D. (1996). *The challenge of pain* (Updated 2nd ed.). London: Penguin.

Mendias, E. P., Clark, M. C., & Guevara, E. B. (2001, April). Women's self-perception and self-care practice: Implications for health care delivery. *Health Care for Women International, 22*, 3.

Menon, A. S., Campbell, D., Ruskin, P., & Hebel, J. R. (2000). Depression, hopelessness, and the desire for life-saving treatments among elderly medically ill veterans. *American Journal of Geriatric Psychiatry, 8*, 333-342.

Merritt, M. M., Bennett, G. G., Sollers, J., Edwards, C. L., & Williams, R. B. (in press). Low educational attainment, John Henryism and cardiovascular reactivity and recovery to personally-relevant stress. *Psychosomatic Medicine*.

Meyer, T. J., & Melvin, M. M. (1995). Effects of psychosocial interventions with adult cancer patients: A meta-analysis of randomized experiments. *Health Psychology, 14*(2), 101-108.

Meyerowitz, B. E., & Chaiken, S. (1987). The effect of message framing on breast self-examination attitudes, intentions, and behavior. *Journal of Personality and Social Psychology, 52*, 500-510.

Meyers, R. J., & Miller, W. R. (2001). *A community reinforcement approach to addiction treatment.* Cambridge, UK: Cambridge University Press.

Micozzi, M. S. (1996). Characteristics of complementary and alternative medicine. In M. S. Micozzi (Ed.), *Fundamentals of complementary and alternative medicine* (pp. 3-8). New York: Churchill Livingstone.

Midence, K., McManus, C., Fuggle, P., & Davies, S. (1996). Psychological adjustment and family functioning in a group of British children with sickle cell disease: Preliminary empirical findings and a meta-analysis. *British Journal of Clinical Psychology, 35*, 439-450.

Miettinen, O. S. (1972). Components of the crude risk ratio. *American Journal of Epidemiology, 96*, 168-172.

Mill, J. S. (1956). *A system of logic, ratiocinative and inductive*. London: Longmans, Green. (Original work published 1843)

Miller, B., & Cafasso, L. (1992). Gender differences in caregiving: Fact or artifact? *Gerontologist, 32*, 498-507.

Miller, G. E., & Cohen, S. (2001). Psychological interventions and the immune system: A meta-analytic review and critique. *Health Psychology, 20*, 47-63.

Miller, N. H., & Taylor, C. B. (1995). *Lifestyle management in patients with coronary heart disease*. Champaign, IL: Human Kinetics.

Miller, S. (1995). Monitoring versus blunting styles of coping with cancer influence the information patients want and need about their disease: Implications for cancer screening and management. *Cancer, 76*, 167-177.

Miller, S., Shoda, Y., & Hurley, K. (1996). Applying cognitive-social theory to health protective behavior: Breast self-examination in cancer screening. *Psychological Bulletin, 119*, 70-94.

Miller, S. M., Mischel, W., O'Leary, A., & Mills, M. (1996). From human papillomavirus (HPV) to cervical cancer: Psychosocial processes in infection, detection, and control. *Annals of Behavioral Medicine, 18*, 219-228.

Miller, S. M., Mischel, W., Schroeder, C. M., Buzaglo, J. S., Hurley, K., Schreiber, P., et al. (1998). *Psychology and Health, 13*, 847-858.

Miller, T. Q., Smith, T. W., Turner, C. W., Guijarro, M. L., & Hallet, A. J. (1996). A meta-analytic review of research on hostility and physical health. *Psychological Bulletin, 119*, 322-348.

Miller, T. R., Romano, E. O., & Spicer, R. S. (2000). The cost of childhood unintentional injuries and the value of prevention. *Future of Children, 10*(1), 137-163.

Miller, W., & Crabtree, B. (1994). Clinical research. In N. Denzin & Y. Lincoln (Eds.), *The handbook of qualitative research* (pp. 340-352). Thousand Oaks, CA: Sage.

Miller, W. R. (Ed.). (1999). *Integrating spirituality into treatment: Resources for practitioners*. Washington, DC: American Psychological Association.

Miller, W. R., & Rollnick, S. (1991). *Motivational interviewing: Preparing people for change*. New York: Guilford.

Miller, W. R., & Rollnick, S. (2002). Motivational interviewing: Preparing people for change (2nd ed.). New York: Guilford.

Minkler, M., & Wallerstein, N. (Eds.). (2003). *Community-based participatory research for health*. San Francisco: Jossey-Bass.

Minor, M. A. (1996). Rest and exercise. In S. T. Wegener, B. L. Belza, & E. P. Gall (Eds.), *Clinical care in the rheumatic diseases* (pp. 73-78). Atlanta, GA: American College of Rheumatology.

Mirowksy, J., & Ross, C. E. (1989). *Social causes of psychological distress*. New York: Aldine de Gruyter.

Mischel, W., & Shoda, Y. (1995). A cognitive-affective system theory of personality: Reconceptualizing situations, dispositions, dynamics, and invariance in personality structure. *Psychological Review, 102*, 246-268.

Mischler, E. (1986). *Research interviewing: Context and narrative*. Cambridge, MA: Harvard University Press.

Misra, D. (Ed.). (2001). *The women's health data book: A profile of women's health in the United States* (3rd ed., pp. 14-45). Washington, DC: Jacobs Institute of Women's Health.

Mittelmark, M. B., Hunt, M. K., Heath, G. W., & Schmid, T. L. (1993). Realistic outcomes: Lessons from community-based research and demonstration programs for the prevention of cardiovascular diseases. *Journal of Public Health Policy, 14*, 437-462.

Mittleman, M. A., Maclure, M., Sherwood, J. B., Mulry, R. P., Tofler, G. H., Jacobs, S. C., Friedman, R., Benson, H., & Muller, J. E. (1995). Triggering of acute myocardial infarction onset by episodes of anger. Determinants of Myocardial Infarction Onset Study Investigators [See comments]. *Circulation, 92*(7), 1720-1725.

Moher, D., Schulz, K. F., & Altman, D. G. (2001). The CONSORT statement: Revised recommendations for improving the quality of reports of parallel-group randomised trials [Comment]. *Lancet, 357*, 1191-1194.

Mohr, D. C., Boudewyn, A. C., Goodkin, D. E., Siskin, L. P., Epstein, L., Cheuk, W., & Lee, L. (2001). Comparative outcomes for individual cognitive-behavioral therapy, supportive-expressive group therapy, and sertraline for the treatment of depression in multiple sclerosis. *Journal of Consulting and Clinical Psychology, 69*, 942-949.

Mohr, D. C., & Cox, D. (2001). Multiple sclerosis: Empirical literature for the clinical health psychologist. *Journal of Clinical Psychology, 57*, 479-499.

Mohr, D. C., Goodkin, D. E., Bacchetti, P., Boudewyn, A. C., Huang, L., Marrietta, P., Cheuk, W., & Dee, B. (2000). Psychological stress and the subsequent appearance of new brain MRI lesions in MS. *Neurology, 55*, 55-61.

Mohr, D. C., Goodkin, D. E., Islar, J., Hauser, S. L., & Genain, C. P. (2001). Treatment of depression is associated with suppression of nonspecific and antigen-specific T(H)1 responses in multiple sclerosis. *Archives of Neurology, 58,* 1081-1086.

Mohr, D. C., Likosky, W., Dick, L. P., Van Der Wende, J., Dwyer, P., Bertagnolli, A. C., & Goodkin, D. E. (2000). Telephone-administered cognitive-behavioral therapy for the treatment of depressive symptoms in multiple sclerosis. *Journal of Consulting and Clinical Psychology, 68*, 356-361.

Molnar, B. E., Buka, S. L., & Kessler, R. C. (2001). Child sexual abuse and subsequent psychopathology: Results from the National Comorbidity Survey. *American Journal of Public Health, 91*, 753-760.

Monastra, V. J., Monastra, D. M., & George, S. (2002). The effects of stimulant therapy, EEG biofeedback and parenting style on the primary symptoms of attention-deficit/hyperactive disorder. *Applied Psychophysiology and Biofeedback, 27*, 231-249.

Monheit, A. C., Wilson, R., & Arnett, R. H. (1998). *Informing American health care policy: The dynamics of medical expenditure and insurance surveys, 1977-1996*. New York: John Wiley.

Montgomery, S. A., & Asberg, M. (1979). A new depression scale designed to be sensitive to change. *British Journal of Psychiatry, 134*, 382-389.

Moos, R. H. (1997). Coping Responses Inventory. In C. P. Zalaquett & R. J. Wood (Eds.), *Evaluating stress: A book of resources* (pp. 51-65). Lanham, MD: Scarecrow.

Morgan, W. P. (Ed.). (1997). *Physical activity and mental health*. New York: Taylor & Francis.

Morin, C. M., Culbert, J. P., & Schwartz, S. M. (1994). Nonpharmacological interventions for insomnia: A meta-analysis of treatment efficacy. *American Journal of Psychiatry, 151*, 1172-1180.

Morris, J. N., Kagan, A., Pattison, D. C., Gardner, M. J., & Raffle, P. A. B. (1966). Incidence and prediction of ischaemic heart-disease in London busmen. *Lancet, 2*, 553-559.

Morrow, L. A., Steinhauer, S. R., Condray, R., & Hodgson, M. (1997). Neuropsychological performance of journeymen painters under acute solvent exposure and exposure-free conditions. *Journal of the International Neuropsychological Society, 3*, 269-275.

Moseley, J. B., O'Malley, K., Petersen, N. J., Menke, T. J., Brody, B., Kuykendall, D. H., et al. (2002). A controlled trial of arthroscopic surgery for osteoarthritis of the knee. *New England Journal of Medicine, 347,* 81-88.

Moser, D. K., & Dracup, K. (1996). Is anxiety early after myocardial infarction associated with subsequent ischemic and arrhythmic events? *Psychosomatic Medicine, 58*(5), 395-401.

Mueller, T., & Leon, A. (1996). Recovery, chronicity, and levels of psychopathology in major depression. *Psychiatric Clinics of North America, 19,* 85-102.

Muldoon, M. F., Waldstein, S. R., Ryan, C. M., Jennings, J. R., Polefrone, J. M., Shapiro, A. P., et al. (2002). Effects of six antihypertensive medications on cognitive performance. *Journal of Hypertension, 20,* 1643-1652.

Mullington, J., & Broughton, R. (1993). Scheduled naps in the management of daytime sleepiness in narcolepsy-cataplexy. *Sleep, 16,* 444-456.

Mulrow, C., & Cook, D. (1998). *Systematic reviews: Synthesis of best evidence for health care decisions.* Philadelphia: American College of Physicians.

Multiple Risk Factor Intervention Trial Research Group. (1982). Multiple Risk Factor Intervention Trial: Risk factor changes and mortality results. *Journal of the American Medical Association, 248,* 1465-1477.

Multiple Risk Factor Intervention Trial Research Group. (1996). Mortality after 16 years for participants randomized to the Multiple Risk Factor Intervention Trial. *Circulation, 94,* 946-951.

Murphy, S. L. (2000). Deaths: Final data for 1998. *National Vital Statistics Report, 48,* 1-105.

Murray, C. J. L., & Lopez, A. D. (Eds.). (1996). *The global burden of disease: A comprehensive assessment of mortality and disability from diseases, injuries, and risk factors in 1990 and projected to 2020.* Boston: Harvard School of Public Health, World Health Organization, and World Bank.

Murtagh, D. R., & Greenwood, K. M. (1995). Identifying effective psychological treatments for insomnia: A meta-analysis. *Journal of Consulting and Clinical Psychology, 63,* 79-89.

Musante, L., Treiber, F. A., Davis, H., Strong, W. B., & Levy, M. (1992). Hostility: Relationship to lifestyle behaviors and physical risk factors. *Behavioral Medicine, 18,* 21-26.

Musgrave, C. F., Allen, C. E., & Allen, G. J. (2002). Spirituality and health for women of color. *American Journal of Public Health, 92,* 557-560.

Myers, L. B. (2000). Identifying repressors: A methodological issue for health psychology. *Psychology and Health, 15,* 205-214.

Myers, L. B., & Brewin, C. R. (1994). Recall of early experience and the repressive coping style. *Journal of Abnormal Psychology, 103,* 288-292.

Myrtek, M. (2001). Meta-analyses of prospective studies on coronary heart disease, Type A personality, and hostility. *International Journal of Cardiology, 79,* 245-251.

Nader, P. R., Stone, E. J., Lytle, L. A., Perry, C. L., Osganian, S. K., Kelder, S., Webber, L. S., Elder, J. P., Montgomery, D., Feldman, H. A., Wu, M., Johnson, C., Parcel, G., & Luepker, R. V. (1999). Three-year maintenance of improved diet and physical activity: The CATCH cohort. *Archives of Pediatrics and Adolescent Medicine, 153*(7), 695-704.

Nahin, R. L., & Straus, S. E. (2001). Research into complementary and alternative medicine: Problems and potential. *British Medical Journal, 322,* 161-164.

Nakajima, A., Hirai, H., & Yoshino, S. (1999). Reassessment of mirthful laughter in rheumatoid arthritis. *Journal of Rheumatology, 26,* 512-513.

Nathan, P. E. (1998). Practice guidelines: Not yet ideal. *American Psychologist, 53,* 290-299.

National Cancer Institute. (n.d.). *Clear & simple: Developing effective print materials for low-literate readers.* Retrieved August 28, 2002, from http://oc.nci.nih.gov/services/clear_and_simple/home.htm

National Center for Chronic Disease Prevention and Health Promotion. (2002). *The burden of chronic diseases and their risk factors: National and state perspectives.* U.S. Department of Health and Human Services. Retrieved from http://www.cdc.gov/nccdphp/burdenbook2002/index.htm

National Center for Complementary and Alternative Medicine. (2002a, May 10). *About NCCAM: General information.* Retrieved from http://nccam.nih.gov/an/general

National Center for Complementary and Alternative Medicine. (2002b, May 11). *For consumers and practitioners: Major domains of complementary and alternative medicine.* Retrieved from http://nccam.nih.gov/fcp/classify

National Center for Health Statistics Vital Statistics System. (2003). *Web-based injury statistics query and reporting system.* Retrieved from http://www.cdc.gov/ncipc/wisqars/

National Center for Health Statistics. (1998). *Health, United States.* Retrieved from www1.oecd.org/std/ others1.html

National Center for Health Statistics. (1999). *National vital statistics report, 47*(19). U.S. Department of Health and Human Services.

National Center for Injury Prevention and Control. (2001). *Injury fact book 2001-2002*. Atlanta, GA: Centers for Disease Control and Prevention.

National Center for Injury Prevention and Control. (2003). *Childhood injury fact sheet*. Retrieved from http://www.cdc.gov/ncipc/factsheets/childh.htm

National Cholesterol Education Program Expert Panel on Detection, Evaluation and Treatment of High Blood Cholesterol in Adults. (2001, May). *Third Report of the National Cholesterol Education Program (NCEP) Expert Panel on Detection, Evaluation and Treatment of High Blood Cholesterol in Adults (ATP-III)*. Retrieved December 2002 from http://www.nhlbi.nih.gov and http://www.guidelines.gov

National Cholesterol Education Program Expert Panel on Detection, Evaluation and Treatment of High Blood Cholesterol in Adults. (2001). Executive summary of the Third Report of the National Cholesterol Education Program (NCEP) Expert Panel on Detection, Evaluation and Treatment of High Blood Cholesterol in Adults (ATP-III). *Journal of the American Medical Association, 285*, 2486-2497.

National Committee for Injury Prevention and Control. (1989). Injury prevention: Meeting the challenge. *American Journal of Preventive Medicine, 5*(3 Suppl.), 1-303.

National Heart, Lung, and Blood Institute, National Institutes of Health. (1998). Clinical guidelines on the identification, evaluation, and treatment of overweight and obesity in adults: The evidence report. *Obesity Research, 6*(Suppl. 2), 51S-209S.

National Institute on Alcohol Abuse and Alcoholism. (2000). *10th Special report to the U.S. Congress on alcohol and health*. NIH Publication No. 00-1583. Rockville, MD: National Institutes of Health.

National Institute of Environmental Health Sciences. (2002, July 25). *NIEHS strategic plan for eliminating environmental health disparities*. Retrieved August 9, 2002, from National Institutes of Health, http://www.niehs.nih.gov/dert/programs/translat/hd/healthdis.htm

National Institute of Mental Health (NIMH) Multisite HIV Prevention Trial Group. (1998). The NIMH multisite HIV prevention trial: Reducing HIV sexual risk behavior. *Science, 280*, 1889-1894.

National Institutes of Health. (1997). *National Asthma Education Program Expert Panel: Clinical Practice Guidelines Expert Panel Report 2: Guidelines for the diagnosis and management of asthma* (DHHS Publication No. 97-4051). Washington, DC: Government Printing Office.

National Research Council. (2001). *New horizons in health: An integrative approach*. Washington, DC: National Academy Press.

National Sleep Foundation. (2002). *Sleep in America poll*. Washington, DC: Author.

Neale, M. C., & Cardon, L. R. (Eds.). (1992). *Methodology for genetic studies of twins and families*. Dordrecht, the Netherlands: Kluwer Academic Press.

Neel, J. V. (1962). Diabetes mellitus: A "thrifty" genotype rendered detrimental by "progress"? *American Journal of Human Genetics, 14*, 353-362.

Nelson, K., Norris, K., & Mangione, C. M. (2002). Disparities in the diagnosis and pharmacologic treatment of high serum cholesterol by race and ethnicity: Data from the Third National Health and Nutrition Examination Survey. *Archives of Internal Medicine, 162*, 929-935.

Ness, R. B., & Kuller, L. H. (Eds.). (1999). *Health and disease among women*. New York: Oxford University Press.

Nestle, M. (2002). *Food politics: How the food industry influences nutrition and health*. Berkeley: University of California Press.

Neugebauer, R. (1999). Mind matters: The importance of mental disorders in public health's 21st century mission. *American Journal of Public Health, 89*, 1309-1311.

Newhouse, J. P. (1993). *Free for all? Lessons from the RAND Health Insurance Experiment*. Cambridge, MA: Harvard University Press.

Nezu, A. M., Nezu, C. M., Friedman, S. H., Faddis, S., & Houts, P. S. (1998). *A problem-solving approach: Helping cancer patients cope*. Washington, DC: American Psychological Association.

Nicassio, P. M., & Greenberg, M. A. (2001). The effectiveness of cognitive-behavioral and psychoeducational interventions in the management of arthritis. In M. H. Weisman & J. Louie (Eds.), *Treatment of rheumatic diseases* (2nd ed., pp. 147-161). Orlando, FL: William Saunders.

Nielson, W. R., Walker, C., & McCain, G. A. (1992). Cognitive behavioral treatment of fibromyalgia syndrome: Preliminary findings. *Journal of Rheumatology, 19*, 98-103.

NIH Consensus Panel. (2000). National Institutes of Health Consensus Development Conference Statement, February 11-13, 1997. *AIDS, 14*(2), S85-S96.

Noll, R. B., Vanatta, K., & Koontz, K. (1996). Peer relationships and emotional well-being of youngsters with sickle cell disease. *Child Development, 67*, 423-436.

Noordenbos, W. (1959). *Pain*. Amsterdam: Elsevier.

Norbeck, J., DeJoseph, J. F., & Smith, R. T. (1996). A randomized trial of an empirically derived social support intervention to prevent low birth weight among African

American women. *Social Science and Medicine, 43,* 947-954.

Norem, J. K. (2001). *The positive power of negative thinking: Using defensive pessimism to harness anxiety and perform at your peak.* New York: Basic Books.

Norris, F. H., Friedman, M. J., & Watson, P. J. (2002). 60,000 disaster victims speak, Part II: Summary and implications of the disaster mental health research. *Psychiatry, 65,* 240-260.

Norris, F. H., Friedman, M. J., Watson, P. J., Byrne, C. M., Diaz, E., & Kaniasty, K. (2002). 60,000 disaster victims speak, Part I: An empirical review of the empirical literature, 1981-2001. *Psychiatry, 65,* 207-239.

Norris, S. L., Nichols, P. J., Caspersen, C. J., Glasgow, R. E., Engelgan, M. M., et al. (2002). Increasing diabetes self-management education in community settings: A systematic review. *American Journal of Preventive Medicine, 22,* 39-66.

Norris, V. K., Stephens, M. P., & Kinney, J. M. (1990). The impact of family interactions on recovery from stroke: Help or hindrance? *Gerontologist, 30,* 535-542.

O'Boyle, C., McGee, H., Hickey, A., O'Malley, K., & Joyce, C. (1992). Individual quality of life in patients undergoing hip replacement. *Lancet 339,* 1088-1091.

Obrist, P. A. (1981). *Cardiovascular psychophysiology: A perspective.* New York: Plenum.

Ockene, J., Emmons, K., Mermelstein, R., Perkins, K., Bonollo, D., Voorhees, C., & Hollis, J. (2000). Relapse and maintenance issues for smoking cessation. *Health Psychology, 19*(Suppl. 1), 17-31.

O'Connor Sauer, W. H., Berlin, J. A., & Kimmel, S. E. (2001). Selective serotonin reuptake inhibitors and myocardial infarction. *Circulation, 104,* 1894-1898.

Office of Behavioral and Social Sciences Research, National Institutes of Health, Department of Health and Human Services. (2003). Retrieved from http://obssr.od.nih.gov/

Office of Disease Prevention and Health Promotion. (2002). *Health communication objectives for Healthy People 2010.* Washington, DC: U.S. Department of Health and Human Services.

Offit, K. (1998). *Clinical cancer genetics: Risk counseling and management.* New York: John Wiley.

Ohman, A. (2000). Fear and anxiety: Evolutionary, cognitive, and clinical perspectives. In M. Lewis & J. M. Haviland-Jones (Eds.), *Handbook of emotions* (2nd ed., pp. 573-593). New York: Guilford.

Okifuji, A., Turk, D. C., Sinclair, J. D., Starz, T. W., & Marcus, D. A. (1997). A standardized manual tender point survey: Development and determination of a threshold point for the identification of positive tender points in fibromyalgia. *Journal of Rheumatology, 24,* 377-383.

Olafson, E., Corwin, D. L., & Summit, R. C. (1993). Modern history of child sexual abuse awareness: Cycles of discovery and suppression. *Child Abuse & Neglect, 17,* 7-24.

Oldridge, N. B., Guyatt, G. H., Fisher, M. E., & Rimm, A. A. (1988). Cardiac rehabilitation after myocardial infarction: Combined experience of randomized clinical trials. *Journal of the American Medical Association, 260,* 945-990.

Olesen, J. C. (1988). Classification and diagnostic criteria for headache disorders, cranial neuralgias, and facial pain: Headache Classification Committee of the International Headache Society. *Cephalalgia, 8*(Suppl. 7).

Ong, L. M. L., de Haes, J. C., Hoos, A. M., & Lammes, F. B. (1995). Doctor-patient communication: A review of the literature. *Social Science and Medicine, 40,* 903-918.

Orleans, C. T. (2000). Promoting the maintenance of health behavior change: Recommendations for the next generation of research and practice. *Health Psychology, 19,* 76-83.

Orleans, C. T., Gruman, J., & Anderson, N. (1999, March). *Roadmaps for the next frontier: Getting evidence-based behavioral medicine into practice.* Paper presented at the Society of Behavioral Medicine, San Diego, CA.

Orleans, C. T., Gruman, J., Ulmer, C., Emont, S. L., & Hollendonner, J. K. (1999). Rating our progress in population health promotion: Report card on six behaviors. *American Journal of Health Promotion, 14,* 75-82.

Orme-Johnson, D., & Walton, K. (1998). All approaches to preventing or reversing effects of stress are not the same. *American Journal of Health Promotion, 12*(5), 297-299.

Orth-Gomér, K., Wamala, S. P., Horsten, M., Schenck-Gustafsson, K., & Mittleman, M. (2000). Marital stress worsens prognosis in women with coronary heart disease: The Stockholm Female Coronary Risk Study. *Journal of the American Medical Association, 284*(23), 3008-3014.

Osler, W. (1892). *Lectures on angina pectoris and allied states.* New York: Appleton.

Osterweis, M. (1985). Bereavement and the elderly. *Aging, 348,* 8-13, 41.

Ostir, G. V., Markides, K. S., Peek, M. K., & Goodwin, J. S. (2001). The association between emotional well-being and the incidence of stroke in older adults. *Psychosomatic Medicine, 63,* 210-215.

Ostrove, J. M., & Adler, N. E. (1998). Socioeconomic status and health. *Current Opinion in Psychiatry, 11*, 649-653.

Overmier, J. B., & Murison, R. (2000). Anxiety and helplessness in the face of stress predisposes, precipitates, and sustains gastric ulceration. *Behavioral Brain Research, 110*, 161-174.

Pablos-Méndez, A. (1994). Letter to the editor. *Journal of the American Medical Association, 271*, 1237-1238.

Paffenbarger, R. S., Jr., Hyde, R. T., Wing, A. L., & Hsieh, C. (1986). Physical activity, all-cause mortality, and longevity of college alumni. *New England Journal of Medicine, 314*, 605-613.

Paffenbarger, R. S., Jr., Hyde, R. T., Wing, A. L., Lee, I-M., Jung, D. L., & Kampert, J. B. (1993). The association of changes in physical activity level and other lifestyle characteristics with mortality among men. *New England Journal of Medicine, 328*, 538-545.

Paffenbarger, R. S., Jr., Wing, A. L., & Hyde, R. T. (1978). Physical activity as an index of heart attack risk in college alumni. *American Journal of Epidemiology, 108*, 161-175.

Palmer, S., & Glass, T. A. (in press). Family function and stroke recovery: A review. *Rehabilitation Psychology*.

Pan American Health Organization. (1996). *Health promotion: An anthology*. Scientific Publication No. 557. Washington, DC: PAHO, World Health Organization.

Panel on Definition and Description, C.R.M.C. (1995). Defining and describing complementary and alternative medicine. *Alternative Therapies in Health and Medicine, 3*(2), 49-57.

Parati, G., DiRienzo, M., Ulian, L., Santucciu, C., Girard, A., Elghozi, J.-L., & Mancia, G. (1998). Clinical relevance of blood pressure variability. *Journal of Hypertension, 16*(Suppl. 3), S25-S33.

Parati, G., & Lantelme, P. (2002). Blood pressure variability, target organ damage and cardiovascular events. *Journal of Hypertension, 20*, 1725-1729.

Parati, G., Omboni, S., & Mancia, G. (1995). Experience with continuous non-invasive finger blood pressure monitoring: A new research tool. *Homeostasis, 36*, 139-152.

Parcel, G. S., O'Hara-Tompkins, N. M., Harrist, R. B., Basen-Engquist, K. M., McCormick, L. K., Gottlieb, N. H., et al. (1995). Diffusion of an effective tobacco prevention program. Part II: Evaluation of the adoption phase. *Health Education Research, 10*, 297-307.

Pargament, K. I. (1997). *The psychology of religion and coping: Theory, research, and practice*. New York: Guilford.

Park, C. L., Cohen, L. H., & Murch, R. (1996). Assessment and prediction of stress-related growth. *Journal of Personality, 64*, 71-105.

Park, C. L., & Folkman, S. (1997). Meaning in the context of stress and coping. *Review of General Psychology, 1*, 115-144.

Parker, J. C., & Wright, G. E. (1995). The implication of depression for pain and disability in rheumatoid arthritis. *Arthritis Care and Research, 8*(4), 279-283.

Parkes, C. M. (1972). *Bereavement: Studies of grief in the adult life*. New York: International Universities Press.

Pasick, R. J. (2001). Response to Kreuter and Skinner. *Health Education Research, 16*, 503-505.

Pasternak, R. C., Smith, S. C., Jr., Bairey-Merz, C. D. N., et al. (2002). ACC/AHA/NHLBI clinical advisory on the use and safety of statins. *Circulation; 106*, 1024-1028.

Patenaude A. F. (in press). *Psychological aspects of cancer genetic testing*. Washington, DC: American Psychological Association.

Paterniti, S., Zureik, M., Ducimetiere, P. J. T., Feve, J. M., & Alperovitch, A. (2001). Sustained anxiety and 4-year progression of carotid atherosclerosis. *Arteriosclerosis Thrombosis and Vascular Biology, 21*, 136-141.

Paterson, D. L., Swindells, S., Mohr, J., Brester, M., Vergis, E., Squier, C., Wagener, M., & Singh, N. (2000). Adherence to protease inhibitor therapy and outcomes in patients with HIV infection. *Annals of Internal Medicine, 133*, 21-30.

Patrick, K., Sallis, J. F., Prochaska, J. J., Lydston, D. D., Calfas, K. J., Zabinski, M. F., et al. (2001). A multicomponent program for nutrition and physical activity change in primary care: PACE+ for adolescents. *Archives of Pediatrics and Adolescent Medicine, 155*, 940-951.

Pavlov, I. P. (1927). *Conditioned reflexes*. London and New York: Oxford University Press.

Payne, A., & Blanchard, E. B. (1995). A controlled comparison of cognitive therapy and self-help support groups in the treatment of irritable bowel syndrome. *Journal of Consulting and Clinical Psychology, 63*, 779-786.

Payne, J. G. (2002). Principles of oral communication for health professionals. In D. Nelson (Ed.), *Health communication*. Washington, DC: American Public Health Association.

Payne, J. G., & Ratzan, S. C. (1993). A thinking globally, acting locally AIDS Action 2000 Plan: The COAST model—Health communication as negotiation. In S. C. Ratzan (Ed.), *AIDS: Effective health communication for the 1990s* (pp. 233-254). Washington, DC: Taylor & Francis.

Pearl, J. (2000). *Causality*. New York: Cambridge University Press.

Pearl, M., Braveman, P., & Abrams, B. (2001). The relationship of neighborhood socioeconomic characteristics to birthweight among 5 ethnic groups in California. *American Journal of Public Health, 91*, 1808-1814.

Pearlin, L. I., & Schooler, C. (1978). The structure of coping. *Journal of Health and Social Behavior, 19*, 2-21.

Pelletier, K. R. (2001). A review and analysis of the clinical- and cost-effectiveness studies of comprehensive health promotion and disease management programs at the worksite: 1998-2000 update. *American Journal of Health Promotion, 16*, 107-116.

Pelto, P. J., & Pelto, G. H. (1978). *Anthropological research: The structure of inquiry* (2nd ed.). Cambridge, UK: Cambridge University Press.

Penaz, J. (1973). Photoelectric measurement of blood pressure, volume, and flow in the finger. In *Digest of the 10th International Conference on Medical and Biological Engineering.* Dresden, Germany.

Pennebaker, J. W. (1989). Stream of consciousness and stress: Levels of thinking. In J. S. Uleman & J. A. Bargh (Eds.), *Unintended thought* (pp. 327-350). New York: Guilford.

Pennebaker, J. W. (1997). *Opening up: The healing power of expressing emotion.* New York: Guilford.

Pennebaker, J. W., & Francis, M. E. (1996). Cognitive, emotional, and language processes in disclosure. *Cognition & Emotion, 10*, 601-626.

Pennebaker, J. W., Francis, M. E., & Booth, R. J. (2001). *Linguistic Inquiry and Word Count (LIWC): A computerized text analysis program.* Mahwah, NJ: Lawrence Erlbaum.

Pennebaker, J. W., Mayne, T. J., & Francis, M. E. (1997). Linguistic predictors of adaptive bereavement. *Journal of Personality & Social Psychology, 72*, 863-871.

Penninx, B., Geerlings, S., Deeg, D., van Eijk, J., van Tilling, W., & Beekman, A. (2001). Minor and major depression and the risk of death in older persons. *Archives of General Psychiatry, 56*, 889-895.

Penninx, B. W., Beekman, A. T., Honig, A., Deeg, D. J., Schoevers, R. A., van Eijk, J. T., & van Tilburg, W. (2001). Depression and cardiac mortality: Results from a community-based longitudinal study. *Archives of General Psychiatry, 58*(3), 221-227.

Penninx, B. W., Guralnik, J. M., Pahor, M., Ferrucci, L., Cerhan, J. R., Wallace, R. B., et al. (1998). Chronically depressed mood and cancer risk in older persons. *Journal of the National Cancer Institute, 90*, 1888-1893.

Penninx, B. W., van Tilburg, T., Kriegsman, D. M., Deeg, D. J., Boeke, A. J., & van Eijk, J. T. (1997). Effects of social support and personal coping resources on mortality in older age: The Longitudinal Aging Study, Amsterdam. *American Journal of Epidemiology, 146*, 510-519.

Pentz, M. A. (1999a). Effective prevention programs for tobacco use. *Nicotine & Tobacco Research, 1*(Suppl. 2), 99-107.

Pentz, M. A. (1999b). Prevention. In M. Galanter & H. Kleber (Eds.), *American Psychiatric Press textbook of substance abuse* (2nd ed., pp. 535-544). Washington, DC: American Psychiatric Press.

Pentz, M. A. (1999c). Prevention aimed at individuals: An integrative transactional perspective In B. S. McCrady & E. E. Epstein (Eds.), *Addictions: A comprehensive guidebook for practitioners.* New York: Oxford University Press.

Pentz, M. A. (in press). Evidence-based prevention: Characteristics, impact, and future direction. *Journal of Psychoactive Drugs.*

Pentz, M. A., Bonnie, R. J., & Shopland, D. S. (1996). Integrating supply and demand reduction strategies for drug abuse prevention. *American Behavioral Scientist, 39*, 897-910.

Pentz, M. A., & Li, C. (2002). The gateway theory applied to prevention. In D. B. Kandel (Ed.), *Stages and pathways of drug involvement: Examining the gateway hypothesis.* Cambridge, UK: Cambridge University Press.

Pentz, M. A., & Trebow, E. (1997). Implementation issues in drug abuse prevention research. *Substance Use and Misuse, 32*, 1655-1660.

Pequegnat, W., & Stover, E. (2000). Behavioral prevention is today's AIDS vaccine! *AIDS, 14*(2), S1-S7.

Pequegnat, W., & Szapocznik, J. (2000). *Working with families in the era of AIDS.* Thousand Oaks, CA: Sage.

Perez, S. (Ed.). (2000). *Moving up the economic ladder: Latino workers and the nation's future prosperity: State of Hispanic America 1999.* Washington, DC: National Council of La Raza.

Perez, M., V. Z., Pettit, J. W., & Joiner, T. E., Jr. (2002). The role of acculturative stress and body dissatisfaction in predicting bulimic symptomatology across ethnic groups. *International Journal of Eating Disorders, 31*(4), 442-454.

Perez-Stable, E. J., Ramirez, A., Villareal, R., Talavera, G. A., Trapido, E., Suarez, L., Marti, J., & McAlister, A. (2001). Cigarette smoking behavior among U.S. Latino men and women from different countries of origin. *American Journal of Public Health, 91*, 1424-1430.

Perkins, K. (1992). Metabolic effects of cigarette smoking. *Journal of Applied Physiology, 72*, 401-409.

Perkins, K. A. (1999). Nicotine self-administration. *Nicotine and Tobacco Research, 1,* S133-S137.

Perry, C. L., Sellers, D. E., Johnson, C., Pedersen, S., Bachman, K. J., Parcel, G. S., Stone, E. J., Luepker, R. V., Wu, M., Nader, P. R., & Cook, K. (1997). The Child and Adolescent Trial for Cardiovascular Health (CATCH): Intervention, implementation, and feasibility for elementary schools in the United States. *Health Education and Behavior, 24*(6), 716-735.

Petersen, R. R. (1996). A re-evaluation of the economic consequences of divorce. *American Sociological Review, 61,* 528-536.

Petersen, T., Dording, C., Neault, N. B., Kornbluh, R., Alpert, J. E., Nierenberg, A. A., et al. (2002). A survey of prescribing practices in the treatment of depression. *Progress in Neuro-Psychopharmacology and Biological Psychiatry, 26,* 177-187.

Peterson, C., Bishop, M. P., Fletcher, C. W., Kaplan, M. R., Yesko, E. S., Moon, C. H., et al. (2001). Explanatory style as a risk factor for traumatic mishaps. *Cognitive Therapy and Research, 25,* 633-649.

Peterson, C., & Bossio, L. M. (1991). *Health and optimism.* New York: Free Press.

Peterson, C., Maier, S. F., & Seligman, M. E. P. (1993). *Learned helplessness: A theory for the age of personal control.* New York: Oxford University Press.

Peterson, C., & Seligman, M. E. P. (1984). Causal explanations as a risk factor for depression: Theory and evidence. *Psychological Review, 91,* 347-374.

Peterson, C., Seligman, M. E. P., & Vaillant, G. E. (1988). Pessimistic explanatory style is a risk factor for physical illness: A thirty-five year longitudinal study. *Journal of Personality and Social Psychology, 55,* 23-27.

Peterson, C., Seligman, M. E. P., Yurko, K. H., Martin, L. R., & Friedman, H. S. (1998). Catastrophizing and untimely death. *Psychological Science, 9,* 127-130.

Peterson, C., & Villanova, P. (1988). An Expanded Attributional Style Questionnaire. *Journal of Abnormal Psychology, 97,* 87-89.

Peterson, J. L., & DiClemente, R. J. (Eds.). (2000). *Handbook of HIV prevention.* New York: Kluwer Academic/Plenum.

Peto, R., Lopez, A. D., Boreham, J., Thun, M., & Heath, C. (1994). *Mortality from smoking in developed countries, 1950-2000: Indirect estimates from national vital statistics.* Oxford, UK: Oxford University Press.

Petraitis, J., & Flay, B. R. (2003). Bridging the gap between substance use prevention theory and practice. In W. Bukoski & Z. Sloboda (Eds.), *Handbook for drug abuse prevention: Theory, science, and practice.* New York: Plenum.

Petraitis, J., Flay, B. R., & Miller, T. Q. (1995). Reviewing theories of adolescent substance abuse: Organizing pieces of the puzzle. *Psychological Bulletin, 117,* 67-86.

Petraitis, J., Flay, B. R., Miller, T. Q., Torpy, E. J., & Greiner, B. (1998). Illicit substance use among adolescents: A matrix of prospective predictors. *Substance Use and Misuse, 33,* 2561-2604.

Pfeffer, J. (1998). *Human equation: Building profits by putting people first.* Boston: Harvard Business School Press.

Pharmaceutical Research and Manufacturers of America. (1999). Facts about diseases/conditions affecting women. *New Medicines in Development for Women,* 29-34.

Phelan, J. C., Link, B. G., Diez-Roux, A., et al. (1999). *Preventability of death and SES gradients in mortality: A fundamental cause perspective.* Presented at the annual meetings of the American Sociological Association, Chicago.

Phillips, K. (1994). Correlates of healthy eating habits in low-income Black women and Latinas. *Preventive Medicine, 23,* 781-787.

Pickens, R. W., & Johanson, C. E. (1992). Craving: Consensus of status and agenda for future research. *Drug and Alcohol Dependence, 30,* 127-131.

Pickering, T. (1997). The effects of environmental and lifestyle factors on blood pressure and intermediary role of the sympathetic nervous system. *Journal of Human Hypertension, 11*(Suppl. 1), S9-S18.

Pickett, K. E., Ahern, J., Selvin, S., & Abrams, B. (2002). Social context, maternal race and preterm birth: A case-control study. *Annals of Epidemiology, 12,* 410-418.

Pickett, K. E., & Pearl, M. (2001). Multilevel analyses of neighbourhood socioeconomic context and health outcomes: a critical review. *Journal of Epidemiology and Community Health, 55,* 111-122.

Picot, S. (1995a). Choice and social exchange theory and the rewards of Black American caregivers. *Journal of the National Black Nurses Association, 7,* 29-40.

Picot, S. (1995b). Rewards, costs and coping of Black American caregivers. *Nursing Research, 44,* 147-152.

Picot, S. J., Debanne, S. M., Namazi, K. H., & Wykle, M. L. (1997). Religiosity and perceived rewards of Black and White caregivers. *Gerontologist, 37,* 89-101.

Pierce, J. P., Fiore, M. C., Novotny, T. E., et al. (1989). Trends in cigarette smoking in the United States: Educational differences are increasing. *Journal of the American Medical Association, 261,* 56-60.

Pimm, T. J., & Weinman, J. (1998). Applying Leventhal's self-regulation model to adaptation and intervention in rheumatic disease. *Clinical Psychology and Psychotherapy, 5,* 62-75.

Piotrowski, C. (1996). Use of the Beck Depression Inventory in clinical practice. *Psychological Reports, 6,* 74-82.

Pirie, P. L., Stone, E. J., Assaf, A. R., Flora, J. A., & Maschewsky-Schneider, U. (1994). Program evaluation strategies for community-based health promotion: Perspectives from the cardiovascular disease community research and demonstration studies. *Health Education Research, 9,* 23-36.

Pittler, M. H. (2001). Complementary and alternative medicine: A European perspective. In E. Ernst (Ed.), *The desktop guide to complementary and alternative medicine: An evidence-based approach* (pp. 388-394). Edinburgh: Harcourt.

Planned Approach to Community Health. (2003). Retrieved from http://www.cdc.gov/nccdphp/patch

Plog, B. (Ed.). (1996). *Fundamentals of industrial hygiene* (4th ed.). Itasca, IL: National Safety Council.

Plomin, R., DeFries, J. C., McClearn, G. E., & Rutter, M. (1997). *Behavior genetics* (3rd ed.). New York: W. H. Freeman.

Poiseuille, J. L. M. (1828). Recherches sur la force du Coeur aortique. Extraits des Theses soutennues dan las Troid Facultes de Medecine de France. *Archives of General Medicine, 18,* 550-555.

Polivy, J., & Herman, C. P. (2002). Causes of eating disorders. *Annual Review of Psychology, 53,* 187-213.

Pollock, M. L., Gaesser, G. A., Butcher, J. D., et al. (1998). The recommended quantity and quality of exercise for developing and maintaining cardiorespiratory and muscular fitness, and flexibility in healthy adults. *Medicine and Science in Sports and Medicine, 30,* 975-991.

Popkin, B. M., Siega-Riz, A. M., & Haines, P. S. (1996). A comparison of dietary trends among racial and socioeconomic groups in the United States. *New England Journal of Medicine, 335,* 716-720.

Portenoy, R. K. (1996). Opioid therapy for chronic nonmalignant pain: A review of the critical issues. *Journal of Pain and Symptom Management, 11*(4), 203-217.

Portes, A., & Rumbaut, R. G. (2000). *Not everyone is chosen: Segmented assimilation and its determinants.* Center for Migration and Development Working Paper Series. Princeton, NJ: Center for Migration and Development, Princeton University.

Portes, A., & Rumbaut, R. G. (2001). Not everyone is chosen: Segmented assimilation and its determinants. In A. Portes & R. G. Rumbaut (Eds.), *Legacies: The story of the immigrant second generation* (pp. 44-69). Berkeley/Los Angeles and New York: University of California Press, Russell Sage Foundation.

Potter, J. D., Finnegan, J. R., Guinard, J.-X., Huerta, E. E., Kelder, S. H., Kristal, A. R., Kumaniyika, S., Lin, R., Motsinger, B. M., Prendergast, F. G., & Sorensen, G. (2000, November). *5 a Day for Better Health Program evaluation report.* NIH Publication No. 01-4904. Bethesda, MD: National Institutes of Health, National Cancer Institute.

Potter, R. I. (1993). Religious themes in medical journals. *Journal of Religious Health, 32,* 217-222.

Powell, L. H., Lovallo, W. R., Matthews, K. A., Meyer, P., Midgley, A. R., Baum, A., Stone, A. A., Underwood, L., McCann, J. J., Janikula Herro, K., & Ory, M. G. (2002). Physiologic markers of chronic stress in premenopausal, middle-aged women. *Psychosomatic Medicine, 64,* 502-509.

Practice guidelines for chronic pain management. A report by the American Society of Anesthesiologists Task Force on Pain Management, Chronic Pain Section. (1997). *Anesthesiology, 86*(4), 995-1004.

President's Advisory Commission on Asian Americans and Pacific Islanders. (2001, January). *A people looking forward: Interim report to the president and the nation.* AAPI White House Initiative. Retrieved from www.aapi.gov

Prislin, R., Suarez, L., Simpson, D. M., & Dyer, J. M. (1998). When acculturation hurts: The case of immunization. *Social Science & Medicine, 47,* 1947-1956.

Prochaska, J. O., DiClemente, C. C., & Norcross, J. C. (1992). In search of how people change: Applications to addictive behaviors. *American Psychologist, 47*(9), 1102-1114.

Prochaska, J. O., DiClemente, C. C., Velicer, W. F., & Rossi, J. S. (1993). Standardized, individualized, interactive, and personalized self-help programs for smoking cessation. *Health Psychology, 12,* 399-405.

Prochaska, J. O., Norcross, J. C., & DiClemente, C. C. (1994). *Changing for good.* New York: William Morrow.

Prochaska, J. O., Redding, C. A., & Evers, K. (2002). The transtheoretical model and stages of change. In K. Glanz, B. K. Rimer, & F. M. Lewis (Eds.), *Health behavior and health education: Theory, research, and practice* (3rd ed., pp. 99-120). San Francisco: Jossey-Bass.

Project MATCH Research Group. (1997). Matching alcoholism treatments to client heterogeneity: Project MATCH posttreatment drinking outcomes. *Journal of Studies on Alcohol, 58,* 7-29.

Puhl, R., & Brownell, K. D. (2001). Bias, discrimination, and obesity. *Obesity Research, 9*, 788-805.

Purcell-Gates, V. (1995). *Other people's words: The cycle of low literacy.* Cambridge, MA: Harvard University Press.

Putnam, R. D. (2000). *Bowling alone: The collapse and revival of American community.* New York: Simon & Schuster.

Rabin, B. S. (1999). *Stress, immune function, and health: The connection.* New York: Wiley-Liss.

Rachman, S. (1977). *Contributions to medical psychology* (Vol. 1 [Vol. 2, 1980, Vol. 3, 1984]). Oxford, UK: Pergamon.

Radloff, L. S. (1977). The CES-D Scale: A self-report depression scale to detect depression in a community sample. *American Journal of Psychiatry, 1*, 385-401.

Rakowski, W. (1999). The potential variances of tailoring in health behavior interventions. *Annals of Behavioral Medicine, 21*, 284-289.

Rakowski, W., & Clark, M. A. (2002). The potential for health care organizations to promote maintenance and change in health behaviors among the elderly. In K. W. Schaie & H. Leventhal (Eds.), *Effective health behavior in the elderly.* New York: Springer.

Ramsay, C., Walker, M., & Alexander, J. (1999). Alternative medicine in Canada: Use and public attitudes. *Public Policy Sources, 21*, 3-31.

Ramsay, R. W. (1977). Behavioral approaches to bereavement. *Behavioral Research and Therapy, 15*, 131-135.

Ransdell, L. B. (1996). Church-based health promotion: A review of the current literature. *American Journal of Health Behavior, 2*, 195-207.

Rasbash, J., et al. (2000). *A user's guide to MLwiN, Version 2.1.* London: Multilevel Models Project, Institute of Education, University of London.

Raskin, A. (1988). Three-Area Severity of Depression Scale. In A. Bellack & M. Hersen (Eds.), *Dictionary of behavioral assessment techniques.* New York: Pergamon.

Ratzan, S. C. (Ed.). (1993). *AIDS: Effective health communication for the 1990s.* Washington, DC: Taylor & Francis.

Ratzan, S. C. (Ed.). (1994, November). Health communication: Challenges for the 21st century [Special issue]. *American Behavioral Scientist, 38*(2).

Ratzan, S. C., Payne, J. G., & Bishop, C. (1996, Spring). Status and scope of health communication. *Journal of Health Communication, 1*(1).

Ratzan, S., Payne, J. G., & Masset, H. (1994, November). Effective health message design: The America Responds to AIDS Campaign. *American Behavioral Scientist, 38*(2), 294-311.

Ratzan, S., Sterans, N., Payne, J. G., Amato, P., & Madoff, M. (1994, November). Education for the health communication professional: A collaborative curricular partnership. *American Behavioral Scientist, 38*(2), 361-380.

Raudenbush, S. W., & Bryk, A. S. (2002). *Hierarchical linear models: Applications and data analysis methods.* Newbury Park, CA: Sage.

Raudenbush, S. W., & Sampson, R. J. (1999). Ecometrics: Toward a science of assessing ecological settings, with application to the systematic social observation of neighborhoods. *Sociological Methodology 29*, 1-41.

RE-AIM Framework. (2003). Retrieved from www.RE-AIM.org

Reason, P., & Rowan, J. (Eds.). (1990). *Human inquiry: A sourcebook of new paradigm research.* New York: John Wiley.

Redfield, R., Linton, R., & Herskovits, M. (1936). Memorandum on the study of acculturation. *American Anthropologist, 38*, 149-152.

Reed, G. M., Kemeny, M. E., Taylor, S. E., Wang, H. Y. J., et al. (1994). Realistic acceptance as a predictor of decreased survival time in gay men with AIDS. *Health Psychology, 13*, 299-307.

Reese, S., et al. (2001, September 7). State-specific trends in high blood cholesterol awareness among persons screened—United States, 1991-1999. *Morbidity and Mortality Weekly Report, 50*, 754-758.

Regier, D. A., Narrow, W., Rae, D., Manderscheid, R. W., Locke, B. Z., & Goodwin, F. K. (1993). The de facto U.S. mental and addictive disorders service system: Epidemiologic Catchment Area prospective 1-year prevalence rates of disorders and services. *Archives of General Psychiatry, 50*, 85-94.

Reis, H. T., & Gable, S. L. (2000). Event sampling and other methods for studying daily experience. In H. T. Reis & C. M. Judd (Eds.), *Handbook of research methods in social and personality psychology* (pp. 190-222). New York: Cambridge University Press.

Reisine, T., & Pasternak, G. (1996). Opioid analgesics and antagonists. In A. Gilman, J. Hardman, & L. Limbird (Eds.), *Goodman and Gilman's: The pharmacological basis of therapeutics* (pp. 521-555). New York: McGraw-Hill.

Resnick, S. M., & Maki P. M. (2001). Effects of hormone replacement therapy on cognitive and brain aging. *Annals of the New York Academy of Sciences, 949*, 203-214.

Resnicow, K. (1997). For the Harlem Health Connection Study Group: A self-help smoking cessation program for inner-city African Americans: Results from the

Harlem Health Connection Project. *Health Education and Behavior, 24,* 201-217.

Resnicow, K. (1999). Cultural sensitivity in public health: Defined and demystified. *Ethnicity and Disease, 9,* 10-21.

Resnicow, K., Jackson, A., Wang, T., De, A. K., McCarty, F., Dudley, W. N., et al. (2001). A motivational interviewing intervention to increase fruit and vegetable intake through Black churches: Results of the Eat for Life trial. *American Journal of Public Health, 91,* 1686-1693.

Revenson, T. A. (2001). Chronic illness adjustment. In J. Worrell (Ed.), *Encyclopedia of women and gender* (Vol. 1, pp. 245-256). San Diego, CA: Academic Press.

Review Panel on Coronary-Prone Behavior and Coronary Heart Disease. (1981). Coronary-prone behavior and coronary heart disease: A critical review. *Circulation, 63,* 1199-1215.

Reynolds, D. V. (1969). Surgery in the rat during electrical analgesia induced by focal brain stimulation. *Science, 164,* 444-445.

Reynolds, W. M. (1994). Assessment of depression in children and adolescents by self-report questionnaires. In W. M. Reynolds & H. F. Johnston (Eds.), *Handbook of depression in children and adolescents: Issues in clinical child psychology* (pp. 209-234). New York: Plenum.

Reynolds, W. M., & Kobak, K. A. (1995). Reliability and validity of the Hamilton Depression Inventory: A paper-and-pencil version of the Hamilton Rating Scale Clinical Interview. *Psychological Assessment, 7,* 472-483.

Reynolds, W. W. (1987). *Reynolds Adolescent Depression Scale: Professional manual.* Odessa, FL: Psychological Assessment Resources.

Rhee, S. H., Parker, J. C., Smarr, K. L., Petroski, G. F., Johnson, J. C., Hewitt, J. E., Wright, G. E., Multon, K. D., & Walker, S. E. (2000). Stress management in rheumatoid arthritis: What is the underlying mechanism? *Arthritis Care and Research, 13,* 435-442.

Rice, B. I. (2001). Mind-body interventions (from research to practice/complementary & integrative medicine). *Diabetes Spectrum, 14,* 213-215.

Rice, R. E., & Katz, J. E. (2001). *The Internet and health communication: Experiences and expectations.* Thousand Oaks, CA: Sage.

Richard, H. W., & Burlew, A. K. (1997). Academic performance among children with sickle cell disease: Setting minimum standards for comparison groups. *Psychological Reports, 81,* 27-34.

Richards, P. S., Baldwin, B. M., Frost, H. A., Clark-Sly, J. B., Berrett, M. E., & Hardman, R. K. (2000). What works for treating eating disorders? Conclusions of 28 outcome reviews. *Eating Disorders, 8,* 189-206.

Rimal, R. N. (2000). Closing the knowledge-behavior gap in health promotion: The mediating role of self-efficacy. *Health Communication, 12,* 219-237.

Rimer, B. K. (2001). Response to Kreuter and Skinner. *Health Education Research, 15,* 503.

Rimer, B. K., & Glassman, B. (1998). Tailoring communication for primary care settings. *Methods of Information in Medicine, 37,* 171-177.

Ringen, K. (2001). Working with labor-management health and welfare funds to provide coverage for smoking cessation treatment. In E. Barbeau, K. Yous, D. McLellan, C. Levenstein, R. Youngstrom, C. E. Siqueira, et al. (Eds.), *Organized labor, public health, and tobacco control policy: A dialogue toward action* [Conference report]. *New Solutions, 11,* 121-126.

Rini, C., Dunkel-Schetter, C., Wadhwa, P. D., & Sandman, C. A. (1999). Psychological adaptation and birth outcomes: The role of personal resources, stress, and sociocultural context in pregnancy. *Health Psychology, 18*(4), 333-345.

Rivara, F. P., & Grossman, D. C. (1996). Prevention of traumatic deaths to children in the United States: How far have we come and where do we need to go? *Pediatrics, 97,* 791-797.

Robert, S. A. (1999). Socioeconomic position and health: The independent contribution of community socioeconomic context. *Annual Review of Sociology, 25,* 489-516.

Robins, J. M. (1998). Correction for non-compliance in equivalence trials. *Statistics in Medicine, 17,* 269-302.

Rodgers, G. B. (1996). The safety effects of child-resistant packaging for oral prescription drugs: Two decades of experience. *Journal of the American Medical Association, 275,* 1661-1665.

Rogers, E. (1983). *Diffusion of innovations.* New York: Free Press.

Rogers, E. (1995). *Diffusion of innovation* (4th ed.). New York: Free Press.

Rogers, E. M., & Shoemaker, F. F. (1971). *Communication of innovations: A cross-cultural approach* (2nd ed.). New York: Free Press.

Rogers, M. P., & Reich, P. (1988). On the health consequences of bereavement. *New England Journal of Medicine, 319,* 510-512.

Rogler, L. H. (1994). International migrations: A framework for directing research. *American Psychologist, 49,* 701-708.

Rohe, W., & Patterson, A. H. (1974). *The effects of varied levels of resources and density on behavior in a day care center.* Paper presented by the Environmental Design Research Association, Milwaukee, WI.

Romano, P. S., Bloom, J., & Syme, S. L. (1991). Smoking, social support, and hassles in an urban African-American community. *American Journal of Public Health, 81,* 1415-1422.

Rook, K. S. (1990). Social relationships as a source of companionship: implications for older adults psychological well being. In B. R. Sarason, T. G. Sarason, & G. R. Pierce (Eds.), *Social support: An interactional view* (pp. 221-250). New York: John Wiley.

Rose, G. (1992). *The strategy of preventive medicine.* Oxford, UK: Oxford University Press.

Rosen, G. (1979). The evolution of social medicine. In H. Freeman, S. Levine, & L. Reeder (Eds.), *Handbook of medical sociology* (3rd ed., pp. 23-50). Englewood Cliffs, NJ: Prentice Hall.

Rosenberg, W., & Donald, A. (1995). Evidence-based medicine: An approach to clinical problem-solving. *British Medical Journal, 310,* 1122-1126.

Rosenfeld, J. P. (1995). A research odyssey: My years in neuroscience. *Biofeedback, 23,* 6-15.

Rosenfeld, J. P. (2000). An EEG biofeedback protocol for affective disorders. *Clinical Electroencephalography, 31,* 7-12.

Rosengren, A., Orth-Gomer, K., Wedel, H., & Wilhelmsen, L. (1993). Stressful life events, social support, and mortality in men born in 1933. *British Medical Journal, 307,* 1102-1105.

Rosenman, R. H., Brand, J. H., Jenkins, C. D., Friedman, M., Straus, R., & Wurm, M. (1975). Coronary heart disease in the Western Collaborative Group Study: Final follow-up experience of 8.5 years. *Journal of the American Medical Association, 233,* 872-877.

Rosenstock, I. M. (1974). The health belief model and preventive health behavior. *Health Education Monographs, 2,* 354-386.

Rosenstock, I. M., Strecher, V. J., & Becker, M. (1988). Social learning theory and the health belief model. *Health Education Quarterly, 15,* 175-183.

Rosenstock, I. M., Strecher, V. J., & Becker, M. H. (1994). The health belief model and HIV risk behavior change. In R. J. DiClemente & J. L. Peterson (Eds.), *Preventing AIDS: Theories and methods of behavioral interventions* (pp. 5-24). New York: Plenum.

Rosenwaike, I., & Shai, D. (1986). Trends in cancer mortality among Puerto Rican-born migrants to New York City. *International Journal of Epidemiology, 15,* 30-35.

Ross, C. E., Mirowksy, J., & Goldsteen, K. (1990). The impact of the family on health: Decade in review. *Journal of Marriage and the Family, 52,* 1059-1078.

Ross, C. E., & Van Willigen, M. (1997). Education and the subjective quality of life. *Journal of Health and Social Behavior, 38,* 277-297.

Ross, R. (1993). The pathogenesis of atherosclerosis: a perspective for the 1990s. *Nature, 362,* 801-809.

Rossi, J. S., Rossi, S. R., Velicer, W. F., & Prochaska, J. O. (1995). Motivational readiness to control weight. In D. B. Allison (Ed.), *Handbook of assessment methods for eating behaviors and weight-related problems: Measures, theory, and research* (pp. 387-430). Thousand Oaks, CA: Sage.

Roter, D. L., & Hall, J. A. (1992). *Doctors talking with patients/patients talking with doctors.* Westport, CT: Auburn House.

Roter, D. L., Hall, J. A., Merisca, R., Nordstrom, B., Cretin, D., & Svarstad, B. (1998). Effectiveness of interventions to improve patient compliance: A meta-analysis. *Medical Care, 36,* 1138-1161.

Roter, D. L., Stewart, M., Putnam, S. M., Lipkin, M., Stiles, W., & Inui, T. S. (1997). Communication patterns of primary care physicians. *Journal of the American Medical Association, 277,* 350-356.

Rothman, K. J. (1977). Epidemiologic methods in clinical trials. *Cancer, 39,* 1771-1775.

Rothman, K. J., & Greenland, S. (1998). *Modern epidemiology* (2nd ed.). Philadelphia: Lippincott.

Rotter, J. B. (1954). *Social learning and clinical psychology.* New York: Prentice Hall.

Rotter, J. B. (1966). Generalized expectancies for internal vs. external control of reinforcement. *Psychological Monographs: General and Applied, 80,* 1-28.

Rowe, J. W., & Kahn, R. L. (1998). *Successful aging.* New York: Pantheon.

Rozanski, A., Blumenthal, J. A., & Kaplan, J. (1999). Impact of psychological factors on the pathogenesis of cardiovascular disease and implications for therapy. *Circulation, 99,* 2192-2217.

Rubin, D. B. (1990). Comment: Neyman and causal inference in experiments and observational studies. *Statistical Science, 5,* 472-480.

Rubin, R. R., & Peyrot, M. (2001). Psychological issues and treatments for people with diabetes. *Journal of Clinical Psychology, 57,* 457-478.

Rudd, R. E. (2002). Health Literacy Action Plan. In Office of Disease Prevention and Health Promotion, *Health communication objectives for Healthy People 2010.* Washington, DC: U.S. Department of Health and Human Services.

Rudd, R. E., Moeykens, B. A., & Colton, T. (2000). Health and literacy: A review of the medical and public health literature. In J. P. Comings, C. Smith, & B. Garner (Eds.), *Annual review of adult learning and literacy* (pp. 158-199). San Francisco: Jossey-Bass.

Rumbaut, R. G. (1996). The crucible within: Ethnic identity, self-esteem and segmented assimilation among children of immigrants. In A. Portes (Ed.), *The new second generation* (pp. 8-29). New York: Russell Sage Foundation.

Runyan, C. W. (1998). Using the Haddon matrix: Introducing the third dimension. *Injury Prevention, 4,* 302-307.

Rush, A. J., Giles, D. E., Schlesser, M. A., & Fulton, C. L. (1985). The Inventory for Depressive Symptomatology (IDS): Preliminary findings. *Psychiatry Research, 18,* 65-87.

Russell, L. B., Gold, M. R., Siegel, J. E., Daniels, N., & Weinstein, M. C. (1996). The role of cost-effectiveness analysis in health and medicine: Panel on Cost-Effectiveness in Health and Medicine. *Journal of the American Medical Association, 276,* 1172-1177.

Sackett, D. L., Rosenberg, W. M., Gray, J. A., Haynes, R. B., & Richardson, W. S. (1996). Evidenced-based medicine: What it is and what it isn't. *British Medical Journal 312,* 71-72.

Sackett, D. L., Straus, S. E., Richardson, W. S., Rosenberg, W., & Haynes, R. B. (2000). *Evidence-based medicine: How to practice and teach EBM* (2nd ed.). Toronto, Ontario, Canada: Churchill Livingstone.

Saelens, B. E., Sallis, J. F., & Frank, L. D. (in press). Environmental correlates of walking and cycling: Findings from the transportation, urban design, and planning literatures. *Annals of Behavioral Medicine.*

Sagan, L. A. (1987). *The health of nations: True causes of sickness and well-being.* New York: Basic Books.

Sallis, J. F., Bauman, A., & Pratt, M. (1998). Environmental and policy interventions to promote physical activity. *American Journal of Preventive Medicine, 15,* 379-397.

Sallis, J. F., Kraft, K., & Linton, L. S. (2002). How the environment shapes physical activity: A transdisciplinary research agenda. *American Journal of Preventive Medicine, 22,* 208.

Sallis, J. F., McKenzie, T. L., Alcaraz, J. E., Kolody, B., Faucette, N., & Hovell, M. F. (1997). The effect of a 2-year physical education program (SPARK) on physical activity and fitness in elementary school students. *American Journal of Public Health, 87,* 1328-1334.

Sallis, J. F., & Owen, N. (1999). *Physical activity and behavioral medicine.* Thousand Oaks, CA: Sage.

Sallis, J. F., & Owen, N. (2002). Ecological models of health behavior. In K. Glanz, B. K. Rimer, & F. M. Lewis (Eds.), *Health behavior and health education: Theory, research, and practice* (3rd ed., pp. 462-484). San Francisco: Jossey-Bass.

Salonen, J. T. (1988). Is there a continuing need for longitudinal epidemiologic research? The Kuopio Ischemic Heart Disease Risk Factor Study. *Annals of Clinical Research, 20,* 46-50.

Sampson, R. J., Morenoff, J. D., & Gannon-Rowley, T. (2002). Assessing "neighborhood effects": Social processes and new directions in research. *Annual Review of Sociology, 28,* 443-478.

Sampson, R. J., Raudenbush, S. W., & Earls, F. (1997). Neighborhoods and violent crime: A multilevel study of collective efficacy. *Science, 277,* 918-924.

Sanders, V. M., & Straub, R. H. (2002). Norepinephrine, the beta-adrenergic receptor, and immunity. *Brain, Behavior, and Immunity, 16*(4), 290-332.

Sandler, I. N., Miller, P., Short, J., & Wolchik, S. A. (1989). Social support as a protective factor for children in stress. In D. Belle (Ed.), *Children's social networks and social supports* (pp. 277-307). New York: John Wiley.

Sapolsky, R. M. (1998). *Why zebras don't get ulcers: An updated guide to stress, stress-related diseases, and coping.* New York: W. H. Freeman.

Sarason, B. R., Sarason, I. G., & Gurung, R. A. R. (2001). Close personal relationships and health outcomes: A key to the role of social support. In B. R. Sarason & S. Duck (Eds.), *Personal relationships: Implications for clinical and community psychology* (pp. 15-41). Chichester, UK: Wiley.

Sartorius, N., & Ban, T. A. (Eds.). (1986). *Assessment of depression.* New York: Springer-Verlag.

Sausen, K. P., Lovallo, W. R., Pincomb, G. A., & Wilson, M. F. (1992). Cardiovascular responses to occupational stress in medical students: A paradigm for ambulatory monitoring studies. *Health Psychology, 11,* 55-60.

Schaefer, J. A., & Moos, R. H. (1992). Life crises and personal growth. In B. Carpenter (Ed.), *Personal coping: Theory, research, and application* (pp. 149-170). Westport, CT: Praeger.

Scheier, I. H., & Cattell, R. B. (1960). *Handbook and test kit for the IPAT 8 Parallel Form Anxiety Battery.* Champaign, IL: Institute for Personality and Ability Testing.

Scheier, M. F., & Bridges, M. W. (1995). Person variables and health: Personality predispositions and acute psychological states as shared determinants for disease. *Psychosomatic Medicine, 57,* 255-268.

Scheier, M. F., Carver, C. S., & Bridges, M. W. (1994). Distinguishing optimism from neuroticism (and trait anxiety, self-mastery, and self-esteem): A reevaluation of the Life Orientation Test. *Journal of Personality and Social Psychology, 67,* 1063-1078.

Scheier, M. F., Matthews, K. A., Owens, J. F., Schulz, R., Bridges, M. W., Magovern, G. J., Sr., et al. (1999). Optimism and rehospitalization following coronary artery bypass graft surgery. *Archives of Internal Medicine, 159,* 829-835.

Schensul, J., Huebner, C., Singer, M., Snow, M., Feliciano, P., & Broomhall, L. (2000). The high, the money and the fame: Smoking bud among urban youth. *Medical Anthropology, 18,* 389-414.

Schensul, S., Schensul, J., & LeCompte, M. (1999). *Essential ethnographic methods. Ethnographer's toolkit: Vol. 2.* Walnut Creek, CA: AltaMira.

Schewe, P. A. (2002). Guidelines for developing rape prevention and risk reduction interventions. In P. A. Schewe (Ed.), *Preventing violence in relationships: Interventions across the lifespan* (pp. 107-121). Washington, DC: American Psychological Association.

Schlosberg, C. (1999-2000). *Immigrant access to health benefits: A resource manual.* Washington, DC: Access Project and the National Health Law Program.

Schmale, A. H., & Iker, H. P. (1971). Hopelessness as a predictor of cervical cancer. *Social Science Medicine, 5,* 95-100.

Schnall, P., Belkic, K., Landsbergis, P., & Baker, D. (2000). The workplace and cardiovascular disease. *Occupational Medicine State of the Art Reviews, 15,* 1-189.

Schneider, K. A. (2002). *Counseling about cancer: Strategies for genetic counseling* (2nd ed.). New York: Wiley-Liss.

Schneider, R. H., Staggers, F., Alexander, C. N., Sheppard, W., Rainforth, M., Kondwani, K., Smith, S., & King, C. G. (1995). A randomized controlled trial of stress reduction for hypertension in older African Americans. *Hypertension, 26*(5), 820-827.

Schneiderman, N. (1987). Psychophysiologic factors in atherogenesis and coronary artery disease. *Circulation, 76*(1 Pt. 2), I41-I47.

Schneiderman, N., Kaufmann, P., & Weiss, S. (Eds.). (1989). *Handbook of research methods in cardiovascular behavioral medicine.* New York: Plenum.

Schneiderman, N., McCabe, P., & Baum, A. (Eds.). (1992). *Perspectives in behavioral medicine: Stress and disease processes.* Hillsdale, NJ: Lawrence Erlbaum.

Schneiderman, N., & Speers, M. A. (2001). Behavioral science, social science, and public health in the 21st century. In N. Schneiderman, M. A. Speers, J. M. Silva, H. Tomes, & J. H. Gentry (Eds.), *Integrating behavioral and social sciences with public health* (pp. 3-28). Washington, DC: American Psychological Association.

Schnurr, P. P., & Green, B. L. (Eds.). (in press). *Physical health consequences of exposure to extreme stress.* Washington, DC: American Psychological Association.

Schochat, T., Croft, P., & Raspe, H. (1994). The epidemiology of fibromyalgia. *British Journal of Rheumatology, 33,* 783-786.

Schorr, E. C., & Arnason, B. G. W. (1999). Interactions between the sympathetic nervous system and the immune system. *Brain, Behavior, and Immunity, 13,* 271-278.

Schrijvers, C. T., Bosma, H., & Mackenbach, J. P. (2002). Hostility and the educational gradient in health: The mediating role of health-related behaviours. *European Journal of Public Health, 12,* 110-116.

Schulberg, H. C., Block, M. R., Madonia, M. J., et al. (1996). Treating major depression in primary care practice. *Archives of General Psychiatry, 53,* 913-919.

Schulkin, J. (2000). Decision sciences and evidence-based medicine: Two intellectual movements to support clinical decision making. *Academic Medicine, 75,* 816-817.

Schulkin, J., McEwen, B. S., & Gold, P. W. (1994). Allostasis, amygdala, and anticipatory angst. *Neuroscience and Biobehavioral Reviews, 18,* 385-396.

Schulman, K., et al. (1999). The effect of race and sex on physicians' recommendations for cardiac catheterization. *New England Journal of Medicine, 244,* 1392-1393.

Schulz, R., & Beach, S. R. (1999). Caregiving as a risk factor for mortality: The Caregiver Health Effects Study. *Journal of the American Medical Association, 282,* 2215-2260.

Schulz, R., Beach, S. R., Ives, D. G., Martire, L. M., Ariyo, A. A., & Kop, W. J. (2000). Association between depression and mortality in older adults: The Cardiovascular Health Study [Comment]. *Archives of Internal Medicine, 160,* 1761-1768.

Schulz, R., Drayer, R., & Rollman, B. (2002). Depression as a risk factor for non-suicide mortality in the elderly. *Biological Psychiatry, 52,* 205-225.

Schulz, R., Martire, L. M., Beach, S. R., & Scheier, M. F. (2000). Depression and mortality in the elderly. *Current Directions in Psychological Science, 9,* 204-208.

Schulz, R., Visintainer, P., & Williamson, G. M. (1990). Psychiatric and physical morbidity effects of caregiving. *Journal of Gerontology, 45,* P181-P191.

Schulz, R., & Williamson, G. M. (1991). A two-year longitudinal study of depression among Alzheimer's caregivers. *Psychology and Aging, 6,* 569-578.

Schuman, H., Steeh, C., Bobo, L., & Krysan, M. (1997). *Racial attitudes in America: Trends and interpretations* (Rev. ed.). Cambridge, MA: Harvard University Press.

Schwartz, J. E., Pieper, C. F., & Karasek, R. A. (1988). A procedure for linking psychosocial job characteristics data to health surveys. *American Journal of Public Health, 78,* 904-909.

Schwartz, M. B., & Brownell, K. D. (2001). Vulnerability to eating disorders in adulthood. In R. E. Ingram & J. M. Price (Eds.), *Vulnerability to psychopathology: Risk across the lifespan* (pp. 412-446). New York: Guilford.

Schwartz, M. D., & Andrasik, F. (Eds.). (2003). *Biofeedback: A practitioner's guide* (3rd ed.). New York: Guilford.

Schwarzer, R., & Leppin, A. (1989). Social support and health: A meta-analysis. *Psychology and Health, 3,* 1-15.

Science Panel on Interactive Communication and Health. (1999). *Wired for health and well-being: The emergence of interactive health communication* (T. R. Eng & D. H. Gustafson, Eds.). Washington, DC: U.S. Department of Health and Human Services, Government Printing Office.

Scribner, R. (1996). Paradox as paradigm: The health outcomes of Mexican Americans [Editorial]. *American Journal of Public Health, 86,* 303-305.

Scribner, R., & Dwyer, J. H. (1989). Acculturation and low birthweight among Latinos in the Hispanic HANES. *American Journal of Public Health, 79,* 1263-1267.

Seeman, T. (1996). Social ties and health: the benefits of social integration. *Annals of Epidemiology, 6,* 442-451.

Seeman, T., Berkman, L., Kohout, F., LaCroix, A., Glynn, R., & Blazer, D. (1993). Intercommunity variation in the association between social ties and mortality in the elderly: A comparative analysis of three communities. *Annals of Epidemiology, 3,* 325-335.

Seeman, T. E. (2000). Health promoting effects of friends and family on health outcomes in older adults. *American Journal of Health Promotion, 14,* 362-370.

Seeman, T. E., Singer, B. H., Rowe, J. W., Horwitz, R. I., & McEwen, B. S. (1997). Price of adaptation—Allostatic load and its health consequences: MacArthur studies of successful aging. *Archives of Internal Medicine, 157,* 2259-2268.

Seeman, T. E., Singer, B., Ryff, C., & Levy-Storms, L. (2002). Psychosocial factors and the development of allostatic load. *Psychosomatic Medicine, 64,* 395-406.

Segall, M., & Wykle, M. (1988-1989). The Black family's experience with dementia. *Journal of Applied Social Sciences, 13,* 170-191.

Seitz, V., & Apfel, N. H. (1999). Effective interventions for adolescent mothers. *Clinical Psychology: Science and Practice, 6,* 50-66.

Seligman, M. E. P. (1975). *Helplessness: On depression, development, and death.* San Francisco: Freeman.

Seligman, M. E. P. (1990). *Learned optimism.* New York: Knopf.

Sells, W. C., & Blum, R. W. (1996). Morbidity and mortality among U.S. adolescents: An overview of data and trends. *American Journal of Public Health, 86,* 513-519.

Selye, H. (1956). *The stress of life.* New York: McGraw-Hill.

Sen, A. (1995). *Inequality re-examined.* New York: Oxford University Press.

Shafer, F. E., & Vichinsky, E. (1994). New advances in the pathophysiology and management of sickle cell disease. *Current Opinion in Hematology, 1,* 125-135.

Shah, S., Peat, J. K., Mazurski, E. J., Wang, H., Sindhusake, D., Bruce, C., et al. (2001). Effect of peer-led programme for asthma education in adolescents: Cluster randomised controlled trial. *British Medical Journal, 322,* 583-585.

Shankar, S., Gutierrez-Mohamed, M. L., & Alberg, A. J. (2000). Cigarette smoking among immigrant Salvadoreans in Washington, DC: Behaviors, attitudes, and beliefs. *Addictive Behaviors, 25,* 275-281.

Shapiro, D., Greenstadt, L., Lane, J. D., & Rubenstein, E. (1981). Tracking-cuff system for beat-to-beat recording of blood pressure. *Psychophysiology, 18,* 129-136.

Shapiro, D., Jamner, L. D., Lane, J. D., Light, K. C., Myrtek, M., Sawada, Y., & Steptoe, A. (1996). Blood pressure publication guidelines: Society for Psychophysiological Research. *Psychophysiology, 33,* 1-12.

Shapiro, D. H., Jr., & Astin, J. A. (1998). *Control therapy: An integrated approach to psychotherapy, health, and healing.* New York: John Wiley.

Sharpe, L., Sensky, T., Timberlake, N., Ryan, B., Brewin, C. R., & Allard, S. (2001). A blind, randomized, controlled trial of cognitive-behavioural intervention for patients with recent onset rheumatoid arthritis: Preventing psychological and physical morbidity. *Pain, 89,* 275-283.

Shea, M. T., Elkin, I., Imber, S. D., Sotsky, S. M., Watkins, J. T., Collins, J. F., et al. (1992). Course of depressive symptoms over follow-up: Findings from the National

Institute of Mental Health Treatment of Depression Collaborative Research Program. *Archives of General Psychiatry, 49*, 782-787.

Shechter, A. L., Lipton, R. B., & Silberstein, S. D. (2001). Migraine comorbidity. In S. D. Silberstein, R. B. Lipton, & D. J. Dalessio (Eds.), *Wolff's headache and other head pain* (7th ed., pp. 108-118). New York: Oxford University Press.

Shekelle, R. B., Hulley, S. B., Neaton, J., Billings, J., Borhani, N., Gerace, T., Jacobs, D., Lassser, N., Mittlemark, M., & Stamler, J. (1985). The MRFIT behavioral pattern study II; Type A behavior pattern and risk of coronary death in MRFIT. *American Journal of Epidemiology, 112*, 559-570.

Sherman, K. A., Montrone, M., & Miller, S. M. (2002, March). *Coping strategies and pregnancy outcome among couples undergoing in-vitro fertilisation* [Abstracts]. Sixtieth Annual Scientific Meeting, American Psychosomatic Society, Barcelona, Spain.

Sherwood, A., Allen, M. T., Fahrenberg, J., Kelsey, R. M., Lovallo, W. R., & van Doornen, L. J. P. (1990). Committee report: Methodological guidelines for impedance cardiography. *Psychophysiology, 27*, 1-23.

Shimp, L. A. (1998). Safety issues in the pharmacologic management of chronic pain in the elderly. *Pharmacotherapy, 18*(6), 1313-1322.

Shumaker, S. A., & Hill, D. R. (1991). Gender differences in social support and physical health. *Health Psychology, 10*, 102-111.

Shumaker, S. A., Schron, E., Ockene, J., & McBee, A. L. (Eds.). (1998). *Handbook of health behavior change* (2nd ed., pp. 491-511). New York: Springer.

Siegel, J. E., Weinstein, M. C., Russell, L. B., & Gold, M. R. (1996). Recommendations for reporting cost-effectiveness analyses: Panel on Cost-Effectiveness in Health and Medicine. *Journal of the American Medical Association, 276*, 1339-1341.

Siegman, A. W. (1993). Cardiovascular consequences of expressing, experiencing, and repressing anger. *Journal of Behavioral Medicine, 16*, 539-569.

Siegman, A. W. (1994). Cardiovascular consequences of expressing and repressing anger. In A. W. Siegman & T. W. Smith (Eds.), *Anger, hostility, and the heart* (pp. 173-197). Hillsdale, NJ: Lawrence Erlbaum.

Siegman, A. W., Dembroski, T. M., & Ringel, N. (1987). Components of hostility and severity of coronary artery disease. *Psychosomatic Medicine, 49*, 127-135.

Siegman, A. W., & Smith, T. W. (Eds.). (1994). *Anger, hostility, and the heart.* Hillsdale, NJ: Lawrence Erlbaum.

Siegrist, J. (1996). Adverse effects of high effort-low reward conditions at work. *Journal of Occupational Health Psychology, 1*, 27-43.

Siegrist, J. (2000). Place, social exchange and health: Proposed sociological framework. *Social Science & Medicine, 51*, 1283-1293.

Silberstein, S. D., & Dongmei, L. (2002). Drug overuse and rebound headache. *Current Pain and Headache Reports, 6*, 240-247.

Silverman, K., Svikis, D., Wong, C. J., Hampton, J., Stitzer, M. L., & Bigelow, G. E. (2002). A reinforcement-based therapeutic workplace for the treatment of drug abuse: three-year abstinence outcomes. *Experimental and Clinical Psychopharmacology, 10*, 228-240.

Simon, R. W. (2002). Revisiting the relationship among gender, marital status, and mental health. *American Journal of Sociology, 107*, 1065-1096.

Simons, J. S., & Carey, M. P. (2001). Prevalence of the sexual dysfunctions: Results from a decade of research. *Archives of Sexual Behavior, 30*, 177-219.

Simonsick, E. M., Wallace, R. B., Blazer, D. G., & Berkman, L. F. (1995). Depressive symptomatology and hypertension-associated morbidity and mortality in older adults. *Psychosomatic Medicine, 57*, 427-435.

Simons-Morton, B. G., Greene, W. H., & Gottlieb, N. H. (1995). *Introduction to health education and health promotion.* Prospect Heights, IL: Waveland.

Sinclair, R. R., & Tetrick, L. E. (2000). Implications of item wording for hardiness structure, relation with neuroticism, and stress buffering. *Journal of Research in Personality, 34*, 1-25.

Sinclair, V. G., Wallston, K. A., Dwyer, K. A., Blackburn, D. S., & Fuchs, H. (1998). Effects of a cognitive-behavioral intervention for women with rheumatoid arthritis. *Research in Nursing and Health, 21*, 315-326.

Singer, A. J., & Clark, R. A. (1999). Cutaneous wound healing. *New England Journal of Medicine, 341*, 738-746.

Singer, B. H., & Ryff, C. D. (Eds.). (2001). *New horizons in health: An integrative approach.* Committee on Future Directions for Behavioral and Social Research at the National Institutes of Health. Washington, DC: National Academy Press.

Singer. J. L. (Ed.). (1990). *Repression and dissociation.* Chicago: University of Chicago Press.

Singh, G., & Siahpush, M. (2001). All-cause and cause-specific mortality of immigrants and native born in the United States. *American Journal of Public Health, 91*, 392-399.

Slade, P., Emery, J., & Lieberman, B. A. (1997). A prospective, longitudinal study of emotions and relationships in

in vitro fertilization treatment. *Human Reproduction,
12*, 183-190.

Slifer, K. J., Cataldo, M. F., Cataldo, M. D., Llorente, A.
M., & Gerson, A. C. (1993). Behavior analysis of
motion control for pediatric neuroimaging. *Journal of
Applied Behavior Analysis, 26,* 469-470.

Smedley, B. D., & Syme, S. L. (Eds.). (2000). *Promoting
health: Intervention strategies from social and behavioral research.* Washington, DC: National Academy
Press.

Smedley, B. D., Stith, A. Y., & Nelson, A. R. (Eds.). (2002).
*Unequal treatment: Confronting racial and ethnic
disparities in health care.* National Academies of
Science. Washington, DC: Institute of Medicine.

Smedley, B. D., Stith, A. Y., & Nelson, A. R. (2003).
*Unequal treatment: Confronting racial and ethnic dis-
parities in health care.* Washington, DC: National
Academies Press.

Smith, J. (1999). Healthy bodies and thick wallets: The dual
relationship between health and socioeconomic status.
Journal of Economic Perspectives, pp. 145-166.

Smith, J. C., Mercy, J. A., & Conn, J. M. (1988). Marital
status and the risk of suicide. *American Journal of
Public Health, 78,* 78-80.

Smith, M. S., Wallston, K. A., & Smith, C. A. (1995). The
development and validation of the Perceived Health
Competence Scale. *Health Education Research: Theory
& Practice, 10*, 51-64.

Smith, M. T., Perlis, M. L., Park, A., Smith, M. S.,
Pennington, J., Giles, D. E., & Buysse, D. J. (2002).
Comparative meta-analysis of pharmacotherapy and
behavior therapy for persistent insomnia. *American
Journal of Psychiatry, 159,* 5-11.

Smith, P. K., & Connolly, K. J. (1977). Social and aggressive behavior in preschool children as a function
of crowding. *Social Science Information, 16,*
601-620.

Smith, T. W. (1992). Hostility and health: Current status of
a psychosomatic hypothesis. *Health Psychology, 11,*
139-150.

Smith, T. W. (1994). Concepts and methods in the study of
anger, hostility, and health. In A. W. Siegman & T. W.
Smith (Eds.), *Anger, hostility, and the heart* (pp. 23-42).
Hillsdale, NJ: Lawrence Erlbaum.

Snijders, T., & Bosker, R. (1999). *Multilevel analysis: An
introduction to basic and advanced multilevel modeling.*
London: Sage.

Snowdon, D. (2001). *Aging with grace: What the Nun Study
teaches us about leading longer, healthier, and more
meaningful lives.* New York: Bantam.

Snyder, C. R. (1994). *The psychology of hope: You can get
there from here.* New York: Free Press.

Social Science Research Council. (1954). Acculturation:
An exploratory formulation. *American Anthropologist,
56*, 973-1002.

Sokejima, S., & Kagamimori, S. (1998). Working hours as
a risk factor for acute myocardial infarction in Japan:
Case-control study. *British Medical Journal, 19*,
775-780.

Solis, J. M., Marks, G., Garcia, M., & Shelton, D. (1990).
Acculturation, access to care, and use of preventive ser-
vices by Hispanics: Findings from HHANES 1982-84.
American Journal of Public Health, 80(Suppl. 11-9).

Sorensen, G. (2001). Worksite tobacco control programs:
The role of occupational health. *Respiration Physiology,
189*, 89-102.

Sorensen, G., Emmons, K., Hunt, M. K., & Johnston, D.
(1998). Implications of the results of community intervention trials. *Annual Review of Public Health, 19*,
379-416.

Sorensen, G., Stoddard, A., Peterson, K., Cohen, N., Hunt,
M. K., Stein, E., et al. (1999). Increasing fruit and vegetable consumption through worksites and families in
the Treatwell 5-A-Day Study. *American Journal of
Public Health, 89*, 54-60.

Sorkin, D., Rook, K. S., & Lu, J. L. (2002). Loneliness,
lack of emotional support, lack of companionship, and
the likelihood of having a heart condition in an elderly
sample. *Annals of Behavioral Medicine, 24*(4), 290-298.

Sorlie, P. D., Backlund, E., Johnson, N. J., & Rogot, E.
(1993). Mortality by Hispanic status in the United
States. *Journal of the American Medical Association,
270*, 2464-2468.

Sorlie, P. D., Backlund, M. S., & Keller, J. B. (1995). U.S.
mortality by economic, demographic, and social characteristics: The National Longitudinal Mortality Study.
American Journal of Public Health, 85, 949-956.

Spalding, A. D. (1995). Racial minorities and other high-
risk groups with HIV and AIDS at increased risk for
psychological adjustment problems in association with
health locus of control orientation. *Social Work in
Health Care, 21*, 81-114.

Spence, J. T., & Spence, K. W. (1966). The motivational
components of manifest anxiety: Drive and drive stimuli. In C. D. Spielberger (Ed.), *Anxiety and behavior*
(pp. 291-326). New York: Academic Press.

Spencer, L., Pagell, F., Hallion, M. E., & Adams, T. B.
(2002). Applying the transtheoretical model to tobacco
cessation and prevention: A review of literature.
American Journal of Health Promotion, 17, 7-71.

Spiegel, D. (1999). *Efficacy and cost-effectiveness of psychotherapy* (1st ed.). Washington, DC: American Psychiatric Press.

Spiegel, D., Bloom, J. R., & Yalom, I. D. (1981). Group support for patients with metastatic cancer: A randomized prospective outcome study. *Archives of General Psychiatry, 38,* 527-533.

Spiegel, D., & Classen, C. (2000). *Group therapy for cancer patients: A research-based handbook of psychosocial care.* New York: Basic Books.

Spielberger, C. D. (1966). Theory and research on anxiety. In C. D. Spielberger (Ed.), *Anxiety and behavior* (pp. 3-20). New York: Academic Press.

Spielberger, C. D. (1972a). Anxiety as an emotional state. In C. D. Spielberger (Ed.), *Anxiety: Current trends in theory and research* (Vol. 1, pp. 24-49). New York: Academic Press.

Spielberger, C. D. (1972b). Current trends in theory and research on anxiety. In C. D. Spielberger (Ed.), *Anxiety: Current trends in theory and research* (Vol. 1, pp. 3-19). New York: Academic Press.

Spielberger, C. D. (1973). *Manual for the State-Trait Anxiety Inventory for Children.* Palo Alto, CA: Consulting Psychologists Press.

Spielberger, C. D. (1977). Anxiety: Theory and research. In B. B. Wolman (Ed.), *International encyclopedia of neurology, psychiatry, psychoanalysis, and psychology.* New York: Human Sciences Press.

Spielberger, C. D. (1979). *Understanding stress and anxiety.* London: Harper & Row.

Spielberger, C. D. (1983). *Manual for the State-Trait Anxiety Inventory: STAI (Form Y).* Palo Alto, CA: Consulting Psychologists Press.

Spielberger, C. D., & Gorsuch, R. L. (1966). The development of the State-Trait Anxiety Inventory. In C. D. Spielberger & R. L. Gorsuch, *Mediating processes in verbal conditioning.* Final report to the National Institutes of Health, U.S. Public Health Service on Grants MH-7229, MH-7446, and HD-947.

Spielberger, C. D., Gorsuch, R. L., & Lushene, R. D. (1970). *STAI: Manual for the State-Trait Anxiety Inventory.* Palo Alto, CA: Consulting Psychologists Press.

Spielberger, C. D., Vagg, P. R., Barker, L. R., Donham, G. W., & Westberry, L. G. (1980). The factor structure of the State-Trait Anxiety Inventory. In I. G. Sarason & C. D. Spielberger (Eds.), *Stress and anxiety* (Vol. 7, pp. 95-109). Washington, DC: Hemisphere.

Spielman, A. J., Caruso, L. S., & Glovinsky, P. B. (1987). A behavioral perspective on insomnia treatment. *Psychiatric Clinics of North America, 10,* 541-553.

Spiteri, M. A., Bianco, A., Strange, R. C., & Fryer, A. A. (2000). Polymorphisms at the glutathione S-transferase, GSTP1 locus: A novel mechanism for susceptibility and development of atopic airway inflammation. *Allergy, 55*(Suppl. 61), 15-20.

Spivak, H., Prothrow-Stith, D., & Hausman, A. (1988). Dying is no accident: Adolescents, violence and intentional injury. *Paediatric Clinics of North America, 35,* 1339-1347.

Spoth, R. L., Redmond, C., Trudeau, L., & Shin, C. (2002). Longitudinal substance initiation outcomes for a universal preventive intervention combining family and school programs. *Psychology of Addictive Behaviors, 16,* 129-134.

Spradley, J. (1979). *The ethnographic interview.* New York: Holt, Rinehart & Winston.

Stables, G., & Heimendinger, J. (Eds.). (2001, September). *5 a Day for Better Health Program monograph.* NIH Publication No. 01-5019. Bethesda, MD: National Institutes of Health, National Cancer Institute.

Stables, G., Subar, A. F., Patterson, B. H., Dodd, K., Heimendinger, J., Krebs-Smith, S. M., Van Duyn, M. A., & Nebeling, L. (2002). Changes in fruit and vegetable consumption and awareness among U.S. adults: Results of the 1991 and 1997 5 a Day for Better Health Program surveys. *Journal of the American Dietetic Association, 102,* 809-817.

Stamler, J., Daviglus, M. L., Garside, D. B., et al. (2000). Relationship of baseline serum cholesterol levels in three large cohorts of younger men to long-term coronary, cardiovascular, and all-cause mortality and to longevity. *Journal of the American Medical Association, 284,* 311-318.

Stanton, A. L., Collins, C. A., & Sworowski, L. A. (2001). Adjustment to chronic illness: Theory and research. In A. Baum, T. A. Revenson, & J. E. Singer (Eds.), *Handbook of health psychology* (pp. 387-403). Mahwah, NJ: Lawrence Erlbaum.

Stark, L. J., Collins, F. L., Osnes, P. G., & Stokes, T. F. (1986). Using reinforcement and cueing to increase healthy snack choices in preschoolers. *Journal of Applied Behavior Analysis, 19,* 367-379.

Steenland, K., Fine, L., Belkic, K., Landsbergis, P., Schnall, P., Baker, D., et al. (2000). Research findings linking workplace factors to CVD outcomes. *Occupational Health, 15,* 7-68.

Steer, R. A., Clark, D. A., Beck, A. T., & Ranieri, W. F. (1999). Common and specific dimensions of self-reported anxiety and depression: The BDI-II vs. the BDI-IA. *Behaviour Research and Therapy, 37,* 183-190.

Stefanatou, A., & Bowler, D. (1997). Depiction of pain in the self-drawings of children with sickle cell disease. *Child Care, Health, and Development, 23,* 135-155.

Stein, M. J., Wallston, K. A., & Nicassio, P. M. (1988). Factor structure of the Arthritis Helplessness Index. *Journal of Rheumatology, 15,* 427-432.

Steinmetz, K. A., & Potter, J. D. (1991). Vegetables, fruit, and cancer II: Mechanisms. *Cancer Causes and Control, 2,* 427-442.

Stepanski, E. J., & Perlis, M. L. (2000). Behavioral sleep medicine: An emerging subspecialty in health psychology and sleep medicine. *Journal of Psychosomatic Research, 49,* 343-347.

Stephens, T. (1988). Physical activity and mental health in the United States and Canada: Evidence from four population surveys. *Preventive Medicine, 17,* 35-47.

Steptoe, A., & Butler, N. (1996). Sports participation and emotional wellbeing in adolescents. *Lancet, 347,* 1789-1792.

Sterling, P., & Eyer, J. (1988). Allostasis: A new paradigm to explain arousal pathology. In S. Fisher & J. Reason (Eds.), *Handbook of life stress, cognition and health* (pp. 629-649). New York: John Wiley.

Stern, M. P., & Wei, M. (1999). Do Mexican Americans really have low rates of cardiovascular disease? *Preventive Medicine, 29,* 90-95.

Sternberg, E. M. (2000). *The balance within: The science connecting health and emotion.* New York: W. H. Freeman.

Sternberg, E. M., & Licino, J. (1995). Overview of neuroimmune stress interactions: Implications for susceptibility to inflammatory disease. In G. P. Chrousos, R. McCarty, K. Pacak, G. Cizza, E. Sternberg, P. W. Gold, & R. Kvetnansky (Eds.), *Stress: Basic mechanisms and clinical implications.* New York: Annals of the New York Academy of Science.

Stetter, F., & Kupper, S. (2002). Autogenic training: A meta-analysis of clinical outcome studies. *Applied Psychophysiology and Biofeedback, 27,* 45-98.

Stewart, B. W., & Kleihues, P. (Eds.). (2003). *World cancer report.* Lyon, France: IARC Press.

Stewart, M., Brown, J. B., Weston, W. W., McWhinney, I. R., McWilliam, C. L., & Freeman, T. R. (1995). *Patient-centered medicine: Transforming the clinical method.* Thousand Oaks, CA: Sage.

Stipek, D. J., Lamb, M. E., & Zigler, E. F. (1981). OPTI: A measure of children's optimism. *Educational and Psychological Measurement, 41,* 131-143.

Stokols, D. (1972). On the distinction between density and crowding: Some implications for future research. *Psychological Review, 79,* 275-277.

Stokols, D., Pelletier, K., & Fielding, J. (1996). The ecology of work and health: Research and policy directions for the promotion of employee health. *Health Education Quarterly, 23,* 137-158.

Stolerman, J. P., & Jarvis, M. J. (1995). The scientific case that nicotine is addictive. *Psychopharmacology, 117,* 2-10.

Stone, A. A., Cox, D. S., Valdimarsdottir, H., & Jandorf, L. (1987). Evidence that secretory IgA antibody is associated with daily mood. *Journal of Personality & Social Psychology, 52,* 988-993.

Stone, A. A., Neale, J. M., Cox, D. S., Napoli, A., Valdimarsdottir, H., & Kennedy-Moore, E. (1994). Daily events are associated with a secretory immune response to an oral antigen in men. *Health Psychology, 13,* 440-446.

Stone, A. A., & Shiffman, S. (1998). Ecological momentary assessment: A new tool for behavioral medicine research. In D. S. Krantz & A. Baum (Eds.), *Technology and methods in behavioral medicine* (pp. 117-131). Mahwah, NJ: Lawrence Erlbaum.

Stone, A. A., & Shiffman, S. (2002). Capturing momentary, self-report data: A proposal for reporting guidelines. *Annals of Behavioral Medicine, 24,* 236-243.

Stone, A. A., Shiffman, S. S., & DeVries, M. W. (1999). Ecological momentary assessment. In D. Kahneman, E. Diener, & N. Schwarz (Eds.), *Well-being: The foundations of hedonic psychology* (pp. 26-39). New York: Russell Sage.

Stoney, C. M. (1992). The role of reproductive hormones in cardiovascular and neuroendocrine function during behavioral stress. In J. R. Turner, A. Sherwood, & K. C. Light (Eds.), *Individual differences in cardiovascular response to stress* (pp. 147-163). New York: Plenum.

Strasburger, V. C. (1997). "Sex, drugs, rock 'n' roll," and the media—Are the media responsible for adolescent behavior? *Adolescent Medicine, 8,* 403-414.

Strategier, L. D., Chwalisz, K., Altmaier, E. M., Russell, D. W., & Lehmann, T. H. (1997). Multidimensional assessment of chronic low back pain: Predicting treatment outcomes. *Journal of Clinical Psychology in Medical Settings, 4,* 91-110.

Straus, M. A. (2001). *Beating the devil out of them: Corporal punishment by American families and its effects on children* (2nd ed.). Somerset, NJ: Transaction.

Strauss, R. S. (2002). Childhood obesity. *Pediatric Clinics of North America, 49,* 175-201.

Strawbridge, W. J., Deleger, S., Roberts, R. E., & Kaplan, G. A. (2002). Physical activity reduces the risk of subsequent depression for older adults. *American Journal of Epidemiology, 156*, 328-334.

Strawbridge, W. J., Wallhagen, M. I., & Cohen, R. D. (2002). Successful aging and well-being: Self-rated compared with Rowe and Kahn. *The Gerontologist, 42*, 727-733.

Strecher, V., Champion, V., & Rosenstock, I. (1997). The health belief model and health behavior. In D. Gochman (Ed.), *Handbook of health behavior research: Vol. I. Personal and social determinants* (pp. 71-92). New York: Plenum.

Strickland, B. R. (1978). Internal-external expectancies and health-related behavior. *Journal of Consulting and Clinical Psychology, 46*, 1192-1211.

Stringer, E. T. (1996). *Action research: A handbook for practitioners*. Thousand Oaks, CA: Sage.

Stroebe, M. S., & Stroebe, W. (1983). Who suffers more? Sex differences in health risks of the widowed. *Psychological Bulletin, 93*, 279-301.

Strong, C. (1984). Stress and caring for elderly relatives: Interpretations and coping strategies in an American Indian and White sample. *Gerontologist, 24*, 251-256.

Stuart, R. B. (1971). A three-dimensional program for the treatment of obesity. *Behaviour Research and Therapy, 9*, 177-186.

Stuber, M. (2002, February). *Humor and immune function*. Lecture presented at the University of California, San Diego, CA.

Stull, D. E., Kosloski, K., & Kercher, K. (1994). Caregiver burden and generic well-being: Opposite sides of the same coin? *Gerontologist, 34*, 88-94.

Subramanian, S. V., Belli, P., & Kawachi, I. (2002). The macroeconomic determinants of health. *Annual Reviews of Public Health, 23*, 287-302.

Subramanian, S. V., Blakely, T., & Kawachi, I. (2003). Income inequality as a public health concern: Where do we stand? *Health Services Research, 38*(1), 153-167.

Subramanian, S. V., Daniels, K., & Kawachi, I. (2002). Social trust and self-rated poor health in U.S. communities: A multilevel analysis. *Journal of Urban Health, 79*(4, Suppl. 1), S21-S34.

Subramanian, S. V., Jones, K., & Duncan, C. (2003). Multilevel methods for public health research. In I. Kawachi & L. F. Berkman (Eds.), *Neighborhood and health* (pp. 65-111). New York: Oxford University Press.

Subramanian, S. V., Kawachi, I., & Kennedy, B. P. (2001). Does the state you live in make a difference? Multilevel analysis of self-rated health in the U.S. *Social Science and Medicine, 53*, 9-19.

Subramanian, S. V., Lochner, K., & Kawachi, I. (2003). Neighborhood differences in social capital in the U.S.: Compositional artifact or a contextual construct. *Health and Place, 9*, 33-44.

Substance Abuse and Mental Health Services Administration, Center for Substance Abuse Prevention, Division of State and Community Systems Development. (1999). *Preventing problems related to alcohol availability: Environmental approaches*. Department of Health and Human Services Publication No. (SMA) 99-3298. Retrieved from http://www.health.org/ govpubs/ PHD822/aar.htm

Sugisawa, H., Liang, J., & Liu, X. (1994). Social networks, social support and mortality among older people in Japan. *Journal of Gerontology, 49*, S3-S13.

Suls, J., Wan, C., & Costa, P. (1995). Relationship of trait anger to resting blood pressure: A meta-analysis. *Health Psychology, 14*, 444-456.

Surwit, R. S., van Tilburg, M. A. L., Zucker, N., McCaskill, C. C., Parekh, P., Feinglos, M. N., et al. (2001). Stress management improves long-term glycemic control in Type 2 diabetes. *Diabetes Care, 25*, 30-34.

Surwit, R. S., Williams, R. B., & Shapiro, D. (1982). *Behavioral approaches to cardiovascular disease*. New York: Academic Press.

Sussman, S., Dent, C. W., Burton, D., Stacy, A. W., & Flay, B. R. (1995). *Developing school-based tobacco use prevention and cessation programs*. Thousand Oaks, CA: Sage.

Svedlund, J., & Sjodin, I. (1985). A psychosomatic approach to treatment in the irritable bowel syndrome and peptic ulcer disease with aspects of the design of clinical trials. *Scandinavian Journal of Gastroenterology* (Suppl. 109), pp. 147-151.

Swindells, S., Mohr, J., Justis, J. C., Berman, S., Squier, C., Wagener, M. M., & Singh, N. (1999). Quality of life in patients with human immunodeficiency virus infection: Impact of social support, coping style and hopelessness. *International Journal of STD and AIDS, 10*, 383-391.

Swisher, J. D., & Clayton, R. (2000). Sustainability in prevention. *Addictive Behaviors, 25*, 965-973.

Syme, S. L. (1979). Psychosocial determinants of hypertension. In E. Oresti & C. Klint (Eds.), *Hypertension determinants, complications, and intervention* (pp. 95-98). New York: Grune & Stratton.

Talbot, E. A., Moore, M., McCray, E., & Binkin, N. J. (2000). Tuberculosis among foreign-born persons in the

United States, 1993-1998. *Journal of the American Medical Association, 284,* 2894-2900.

Talo, S., Forssell, H., Heikkonen, S., & Puukka, P. (2001). Integrative group therapy outcome related to psychosocial characteristics in patients with chronic pain. *International Journal of Rehabilitation Research, 24,* 25-33.

Tarter, R. E., Butters, M., & Beers, S. R. (Eds.). (2001). *Medical neuropsychology* (2nd ed.). New York: Kluwer Academic/Plenum.

Task Force of the European Society of Cardiology and the North American Society of Racing and Electrophysiology. (1996). Heart rate variability: Standards of measurement, physiological interpretation, and clinical use. *Circulation, 93,* 1043-1065.

Taylor, C. B., Winzelberg, A., & Celio, A. (2001). Use of interactive media to prevent eating disorders. In R. Striegel-Moor & L. Smolak (Eds.), *Eating disorders: New direction for research and practice* (pp. 255-270). Washington, DC: American Psychological Association.

Taylor, J. A. (1951). The relationship of anxiety to the conditioned eyelid response. *Journal of Experimental Psychology, 41,* 81-92.

Taylor, J. A. (1953). A personality scale of manifest anxiety. *Journal of Abnormal Social Psychology, 48,* 285-290.

Taylor, R. R., & Jason, L. A. (1998). Comparing the DIS with the SCID: Chronic fatigue syndrome and psychiatric comorbidity. *Psychology and Health: The International Review of Health Psychology, 13,* 1087-1104.

Taylor, S. E. (1983). Adjustment to threatening events: A theory of cognitive adaptation. *American Psychologist, 38,* 1161-1173.

Taylor, S. E., & Brown, J. D. (1988). Illusion and well-being: A social psychological perspective on mental health. *Psychological Bulletin, 103,* 193-210.

Taylor, S. E., & Brown, J. D. (1994). Positive illusions and well-being revisited: Separating fact from fiction. *Psychological Bulletin, 116,* 21-27.

Taylor, S. E., Kemeny, M. E., Reed, G. M., Bower, J. E., & Gruenewald, T. L. (2000). Psychological resources, positive illusions, and health. *American Psychologist, 55,* 99-109.

Tedeschi, R. G., Park, C. L., & Calhoun, L. G. (Eds.). (1998). *Posttraumatic growth: Positive changes in the aftermath of crisis.* Mahwah, NJ: Lawrence Erlbaum.

Tennen, H., Affleck, G., Urrows, S., Higgins, P., & Mendola, R. (1992). Perceiving control, construing benefits, and daily processes in rheumatoid arthritis. *Canadian Journal of Behavioral Science, 242,* 186-203.

Terry, D. J., Gallois, C., & McCamish, M. (1993). *The theory of reasoned action: Its application to AIDS-preventive behavior.* Oxford, UK: Pergamon.

The Community Guide. (2003). *Guide to community preventive services.* Retrieved from www.TheCommunity Guide.org

The Third National Health and Nutrition Examination Survey (NHANES III) (1988-1994). (2002). Retrieved December 2002 from http://www.cdc.gov/nchs/about/major/nhanes/datatblelink.htm

Therrien, M., & Ramirez, R. R. (2001). *Current population reports: The Hispanic population in the United States, population characteristics March 2000.* Washington, DC: U.S. Census Bureau, Department of Commerce.

Thoits, P. (1995). Stress, coping, and social support processes: where are we? What next? *Journal of Health and Social Behavior* [Extra issue], pp. 53-79.

Thoits, P. A. (1986). Social support as coping assistance. *Journal of Consulting and Clinical Psychology, 54,* 416-423.

Thompson, S. C., Sobolew-Shubin, A., Graham, M. A., & Janigian, A. S. (1989). Psychosocial adjustment following a stroke. *Social Science & Medicine, 28,* 239-247.

Thorogood, M., Cowen, P., Mann, J., Murphy, M., & Vessey, M. (1992). Fatal myocardial infarction and use of psychotropic drugs in young women. *Lancet, 340,* 1067-1068.

Thune, I., & Furberg, A. (2001). Physical activity and cancer risk: Dose-response and cancer, all sites and site specific. *Medicine and Science in Sports and Exercise, 33,* S530-S550.

Tienda, M. (1991). Poor people and poor places: Deciphering neighborhood effects on poverty outcomes. In J. Huber (Ed.), *Macro-micro linkages in sociology* (pp. 244-262). Newbury Park, CA: Sage.

Timio, M., Verdecchia, P., Venanzi, S., Genteli, S., Ronconi, M., Francucci, B., Montanari, M., & Bichisao, E. (1988). Age and blood pressure changes: A 20-year follow-up study in nuns in a secluded order. *Hypertension, 12*(4), 457-461.

Tobler, N. S. (1997). *Meta-analysis of adolescent drug prevention programs: Results of the 1993 meta-analysis.* NIDA Research Monograph, 170, 5-68.

Tornieporth, N. G., Ptachewich, Y., Poltoraskaia, N., Ravi, B. S., Katapadi, M., Berger, J. J., et al. (1997). Tuberculosis among foreign-born persons in New York City, 1992-1994: Implications for tuberculosis control.

International Journal of Tuberculosis and Lung Disease, 1, 528-535.

Tornstam, L. (1994). Gero-transcendence: A theoretical and empirical exploration. In L. E. Thomas & S. A. Eisenhandler (Eds.), *Aging and the religious dimension* (pp. 203-225). Westport, CT: Auburn House.

Toseland, R. W., & Rossiter, C. M. (1989). Group interventions to support family caregivers: A review and analysis. *The Gerontologist, 29*(4), 438-448.

Tran, P. V., Bymaster, F. P., McNamara, R. K., & Potter, W. Z. (2003). Dual monoamine modulation for improved treatment of major depressive disorder. *Journal of Clinical Psychopharmacology, 23*(1), 78-86.

Treiber, F. A., Kamarck, T., Schneiderman, N., Sheffield, D., Kapuku, G., & Taylor, T. (2003). Cardiovascular reactivity and development of preclinical and clinical disease states. *Psychosomatic Medicine, 65,* 46-62.

Tremblay, R. E., Pagani-Kurtz, L., Masse, L. C., Vitaro, F., & Pihl, R. O. (1995). A bimodal preventive intervention for disruptive kindergarten boys: Its impact through mid-adolescence. *Journal of Consulting Clinical Psychology, 63,* 560-568.

Triandis, H. C. (1996). The psychological measurement of cultural syndromes. *American Psychologist, 51,* 407-415.

Trivedi, M. H., & Kleiber, B. A. (2001). Algorithm for the treatment of chronic depression. *Journal of Clinical Psychiatry, 62* (Suppl 6), 22-29.

Troiano, R. P., & Flegal, K. M. (1998). Overweight children and adolescents: Description, epidemiology, and demographics. *Pediatrics, 101,* 497-504.

Troiano, R. P., & Flegal, K. M. (1999). Overweight prevalence among youth in the United States: Why so many different numbers? *International Journal of Obesity and Related Metabolic Disorders, 23*(Suppl. 2), S22-S27.

Tugade, M. M., & Fredrickson, B. L. (2002). Positive emotions and emotional intelligence. In L. Feldman Barrett & P. Salovey (Eds.), *The wisdom of feelings: Psychological processes in emotional intelligence* (pp. 319-340). New York: Guilford.

Tugade, M. M., & Frederickson, B. L. (in press). Resilient individuals use positive emotions to bounce back from negative emotional experiences. *Journal of Personality and Social Psychology.*

Tugwell, P., Bombardier, C., Buchanan, W. W., Goldsmith, C. H., Grace, E., & Hanna, B. (1987). The MACTAR Patient Preference Disability Questionnaire. *Journal of Rheumatology, 14,* 446-451.

Turk, D. (1996). Biopsychosocial perspective on chronic pain. In R. Gatchel & D. Turk (Eds.), *Psychological approaches to pain management: A practitioner's handbook.* New York: Guilford.

Turk, D. C. (1990). Customizing treatment for chronic pain patients: Who, what, and why. *Clinical Journal of Pain, 6,* 255-270.

Turk, D. C., & Flor, H. (1989). Primary fibromyalgia is more than tender points: Toward a multiaxial taxonomy. *Journal of Rheumatology, 16,* 80-86.

Turk, D. C., Okifuji, A., Sinclair, J. D., & Starz, T. W. (1996). Pain, disability, and physical functioning in subgroups of patients with fibromyalgia. *Journal of Rheumatology, 23,* 1255-1262.

Turk, D. C., Okifuji, A., Sinclair, J. D., & Starz, T. W. (1998). Interdisciplinary treatment for fibromyalgia syndrome: Clinical and statistical significance. *Arthritis Care and Research, 11,* 186-195.

Turk, D. C., Okifuji, A., Starz, T. W., & Sinclair, J. D. (1996). Effects of type of symptom onset on psychological distress and disability in fibromyalgia syndrome patients. *Pain, 68,* 423-430.

Turk, D. C., Okifuji, A., Starz, T. W., & Sinclair, J. D. (1998). Differential responses by psychosocial subgroups of fibromyalgia syndrome patients to an interdisciplinary treatment. *Arthritis Care and Research, 11,* 397-404.

Turk, D. C., & Rudy, T. E. (1988). Toward an empirically derived taxonomy of chronic pain states: An integration of psychological assessment data. *Journal of Consulting and Clinical Psychology, 56,* 233-238.

Turk, D. C., & Rudy, T. E. (1990). The robustness of an empirically derived taxonomy of chronic pain patients. *Pain, 42,* 27-35.

Turk, D. C., Rudy, T. E., Kubinski, J. A., Zaki, H. S., & Greco, C. M. (1996). Dysfunctional TMD patients: Evaluating the efficacy of a tailored treatment protocol. *Journal of Consulting and Clinical Psychology, 64,* 139-146.

Turk, D. C., & Sherman, J. J. (2002). Treatment of patients with fibromyalgia syndrome. In D. C. Turk & R. J. Gatchel (Eds.), *Psychological approaches in pain management: A practitioner's handbook* (2nd ed.). New York: Guilford.

Turner, J. R. (1994). *Cardiovascular reactivity and stress patterns of physiological response.* New York: Plenum.

Turner, J. R., Hewitt, J. K., & Cardon, L. R. (1995). *Behavior genetic approaches in behavioral medicine.* New York: Plenum.

Turner, J. R., Sherwood, A., & Light, K. C. (Eds.). (1992). *Individual differences in cardiovascular response to stress.* New York: Plenum.

Turner, R. J., Wheaton, B., & Lloyd, D. (1995). The epidemiology of social stress. *American Sociological Review, 60*, 104-125.

TV Turnoff Network. (2002). Retrieved October 15, 2002, from www.tvturnoff.org

U.S. Bureau of the Census. (2000). *Projections of the total resident population by 5-year age groups, race, and Hispanic origin with special age categories: Middle series 1999-2000; Middle series 2050-2070.* Retrieved June 5, 2002, from http://www.census.gov/population/projections/ nation/summary/np-t4-a.txt

U.S. Department of Health and Human Services, Administration on Children, Youth and Families. (1999). *Child maltreatment 1999.* Washington, DC: Government Printing Office.

U.S. Department of Health and Human Services. (1989a). *Making health communication programs work* (NIH Publication No. 89-1493). Office of Cancer Communications, National Cancer Institute. Rockville, MD: Author.

U.S. Department of Health and Human Services. (1989b). *Reducing the health consequences of smoking: 25 years of progress. A report of the surgeon general.* DHHS Publication No. (CDC) 89-8411. Rockville, MD: U.S. Department of Health and Human Services, Public Health Service, Centers for Disease Control, Center for Chronic Disease Prevention and Health Promotion, Office on Smoking and Health.

U.S. Department of Health and Human Services. (1994). *Preventing tobacco use among young people. A report of the Surgeon General.* Atlanta, GA: Public Health Service, Centers for Disease Control and Prevention, Office on Smoking and Health. (No S/N 017-001-00491-0)

U.S. Department of Health and Human Services. (1996). *Physical activity and health: A report of the surgeon general.* Atlanta, GA: U.S. Department of Health and Human Services, Centers for Disease Control and Prevention, National Center for Chronic Disease Prevention and Health Promotion.

U.S. Department of Health and Human Services. (2001). *Women and smoking: A report of the surgeon general.* Atlanta, GA: U.S. Department of Health and Human Services, Public Health Service, Centers for Disease Control and Prevention, National Center for Chronic Disease Prevention and Health Promotion, Office on Smoking and Health.

U.S. Department of Health and Human Services. (2000). *Healthy People 2010* (2nd ed.). *With understanding and improving health and objectives for improving health* (2 vols.). Washington, DC: Government Printing Office.

U.S. Department of Health and Human Services. (in press). *The health consequences of tobacco use: A report of the surgeon general.* Atlanta, GA: U.S. Department of Health and Human Services, Public Health Service, Centers for Disease Control and Prevention, National Center for Chronic Disease Prevention and Health Promotion, Office on Smoking and Health.

U.S. Preventive Services Task Force. (2000-2003). *Guide to clinical preventive services* (3rd ed.). Retrieved from http://www.ahcpr.gov/clinic/cps3dix.htm

U.S. Task Force on Community Preventive Services. (2001). Tobacco use and exposure to environmental tobacco smoke. *American Journal of Preventive Medicine, 20*(2S), 10-15.

Udry, J. R., Morris, N. M., & Kovenock, J. (1995). Androgen effects on women's gendered behaviour. *Journal of Biosocial Science, 3,* 359-368.

UK ECT Review Group. (2003). Efficacy and safety of electroconvulsive therapy in depressive disorders: A systematic review and meta-analysis. *Lancet, 361,* 799-808.

Umberson, D. (1992). Gender, marital status and the social control of health behavior. *Social Science and Medicine, 34,* 907-917.

Umetsu, D. T., McIntire, J. J., Akbari, O., Macaubas, C., & DeKruyff, R. H. (2002). Asthma: An epidemic of dysregulated immunity. *Nature Immunology, 3*(8), 715-720.

Unden, A. L., & Orth-Gomér, K. (1989). Development of a social support instrument for use in population surveys. *Social Science and Medicine, 29*(12), 1387-1392.

University of Michigan Health System. (2003). Retrieved from www.med.umich.edu

Updegraff, J. A., & Taylor, S. E. (2000). From vulnerability to growth: Positive and negative effects of stressful life events. In J. H. Harvey & E. D. Miller (Eds.), *Loss and trauma: General and close relationship perspectives* (pp. 3-28). Philadelphia: Brunner-Routledge.

Utsey, S. O. (1991). Vocational rehabilitation and counseling approaches with sickle cell anemia. *Journal of Applied Rehabilitation Counseling, 22,* 29-31.

Vaillant, G. E. (2002). *Aging well: Surprising guideposts to a happier life.* Boston: Little, Brown.

van Diest, R., & Appels, A. (1991). Vital exhaustion and depression: A conceptual study. *Journal of Psychosomatic Research, 35,* 535-544.

Van Houdenhove, B., Neerinckx, E., Onghena, P., Vingerhoets, A., Lysens, R., & Vertommen, H. (2002). Daily hassles reported by chronic fatigue syndrome and fibromyalgia patients in tertiary care: A controlled quantitative and qualitative study. *Psychotherapy and Psychosomatics, 71,* 207-213.

Vanable, P. A., Ostrow, D. G., McKirnan, D. J., Taywaditep, K. J., & Hope, B. A. (2000). Impact of combination therapies on HIV risk perceptions and sexual risk among HIV-positive and HIV-negative gay and bisexual men. *Health Psychology, 19*, 134-145.

Varshney, A. (2002). *Ethnic conflict and civic life.* New Haven, CT: Yale University Press.

Velicer, W., Fava, J., Prochaska, J., Abrams, D., Emmons, K., & Piere, J. (1995). Distribution of smokers by stage in three representative samples. *Preventive Medicine, 24*, 401-411.

Velicer, W. F., Prochaska, J. O., Bellis, J. M., DiClemente, C. C., Rossi, J. S., Fava, J. H., et al. (1993). An expert system intervention for smoking cessation. *Addictive Behaviors, 18*, 269-290.

Verbrugge, L. M. (1989). The twain meet: Empirical explanations of sex differences in health and mortality. *Journal of Health and Social Behavior, 30*(3), 282-304.

Verbrugge, L. M., Lepowski, J. M., & Konkol, L. L. (1991). Levels of disability among U.S. adults with arthritis. *Journal of Gerontology: Social Sciences, 46*(2), 571-583.

Vernon, S. W., & Buffler, P. A. (1988). The status of status inconsistency. *Epidemiologic Reviews, 10*, 65-86.

Verrier, R. L., & Mittleman, M. A. (1996). Life-threatening cardiovascular consequences of anger in patients with coronary heart disease. *Cardiology Clinics, 14,* 289-307.

Virchow, R. (1848). The Public Health Service [in German]. *Medizinische Reform, 5*, 21-22.

Vitaliano, P. P., Scanlan, J. M., & Zhang, J. (in press). Is caregiving hazardous to one's physical health? A meta-analysis. *Psychological Bulletin.*

Vitaliano, P. P., Scanlan, J. M., Zhang, J., Savage, M. V., Hirsch, I., & Siegler, I. C. (2002). A path model of chronic stress, the metabolic syndrome, and coronary heart disease. *Psychosomatic Medicine, 64*, 418-435.

Vitiello, B., & Lederhendler, I. (2000). Research on eating disorders: Current status and future prospects. *Biological Psychiatry, 47*, 777-786.

Vlaeyen, J. W. S., Nooyen-Haazen, I. W. C. J., Boossens, M. E. J. B., van Breukelen, G., Heuts, P. H. T. G., & The, H. G. (1997). The role of fear in the cognitive-educational treatment of fibromyalgia. In T. S. Jensen, J. A. Turner, & Z. Wiesenfeld-Hallin (Eds.), *Proceedings of the 8th World Congress on Pain: Vol. 8. Progress in pain research and management* (pp. 693-704). Seattle, WA: IASP Press.

Von Baak, M. A. (1998). Exercise and hypertension: facts and uncertainties. *British Journal of Sports Medicine, 32*(1), 6-10.

Vrijkotte, T., van DoorNen, L., & de Geus, E. (2000). Effect of work stress on ambulatory blood pressure, heart rate, and heart rate variability. *Hypertension, 35,* 880-886.

Wack, J., & Rodin, L. (1982). Smoking and its effects on body weight and the systems of caloric regulation. *American Journal of Clinical Nutrition, 35,* 366-380.

Wadden, T. A., Brownell, K. D., & Foster, G. D. (2002). Obesity: Responding to the global epidemic. *Journal of Consulting and Clinical Psychology, 70,* 510-525.

Wadden, T., & Stunkard, A. J. (Eds.). (2002). *Handbook of obesity treatment.* New York: Guilford.

Wagner, E. H., Austin, B. T., & Von Korff, M. (1996a). Improving outcomes in chronic illness. *Managed Care Quarterly, 4,* 12-25.

Wagner, E. H., Austin, B. T., & Von Korff, M. (1996b). Organizing care for patients with chronic illness. *Milbank Quarterly, 74,* 511-544.

Wagstaff, A., & van Doorslaer, E. (2000). Income inequality and health: what does the literature tell us? *Annual Reviews of Public Health, 21,* 543-567.

Waite, L. J., & Gallagher, M. (2000). *The case for marriage: Why married people are happier, healthier and better off financially.* New York: Doubleday.

Walco, G. A., & Dampier, C. D. (1990). Pain in children and adolescents with sickle cell disease: A descriptive study. *Journal of Pediatric Psychology, 15,* 643-658.

Waldstein, S. R. (2000). Health effects on cognitive aging. In P. C. Stern & L. L. Carstensen (Eds.), *The aging mind: Opportunities in cognitive research* (pp. 189-217). Committee on Future Directions for Cognitive Research on Aging. Commission on Behavioral and Social Sciences and Education. Washington, DC: National Academy Press.

Waldstein, S. R., & Elias, M. F. (Eds.). (2001). *Neuropsychology of cardiovascular disease.* Mahwah, NJ: Lawrence Erlbaum.

Waldstein, S. R., Tankard, C. F., Maier, K. J., Pelletier, J. R., Snow, J., Gardner, A.W., et al. (in press). Peripheral arterial disease and cognitive function. *Psychosomatic Medicine.*

Walker, J. (2001). *Control and the psychology of health.* Buckingham, UK: Open University Press.

Wall, P. D., & Melzack, R. (Eds.). (1999). *Textbook of pain.* Edinburgh: Churchill Livingstone.

Wallerstein, N. (1992). Health and safety education for workers with low-literacy or limited English skills. *American Journal of Industrial Medicine, 22,* 751-765.

Wallston, B. S., Wallston, K. A., Kaplan, G. D., & Maides, S. A. (1976). The development and validation of the health related locus of control (HLC) scale. *Journal of Consulting and Clinical Psychology, 44,* 580-585.

Wallston, K. A. (1989). Assessment of control in health care settings. In A. Steptoe & A. Appel (Eds.), *Stress, personal control and health* (pp. 85-105). Chicester, UK: Wiley.

Wallston, K. A. (1992). Hocus-pocus, the focus isn't strictly on locus: Rotter's social learning theory modified for health. *Cognitive Therapy and Research, 16*, 183-199.

Wallston, K. A. (1997). A history of the Division of Health Psychology: Healthy, wealthy, and Weiss. In D. E. Dewsbury (Ed.), *Unification through division: Histories of the Divisions of the American Psychological Association* (Vol. 2, pp. 239-267). Washington, DC: American Psychological Association.

Wallston, K. A. (2001a). Conceptualization and operationalization of perceived control. In A. Baum, T. Revenson, and J. E. Singer (Eds.), *The handbook of health psychology* (pp. 49-58). Mahwah, NJ: Lawrence Erlbaum.

Wallston, K. A. (2001b). Control beliefs. In N. J. Smelser & P. B. Baltes (Eds.), *International encyclopedia of the social and behavioral sciences.* Oxford, UK: Elsevier Science.

Wallston, K. A., Malcarne, V. L., Flores, L., Hansdottir, I., Smith, C. A., Stein, M. J., et al. (1999). Does God determine your health? The God Locus of Health Control scale. *Cognitive Therapy and Research, 23*, 131-142.

Wallston, K. A., & Smith, M. S. (1994). Issues of control and health: The action is the interaction. In G. Penny, P. Bennett, & M. Herbert (Eds.), *Health psychology: A lifespan perspective* (pp. 153-168). Chur, Switzerland: Harwood.

Wallston, K. A., Stein, M. J., & Smith, C. A. (1994). Form C of the MHLC Scales: A condition-specific measure of locus of control. *Journal of Personality Assessment, 63*, 534-553.

Wallston, K. A., & Wallston, B. S. (1981). Health locus of control scales. In H. Lefcourt (Ed.), *Research with the locus of control construct* (Vol. 1). New York: Academic Press.

Wallston, K. A., & Wallston, B. S. (1982). Who is responsible for your health: The construct of health locus of control. In G. Sanders & J. Suls (Eds.), *Social psychology of health and illness* (pp. 65-95). Hillsdale, NJ: Lawrence Erlbaum.

Wallston, K. A., Wallston, B. S., & DeVellis, R. (1978). Development of the multidimensional health locus of control (MHLC) scales. *Health Education Monographs, 6*, 160-170.

Wamala, S. P. (2001). Large social inequalities in coronary heart disease risk among women: Low occupational status and family stress are crucial factors. *Swedish Journal of Medicine, 98*(3), 177-180.

Wamala, S. P., & Lynch, J. (Eds.). (2002). *Gender and social inequalities in health: A public health issue.* Lund, Sweden: Studentlitteratur.

Ware, J., & Sherbourne, C. (1992). The MOS 36-item Short Form health survey (SF-36) 1: Conceptual framework and item selection. *Medical Care 30,* 473-483.

Ware, J. E., Davies-Avery, A., & Donald, C. A. (1978). *Conceptualization and measurement of health for adults in the health insurance study: Vol. 5. General health perceptions.* RAND Corporation Report R-1987/5-HEW. Santa Monica, CA: RAND.

Warshauer, M. E., Silverman, D. T., Schottenfeld, D., & Pollack, E. S. (1986). Stomach and colorectal cancers in Puerto Rican-born residents of New York City. *Journal of the National Cancer Institute, 76,* 591-595.

Wasilewski, Y., Clark, N., Evans, D., Feldman, C. H., Kaplan, D., Rips, J., et al. (1988). The effect of paternal social support on maternal disruption caused by childhood asthma. *Journal of Community Health, 13,* 33-42.

Way, D., & Jones, L. (2000). *Implementation strategies: Collaboration in primary care—Family doctors & nurse practitioners delivering shared care.* Unpublished manuscript, Ontario College of Family Physicians, Toronto, Ontario.

Wechsler, H., Davenport, A., Dowdall, G., Moeykens, B., & Castillo, S. (1994). Health and behavioral consequences of binge drinking in college: A national survey of students at 140 campuses. *Journal of the American Medical Association, 272,* 1672–1677.

Wechsler, H., Dowdall, G. W., Davenport, A., & Castillo, S. (1995). Correlates of college student binge drinking. *American Journal of Public Health, 85,* 921-926.

Wechsler, H., Lee, J. E., Hall, J., Wagenaar, A. C., & Lee, H. (2002). Secondhand effects of student alcohol use reported by neighbors of colleges: The role of alcohol outlets. *Social Science and Medicine, 55,* 425-435.

Wechsler, H., Lee, J. E., Kuo, M., Seibring, M., Nelson, T. F., & Lee, H. (2002). Trends in alcohol use, related problems and experience of prevention efforts among U.S. college students 1993-2001: Results from the 2001 Harvard School of Public Health College Alcohol Study. *Journal of American College Health, 50,* 203-217.

Wechsler, H., & Nelson, T. F. (2001). Binge drinking and the American college student: What's five drinks? *Psychology of Addictive Behaviors, 15,* 287-291.

Weihs, K. L., Enright, T. M., Simmens, S. J., & Reiss, D. (2000). Negative affectivity, restriction of emotions, and the site of metastases predict mortality in recurrent breast cancer. *Journal of Psychosomatic Research, 49*(1), 59-68.

Weinberg, C. R. (1986). Applicability of simple independent-action model to epidemiological studies involving two factors and a dichotomous outcome. *American Journal of Epidemiology, 123,* 162-173.

Weinberger, D. A., Schwartz, G. E., & Davidson, R. J. (1979). Low-anxious, high-anxious and repressive coping styles: Psychometric patterns and behavioral responses to stress. *Journal of Abnormal Psychology, 88,* 369-380.

Weiner, H. (1991a). From simplicity to complexity (1950-1990): The case of peptic ulceration: I. Human studies. *Psychosomatic Medicine, 53,* 467-490.

Weiner, H. (1991b). From simplicity to complexity (1950-1990): The case of peptic ulceration: II. Animal studies. *Psychosomatic Medicine, 53,* 491-516.

Weinhardt, L. S., Carey, M. P., Johnson, B. T., & Bickham, N. L. (1999). Effects of HIV counseling and testing on sexual risk behavior: A meta-analytic review of the published research, 1985-1997. *American Journal of Public Health, 89,* 1397-1405.

Weinhardt, L. S., Forsyth, A. D., Carey, M. P., Jaworkski, B. C., & Durant, L. E. (1998). Reliability and validity of self-report measures of HIV-related sexual behavior: Progress since 1990 and recommendations for research and practice. *Archives of Sexual Behavior, 27,* 155-180.

Weinstein, M. C., Siegel, J. E., Gold, M. R., Kamlet, M. S., & Russell, L. B. (1996). Recommendations of the Panel on Cost-Effectiveness in Health and Medicine. *Journal of the American Medical Association, 276,* 1253-1258.

Weinstein, N. (1993). Testing four competing theories of health-protective behavior. *Health Psychology, 12,* 324-333.

Weinstein, N. D. (1980). Unrealistic optimism about future life events. *Journal of Personality and Social Psychology, 39,* 806-820.

Weinstein, N. D., & Sandman, P. M. (2002). The precaution adoption process model and its application. In R. J. DiClementi, R. A. Crosby, & M. C. Kegler (Eds.), *Emerging theories in health promotion practice and research: Strategies for improving public health* (pp. 16-39). San Francisco: Jossey-Bass.

Weiss, J. M. (1968). Effects of coping on stress. *Journal of Comparative and Physiological Psychology, 65,* 251-260.

Weiss, J. M. (1984). Behavioral and psychological influences on gastrointestinal pathology: experimental techniques and findings. In W. Doyle Gentry (Ed.), *Handbook of behavioral medicine* (pp. 174-221). New York: Guilford.

Weller, E. B., Weller, R. A., Rooney, M. T., & Fristad, M. A. (1999). *ChIPS: Children's Interview for Psychiatric Syndromes.* Washington, DC: American Psychiatric Press.

Wenger, N. K. (1999). Cardiac rehabilitation: A guide to practice in the 21st century. New York: Marcel Dekker.

Wenger, N. K., Froehlicher, E. S., Smith, L. K., Ades, P. A., et al. (1995). *Cardiac rehabilitation: Clinical practice guidelines.* Rockville, MD: Agency for Health Care Policy and Research and the National Heart, Lung, and Blood Institute.

Werner, E., & Smith, R. S. (1992). *Overcoming the odds: High-risk children from birth to adulthood.* Ithaca, NY: Cornell University Press.

Werner, O., & Schoepfle, M. (1987). *Systematic fieldwork: Foundations of ethnography and interviewing.* Newbury Park, CA: Sage.

West, C. (1984). *Routine complications: Troubles with talk between doctors and patients.* Bloomington: Indiana University Press.

Wethington, E., & Kessler, R. C. (1986). Perceived support, received support, and adjustment to stressful events. *Journal of Health and Social Behavior, 27,* 78-89.

Wheaton, B. (1985). Models for the stress-buffering function of coping resources. *Journal of Health and Social Behavior, 26,* 352-364.

Wheaton, B. (1999). The nature of stressors. In A. V. Horwitz & T. L. Scheid (Eds.), *A handbook of the study of mental health: Social contexts, theories, and symptoms.* New York: Cambridge University Press.

Whelton, S. P., Chin, A., Xin, X., & He, J. (2002). Effect of aerobic exercise on blood pressure: A meta-analysis of randomized, controlled trials. *Annals of Internal Medicine, 136,* 493-503.

White, D., & Pitts, M. (1998). Educating young people about drugs: A systematic review. *Addiction, 93,* 1475-1487.

White, R. W. (1959). Motivation reconsidered: The concept of competence. *Psychological Review, 66,* 297-333.

Whiting, P., Bagnall, A.-M., Sowden, A. J., Cornell, J. E., Mulrow, C. D., & Ramirez, G. (2001). Interventions for the treatment and management of chronic fatigue syndrome. *Journal of the American Medical Association, 286,* 1360-1368.

Whitlock, E. P., Orleans, C. T., Pender, N., & Allan, J. (2002). Evaluating primary care behavioral counseling interventions: An evidence-based approach. *American Journal of Preventive Medicine, 22,* 267-284.

Whitt, H. P. (1983). Status inconsistency: A body of negative evidence or a statistical artifact? *Social Forces, 62,* 201-233.

Whorwell, P. J., Prior, A., & Faragher, E. B. (1984). Controlled trial of hypnotherapy in the treatment of severe refractory irritable-bowel syndrome. *Lancet*, 1232-1234.

Wiecha, J. M., Lee, V., & Hodgkins, J. (1998). Patterns of smoking, risk factors for smoking, and smoking cessation among Vietnamese men in Massachusetts (United States). *Tobacco Control, 7*, 27-34.

Wilhelmsen, I., Tangen, T., Ursin, H., & Berstad, A. (1994). Effect of short-term cognitive psychotherapy on recurrence of duodenal ulcer: A prospective randomized trial. *Psychosomatic Medicine, 56*, 440-448.

Willemsen, M., de Vries, H., van Breukelen, G., & Genders, R. (1998). Long-term effectiveness of two Dutch work site smoking cessation programs. *Health Education and Behavior, 25*, 418-435.

Willett, W. C. (1998). *Nutritional epidemiology* (2nd ed.). New York: Oxford University Press.

Willett, W. C. (2001). Diet and cancer: One view at the start of the millennium. *Cancer Epidemiology, Biomarkers, and Prevention, 10*, 3-8.

Williams, D. R. (1996). Racism and health: A research agenda. *Ethnicity & Disease, 6*, 1-6.

Williams, D. R. (1999). Race, socioeconomic status, and health: The added effects of racism and discrimination. In N. E. Adler, M. Marmot, B. S. McEwen, & J. Stewart (Eds.), *Socioeconomic status and health in industrial nations: Social, psychological, and biological pathways* (Vol. 896, pp. 173-188). New York: New York Academy of Sciences.

Williams, D. R. (2001). Racial variations in adult health status: Patterns, paradoxes, and prospects. In N. J. Smelser, W. J. Wilson, & F. Mitchell (Eds.), *America becoming: Racial trends and their consequences* (Vol. 2, pp. 371-410). Washington, DC: National Academy Press.

Williams, D. R., & Neighbors, H. W. (2002). Racism, discrimination, and hypertension: Evidence and needed research. *Ethnicity & Disease, 11*(4), 800-816.

Williams, D. R., Neighbors, H. W., & Jackson, J. S. (2003). Racial/ethnic discrimination and health: Findings from community studies. *American Journal of Public Health, 93*, 200-208.

Williams, D. R., & Williams-Morris, R. (2000). Racism and mental health: The African American experience. *Ethnicity & Health, 5*, 243-268.

Williams, D. R., Yu, Y., Jackson, J., & Anderson, N. (1997). Racial differences in physical and mental health: Socioeconomic status, stress, and discrimination. *Journal of Health Psychology, 2*, 335-351.

Williams, J. E., Nieto, F. J., Sanford, C. P., Couper, D. J., & Tyroler, H. A. (2002). The association between trait anger and incident stroke risk: The Atherosclerosis Risk in Communities (ARIC) Study. *Stroke, 33*, 13-20.

Williams, J. E., Paton, C. C., Siegler, I. C., Eigenbrodt, M. L., Nieto, F. J., & Tyroler, H. A. (2000). Anger proneness predicts coronary heart disease risk: Prospective analysis from the Atherosclerosis Risk in Communities (ARIC) Study. *Circulation, 101*, 2034-2039.

Williams, J. K. (2001). Understanding evidence-based medicine: A primer. *American Journal of Obstetrics and Gynecology, 185*, 275-278.

Williams, R. B. (1987). Redefining the Type A hypothesis: Emergence of the hostility complex. *American Journal of Cardiology, 60*, 27J-32J.

Wilson, G. T., & Fairburn, C. G. (2002). Treatments for eating disorders. In P. E. Nathan and J. M. Gorman (Eds.), *A guide to treatments that work* (2nd ed., pp. 559-592). London: Oxford University Press.

Wilson, P. W., D'Agostino, R. B., Levy, D., et al. (1998). Prediction of coronary heart disease using risk factor categories. *Circulation, 97*, 1837-1847.

Wincze, J. P., & Carey, M. P. (2001). *Sexual dysfunction: Guide for assessment and treatment* (2nd ed.). New York: Guilford.

Wing, R. R., Goldstein, M. G., Acton, K. J., Birch, L. L., Jakicic, J. M., Sallis, J. F., et al. (2001). Behavioral science research in diabetes: Lifestyle changes related to obesity, eating behavior, and physical activity. *Diabetes Care, 24*, 117-123.

Wing, S., Barnett, E., Casper, M., & Tyroler, H. A. (1992). Geographic and socioeconomic variation in the onset of decline of coronary heart disease mortality in White women. *American Journal of Public Health, 82*, 204-209.

Winkleby, M. A. (1994). The future of community-based cardiovascular disease intervention studies. *American Journal of Public Health, 84*, 1369-1372.

Winkleby, M. A., Feldman, H. A., & Murray, D. M. (1997). Joint analysis of three U.S. community intervention trials for reduction of cardiovascular disease risk. *Journal of Clinical Epidemiology, 50*, 645-648.

Winn, M. (1985). *The plug-in drug: Television, children, and the family.* New York: Viking.

Wiseman, V. L. (1999). Culture, self-rated health and resource allocation decision-making. *Health Care Analysis, 7*, 207-223.

Wissler, C. (1923). *Man and culture.* New York: Thomas Y. Crowell.

Wolf, S., & Wolff, H. G. (1947). *Human gastric function: An experimental study of a man and his stomach.* New York: Oxford University Press.

Wolfe, F., Smythe, H. A., Yunus, M. B., Bennett, R. M., Bombardier, C., Goldenberg, D., Tugwell, P., Campbell, S. M., Abeles, M., Clark, P., Fam, A. G., Farber, S. J., Fiechtner, J. J., Franklin, C. M., Gatter, R. A., Hamaty, D., Lessard, J., Lichtbroun, A. S., Masi, A. T., McCain, G. A., Reynolds, W. J., Romano, T. J., Russell, I. J., & Sheon, R. P. (1990). The American College of Rheumatology 1990 criteria for the classification of fibromyalgia: Report of the Multicenter Criteria Committee. *Arthritis and Rheumatism, 36,* 160-172.

Wolff, T. (2001). A practitioner's guide to successful coalitions. *American Journal of Community Psychology 29,* 173-191.

Wolff, T., & Kaye, G. (1991). *From the ground up! A workbook on coalition building and community development.* Amherst, MA: AHEC/Community Partners.

Wolpaw, J. R. (Guest editor), Birbaumer, N., Heetderks, W. J., McFarland, D. J., Peckham, P. H., Schalk, G., Donchin, E., Quatrano, L. A., Robinson, C. J., & Vaughan, T. M. (2000). Brain-computer interface technology: A review of the first international meeting. *IEEE Transactions on Rehabilitation Engineering, 8,* 164-173.

Wood, J. B., & Parham, I. A. (1990). Coping with perceived burden: Ethnic and cultural issues in Alzheimer's family caregiving. *Journal of Applied Gerontology, 9,* 325-339.

Woolf, S. H., & Atkins, D. (2001). The evolving role of prevention in health care contributions of the U.S. Preventive Services Task Force. *American Journal of Preventive Medicine, 20*(3S), 13-20.

Worden, J. K., & Flynn, B. S. (2000). Effective use of mass media to prevent cigarette smoking. *Journal of Public Health Management and Practice, 6,* vii-viii.

Worell, J. (Ed.). (2001). *Encyclopedia of women and gender: Sex similarities and differences and the impact of society on gender.* London: Academic Press, Harcourt Place.

World Cancer Research Fund and American Institute for Cancer Research. (1997). *Food, nutrition and the prevention of cancer: A global perspective.* Washington, DC: American Institute for Cancer Research.

World Health Organization. (1992, January). *Informal expert group meeting on the craving mechanism, report 1992.* Proceedings of the Meeting of the United Nations International Drug Control Programme, World Health Organization, Vienna, Austria. Geneva, Switzerland: Author.

World Health Organization. (1997). *Tobacco or health: A global status report.* Geneva: Author.

World Health Organization. (1999). *The World Health report: Making a difference.* Geneva, Switzerland: Author.

World Health Organization. (2000). *Obesity: Preventing and managing the global epidemic: Report of a WHO consultation* (WHO Tech. Rep. Ser. 894), 1-253.

Wright, R. J., & Fisher, E. B. (in press). Putting asthma into context: Influences on risk, behavior, and intervention. In I. Kawachi & L. F. Berkman (Eds.), *Neighborhoods and health.* New York: Oxford University Press.

Wright, R., Rodriguez, M., & Cohen, S. (1998). Review of psychosocial stress and asthma: An integrated biopsychosocial approach. *Thorax, 53,* 1066-1074.

Wright, R., & Steinbach, S. (2001). Violence: An unrecognized environmental exposure that may contribute to greater asthma morbidity in high risk inner-city populations. *Environmental Health Perspectives, 109,* 1085-1089.

Wright, R., & Weiss, S. (2000). Epidemiology of allergic disease. In S. Holgate, M. Church, & L. Lichtenstein (Eds.), *Allergy* (2nd ed.). London: Harcourt.

Writing Group for the Activity Counseling Trial Research Group. (2001). Effects of physical activity counseling in primary care. *Journal of the American Medical Association, 286,* 677-687.

Wulsin, L. R., Vaillant, G. E., & Wells, V. E. (1999). A systematic review of the mortality of depression. *Psychosomatic Medicine, 61,* 6-17.

Wykle, M., & Segall, M. (1991). A comparison of Black and White family caregivers' experience with dementia. *Journal of the National Black Nurses Association, 5,* 29-41.

Yanek, L. R. (2001). Project Joy: Faith-based cardiovascular health promotion for African American women. *Public Health Reports, 1,* 68-81.

Yee, B. W. K., Mokuau, N., & Kim, S. (Eds.). (1999). *Developing cultural competence in Asian American and Pacific Islander communities: Opportunities in primary health care and substance abuse prevention.* Cultural Competence Series, Vol. 5 (DHHS Pub. No. (SMA)98-3193), Special Collaborative Edition. Washington DC: Center for Substance Abuse Prevention (SAMSHA), Bureau of Primary Health Care (HRSA), and Office of Minority Health (DHHS).

Yee, J. L., & Schulz, R. (2000). Gender differences in psychiatric morbidity among family caregivers: A review and analysis. *Gerontologist, 40,* 147-164.

Yesavage, J., Brink, T., Rose, T., Lum, O., Huang, V., Adey, M., et al. (1983). Development and validation of a geriatric depression screening scale: A preliminary report. *Journal of Psychiatric Research, 17,* 37-49.

Yin, R. K., Kaftarian, S. J., Yu, P., & Jansen, M. A. (1997). Outcomes from CSAP's Community Partnerships Program: Findings from the National Cross-Site Evaluation. *Evaluation and Program Planning, 20,* 345-356.

Yonkers, K. A., & Samson, J. (2000). Mood disorders measures. In American Psychiatric Association (Ed.), *Handbook of psychiatric measures* (pp. 515-548). Washington, DC: American Psychiatric Association.

Yule, G. U. (1903). Notes on the theory of association of attributes in statistics. *Biometrika, 2,* 121-134.

Zambrana, R. E., & Carter-Pokras, O. (2001). Health data issues for Hispanics: Implications for public health research. *Journal of Health Care for the Poor and Underserved, 12, 1,* 20-34.

Zane, N. W. S., Takeuchi, D. T., & Young, K. N. J. (Eds.). (1994). *Confronting critical health issues of Asian and Pacific Islander Americans.* Thousand Oaks, CA: Sage.

Zarit, S. H. (1994). Methodological considerations in caregiver intervention and outcome research. In E. Light, G. Niederehe, & B. D. Lebowitz (Eds.), *Stress effects on family caregivers of Alzheimer's patients* (pp. 351-369). New York: Springer.

Zautra, A. J., Smith, B. W., & Yocum, D. (2002). Psychosocial influences on arthritis-related disease activity. In T. Sivik, D. Byne, D. R. Lipsitt, G. N. Christodoulou, & H. Dienstfrey (Eds.), *Psycho-neuro-endocrino-immunology (PNEI): A common language for the whole human body. Proceedings of the 16th World Congress on Psychosomatic Medicine.* Amsterdam: Elsevier.

Zeidner, M., & Endler, N. S. (Eds.). (1996). *Handbook of coping.* New York: John Wiley.

Zenilman, J. (1996). Gonococcal susceptibility to antimicrobials in Baltimore, 1988-1994. What was the impact of ciprofloxcin as first-line therapy for gonorrhea? *Sexually Transmitted Diseases, 23,* 213-218.

Zenz, C. (Ed.). (1994). *Occupational medicine* (3rd ed.). St. Louis, MO: C. V. Mosby.

Zigmond, A. S., & Snaith, R. P. (1983). The Hospital Anxiety and Depression Scale. *Acta Psychiatrica Scandinavica, 67,* 361-370.

Zuckerman, M. (1960). The development of an Affect Adjective Check List for the measurement of anxiety. *Journal of Consulting Psychology, 24,* 457-462.

Zuckerman, M., & Lubin, B. (1965). *Manual for the Multiple Affect Adjective Checklist.* San Diego, CA: Educational and Industrial Testing Service.

Zuckerman, M., & Lubin, B. (1998). *Manual for the Multiple Adjective Check List* (3rd ed.). San Diego, CA: Educational and Industrial Testing Service.

Zung, W. W. K. (1965). A self-rating depression scale. *Archives of General Psychiatry, 12,* 63-70.

Author Index

Abel, G. G., 725
Abeles, M., 329, 333
Abrams, D., 737
Ackerman, M. D., 317
Adams, J. E., 180
Adams, J. S., 296
Adams, L. A., 729
Adey, M., 231
Adler, N. E., 345, 768
Affleck, G., 307
Ahlbom, A., 108, 562, 563, 564
Aiello, J. R., 227
Aitkin, M., 603
Ajzen, I., 218, 476, 549, 793, 796, 799
Akerstedt, T., 820
Alberg, A. J., 3
Alcaraz, J. E., 660, 661
Alderman, E. L., 711
Aldwin, C. M., 92
Alexander, C. N., 111
Alexander, J., 211
Allan, J., 320
Allen, A. J., 201, 203
Allensworth, D., 704, 705, 706
Alperovitch, A., 58
Alpert, J. E., 239
Altmaier, E. M., 337
Altman, D. G., 696
Altman, I., 226
Amaro, H., 2
Amick, B. C., III, 562, 563, 564
Amir, N., 56
Andersen, R. R., 210
Anderson, D., 603
Anderson, I. M., 239
Anderson, J., 4
Anderson, L. M., 2
Anderson, N. B., 255, 257, 258, 322
Anderson, R. M., 720
Andrasik, F., 98
Andrews, L., 21, 22
Antonovsky, A., 344, 345
Antonuccio, D. O., 237

Apfel, N. H., 674
Appel, L. J., 102
Arcia, E., 2, 579
Arconad, M., 237
Ariyo, A. A., 303
Armstead, C. A., 257
Armstrong, F. D., 725
Arnett, D., 145
Arsianian, S. A., 704
Asberg, M., 231
Ascher, J., 740
Ascherio, A., 504, 755
Ashby, F. G., 308
Aspinwall, L. G., 307
Aspnes, A., 13
Assaf, A. R., 142
Astin, J. A., 69, 211, 219
Atienza, A. A., 143
Atkins, D., 320
Austin, B. T., 171, 173, 174
Austin, J., 28
Avorn, J., 28

Babbar, R., 110
Bacchetti, P., 82
Bachman, K. J., 706, 707
Backlund, M. S., 344
Badger, G. J., 267
Bahr, G. R., 28
Bailey, D., 2, 579
Bailey, W., 737, 738, 739, 740
Baker, D., 108, 562
Baker, J. E., 174
Balcazar, H., 2
Balch, G. I., 340
Baldwin, J. M., 502
Ban, T. A., 231
Bandura, A., 10, 27, 218, 340, 475, 549, 709, 710, 713, 720
Barbarin, O., 725
Barefoot, J. C., 307, 308, 309, 527
Barerra, M., Jr., 780
Barker, H., 502
Barker, L. R., 61

Barlow, B., 550
Barlow, D. H., 56, 317
Barlow, J., 175
Barnes, D. E., 732
Baron-Epel, O., 715, 716
Barrett, D. J., 291, 725
Bartlett, J. A., 23
Basbaum, A. I., 356
Basmajian, J. V., 100
Bassi, L., 562
Bassuk, S., 757
Baum, A., 227
Baumstark, K. E., 333
Bausell, R. B., 212
Beach, S. R., 208, 303
Beaglehole, R., 345
Beck, A. T., 231, 232, 236, 522
Beck, J. S., 232
Becker, A. B., 145, 200, 201, 202, 203
Becker, M. H., 475, 476, 720
Beckett, L. A., 208
Beckham, E. E., 231
Beckner, W., 69
Bedi, M., 110
Beekman, A. T., 208
Beers, S. R., 199
Begg, D. J., 551
Beilenson, P. L., 551
Belgrave, F., 725
Belkic, K., 562
Bellamy, N., 686
Bellis, J. M., 790
Benbasal, J., 740
Bendtsen, L., 331
Benin, M. B., 2
Benjamin, B., 821
Benjamini, L. S., 364
Bennett, G. G., 567
Bennett, N., 603
Bennett, P., 673
Bennett, R. M., 329, 333
Benotsch, E. G., 22, 28
Benson, H., 58
Benyamini, Y., 717, 718
Berg, M. A., 335
Berger, W. E., III, 710
Bergman-Losman, B., 364
Bergner, M., 686
Berkman, L. F., 208, 363, 587, 753, 754, 755, 756, 757
Berman, B. M., 69, 212
Berman, S., 522
Bernard-Bonnin, A., 76
Bernard, H. R., 569
Berne, R. M., 102

Bernstein, B. M., 28
Berntson, G. G., 587
Bero, L. A., 732
Besson, J. M., 356
Best, K. M., 309
Bichisao, E., 107
Bien, T., 743
Bigelow, G. E., 267
Billings, J., 520
Birbaumer, N., 101
Black, D., 345
Blackburn, D. S., 219
Blakely, T., 539
Blanchard, E. B., 554, 557
Blazer, D. G., 208, 235, 755
Block, J., 309
Block, M. R., 209
Blumenthal, J. A., 110, 304, 364, 527
Bobbitt, R. A., 686
Bobo, J., 743
Bobo, L., 254
Boeke, A. J., 755
Bogden, J. F., 704
Bogurt, L. M., 22
Bolan, G., 27
Boles, S. M., 321
Bolger, N., 781
Bombardier, C., 329, 333, 687
Bonds, S., 725
Bonnin, D., 76
Bonollo, D., 740, 743
Boreham, J., 730
Borhani, N., 520
Borkum, J., 467, 469
Bosschieter, E. B., 502
Bossé, R., 93
Botvin, G. J., 3
Boudewyun, A. C., 82
Bouknight, R. R., 174
Bower, J. E., 307
Bowie, W. R., 202
Bowlby, J., 93
Bowling, A. C., 502
Boyce, T., 345, 768
Bracht, N., 143
Brady, J. V., 350
Brand, J. H., 519
Brand, R., 755
Branigan, C. A., 308
Brasfield, T. L., 28, 721
Brennan, L., 70, 789
Brester, M., 21, 22, 23
Brewin, C. R., 694
Brickman, P., 460

Brink, T., 231
Brody, B., 319
Broomhall, L., 570
Bross, I. D. J., 215
Broughton, R., 729
Brown, G. E., 151
Brown, G. K., 231, 232
Brown, J. B., 210
Brown, J. D., 217, 307
Brown, P. C., 364
Brown, R. T., 725, 739
Brown, V., 14
Browning, S. R., 565
Brownley, K. A., 566, 567
Bruce, C., 175
Brumback, B. A., 215, 294
Brunner, E., 768
Buchanan, W. W., 686, 687
Buchholz, W. M., 522
Buckelew, S. P., 333
Buckles, J., 28
Budney, A. J., 267, 269
Buffington, A., 13
Bultman, L., 674
Bunce, A., 4
Bunker, C. H., 566
Burg, M. M., 363, 364
Burge, R., 743
Burleson, M. H., 587
Burlew, A. K., 725
Burt, R. S., 756
Bush, J. W., 223
Buss, A. H., 528
Butters, M., 199
Butts, E., 4
Buysse, D. J., 728
Buzaglo, J. S., 544
Bye, L. L., 713
Byers, R. H., 27
Bymaster, F. P., 239
Byrne, D. G., 363

Cabana, M. D., 173
Cacioppo, J. T., 586, 587
Caetano, R., 2
Cage, M., 28
Caine, E. D., 208
Calkins, D. R., 210
Cameron, N., 60
Campbell, D., 522
Campbell, J., 686
Campbell, J. K., 470
Campbell, R. S., 327
Campbell, S. M., 329, 333

Cannon, W. B., 146, 151, 366
Caplin, D. L., 174
Cappelli, P., 562
Carels, R. A., 364
Carey, M. P., 25, 26, 27, 316, 317, 712
Carlaw, R., 143
Carleton, R. A., 142
Carlson, B., 469, 470
Carroll, D., 154
Carson, J., 13
Caruso, L. S., 728
Carver, C. S., 307, 308, 641, 775
Carver, M. D., 586
Carye, K. B., 712
Case, A., 769
Casey, K. L., 355
Casper, M., 144
Caspersen, C. J., 175, 660
Cassel, J. C., 766, 780
Cassidy, A., 206
Catanzaro, S. J., 307
Cattell, R. B., 60
Catz, S. L., 22
Celio, A., 713
Cerhan, J. R., 303
Chae, C. U., 103
Chaiken, S., 712
Chambless, L., 145
Champeau, D., 267
Chaney, E. F., 266
Chang, H., 562, 564
Chapagne, M. A., 711
Charette, C., 76
Chastain, R., 218
Chen, M. S., Jr., 4
Chen, X., 2
Chesney, A., 345
Chesney, M. A., 22, 768, 813
Cheuk, W., 82
Chevron, E. S., 235
Chobanian, A. V., 103
Chong, Y., 2
Chorousos, G. P., 178, 333
Chung, R. C. -Y., 75
Chwalisz, K., 337
Clair, J. M., 15
Clapp, D., 544
Clark, D. A., 231
Clark, L. A., 231
Clark, M., 710
Clark, M. A., 790
Clark, M. C., 580
Clark, N. M., 170, 171, 172, 173, 174
Clark, P., 329, 333

Clark, R., 255, 257
Clark, V. R., 255
Clauw, D. J., 178, 331, 333
Clayton, D., 214
Cleary, P. D., 28
Clifford, J., 570
Clore, G. L., 308
Coakley, E. H., 563
Coates, D., 460
Coates, T. J., 28
Cobain, M. J., 317
Cobas, J. A., 2
Cobb, S., 780
Cochran, S. D., 258
Coe, C. L., 679
Coffman, G., 2
Cohen, R., 755
Cohen, R. D., 522
Cohen, S., 178, 226, 227, 257, 258, 363, 364, 737, 738,
    739, 740, 754, 768, 780, 781
Colditz, G. A., 501, 504, 518, 563, 755
Cole, J., 740
Coleman, J. S., 751
Colin, J. -N., 740
Collins, J. F., 239
Condray, R., 199
Conn, J. M., 260
Connolly, K. J., 227
Connor, J. T. H., 210
Cook, D., 696
Cook, K., 706, 707
Cook, W. W., 528
Cooper-Patrick, L., 173
Corbett, M., 257
Corcoran, J., 672, 673, 674
Cordingley, G. E., 469, 470
Correa, V., 2, 579
Coulander, C., 501
Couper, D. J., 304
Cousins, N., 306, 781
Covey, L., 743
Cowen, P., 57
Cox, C., 208
Cox, D. S., 307
Cox, V. C., 226
Crabtree, B., 569, 570
Cram, J. R., 100
Creed, F., 555
Creer, T. L., 174
Creet, T. L., 170
Crellin, J. K., 210
Cretin, D., 173
Crofford, L. J., 330
Croft, P., 333

Cronin-Stubbs, D., 208
Crowson, J. J., Jr., 522
Csikszentmihalyi, M., 291
Culbert, J. P., 728
Cummins, S., 622
Cutrona, C. E., 781

Dabelea, D., 704
Daniel, M., 202
Daniels, K., 753
Daniels, N., 224
Dannenberg, A. L., 551
Danner, D. D., 307, 462
Dantona, R. L., 267
Dantzer, R., 679
Darwin, C., 59
D'Atri, D. A., 107
Daubman, K. A., 308
Davey-Smith, G., 359, 768
Davidson, K. W., 322
Davidson, L. L., 550
Davidson-Katz, K., 306
Davies, S., 725
Davies-Avery, A., 714
Davis, C. G., 307
Davison, R. J., 693
Dawson, D., 555
deBacker, G., 821
Debski, T. T., 153
DeBusk, R. F., 710
Dee, B., 82
Deeg, D. J., 208, 755
de Geus, E., 298
dela Cruz, F. A., 4
Delbanco, T. L., 210
Dember, W. N., 642
Dembroski, T. M., 527, 528
De Meyer, G. R. Y., 103
Demitrack, M. A., 330
Demyttenaere, K., 173
Dennis, C. A., 710
Der, G., 768
Derogatis, L. R., 232
DeRubeis, R. J., 239
DeVellis, R., 218
De Vries, H., 790
DeVries, M. W., 291, 292, 307
DeWalt, B., 569
DeWalt, K., 569
Dewsbury, D. E., 473
Diaz, T., 3
Diaz, Y. E., 721
Dickenson, A. H., 356
DiClemente, C. C., 340, 737, 790, 803

Diderichsen, F., 563, 564
Diener, E., 460
Diez-Roux, A. V., 145, 346
DiFonzo, K., 28
DiGuiseppi, C., 550
Dijkstra, A., 790
Ding, Y., 103
Dion, K. L., 255
DiRienzo, M., 103
Disselhorst-Klug, C., 100
Dobbins, J. G., 177
Dobson, K. S., 239
Doka, K. J., 92
Domar, A. D., 544
Donald, A., 319
Donald, C. A., 714
Donatelle, R., 267
Donchin, E., 101
Doner, L., 340
Dongmei, L., 468
Donham, G. W., 61
Dording, C., 239
Dorfman, S., 737, 738, 739, 740
Douglas, J. C., 103
Douglas, J. M., 27
Dracup, K., 57
Dramaix, M., 821
Dressler, W. W., 108, 765
Druss, B. G., 211
Ducimetiere, P. J. T., 58
Duncan, G., 562, 564
Duncan-Jones, P., 363
Dunham, J., 299
Dunkel Schetter, C., 670
Dunn, J., 821
Durant, L. E., 26
Durkee, A., 528
Durkin, M. S., 550
Duzey, O., 170
Dwyer, J. H., 2, 3
Dwyer, K. A., 219
Dyer, J. M., 3
Dzewaltowski, D. A., 661

Eakin, E. G., 170
Earls, F., 752
Ebel, B. E., 173
Ebrahim, S., 111, 359
Eckenrode, J. E., 781
Eckman, J. R., 725
Edwards, C. L., 13, 14, 567
Eigenbrodt, M. L., 304
Eisenberg, D. M., 210
Ekman, P., 308

Elder, J. P., 706, 707, 708
Elghozi, J. -L., 103
Elias, M. F., 199
Elkin, I., 239
Ellaway, A., 622, 768
Elo, I. T., 768
Emery, C. F., 198
Emery, G., 236
Emmons, K., 737, 740, 743
Engel, B. T., 111
Engel, G. L., 498, 583
Engelgan, M. M., 175
Enright, T. M., 57
Enzlin, P., 173
Epstein, J. A., 3
Erbaugh, J., 232
Erlen, J. A., 22, 23
Ernst, J. M., 586, 587
Eshleman, S., 208, 768
Estabrooks, P. A., 661
Estrada, C. A., 308
Evans, D., 170, 171, 172, 173
Evans, G. W., 226, 227, 768
Everson, S. A., 522
Ewart, C. K., 9, 11

Fagerstrom, K., 737
Fahey, J. L., 92
Fair, J. M., 711
Fairhurst, S., 737
Fam, A. G., 329, 333
Faragher, E. B., 554
Farber, S. J., 329, 333
Farquhar, J. W., 143, 711
Farrell, D., 789, 790
Faucette, N., 660, 661
Fava, J. H., 737, 790
Fawzy, F. I., 781
Fawzy, N. W., 781
Fazio, R. H., 796
Feeney, A., 768
Feighner, J., 740
Feikje, G., 344
Feinleib, M., 519
Feldman, C. H., 170, 171, 173
Feldman, H. A., 143, 144, 706, 707, 708
Feldman, L., 361
Feldman Barrett, L., 291
Feliciano, P., 570
Ferber, R., 729
Ferguson, S. A., 551
Ferrari, M. D., 467, 468
Ferris, R., 740
Ferrucci, L., 303

Feuerstein, M., 498
Feve, J. M., 58
Fibiger, H., 740
Fiechtner, J. J., 329, 333
Fielden, H., 502
Fields, H. L., 356
Fiester, S., 737, 743
Finch, B., 2
Fiore, M. C., 345, 737, 738, 739, 740
First, M. B., 232
Firzgerald, E. F., 107
Fischer, C. S., 756
Fischer, M., 570
Fishbein, M., 27, 476, 720, 796, 797, 799
Fisher, J. D., 781
Fisher, L. D., 260, 710
Fisher, R. A., 214, 216
Fishman, B., 15
Fitzpatrick, T. R., 93, 94
Fix, M., 254
Flay, B. R., 799
Flegal, K. M., 704
Flor, H., 336
Flora, J. A., 143, 712
Flores, L., 218
Foege, W. H., 127
Folkman, S., 307, 367, 768, 775
Foner, N., 1
Fong, G. T., 26
Fontana, A., 570
Ford, D. E., 208
Ford, G., 768
Forssell, H., 337
Forsyth, A. D., 26
Fortmann, S. P., 143
Foster, C., 210
Fox, L., 13
Foxx, R., 739
France, K. G., 729
Francis, M. E., 307
Francucci, B., 107
Frank, E., 236
Frankenhaeuser, M., 363, 364
Frankish, C. J., 202
Franklin, C. M., 329, 333, 672, 673, 674
Franklin, S. S., 103
Franzini, L., 3
Frasure-Smith, N., 208
Fredrickson, B. L., 306, 307, 308, 309
Fredrikson, M., 364
Freeman, T. R., 210
Freriks, B., 100
Freud, S., 59, 60, 93
Frey, J. H., 570

Friedland, G., 21, 22
Friedman, H. S., 325
Friedman, M., 49, 518, 519, 520, 524
Friedman, R., 58
Fries, J. F., 68
Friesen, W. V., 307, 308, 462
Frijda, N. H., 56
Fristad, M., 232
Fromhout, D., 502
Froom, P., 740
Fuchs, H., 219
Fuggle, P., 725
Fukuda, K., 177
Furberg, A., 123
Furnham, A., 211

Gaarder, K. R., 111
Gable, S. L., 291
Gallagher, M., 260
Gallo, L. C., 10, 305, 769
Gantz, N. M., 177
Garcia, M., 2, 3
Gardner, A. W., 199
Gardner, M. J., 656
Garg, A. X., 8, 22
Garmezy, N., 309
Garrett, J. M., 565
Gasper, K., 308
Gass-Sternas, K. A., 92
Gatchel, R. J., 227
Gatsonis, C., 103
Gatter, R. A., 329, 333
Gaudry, E., 61
Gee, D., 710
Geleziunas, R., 21
Gelfand, L. A., 239
Genain, C. P., 83
Genteli, S., 107
George, M. A., 202
Georgiades, A., 110
Gerace, T., 520
Gerson, K., 756
Ghandour, G., 520, 710
Gibbon, M., 232
Gibrar, O., 57
Gielen, A. C., 551
Gilchrist, V., 569
Giles, D. E., 232, 728
Gill, J. J., 520
Gilson, B., 686
Giovannucci, E., 755
Giovengo, S. L., 332
Girard, A., 103
Girdler, S. S., 566, 567

Glantz, S. A., 732
Glaser, R., 260, 302, 303, 305, 364, 588
Glasgow, M. S., 111
Glasgow, R. E., 170, 175, 321
Glass, J. M., 335
Glass, R., 717, 752
Glass, T., 754, 756, 757
Glassman, A. H., 303, 743
Glassman, B., 789
Glickman-Weiss, E., 153
Glovinsky, P. B., 728
Glynn, R. J., 103, 755
Gner, R., 100
Goadsby, P. J., 467, 468
Goff, D. V., 502
Gold, M. R., 224
Goldberg, D. E., 522
Golden, R., 740
Goldenberg, D., 329, 333
Goldman, D. P., 769
Goldman, S. L., 307
Goldsmith, C. H., 686
Goldsteen, K., 260
Goldstein, M., 322, 737, 738, 739, 740, 743
Gong, M., 171, 172, 173
Goodkin, D. E., 82, 83
Goodkin, K., 15
Goodwin, F. K., 208
Goodwin, J., 307
Gordon, M., 1
Gore, S., 781
Gorsuch, R. L., 60, 61
Gottlieb, B., 754, 781
Gove, W. R., 227
Grace, G. M., 335
Graham, J., 28
Grahl, C., 6
Granovetter, M., 758
Grant, D., 674
Grant, E., 751
Gray, J. A., 696
Gray, R., 470
Graziano, S., 27
Greco, C. M., 337
Green, L. E., 549
Green, L. W., 202
Greene, E., 93
Greene, W. C., 21
Greenland, S., 213, 215, 216, 294
Greenstadt, L., 103
Greenwood, G., 307
Greenwood, K. M., 728
Gritz, E., 737, 738, 739, 740
Groessl, E. J., 226

Gross, J. J., 308
Grosscup, S. J., 235, 237
Grossman, D. C., 548
Grossman, W., 206
Groves, E. R., 215
Gruenewald, T. L., 307
Gruman, J., 322
Guevara, E. B., 580
Guijarro, M. L., 304, 526, 528
Guile, C. A., 174
Gullette, E. C. D., 110
Gumnick, J. F., 238, 239, 240
Guralnik, J. M., 103, 303
Gurung, R. A., 670
Guthrie, E., 555
Guthrie, R., 4
Gutierrez-Mohamed, M. L., 3
Gutmann, M. C., 1, 4
Guy, W., 232
Guzman, J. R., 201, 203
Gybels, J. M., 356

Haan, M. N., 199
Haddon, W., Jr., 549
Haffner, S. M., 4
Hagg, G., 100
Hahn, B. A., 260
Haines, A. P., 56
Haines, P. S., 345
Hainsworth, J., 175
Hall, A., 755
Hall, J. A., 173
Hall, S., 255
Hallet, A. J., 304, 526, 528
Hallqvist, J., 563, 564
Hamaty, D., 329, 333
Hamburg, D. A., 180
Hamelsky, S. W., 466
Hamilton, M., 231, 232
Hampton, J., 267
Hanauer, P., 732
Handsdottir, I., 218
Haney, T. L., 307, 308, 309, 527
Harpham, T., 751
Harrell, J., 255
Harris, K. M., 2
Harris, M. B., 672, 673, 674
Hartnett, S. A., 16, 565
Haskell, W. L., 143, 711
Hasselblad, V., 470
Hathaway, S. R., 60, 232, 600
Hatsukami, D., 740
Hauck, E. R., 198
Haug Ogden, D., 267

Hauser, S. L., 83
Hauth, A. C., 721
Hawkley, L. C., 587
Haynes, R. B., 8, 22, 319, 696
Haynes, S. G., 519
Hays, R. D., 208
Hayward, R. A., 174
Hazuda, H. P., 4
Head, J., 768
Heagarty, M. C., 550
Heath, C., 730
Heath, G. W., 143
Hebel, J. R., 522
Heck, K., 346
Heckman, T. G., 15
Hedman, M., 364
Heeren, T., 2
Heetderks, W. J., 101
Heikkonen, S., 337
Heiman, J. R., 319
Heisler, M., 174
Helgeson, V., 781
Heller, R. S., 710
Helms, M. J., 307, 308, 309
Henderson, S., 363
Hennekens, C. H., 103, 501, 504, 518
Herbert, C. J., 202
Herman, A. G., 103
Hermens, H., 100
Herskovits, M., 1
Herzog, A. R., 345
Hester, R. K., 266, 268
Heuts, P. H. T. G., 335
Heyman, R., 737, 738, 739, 740
Hickey, A., 687
Hickie, I., 177
Higgins, S. T., 267, 268, 269
Hill, D. R., 363
Hills, M., 214
Hilton, J. L., 254
Hinde, J., 603
Hinderliter, A. L., 566, 567
Hines, E. A., 151
Hirschfeld, R. M., 231
Hitchcock, P. J., 720
Hoberman, H. M., 363
Hobson, J. A., 587
Hochberg, M. C., 69
Hodgkins, J., 2
Hodgson, M., 199
Holbrook, J., 737, 738, 739, 740
Hollis, J., 740, 743
Holman, H. R., 174, 218
Holmes, G. P., 177
Holroyd, K. A., 467, 468, 469, 470

Honig, A., 208
Hope, B. A., 28
Hopkins, M., 335
Hopper, J., 260
Horsten, M., 364
Horwitz, A. V., 260
Horwitz, W. L., 725
Houck, E., 14
House, J. S., 344, 345, 755, 781
Houseworth, S. J., 527
Houts, A. c., 729
Hovell, M. F., 660, 661
Howe, S., 642
Howell-White, S., 260
Hoxworth, T., 27
Hsieh, C., 656
Hsieh, C. -C., 123
Hu, F. B., 501, 504
Huang, L., 82
Huang, V., 231
Hudson, L. D., 267
Hudson, S. M., 729
Huebner, C., 570
Hugdahl, K., 587
Hughes, E. C., 764
Hughes, J., 737, 740, 743
Hughes, M., 208, 227, 768
Hulley, S. B., 520
Hummer, M. K., 642
Hunt, K., 359, 768
Hunt, L. M., 1, 2, 4
Hunt, M. K., 143
Hunt, S., 686
Hurwitz, M. E., 171, 172, 173
Hyde, R. T., 656

Iatesta, M., 27
Idler, E. L., 717, 718
Iker, H. P., 522
Illsley, R., 345
Imber, S. D., 239
Imeson, J. D., 56
Inui, T. S., 208
Irving, L. M., 522
Isen, A. M., 308
Islar, J., 83
Ismail, A. L., 3
Israel, A. C., 174
Israel, B. A., 145, 200, 201, 202, 203
Istvan, J., 743
Ives, D. G., 303

Jackson, J. S., 255, 256, 257, 258
Jackson, R. M., 756
Jacob, R. G., 103

Jacobs, D. R., Jr., 143, 520
Jacobs, S. C., 58
Jaen, C., 737, 738, 739, 740
Jagust, W. J., 199
Jahoda, M., 459
James, S. A., 16, 565, 568
Jamner, L. D., 103
Janoff-Bulman, R., 460
Janz, N. K., 475
Jason, L. A., 177
Jaworkski, B., 26
Jemmott, J. B., 26
Jemmott, L. S., 26
Jenkins, A. L., 502
Jenkins, C. D., 519, 766
Jenkins, D. J., 502
Jennings, J. R., 153, 199
Jensen, R., 331
Joffe, A., 551
Johnson, B. T., 27
Johnson, C. A., 2
Johnson, C. C., 706, 707, 708
Johnson, D. W., 200
Johnson, F. P., 200
Johnson, J. V., 563, 564
Johnson, K., 206
Johnson, M. M. S., 308
Johnson, P. S., 153
Johnson, V. E., 317
Johnston, C., 340
Johnston, J. A., 661
Johnstone, I. M., 711
Joiner, T. E., Jr., 2, 309
Joleen, B., 100
Jolly, J., 232
Jonas, W., 211
Jones, A. L., 550
Jones, D. W., 102
Jones, K. L., 704
Jones, L., 212
Jones, W. H., 586
Jonsson, B. G., 820
Joyce, C., 687
Julius, S., 102
Justic, J. C., 522

Kaciroti, N., 171, 172, 173
Kagan, A., 656
Kahn, B. E., 308
Kahn, R. L., 768, 784
Kalichman, S. C., 15, 28
Kalish, R., 91, 92
Kalman, D., 743
Kalsbeek, W. D., 16, 565

Kamarck, T. W., 153, 363
Kamb, M. L., 27
Kamlet, M. S., 224
Kanani, R., 22
Kanfer, F. H., 170
Kannel, W. B., 519
Kanner, A. D., 307
Kantrowitz, E., 768
Kaplan, D., 171, 173
Kaplan, G., 715, 716, 755
Kaplan, G. A., 522, 572
Kaplan, G. D., 217
Kaplan, J., 304
Kaplan, J. E., 177
Kaplan, J. R., 513
Kaplan, R. M., 223, 226, 322
Kapuku, G., 153
Karasek, R. A., 108, 296, 562, 563
Karlovac, M., 226
Karoly, P., 170
Kasl, S. K., 107
Kasl, S. V., 563
Kasman, G., 100
Katz, H., 562
Katz, M. M., 231
Kaufmann, P. G., 322
Kawachi, I., 57, 58, 302, 304, 307, 518, 539,
    563, 717, 751, 752, 753, 755
Keddie, A. M., 3
Keefe, F., 13
Keenan, N. I., 565
Keith, V. M., 2
Kelder, S. H., 706, 707, 708
Keller, J. B., 344
Kelly, J. A., 22, 27, 28, 721
Kemeny, M. E., 92, 307, 522, 781
Kendler, K. S., 768
Kennedy, B. P., 717, 751
Kennedy, S., 588
Kent, C., 27
Kerns, R. D., 336
Kerr, E. A., 174
Kessel, B., 544
Kessler, R. C., 208, 210, 235, 257, 258, 259, 345,
    768, 780
Keys, A., 501
Khan, S. A., 103
Khoshaba, D. M., 463, 464
Kiecolt-Glaser, J. K., 260, 302, 303,
    305, 364, 588
Killough, A. L., 14
King, A. C., 143, 663
King, C., 111
King, D. A., 208
King, R., 821

Kinkle, L. F., Jr., 821
Kirby, D., 674
Kitagawa, E. M., 215
Kittel, F., 821
Klassen, T. P., 550
Kleiber, B. A., 240
Klerman, G. L., 235, 236
Klohnen, E. C., 309
Klonoff, E. A., 14
Knatterud, G. L., 322
Knickman, J. R., 769
Knoke, D., 562
Knutsson, A., 820
Kobak, K. A., 232
Kobasa, S. C., 463
Kockman, A., 15
Koepsell, T. D., 550
Kohout, F., 755
Kolody, B., 2, 660, 661
Komaroff, A. L., 177
Kondwani, K., 111
Koob, J. J., 28
Koontz, K., 725
Kop, W. J., 303
Kornbluh, R., 239
Kornitzer, J., 821
Kottke, T., 737, 738, 739, 740
Kovacs, M., 232
Kovenock, J., 363
Kowalewski, R., 587
Kozak, M. J., 56
Kraemer, D. T., 307
Kraemer, H. C., 710
Krauss, R. M., 711
Kremen, A. M., 309
Kressel, S., 686
Kressin, N. R., 93
Kreuter, M. W., 549, 789, 790
Krieger, N., 2, 255, 256, 257, 292, 293
Kriegsman, D. M., 755
Krysan, M., 254
Kubinski, J. A., 337
Kubzansky, L. D., 57, 58, 302, 304, 307
Kuczmierczyk, A. R., 498
Kueneman, K., 306
Kuhn, L., 550
Kulik, J. A., 497
Kuller, L. H., 58, 199, 566
Kumpfer, K. L., 309
Kunn, P., 4
Kuno, R., 28
Kunst, A. E., 344
Kuykendall, D. H., 319
Kyomugisha, F., 28

Labbe, E. E., 498
LaCroix, A., 755
Lakey, B., 780
Lamb, M. E., 643
Lambert, J. A., 260, 261
Lando, H., 737, 738, 739, 740
Landrine, H., 14
Landro, N. I., 335
Landsbergis, P., 562
Lane, J. D., 103
Langley, J. D., 551
Lantelme, P., 103
Lantz, P. M., 203, 344, 345
LaPiere, R. T., 795
Larkin, G., 309
Larson, A. A., 332
Larson, J., 307
Larson, M. G., 103
Lasater, T. M., 142
Laska, M. K., 15
Lasser, N., 520
Last, J. M., 210
Laumann, E. O., 316
Lavoie, J. P., 781
Lawlor, D. A., 359
Lawson, E., 704, 705, 706
Lazarus, R. S., 307, 308, 367, 774, 775
Leaf, W. A., 551
Le Bars, D., 356
Leber, W. R., 231
LeCompte, M., 569, 571
Lee, I. -M., 123
Lee, V., 2
Lefcourt, H. M., 306, 307
Lefebvre, R. C., 142, 340
Lehman, E. Q., 821
Lehmann, T. H., 337
Lemanek, K. L., 725
Lenfant, C., 102
Lentz, A., 27
Lepore, S. J., 227, 781
Lepowski, J. M., 344, 345
Leppin, A., 780, 781
Lerner, D. J., 563
Lesperance, F., 208
Lessard, J., 329, 333
Levenson, H., 218
Levenson, R. W., 308
Leventhal, H., 476
Levin, K. D., 27
Levine, S., 563
Levison, M. J., 170
Levstek, D. A., 170, 174
Levy, D., 103, 203

Levy, M. N., 102
Lew, H. T., 710
Lewin, K., 474
Lewinsohn, P. M., 235, 237
Liang, J., 755
Lichtebroun, A. S., 329, 333
Lichtenstein, B., 15
Lichtenstein, R., 203
Lieberson, S., 345
Liebert, R. M., 729
Liebeskind, J. C., 355
Light, K. C., 103, 516, 566, 567
Lillard, L. A., 260
Lin, A., 82
Lindemann, E., 93
Lindsey, L. L., 363
Link, B. G., 143, 345, 346
Linton, R., 1
Lipchik, G. L., 467, 469, 470
Lipkin, M., 208
Lipton, R. B., 466, 467, 468
Littlefield, C. H., 93
Liu, X., 755
Livingston, W. K., 355
Lloyd, D., 345
Lobel, M., 670
Lochner, K., 751, 752
Locke, B. Z., 208
Loeser, J. D., 356
Logan, P. D. L., 345
Lopez, A. D., 208, 730
Lorig, K. R., 68, 174, 218
Lotufo-Neto, F., 238
Loue, S., 4
Loughrey, K., 340
Lu, J. L., 587
Lubach, G. R., 679
Lubin, B., 60, 232
Luepker, R. V., 143, 145, 660, 706, 707, 708
Luke, W., 28
Lum, O., 231
Lumley, M. A., 13
Lundberg, U., 363, 364
Lushene, R. D., 60, 61
Lynch, J., 360
Lyness, J. M., 208
Lytle, L. A., 708

MacDougall, J. M., 527
MacIntyre, N. R., 198
Macintyre, S., 359, 622, 768
MacKay, J. M., 550
Mackenback, J. P., 344
Mackey, S. F., 711

Macklem, D. J., 13
MacLennan, A. H., 211
Maclure, M., 58
Maddi, S. R., 463, 464
Madonia, M. J., 209
Maes, M., 82
Mahler, H. I. M., 497
Maibach, E., 712
Maides, S. A., 217
Maier, K. J., 199
Maiman, L. A., 171, 172, 173
Maki, P. M., 198
Malarkey, W. B., 364, 587
Malcarne, V. I., 218
Malotte, K., 27
Mancia, G., 102, 103
Mancuso, R. A., 308
Manderscheid, R. W., 208
Mann, J., 57
Manolio, T. A., 199
Manson, F., 59
Manson, J. E., 501, 504, 518
Manuck, S. B., 103, 151, 153, 513
Mararazzo, J. D., 497
Marcus, D. A., 333
Marcus, G., 570
Marin, B. V., 3
Marin, G., 3
Markides, K. S., 307
Markovic, N., 566
Markovitz, J. H., 58
Markowitz, J. C., 15
Marks, G., 2, 3
Marks, N. F., 260
Marlatt, G. A., 266
Marmot, M. G., 298, 768
Maron, D. J., 711
Marottoli, R., 757
Marrietta, P., 82
Marris, P., 93
Marsella, A. J., 231
Marsh, K. L., 27
Marti, J., 2
Martin, L. R., 325
Martin, P., 740
Martin, R., 528
Martin, S., 642
Martire, L. M., 208, 303
Marx, E., 705, 706
Marxer, F., 108
Masi, A. T., 329, 333
Massing, M., 145
Masten, A. S., 309
Masten, J., 15

Masters, W. H., 317
Matarazzo, J., 743
Mathieu, C., 173
Matthews, K. A., 10, 58, 305, 514, 769
May, R. M., 59, 720
Maynard, K. E., 307, 308, 309, 527
Mayne, T. J., 302, 307
Mays, V. M., 258
Mazonson, P. D., 174, 218
Mazur, A., 260
Mazurski, E. J., 175
McAdams, D. P., 327
McAlister, A. L., 2, 713
McAuliffe, T. L., 22
McCabe, M. P., 317
McCain, G. A., 226, 329, 333, 337
McClintock, M. K., 587
McCrory, D., 470
McDonald, H. P., 8, 22
McDonough, P., 562, 564
McEwen, B. S., 769
McEwen, J., 686
McFarland, D. J., 101
McGee, H., 687
McGinnis, J. M., 127, 769
McGonagle, K. A., 208, 768
McGranaghan, R., 203
McGuire, L., 302, 303, 305
McKay, G., 781
McKenna, S., 686
McKenzie, T. L., 660
McKetney, E. C., 566
McKibbon, K. A., 22
McKinlay, S. M., 142, 145, 660, 706, 707
McKinley, J. C., 60, 232, 600
McKirnan, D. J., 28
McKusick, L., 28
McManus, C., 725
McMullen, W., 28
McNamara, R. K., 239
McNeilly, M. D., 257
McTiernan, A., 123
McWhinney, I. R., 210
McWilliam, C. L., 210
Meade, T. W., 56
Means, B., 308
Mecklenburg, R., 737, 738, 739, 740
Medley, D. M., 528
Meilahn, E. N., 58
Melamed, S., 740
Melin, B., 364
Mellors, M. P., 22, 23
Melton, R., 642
Melzack, R., 355, 356, 357, 646

Mendelson, M., 232
Mendes de Leon, C. F., 208, 757
Mendias, E. P., 580
Menke, T. J., 319
Menon, A. S., 522
Mercy, J. A., 260
Merisca, R., 173
Merkin, S. S., 145
Merletti, R., 100
Mermelstein, R., 363, 740, 743
Merritt, M. M., 567
Merritt, R. K., 660
Mertz, E., 308
Meston, C. M., 319
Metzner, H., 755
Meyerowitz, B. E., 712
Meyers, R. J., 268, 269
Michalek, J., 260
Micozzi, M. S., 210
Middlestadt, S. E., 720
Midence, K., 725
Miettinen, O. S., 215
Mill, J. S., 214
Miller, G. E., 178
Miller, N. H., 710
Miller, P., 781
Miller, S. M., 476, 544, 545
Miller, T. Q., 304, 526, 528, 799
Miller, T. R., 548
Miller, W. R., 266, 268, 269, 569, 570, 602
Minkler, M., 202
Mirowksy, J., 260
Mischel, W., 544
Mischler, E., 569
Mitleman, M. A., 58
Mittelmark, M. B., 143
Mittleman, A. M., 364
Mittlemark, M., 520
Mock, J., 232
Moeschberger, M., 4
Moher, D., 550, 696
Mohr, D. C., 82, 83
Mohr, J., 21, 22, 23, 522
Molock, S., 725
Montague, P., 8
Montanari, M., 107
Montgomery, D., 708
Montgomery, S. A., 231
Montrone, M., 545
Moos, R. H., 307, 775
Mora, M. E., 2
Morgan, M. G., 28
Morgenstern, H., 213
Morin, C. M., 728

Morin, M., 22
Morris, J. N., 345, 656, 686
Morris, N. M., 363
Morrow, L. A., 199
Moseley, J. B., 319
Moser, D. K., 57
Moskowitz, J. T., 307
Muldoon, M. F., 103, 199
Mullen, K., 345
Mullen, P., 737, 738, 739, 740
Muller, J. E., 58
Mullington, J., 729
Mulrow, C., 696
Mulry, R., 58
Murison, R., 351, 353
Murphy, D. A., 28
Murphy, M., 57
Murray, C. J. L., 208
Murray, D. M., 143, 144
Murtagh, D. R., 728
Myers, L. B., 694
Myrsten, A. L., 364
Myrtek, M., 103

Nader, P. R., 145, 660, 706, 707, 708
Nadler, A., 781
Nahin, R. L., 212
Napoli, A., 307
Narrow, W., 208
Nash, J. M., 467, 469
Nass, C., 712
Neale, J. M., 307
Neaton, J., 520
Neault, N. B., 239
Neighbors, H. W., 108, 255, 256, 257
Nelson, A. R., 254, 579
Nelson, C. B., 208, 768
Nemeroff, C. B., 238, 239, 240
Nett, L., 737, 738, 739, 740
Neugebauer, R., 207
Newman, H., 502
Nicassio, P. M., 219
Nichols, P. J., 175
Nicholson, L., 704, 705, 706
Nielson, W. R., 335, 337
Nierenberg, A. A., 239
Nieto, F. J., 145, 304
Nolen-Hoeksema, S., 307
Noll, R. B., 725
Noordenbos, W., 355
Noossens, M. E. J. B., 335
Nooyen-Haazen, I. W. C. J., 335
Norcross, J. C., 340
Nordstrom, B., 173

Norem, J. K., 642
Norlock, F. E., 210
Norregaard, J., 331
Norris, S. L., 175
North, F., 768
Northridge, M., 345
Northrop, D., 705, 706
Nothwehr, F., 171, 172, 173
Novotny, T. E., 345
Nowicki, G. P., 308

O'Boyle, C., 687
Obrist, P. A., 510
Ockene, J., 740, 743
O'Connor, P., 550
O'Dell, P., 674
O'Donnell, F. J., 469, 470
Ogburn, W. F., 215
Ogrocki, P., 260
Ohene-Frempong, K., 725
Ohman, A., 308
Okifuji, A., 333, 336, 337
O'Leary, M. R., 266
Olesen, J. C., 331, 466
Olevitch, L., 789, 790
O'Malley, K., 319, 687
Omboni, S., 102
Orav, J., 544
Orlandi, M., 713
Orleans, C. T., 320, 322
Orth-Gomér, K., 363, 364, 780, 820
Osganian, S. K., 708
Osterman, P., 562
Osterweis, M., 92
Ostfeld, A. M., 107
Ostir, G. V., 307
Ostrove, J. M., 768
Ostrow, D. G., 28
Overmier, J. B., 351, 353
Owen, N., 662
Ozer, E. M., 813

Padawer, W., 729
Padilla, G. V., 4
Paffenbarger, R. S., Jr., 123, 656
Pahor, M., 303
Paik, A., 316
Panis, C., 260
Parati, G., 102, 103
Parcel, G. S., 145, 660, 706, 707, 708
Paré, W. P., 353
Park, A., 728
Park, C. L., 307
Park, D. C., 335

Parker, E. A., 145, 200, 201, 202, 203
Parkes, C. M., 91, 92, 93
Pasick, R. J., 790
Paterniti, S., 58
Paterson, D. L., 21, 22, 23
Paton, C. C., 304
Patrick, K., 661
Patrick, R., 766
Patterson, A. H., 227
Pattison, D. C., 656
Paul, L. A., 355
Paulsen, A., 587
Paulus, P. B., 226, 227
Pavlov, I. P., 59, 350, 668
Paxson, C., 769
Payne, A., 557
Pearl, J., 213, 215, 216, 294
Pearlin, I. I., 781
Pearlin, L. I., 218
Peat, J. K., 174
Peckham, P. H., 101
Pedersen, S., 706, 707
Peek, M. K., 307
Pelletier, J. R., 199
Pelto, G. H., 569
Pelto, P. J., 569
Pender, N., 320
Pennebaker, J. W., 307, 327
Pennington, J., 728
Penninx, B. W., 208, 303, 755
Penzien, D. B., 470
Pequegnat, W., 721
Perez, M. V. Z., 2
Perez-Stable, E. J., 2, 3
Perkins, K., 740, 743
Perlis, M. L., 726, 728
Perry, C. L., 145, 660, 706, 707, 708
Perry, M., 528
Petel, C., 768
Peterman, T. A., 27
Petersen, N. J., 319
Petersen, R. R., 260
Petersen, T., 239
Peterson, C., 325, 642
Peto, R., 730
Petraitis, J., 799
Pettit, J. W., 2
Pettitt, D. J., 704
Pfeffer, J., 299
Phelan, J. C., 143, 345, 346
Phillips, K., 582
Pickering, T., 108
Pieper, C. F., 562, 563, 564
Pierce, J. P., 345

Piere, J., 737
Pinderton, S., 28
Pindyck, J., 28
Piotrowski, C., 231
Pittler, M. H., 211
Plat, A. F., 725
Poiseuille, J. L. M., 102
Polefrone, J. M., 199
Polissar, L., 550
Pollard, W. E., 686, 725
Popkin, B. M., 345
Portes, A., 1, 2
Potter, J. D., 120, 123
Potter, W. Z., 239, 740
Powe, N. R., 173
Preston, S. H., 768
Preusser, D. F., 551
Prior, A., 554
Prislin, R., 3
Prochaska, J. O., 340, 476, 737, 790, 803
Prothrow-Stith, D., 752
Prows, S. L., 267
Pukkala, E., 522
Puska, P., 713, 755
Putnam, R. D., 751, 752
Putnam, S. M., 208
Puukka, P., 337

Quatrano, L. A., 101

Rachman, S., 593
Radloff, L. S., 231
Rae, D., 208
Raffle, P. A. B., 656
Ragland, D. R., 566
Rainforth, M., 111
Rakowski, W., 790
Ramirez, A., 2
Ramsay, C., 211
Ramsay, R. W., 93
Ramsay, T. B., 781
Ramsey, D. L., 568
Rand, C. S., 173
Ranieri, W. F., 231
Raskin White, H., 260
Raspe, H., 333
Raudenbush, S. W., 752
Reason, P., 570
Reaven, G., 594
Redfield, R., 1
Reed, G. M., 307, 522
Regier, D. A., 208
Reich, P., 93
Reis, H. T., 291

Reiss, D., 57
Resnick, M., 737, 743
Resnick, S. M., 198
Reuterwall, C., 563, 564
Reynolds, D. V., 355
Reynolds, R. C. V., 170, 174
Reynolds, W. J., 329, 333
Reynolds, W. M., 231, 232
Rhodes, F., 27
Ribble, J. C., 3
Richard, H. W., 725
Richardson, W. S., 319
Richelson, E., 740
Rickert, V. I., 729
Rimal, R. N., 712
Rimer, B. K., 789, 790
Rimm, E., 501, 504, 755
Ringel, N., 528
Rips, J., 171, 173
Rivara, F. P., 548, 550
Robbins, C., 755
Roberts, I. G., 550
Robins, J. M., 215, 216
Robinson, C. J., 101
Robinson, E. L., 257
Robinson, G., 308
Robinson, L., 737, 738, 739, 740
Robles, T. F., 302, 303, 305
Rocella, E. J., 102
Rock, N., 737, 743
Rodgers, G. B., 551
Rogers, E. E., 721
Rogers, J., 27
Rogers, M. P., 93
Rogers, T. F., 28
Rogers, W. H., 208, 562, 564
Rohe, W., 227
Rollnick, S., 602
Roloff, D., 171, 173
Romano, E. O., 548
Romano, T. J., 329, 333
Rompa, D., 28
Rompf, J., 710
Ronconi, M., 107
Rook, K. S., 587, 757
Rooney, M. T., 232
Rose, T., 231
Rosen, G., 344, 345
Rosen, R. C., 316
Rosenberg, W. M., 319, 696
Rosengran, A., 780
Rosenheck, R. A., 211
Rosenman, R. H., 49, 518, 519, 524
Rosenstock, I. M., 476, 549, 720

Rosenzweig, A. S., 308
Rosner, B. A., 501, 504, 518
Ross, C. E., 260, 716
Rossi, J. S., 737, 790
Rossiter, C. M., 781
Roter, D. L., 173, 208
Rothman, K. J., 213, 216, 294
Rotter, J. B., 217
Rouleau, J. L., 725
Rounsaville, B. J., 235, 236
Rousseau, E., 76
Rowan, J., 570
Rowe, J. W., 307, 784
Rozanski, A., 304
Rubenstein, E., 103
Rubin, D. B., 294
Rubin, H. R., 173
Rudy, T. E., 336, 337
Rumbaut, R. G., 1, 2, 3
Runyan, C. W., 551
Rush, A. J., 232, 236
Rushton, J. P., 93
Ruskin, P., 522
Russell, D. W., 337, 781
Russell, I. J., 329, 332, 333
Russell, L. B., 224
Ryan, C. M., 199

Sackett, D. L., 319, 696
Sacks, F. M., 504
Sagan, L. A., 521
Sallis, J. F., 660, 661, 662
Salonen, J. T., 522, 572, 755
Salovey, P., 307
Sampson, R. J., 752
Samson, J., 231
Sanders, V. M., 679
Sandler, I. N., 781
Sandman, P. M., 549
Sanford, C. P., 304
Santucciu, C., 103
Sapolsky, R. M., 599
Sartorius, N., 231
Sawada, Y., 103
Schaefer, J. A., 307
Schalk, G., 101
Schatzkin, A., 346
Scheien, R. L., 198
Scheier, I. H., 60
Scheier, M. F., 208, 307, 641, 775
Schenck-Gustafsson, K., 364
Schensul, J., 569, 570, 571
Schensul, S., 569, 571
Scherwitz, L. W., 527

Schmale, A. H., 522
Schmid, T. L., 143
Schnall, P., 562
Schneider, M., 227
Schneider, R. H., 111
Schneider, S., 92
Schneiderman, N., 58, 153
Schochat, T., 333
Schoepfle, M., 569
Schoevers, R. A., 208
Scholler, C., 781
Schooler, C., 218
Schork, M. A., 171, 173
Schroeder, C. M., 544
Schulberg, H. C., 209
Schulz, A. J., 145, 200, 201, 202, 203
Schulz, K. F., 696
Schulz, R., 208, 303
Schuman, H., 254
Schwartz, G. E., 693
Schwartz, J. E., 563
Schwartz, M. D., 98
Schwartz, S. M., 728
Schwarzer, R., 780, 781
Scott, R., 363
Scott-Sheldon, L. A. J., 27
Scribner, R., 2, 3
Seeman, T. E., 363, 364, 587, 754, 755
Seitz, V., 674
Seligman, M. E. P., 219, 325, 352, 460, 641
Sellers, D. E., 706, 707
Selye, H., 366
Sen, A., 360
Shah, R. V., 710
Shah, S., 175
Shankar, S., 3
Shapiro, A. P., 199
Shapiro, D., 103
Shapiro, D. H., Jr., 219
Shapiro, P. A., 303
Sharpe, M. C., 177
Shaw, B. F., 236
Shea, M. T., 239
Sheasby, J., 175
Shechter, A. L., 468
Sheffield, D., 153
Shekelle, R. B., 520
Shelton, D., 2, 3
Shemanski, L., 199
Sheon, R. P., 329, 333
Sheppard, W., 111
Sheps, S. G., 102
Sherbourne, C. D., 2, 208, 686
Sheridan, J. F., 364
Sherman, J. J., 334

Sherman, K. A., 545
Sherr, L., 22
Sherwood, A., 110, 364, 566, 567
Sherwood, J. B., 58
Shiffman, S. S., 291, 292, 307
Shipton-Levy, R., 28
Shoor, S., 218
Short, J., 781
Shumaker, S. A., 363
Sidney, S., 256
Siega-Riz, A. M., 345
Siegel, J. E., 224
Siegler, I. C., 304, 307, 308, 309
Siegman, A. W., 528
Siegrist, J., 295, 298, 299
Sikkema, K. J., 15
Silberstein, S. D., 468
Silver, R. C., 781
Silverman, K., 267, 268
Silverman, W. K., 174
Simmens, S. J., 57
Simon, R. W., 260, 261
Simons, A. D., 239
Simons, J. S., 316
Simonsick, E. M., 208
Simpson, D. M., 3, 28
Sinclair, J. D., 333, 336, 337
Sinclair, R. R., 463
Sinclair, V. G., 219
Sindhusake, D., 175
Singer, E., 28
Singer, M., 570
Singh, N., 21, 22, 23, 522
Skinner, C. S., 790
Skinner, M., 2, 579
Slade, J., 732
Slate, S., 123
Slawsby, E., 544
Sletvold, H., 335
Smedley, B. D., 254, 579
Smith, B. W., 82
Smith, C., 345
Smith, C. A., 218
Smith, D. M., 174
Smith, G. D., 111
Smith, J. C., 260
Smith, J. P., 769
Smith, M. S., 218, 728
Smith, M. T., 728
Smith, P. K., 227
Smith, R. S., 309
Smith, S., 111
Smith, T. W., 304, 364, 526, 528
Smithe, J., 769
Smythe, H. A., 329, 333

Snaith, R. P., 232
Snow, J., 199
Snow, M., 570
Snowdon, D. A., 307, 462, 785
Snyder, C. R., 522, 523
Soeken, K., 69
Softley, D., 203
Solis, J. M., 2
Sollers, J., 567
Song, C., 82
Sorkin, D., 587
Sorlie, P. D., 344
Sotsky, S. M., 239
Sparrow, D., 57, 58, 304, 307
Speicher, C. E., 260
Speigelman, D., 504
Speizer, F. E., 504, 518
Spence, J. T., 60
Spence, K. W., 60
Spicer, R. S., 548
Spiegel, D., 222, 587
Spielberger, C. D., 60, 61
Spielman, A. J., 728
Spielman, L. A., 15
Spiro, A., III, 93, 304
Spitzer, R. L., 232
Spradley, J., 570
Spritzer, K., 208
Squier, C., 21, 22, 23, 522
Stachenko, S., 76
Staggers, F., 111
Stamler, J., 520
Stampfer, M. J., 501, 504, 518, 755
Stansfeld, S., 768
Starz, T. W., 333, 336, 337
Steeh, C., 254
Steer, R. A., 231, 232, 522
Steffey, D., 13
Stegeman, D., 100
Steilen, M., 28
Stein, M. J., 218, 219
Steinhauer, S. R., 199
Steinmetz, K. A., 120
Stensland, M., 469, 470
Stepanski, E. J., 726
Stephens, T., 660
Steptoe, A., 103
Stern, M. P., 4, 579
Stetner, F., 743
Steuve, C. A., 756
Stevenson, L. Y., 28, 721
Stewart, M., 208, 210
Stewart, W. A., 466
Stewart, W. F., 563, 564
Stiles, T. C., 335

Stiles, W., 208
Stipek, D. J., 643
Stites, D. P., 28
Stith, A. Y., 254, 579
Stitt, L. E., 686
Stitzer, M. L., 267, 737, 738, 739, 740
St. Lawrence, J. S., 28, 721
Stokols, D., 226
Stone, A. A., 291, 292, 307
Stone, E. J., 145, 660, 706, 707, 708
Stoney, C. M., 155
Stout, J. C., 260
Stover, E., 721
Strategier, L. D., 337
Straub, R. H., 679
Straus, R., 519
Straus, S. E., 177, 212, 319
Strauss, R. S., 627
Strecher, V. J., 476, 720, 789
Strickland, B. R., 217
Stroebe, M. S., 92, 93
Stroebe, W., 92, 93
Strogatz, D. S., 565, 568
Struyk, R. J., 254
Stuart, A., 28
Stuber, M., 307
Studts, J., 13
Suarez, L., 2, 3
Subramanian, S. V., 539, 752, 753
Suchday, S., 11
Sugisawa, H., 755
Sullivan, M., 15
Superko, H. R., 710, 711
Sutton, S. M., 340
Svarstad, B., 173
Svikis, D., 267
Swartz, N., 235
Swindells, S., 21, 22, 23
Swindells, S., 522
Syme, L., 768
Syme, S. L., 363, 565, 587, 755
Szapocznik, J., 721
Szczepanski, R., 364
Szpunar, S. M., 3

Takeucki, D. T., 73
Talajic, M., 208
Talavera, G., 2
Taliaferro, J., 255
Talo, S., 337
Tamres, L., 103
Tang, T. Z., 239
Tankard, C. F., 199
Tarter, R. E., 199
Tasker, R. R., 356

Taylor, A. W., 211
Taylor, C. B., 143, 710, 713
Taylor, J. A., 60
Taylor, J. O., 103
Taylor, R. H., 502
Taylor, R. R., 177
Taylor, S. E., 92, 217, 307, 522
Taylor, T., 153
Taywaditep, K. J., 28
Tennen, H., 307
Tetrick, L. E., 463
Thase, M. E., 236, 238
Thayer, J. F., 103
The, H. G., 335
Theorell, T., 108, 296, 298, 562, 563, 564
Thoits, P. A., 757, 780, 781
Thomas, E., 751
Thomas, R. J., 710
Thomas, S., 307
Thompson, D., 227
Thoresen, C. E., 520
Thorogood, M., 57
Thun, M., 730
Thune, I., 123
Timio, M., 107
Tofler, G. H., 58
Tomenson, B., 555
Tommasello, A., 737, 738, 739, 740
Tornstam, L., 785
Toseland, R. W., 781
Toumisto, M., 364
Tran, P. V., 239
Trapido, E., 2
Treiber, F. A., 153
Triandis, H. C., 229
Trivedi, M. H., 238, 240
Troiano, R. P., 704
Tugade, M. M., 308, 309
Tugwell, P., 329, 333, 687
Tuomilehto, J., 522
Turk, D. C., 333, 334, 336, 337
Turken, A. U., 308
Turner, A., 175
Turner, C. W., 304, 526, 528
Turner, J. R., 151, 566, 567
Turner, R. J., 345
Tweedy, D., 110
Tyroler, H. A., 144, 304

Udry, J. R., 363
Ukoli, F. A., 566
Ulian, L., 103
Ulrich, C., 123

Umberson, D., 260
Underwood, L. G., 257, 258, 781
Underwood, S., 754
Ung, E., 218
Unger, J. B., 2
Useem, M., 562
Utsey, S. O., 725

Vagg, P. R., 61
Vaillant, G. E., 303, 784
Vallareal, R., 2
van Breukelen, G., 335
Van Devanter, N., 28
van DoorNen, L., 298
van Eijk, J. T., 208, 755
van Tilburg, W., 208, 755
Van Willigen, M., 716
Vanable, P. A., 25, 28
Vanatta, K., 725
Varshney, A., 753
Varshney, V. P., 110
Vaughan, T. M., 101
Vega, W., 2
Velasquez, M., 737
Velicer, W. F., 737, 790
Venanzi, S., 107
Verbrugge, L. M., 358
Verdecchia, P., 107
Vergis, E., 21, 22, 23
Vessey, M., 57
Villanova, P., 642
Villejo, L., 737, 738, 739, 740
Virchow, R., 344
Viruell-Fuentes, E., 203
Visscher, B., 92
Vlaeyen, J. W. S., 335
Vogt, T. M., 321
Vokonas, P., 304, 307
von Hippel, W., 254
Von Korff, M., 171, 173, 174
Voorhees, C., 740, 743
Vrijkotte, T., 298

Wadhwa, P., 670
Wagenaar, A. C., 551
Wagener, D., 346
Wagener, M., 21, 22, 23
Wagener, M. M., 522
Wagner, E. H., 171, 173, 174
Waite, L. J., 260
Waldstein, S. R., 198, 199
Walker, A., 550
Walker, C., 337

Walker, J., 217, 219
Walker, M., 211
Wall, E. M., 470
Wall, P. D., 355, 356, 646
Wallace, R. B., 208, 303
Wallerstein, N., 202
Wallin, L., 364
Wallston, B. S., 217, 218
Wallston, K. A., 217, 218, 219, 473
Wamala, S. P., 360, 364
Wan, C. K., 528
Wang, H., 175
Wang, H. Y. J., 522
Ward, C. H., 232
Ware, J. E., 686, 714
Wasilewski, Y., 170, 171, 173
Watkins, J. T., 239
Watson, D., 231, 528
Waugh, C. E., 309
Way, D., 212
Wayment, H., 781
Webber, L. S., 706, 707, 708
Webster, W., 14
Wedel, H., 780
Wei, M., 579
Weihs, K. L., 57
Weinberg, C. R.295
Weinberger, D. A., 693
Weiner, H., 92
Weinhardt, L. S., 26
Weinstein, M. C., 224
Weinstein, N. D., 476, 549, 642
Weintraub, J. K., 775
Weiss, J. M., 352
Weiss, S. T., 57, 58, 304
Weissman, M. M., 235, 236
Weller, E. B., 232
Weller, R. A., 232
Wellman, B., 755
Wells, K. B., 208
Wells, V. E., 303
Werner, E., 309
Werner, O., 569
Westberry, L. G., 61
Weston, W. W., 210
Wethington, E., 780, 781
Wewers, M. E., 4, 737, 738, 739, 740
Wheaton, B., 93, 257, 345
Whitaker, R., 2
Whitcher-Alagna, S., 781
White, H., 260
White, I., 768
White, P. D., 465

White, R. W., 218
Whitlock, E. P., 320
Whitney, L. H., 821
Whitt, H. P., 765, 766
Whitten, C., 725
Whorwell, P. J., 554
Wiecha, J. M., 2
Wilhelmsen, L., 780
Willett, W. C., 501, 504, 518
Williams, A. F., 551
Williams, D. R., 103, 108, 254, 255, 256, 257,
    258, 345, 581, 769
Williams, J. B. W, 232
Williams, J. E., 304
Williams, P. T., 143, 711
Williams, R. B., 527, 567
Williams-Morris, R., 254, 255
Williams-Russo, P., 769
Wills, T. A., 780, 781
Wilson, D. H., 211
Wilson, M. H., 551
Wincze, J. P., 317
Wing, A. L., 656
Wing, R. R., 58
Wing, S. B., 144, 568
Winkleby, M. A., 143, 144
Winzelberg, A., 713
Wiseman, V. L., 716
Wisotzek, I. E., 725
Wittchen, H. U., 768
Wolchik, S. A., 781
Wolever, T. M., 502
Wolf, S., 100, 350
Wolfe, F., 329, 333
Wolff, H. G., 350
Wolpaw, J. R., 101
Wong, C. J., 267
Wong, N. D., 103
Wood, D. L., 2
Wooley, S. F., 705, 706
Woolf, S. H., 320
Wortman, C. B., 781
Wright, C., 175
Wu, M., 706, 707, 708
Wulsin, L. R., 303
Wurm, M., 519
Wyche, J., 704, 705, 706

Yesavage, J., 231
Yocum, D., 82
Yoediono, Z., 208
Yonkers, K. A., 231
Young, K. N. J., 73

Young, M. J., 308
Youngren, M. A., 235, 237
Yu, Y., 257, 258
Yule, G. U., 215
Yunus, M. B., 329, 333
Yurko, K. H., 325

Zaki, H. S., 337
Zane, N. W. S., 73
Zautra, A. J., 82

Zbylot, P., 713
Zenilman, J., 27, 722
Zhao, S., 208, 235, 768
Ziedonis, D., 737, 743
Zigler, E. F., 643
Zigmond, A. S., 232
Zuckerman, A., 781
Zuckerman, M., 60, 232
Zung, W. W. K., 231
Zureik, M., 58

Subject Index

Abuse. *See* Child abuse/neglect; Sexual abuse
Access to health care, 2
    cancer screening, 133
    gender differences and, 359-360
    genetic testing and, 370-371
    health disparities and, 492
    immigrant populations and, 535
    language proficiency and, 3, 535, 579
    Latinos, 576
    socioeconomic status and, 769
Acculturation theory, 1-2
    access to health care and, 3
    bidirectionality of acculturation, 1, 4
    epidemiologic paradox, acculturation hypothesis
      and, 3
    gender effects, 3
    health outcomes and, 2
    measures/scales of, 3-4
    modernization associations, 4
    research limitations, 4
    socioeconomic status and, 3
    stress and, 2
ACTION Trial, 507
Activities of daily living (ADLs), 45, 159, 184,
    506, 717
Activity Counseling Trial (ACT), 664
Adaptation. *See* General adaptation syndrome
Addictive behavior:
    motivational interviewing and, 602
    See also Alcohol abuse; Drug abuse
Adherence, 6
    dosage modifications, 7
    exercise programs, 508-509
    HIV/AIDS treatment, 19, 20, 21-23
    improvement strategies, 8, 22
    measures of, 7-8
    missed dosages, 6-7
    negative patterns of, 6-7
    performance errors and, 7
    problems with, 6
    sleep disorders and, 729
    treatment initiation/cessation, 6
Adjustment disorders, 20

Adolescent health:
    diabetes mellitus and, 245-246
    physical activity interventions, 661-662
    safer-sex interventions and, 26
    youth violence prevention, 807-808
    See also Bogalusa Heart Study; Pregnancy
      prevention-adolescents; Smoking
      prevention-adolescents
Adolescent Health Survey, 4
Adoption of health behaviors, 9-12
Adrenocorticotropic hormone (ACTH), 313, 676, 680, 777
Adult Treatment Panel (ATP), 615
Affect Adjective Check List (AACL), 60
Affect. *See* Emotional states
African Americans, 1, 12
    blood pressure, control of, 103
    caregiving coping strategies, 159-160
    disease etiology, behavioral/sociocultural factors, 15
    disease-related coping styles, 15, 16-17
    equality concept and, 13
    future medical treatment of, 16-17
    genetic research and, 13
    historical context of, 12-13, 15
    HIV/AIDS and, 13-15
    hostility, glucose metabolism and, 525
    hypertension in, 108
    John Henryism and, 16-17
    low birth weight infants and, 590-591
    one drop rule, 12
    patient-doctor interactions and, 14-15
    sickle cell disease and, 15-16
    social environment and, 14, 108
    treatment compliance and, 14
    See also Bogalusa Heart Study; Discriminatory
      practices; Health disparities
Age:
    cardiovascular reactivity and, 155
    effort-reward imbalance and, 298
    successful aging, 784-785
Agency for Health Care Policy and Research
    (AHCPR), 188
Agency for Healthcare Research and Quality (AHRQ),
    139, 320, 375, 469, 470, 697, 737, 829

Agency for Toxic Substances and Disease Registry
    (ATSDR), 165
Aggression Questionnaire (AQ), 528
AIDS. *See* HIV/AIDS; HIV/AIDS prevention; HIV/AIDS
    stress management; HIV/AIDS treatment adherence
Air pollution, 80, 749
Alameda County Study, 31-32, 363-364, 587, 666, 755
Alan Guttmacher Institute, 375, 829
Alcohol abuse, 2, 32
    abuse/dependence, definition of, 32-33
    accidental injury and, 35
    behavioral skills training and, 266
    biological variables and, 33
    biphasic effect of alcohol, 34
    cancer risk and, 36, 120-121, 128
    cardiovascular disease and, 35-36
    child/adolescent use, 113
    cognitive/motor functioning and, 34
    demographic characteristics and, 33-34
    erectile dysfunction and, 316
    fetal alcohol syndrome and, 37
    health disparities and, 490
    immune function and, 35
    liver disease and, 35, 36-37
    long-term effects of, 35-37
    pessimism and, 639
    prevalence survey, 32
    psychological variables and, 33
    reproductive function and, 37
    short-term effects of, 34-35
    smoking cessation and, 743
    social/environmental variables and, 33
    violent behavior and, 34-35
    See also Binge drinking
Alcohol abuse treatment, 37
    behavior therapy techniques, 38-39
    brief interventions, 38
    cognitive approaches to, 39
    cognitive-behavioral treatments, 39-40
    community reinforcement approach, 39-40
    outpatient treatment, 38-40
    pharmacotherapies, 39
    professional treatment, 38-40
    relapse prevention approach, 39
    relationship therapies, 39
    self-help, 38
    treatment modality selection, 40
Alcoholics Anonymous (AA), 38, 265
Allostasis/allostatic load, 40-41
    allostatic states and, 41, 42
    brain function in, 43, 44
    caregiving duties and, 46
    definition of, 41
    homeostasis and, 41, 42

hypothalamic-pituitary-adrenal (HPA) axis and, 41-42
    load/overload process, 42-43
    measurement of, 43-44
    mediators of, 42, 43
    prolonged/inadequate response profiles and, 42
    stress and, 41-42
Alternative medicine. *See* Complementary/alternative
    medicine (CAM)
Alzheimer's Association, 375, 829
Alzheimer's disease (AD), 45, 460
    activities of daily living and, 45
    caregiving duties and, 45-48
    diagnosis criteria, 45
    lipid disturbances and, 596
    physical health implications of, 46-47
    psychosocial implications of, 45-46
American Academy of Child and Adolescent Psychiatry
    (AACAP), 375, 829
American Academy of Nursing, 376, 830
American Academy of Pediatrics (AAP), 376, 830
American Academy of Sleep Medicine, 727
American Association of Cardiovascular and Pulmonary
    Rehabilitation (AACVPR), 139
American Association of Colleges of Nursing
    (AACN), 376, 830
American Association of Spinal Cord Injury Psychologists
    and Social Workers (AASCIPSW), 376, 830
American Association of Suicidology (AAS), 376, 830
American Cancer Society (ACS), 143, 339, 376, 830
American College of Cardiology (ACC), 140
American College of Occupational and Environmental
    Medicine (ACEOM), 636
American College of Preventive Medicine (ACPM),
    376, 830
American Counseling Association (ACA), 377, 831
American Diabetes Association, 377, 831
American Heart Association (AHA), 139, 143, 377, 831
American Institute of Stress, 377, 831
American Lung Association, 749
American Psychiatric Association, 377, 831
American Psychiatric Association Practice Guideline
    for the Treatment of Patients With Nicotine
    Dependence, 737
American Psychological Association (APA), 377, 381,
    473, 696, 831, 835
American Psychological Society (APS), 377, 831
American Psychosocial Oncology Society, 378, 832
American Psychosomatic Society (APS), 378, 473-474, 832
American Public Health Association (APHA), 378, 832
American Sleep Disorders Association, 726
American Social Health Association, 378, 832
American Society for Clinical Nutrition (ASCN), 378, 832
American Society for Nutritional Sciences, 378, 832
American Sociological Association (ASA), 378, 832

Anger:
    anger-in/anger-out, 51, 531-532
    anger-suppression hypothesis, 51
    biological mechanisms in, 50
    cardiovascular disease and, 49-50, 304, 524-525
    cardiovascular reactivity and, 156
    caregiver health and, 48
    epidemiological evidence of effects, 49-50
    hostility, 304
    hypertension and, 50-52
    morbidity/mortality and, 304
    pain experience and, 649
    prevention programs and, 50
    See also Hostility; Hostility measurement; Hostility
        psychophysiology
Anger Expression Scale, 525
Anger-in Scale, 51, 53
Anger measurement, 52
    anger/hostility dimensions, 53
    covert anger, 53
    heart disease outcomes and, 53
    interpersonal analogue assessment and, 54
    overt anger, 53-54
Anorexia nervosa (AN), 279, 280 (table)
    etiology of, 283-284
    treatment of, 286
Antidepressant medications, 237
    bulimia nervosa and, 116-117
    chronic pain management and, 192
    current generation of, 238-239
    headache treatment and, 468
    monoamine oxidase inhibitors, 237-238
    obesity treatment and, 634
    selective serotonin reuptake inhibitors, 237, 238
    tricyclic antidepressants, 238
Antiretroviral treatment, 19, 21-23
Anxiety, 15, 55
    acute anxiety, 58
    cancer-related distress, 135
    coronary heart disease and, 55, 56-58, 304
    definition of, 59-60
    disease development and, 56-57
    disease prognosis and, 57
    dose-response effect and, 57
    generalized anxiety disorder, 500
    headaches and, 468
    heart rate variability and, 58
    HIV/AIDS diagnosis and, 20
    hypertension and, 58
    injection anxiety, 612
    lipids and, 584-585
    loneliness and, 586
    measurement of, 59-61
    morbidity/mortality and, 57-58, 304

    nature of, 55-56
    pain experience and, 649
    physical effects of, 57-58
    psychiatric disorders and, 57
    threat response of, 41-42
    trait/state anxiety, 60-61
    white-coat effect, 51-52, 103
Anxiety Scale Questionnaire (ASQ), 60
Apnea, 199, 500, 727, 729
Applied behavior analysis, 62
    adherence motivation and, 63
    adjunct to interventions, 64
    antecedent stimuli and, 63
    healthy behaviors, motivation for, 64-65
    medical diagnostic procedures and, 63
    negative reinforcement, 62
    operant conditioning and, 62-63
    punishers, 62-63
    unhealthy behaviors, reduction of, 64
Arteriosclerosis. See Bogalusa Heart Study
Arthritis, 65
    assertiveness, communication and, 67, 68
    attention diversion and, 68
    behavioral therapy and, 66-67
    cognitive-behavioral treatment of, 65-66
    cognitive restructuring and, 68
    cognitive therapy and, 67-68
    depression incidence and, 72
    operant programs and, 66
    pacing/goal-setting and, 66
    pain, culture and, 71-72
    physical disability and, 72
    problem-solving and, 66
    psychoeducational programs on, 68-69
    psychosocial aspects of, 71-72
    relaxation/biofeedback strategies and, 67
    self-management approaches, 66-67
    stress management and, 69
    supportive counseling/psychotherapy and, 69
    treatment effectiveness, 69-70
    treatment-related changes, 70
    treatments, administration modes, 69
Arthritis Impact Measurement Scale (AIMS), 687
Asian Americans, 2
    acculturation scales for, 4
    alcohol abuse and, 34
    sickle cell disease and, 15
    See also Discriminatory practices
Asian Americans/Pacific Islanders (AAPIs), 72-73,
        73 (table)
    alcohol intake and, 75
    dietary patterns, 74
    epidemiology of, 73, 74 (table)
    exercise patterns, 75

health status, cultural influences on, 73-75
   religious practices and, 74
   smoking rates and, 74-75
   traditional health practices, health care decisions and, 75
   See also Health disparities
Assimilation theory, 1-2
Assisted reproduction. *See* Infertility
Association for the Advancement of Behavior Therapy
   (AABT), 379, 833
Association for Applied Psychophysiology and
   Biofeedback (AAPB), 378-379, 832-833
Association of Behavior Analysis, 379, 833
Association of State and Territorial Directors of Health
   Promotion and Public Health Education
   (ASTDHPPHE), 379, 833
Association of Teachers of Preventive Medicine (ATPM),
   379, 833
Asthma, 75-76
   autonomic control in, 78-79
   behavioral management of, 76-77
   biofeedback methods and, 99
   cognitive-behavioral interventions and, 76
   cognitive functioning and, 199
   current disease paradigm, 77-78
   education programs and, 76
   endocrine system function and, 78
   environmental stress and, 80, 81
   immune function and, 79
   integrated management of, 76-77
   life stress and, 77, 80, 81
   oxidative stress and, 80
   psychological distress and, 78, 80
   psychosocial interventions and, 76
   repressive coping and, 695
   respiratory infection and, 79
   self-management of, 78, 80
   social connectedness and, 80
   socioeconomic status/race and, 80
   stress and, 77-81
Atherosclerosis, 58, 139, 154, 302, 679
Atherosclerosis Risk in Communities (ARIC) Study,
   49, 304
Attention deficit disorder (ADD), 100, 101
Attitudes. *See* Health beliefs/attitudes
Attributional Style Questionnaire (ASQ), 323, 640, 641-642
Autogenic training, 692
Autoimmune diseases, 81
   anti-inflammatory hormones and, 82
   cognitive functioning and, 199
   emotional expression and, 82-83
   mind-body relations and, 83
   pro-inflammatory processes and, 82, 83
   psychosocial interventions and, 82, 83
   social stress and, 82-83

   social support and, 82, 83
   supportive-expressive group therapy, 83
Autonomic nervous system (ANS), 42
   airway control, stress and, 78-79
   blood pressure, control of, 102-103
   chronic fatigue syndrome and, 178
   fibromyalgia syndrome and, 331
   immune system function and, 675-676
   lipid metabolism and, 585
   negative emotions and, 308
   stress, cardiovascular responses to, 148-149
   stress response and, 777

Beck Depression Inventory, 190, 231, 232
Behavioral assimilation. *See* Acculturation
Behavioral genetics, 85
   additive genetic variation, traits and, 85-86
   cancer incidence and, 87-88
   cardiovascular disease and, 87
   diabetes and, 88
   eating disorders and, 284
   environmental influences and, 86
   health studies and, 87-88
   hypertension and, 88
   integrated/interdisciplinary approaches to health and,
      88-89
   model fitting and, 86-87
   obesity and, 88
   research methodology in, 85-87
   structural equation modeling and, 86
   tobacco use and, 88, 736
   twin studies and, 86-87, 87 (figure)
   See also Genetic testing
Behavioral medicine. *See* Evidence-based behavioral
   medicine (EBBM); Health psychology;
   Psychophysiology
Behavioral Risk Factor Surveillance System (BRFSS),
   89-90, 165
   behavioral surveillance history, 90
   health promotion activities and, 90
   population-based data and, 90
   prevalence estimates and, 90, 616-617
   social capital, health ranking and, 752
   successes of, 90-91
Behavioral and Social Sciences Working Group
   (BSSWG), 165
Behavioral therapy (BT), 237
Behavioral treatment models, 15-16
   alcohol abuse treatments, 38-40
   arthritis and, 66-67
   asthma, 75-77
   behavioral shaping, 317
   community reinforcement approach, 39-40
   erectile dysfunction and, 317, 319

headaches and, 468
HIV/AIDS and, 19, 23
hypertension and, 110-111
John Henryism and, 16-17
marital therapy, 267-268
See also Drug abuse-behavioral treatment
Behavior change theories, 271, 288, 509, 720
See also Social marketing; Transtheoretical model
(TTM) of behavior change
Behavior contracts, 267
Behavior OnLine, 379, 833
Behaviors. *See* Applied behavior analysis; Health
behaviors
Beliefs. *See* Control beliefs; Health beliefs/attitudes;
Hopelessness; Self-efficacy
Bell Telephone Company cohort study, 463, 821
Benefit-finding, 775
Benefit reminding, 775
Bereavement, 30, 31, 91
Alzheimer's disease and, 46
bulimic symptoms and, 116
child's death, 92
cognitive restructuring and, 93
disenfranchised grief, 92
friend's death, 92
gender effects and, 92-93
health disadvantage and, 94
infertility and, 544
parent's death, 92
predictability, restoration of, 93
role transition and, 91
separation anxiety and, 93
sibling's death, 92
social supports, stress and, 93-94
sociobiological perspective on, 93
spouse's death, 91-92
Biculturalism, 2, 4
Binge drinking, 36, 94-95
environmental factors in, 96-97
high-risk students, 96
prevention interventions, 97-98
secondhand effects of, 96
study of, 95-96, 95 (table)
Binge eating disorder (BED), 280 (table), 281
etiology of, 284-286
treatment of, 287
Biofeedback, 66, 67, 98
blood pressure and, 99
cancer treatments and, 130
cardiorespiratory biofeedback, 98-100
diabetes mellitus and, 243-244
headaches and, 469
heart rate/rate variability and, 99
musculoskeletal activity and, 100

neurofeedback and, 100-101
Raynaud's disease and, 692
respiratory parameters and, 99-100
thermal feedback, 98-99
Biofeedback-assisted relaxation (BAR), 111, 243-244
Biological variables:
alcohol abuse and, 33
allostasis/allostatic load, measurement of, 43-44
anger, cardiovascular disease and, 50
biobehavioral stress reactivity, 108-110
depression treatments, 237-239
See also Behavioral genetics
Bipolar disease, 208
Bladder cancer, 125, 127
Blood pressure (BP):
assessment of, 102
cardiac output, 102
hostility and, 529-530, 531
Korotkoff sounds and, 103, 147
measurement of, clinical/research settings, 103
physical activity, response to, 104-106
physiological basis of, 102-103
variability in, shear stress and, 103
See also Hypertension
Blood supply safety, 24
Body dissatisfaction, 2, 283
Body mass index (BMI), 627, 631
Body weight:
cancer risk and, 122, 128
cardiovascular risk and, 140
health disparities and, 490-491
smoking cessation and, 740, 743
See also Eating disorders; Metabolic syndrome;
Obesity
Bogalusa Heart Study, 112-113
accomplishments of, 113
dietary intake/eating patterns, 113-114
protocols for, 113
psychosocial factors, 114
tobacco/alcohol use, 113
Bortner Rating Scale Type, 519
Boys and Girls Clubs, 274
Brain cancer, 125
Brain function:
allostatic load/overload and, 43, 44
endogenous opioids and, 315
migraine headaches and, 467
neuromatrix theory of pain, 356-357
See also Gate control theory;
Psychoneuroimmunology
Breast cancer, 124, 127, 133
genetic testing and, 369, 370
personality characteristics and, 525
risk perceptions and, 134

British Regional Heart Study, 506
Broaden-and-build theory, 306, 307-308
Bulimia nervosa (BN), 2, 115, 279, 280 (table), 281
    antidepressant medication and, 116-117
    binge-starve cycle in, 115
    cognitive-behavioral therapy and, 115
    dialectical behavior therapy and, 116
    etiology of, 283-284
    interpersonal psychotherapy and, 115-116
    laxative abuse, 115, 279
    loneliness and, 587
    psychotherapeutic approaches to, 115-116
    treatment settings for, 117
    treatments for, 286
Bullying Prevention Program (BPP), 808
Buss-Durkee Hostility Inventory (BDHI), 49, 524, 528

CA125 blood test, 133
Caerphilly Study, 49, 525
Campañeros el la Salud, 196
Campbell Collaboration, 320
Cancer:
    alcohol abuse and, 36
    behavioral genetics and, 87-88
    breast cancer, 124
    cognitive functioning and, 199
    colon cancer, 122, 124
    esophageal cancer, 122
    health disparities and, 488
    Kaposi's sarcoma, 19, 30
    kidney cancer, 122
    prostate cancer, 122, 124-125
    psychoneuroimmunology and, 680-681
    rectal cancer, 124
    repressive coping and, 694
    stomach cancer, 74
    tobacco use and, 137-138
Cancer-diet relationship, 119
    alcohol use and, 120-121
    body weight and, 122
    fiber ingestion and, 128
    fruits/vegetables and, 120
    macro/micronutrients and, 121
    physical activity and, 121-122
    prevention strategies and, 128
    red meats and, 120
    whole foods and, 119-120
Cancer-physical activity relationship, 121-122, 123
    breast cancer and, 124
    colon/rectal cancer and, 124
    methodological issues and, 125-126
    overall cancer risk and, 123-124, 125
    physiological mechanisms in, 124
    post-diagnosis exercise and, 125

    prostate cancer and, 124-125
    public health recommendations, 126
    site-specific cancer and, 125
Cancer prevention, 126-127
    alcohol use/abuse and, 128
    chemopreventive measures, 128
    dietary modifications and, 128
    exercise/weight control and, 128
    genetic susceptibility and, 127
    mortality rates and, 127, 129
    occupational/environmental exposures and, 129
    personal approach to, 127-128
    sun exposure and, 128
    tobacco use and, 127-128
    vaccinations, 128-129
Cancer-psychosocial treatment, 129-130
    anticipatory nausea and, 130
    cancer prevention strategies and, 132
    cognitive-behavioral interventions, 130-131, 132
    educational interventions, 130
    emotional distress and, 130-131
    family involvement in, 131
    group therapy approaches, 131
    health outcomes and, 131
    immune functioning and, 131-132
    pain and, 130
Cancer screening, 133
    adherence factors in, 133-135
    cancer-related distress, 135
    cancer-related expectancies/beliefs and, 134
    cancer-related knowledge, risk perceptions and, 133-134
    cognitive-social behavior model and, 133
    cultural values and, 134
    elderly patients and, 134
    fatalistic beliefs and, 134
    long-term adherence issues, 133
    media exposure and, 134
    psychosocial interventions, adherence and, 135-136
    self-examination procedures, 134, 135
    self-regulatory skills and, 135
Cardiac rehabilitation, 138-139
    case example, 141
    education/clinical monitoring, 139
    exercise and, 139-140
    guidelines for, 139
    lifestyle-related risk factors and, 140
    multifactorial risk reduction and, 140-141
    psychosocial aspects of, 141
    serum lipid levels and, 140
    setting/personnel in, 140
    tobacco use and, 140
    treadmill testing, 139
    walking/stationary bicycling and, 139-140
    weight control and, 140

Cardiovascular disease (CVD), 0
    alcohol use and, 35-36, 121
    allostatic overload and, 44
    anger and, 49-50
    anxiety and, 304
    behavioral genetics and, 87
    carotid atherosclerosis, 154
    cognitive functioning and, 199
    depression and, 303
    health disparities and, 487, 492
    hypertension and, 106
    left ventricular mass, 154, 514
    negative emotions and, 302-305
    opioid dysfunction in, 314
    psychoneuroimmunology and, 679
    repressive coping and, 695
    shift work and, 821
    women and, 814
    See also Anger; Anxiety; Coronary heart disease
        (CHD); Metabolic syndrome
Cardiovascular disease prevention-community
        interventions, 142
    analysis of, 143, 144 (table)
    environmental factors, health behaviors and, 145
    future of, 144-145
    outcome shortfall, 143-144
    risk reduction education programs, 142
    trial results, 142-143
Cardiovascular psychophysiology measures, 146
    ambulatory monitoring studies, 149-150
    autonomic nervous system and, 148-149
    baroreceptor sensitivity and, 149
    blood pressure, 147, 149-150
    cardiac output, systemic vascular resistance and, 148
    cardiovascular reactivity lab studies, 146-149
    catecholamine levels, 148-149, 150
    heart rate, 147, 149, 150
    hemodynamics monitoring, 150
    impedance cardiography monitoring, 150
    limb blood flow, 148
    stress reactions, 148-149
    ultrasound imaging and, 149
Cardiovascular reactivity, 151
    active vs. passive coping strategies and, 154-155
    age effects and, 155
    clinical/subclinical endpoints prediction, 153-154
    current research on, 157
    family history and, 155
    gender effects and, 155
    hostility-anger dimensions and, 156
    hypertension prediction and, 153
    hypothesis limitations, 157
    laboratory studies of, 146-149, 152, 152 (figure)
    laboratory-to-life generalizability, 153

    menopause and, 155
    menstrual cycle and, 155
    mental/emotional stressors and, 152
    race effects and, 155-156
    reactivity model, origins of, 151-157
    situational determinants of, 156-157
    stress concept and, 151, 778
    test-retest reliability and, 153
    trait conceptualization of, 152
    twin studies and, 155
    type A behavior personality and, 156
    See also Heart disease-reactivity
Caregivers:
    Alzheimer's patients and, 45-48
    anger and, 48
    cancer interventions and, 131
    demographic variables and, 47
    depression and, 46, 47-48
    ethnicity and, 47
    health outcomes and, 47, 48
    illness incidence and, 46
    life satisfaction and, 460
    physiological functioning and, 46-47
    pre-existing comorbidities and, 48
    resources of, 48
    sandwich generation, 46
    theoretical explanatory models and, 47
    vulnerabilities of, 47-48
Caregiving stress, 158
    appraisal and, 160
    chronic illness/disability and, 159
    coping mechanisms and, 159-160
    situational stress, 159
    social supports and, 160
    spirituality and, 160
    stress, definition of, 158-159
Care Need Index (CNI), 717
Carrera program, 674
Caucasian Americans, 13, 14, 15
    caregiving coping strategies, 159-160
    hostility, glucose metabolism and, 525
    See also Bogalusa Heart Study; Discriminatory
        practices
Celexa, 238, 500
Center for the Advancement of Health, 162, 380, 834
    additional publications of, 163
    Health Behavior News Service, 163
    health views, expansion of, 162-163
Center for Behavioral Neuroscience, 379, 833
Center for Communication Programs (CCP), 379-380,
        833-834
Center for Epidemiologic Studies Depression Scale
        (CES-D), 231, 255
Center for Health Statistics, 671

Center for Medicare and Medicaid Services
    (CMS), 478
Centers for Disease Control and Prevention (CDC), 18,
    27, 89, 380, 834
    administrative functions of, 165
    adolescent pregnancy rates, 671
    behavioral/social science disciplines and, 165
    Community Preventive Services Task Force, 289
    dietary behavior change and, 339
    mission of, 164
    organizational components of, 164-165
    research activities of, 165
    school-based health promotion, 705-706
    sexually transmitted disease treatment, 722
Central nervous system (CNS), 0
    endogenous opioids and, 315
    gate control theory of pain and, 355
    tension-type headaches and, 467
    See also Multiple sclerosis
Cerebrovascular disease, 49, 166
    health disparities and, 487
    post-stroke interventions, 167
    psychosocial factors, stroke onset and, 166
    social support, functional recovery and, 166
    stroke course, 166
    stroke impact, psychosocial functioning and, 166
Cervical cancer, 128-129, 133, 522
Chernobyl nuclear accident, 253
Child abuse/neglect, 167-168
    emotional abuse, 169
    mental health/behavioral problems and, 169-170
    mortality rates and, 168
    neglect, 169
    physical abuse, 168
    physical consequences of, 169
    pre-natal drug abuse and, 169
    prevention programs, 808
    seduction theory and, 168
    sexual abuse, 168-169
Child Abuse Prevention and Treatment Act
    (CAPTA), 168
Child and Adolescent Trial for Cardiovascular Health
    (CATCH), 145, 660, 706-708
Child health, 2
    diabetes mellitus and, 245-246
    injury prevention, 547-553
    maternal-child HIV transmission, 25
    physical activity interventions, 660-661
    sleep disorders and, 729
    See also Adolescent health; Bogalusa Heart Study;
        Infant health; Obesity in children
Child Health Insurance Plan (CHIP), 536
Children's Aid Society, 674
Children's Depression Inventory (CDI), 232

Children's Interview for Psychiatric Syndromes, 232
Chinese Exclusionary Act of 1882, 533
Cholesterol counts:
    alcohol abuse and, 36
    allostatic overload measures, 44
    high-density lipoprotein cholesterol, 343, 503
    low density lipoprotein cholesterol, 502, 503
    See also Heart disease-dietary factors; Lipids;
        Metabolic syndrome; National Cholesterol
        Education Program (NCEP)
Chronic disease, 179-180
    adaptive tasks and, 180
    adherence-promoting interventions and, 22
    adjustment determinants, 181-182
    adjustment process, 180-181
    cognitive appraisals of, 181
    coping processes and, 181
    John Henryism model and, 16
    life-contextual adjustments, 181
    macrolevel contextual factors and, 182-183
    personality factors, 181-182
    positive adjustment outcomes and, 180
    social supports and, 182
    stress appraisal and, 108
Chronic disease management, 170
    circles of influence in, 171-172, 171 (figure)
    communication/counseling and, 173
    community programs/policies and, 174-175
    expressive writing and, 326-327
    family role in, 171
    financial policies and, 175
    health care organizations/systems and, 174
    health professionals and, 173-174
    human/economic costs and, 172
    improvement of, 175
    information, provision of, 173-174
    management tasks, self-regulation and, 172
    patient/family tasks in, 172-173
Chronic fatigue syndrome (CFS), 176-177
    biopsychosocial model of, 177-178
    case definition of, 177
    epidemiological studies of, 178
    etiology of, 177-178
    non-pharmacological interventions, 178-179
    psychiatric instruments use and, 177
    See also Fibromyalgia syndrome (FMS)
Chronic illness. See Chronic disease
Chronic obstructive pulmonary disease (COPD), 183-184
    anxiety and, 185
    behavioral functioning and, 185-187
    cognitive functioning and, 185, 199
    definition of, 184
    demographic/symptom profile in, 184
    depression and, 185

hypoxia and, 184
medical treatment of, 184
medication compliance in, 185-186
nutritional status and, 186
physical exercise and, 186-187
psychosocial distress and, 184-185
pulmonary rehabilitation programs, 186
smoking cessation and, 186
social functioning and, 185
treatment strategies in, 186
Chronic pain:
arthritis and, 71-72
biopsychosocial model of, 646
endogenous opioids and, 314
fibromyalgia syndrome and, 331-332
HIV/AIDS and, 21
sickle cell disease and, 15-16
See also Gate control theory; Pain
Chronic pain management, 187-188
adjuvant therapies and, 192
alternative/complementary techniques, 192
clinical pain, differences in, 188-189
education and, 191
guidelines for, 188, 189
manifestations of pain, 189
manual therapy and, 192
nerve blocks and, 192
non-opioid analgesics and, 191
opioid analgesics and, 191, 313
pain assessment, 189-190
pain impact, 188, 188 (figure)
patient self-report guidelines, 190-191
psychological counseling and, 192-193
referrals and, 193
therapeutic modalities in, 191
treatments for, 191-193
Church-based interventions, 194
behavior change programs and, 194
church facilities, use of, 195
cultural sensitivity and, 196-197
minority population and, 194
program recruitment function, 195
research partnerships and, 195
research studies, 195-197, 196 (table)
results, publishing of, 197
separation of church and state, 194
spiritual/scriptural components in, 197
volunteerism in, 194-195
See also Community-based participatory research;
Spirituality
Civil Rights Act of 1964, 535
Clinical practice, 696
constraints on treatment, 696
evidence-based movement and, 696

research base of, 696
research-practice gap and, 697
treatment decision-making, 696-697
Clinical trials, 6
Cochrane Collaborative Group, 175, 320, 696, 697
Cognitive-behavioral treatment (CBT), 15-16, 27
alcohol abuse treatments, 39-40
arthritis and, 65-68
asthma, 76
autoimmune diseases and, 83
cancer treatments, 130-131
chronic fatigue syndrome and, 178
diabetes mellitus and, 243
eating disorders and, 115, 286-287
fibromyalgia syndrome and, 333-337
guided imagery, 130-131, 335
headaches and, 469
problem-solving therapy, 130, 131
rheumatoid arthritis and, 700-701
stress management, 31
See also Arthritis
Cognitive functioning, 197-198
age factors in, 198
allostatic overload and, 44
Alzheimer's disease and, 45, 198
chronic obstructive pulmonary disease and, 185
environmental/occupational toxins and, 199
genetic factors in, 198-199
hormonal factors in, 198
learned helplessness, 114
lifestyle factors in, 198
medical diseases and, 199
metabolic syndrome and, 596
See also Multiple sclerosis
Cognitive psychotherapy, 236
Cognitive restructuring, 68, 93, 130, 318-319
Cognitive-Social Health Information Processing (C-SHIP)
model, 133, 476, 546
Cognitive-transactional model, 367-368
College on Problems of Drug Dependence (CPDD), 380, 834
College students:
examination stress, 538-539
loneliness and, 587
physical activity interventions, 661-662
See also Binge drinking
Colon cancer, 122, 124, 128, 133
cancer screening, 135
familial adenomatous polyposis, 371
Colonoscopy, 133, 134
Commission on Accreditation of Rehabilitation Facilities
(CARF), 380, 834
Communication network theories, 273
See also Health communication; Tailored
communications

Community-based organizations, 19
    drug abuse prevention and, 272, 274-275
    intervention dissemination, 27
    See also Cardiovascular disease prevention-community
        interventions
Community-based participatory research
        (CBPR), 200
    case example, 202-203
    practice recommendations, 203-204
    principles of, 200-202
    rationale for, 202
Community coalitions, 204
    action planning/implementation, 206
    collaborative interaction processes and, 106
    development stages, 204-205
    evaluation of, 206-207
    institutionalization/sustainability and, 207
    integration, level of, 205-206
    membership of, 205
    pre-formation considerations, 205
    See also Community-based participatory research
Community Preventive Services Task Force, 289
Community Reinforcement Approach (CRA), 268
Community Reinforcement and Family Training
        (CRAFT), 269
Community Survey of the Project on Human Development
        in Chicago Neighborhoods, 751
Comorbid disorders, 207
    depression/anxiety and, 207-208
    headaches, psychiatric disorders and, 468
    heart disease and, 208
    interventions and, 208-209
    research needs on, 209
Complementary/alternative medicine (CAM), 209-210
    choice of, 211
    conventional medicine and, 210
    evidence-based practice of, 211-212
    future of, 212
    integrated medicine and, 212
    utility of, 210-211
Compliance. *See* Adherence
Computed tomography (CT) scans, 646
Conditioning theory, 62-63, 130, 668-669, 676
Confounding, 213
    adjustment for, 216
    effect estimation, bias in, 214
    factors in, 215
    potential-outcome model and, 214-215
    prevention of, 215-216
Congestive heart failure (CHF), 507
Consolidated Standards of Reporting Trials (CONSORT)
        guidelines, 321, 322, 696
Consortium of Social Science Associations (COSSA),
        380, 834

Content Analysis of Verbatim Explanations (CAVE),
        323-324, 642
Contingency management (CM), 266-267
Control beliefs, 217, 793
    altering control, 219
    desire for control and, 219
    job decision latitude, 561-562
    learned helplessness and, 218-219
    locus of control and, 217-218
    perceived competence/mastery, self-efficacy
        and, 218
Convulsive disorders, 101
Cook-Medley Hostility (HO) Scale, 49, 53, 524,
        528, 529-530
COPE measures, 775
Coping in Health and Illness Project (CHIP), 29-30
Coping Responses Inventory (CRI), 775
Coping strategies, 774-775
    active vs. passive coping, 154-155
    coping dimensions, 775
    cultural factors and, 229
    diabetes management and, 246
    disease management, 15
    drug abuse and, 266
    HIV infection and, 28
    immune response and, 31
    John Henryism and, 16-17, 565-568
    meaning-focused coping, 775
    measures of coping, 775-776
    negative emotions and, 302
    pain control, 648
    physiological mechanisms, 42
    positive emotions and, 309
    psychosocial factors and, 15-16
    rheumatoid arthritis and, 700
    spiritual coping methods, 773
    stress appraisal, hypertension and, 108
    See also Caregiving stress; Explanatory style;
        Happiness; Repressive coping
CORE survey, 95
Cornell Heart Study, 562
Coronary artery bypass surgery, 139
Coronary artery disease (CAD), 0
    anger/hostility and, 54
    anxiety and, 58
    depression and, 208
    psychophysiological pathways in, 499
    See also Bogalusa Heart Study
Coronary heart disease (CHD), 0
    anger/hostility and, 49, 53, 54, 304
    anxiety and, 55, 56-58
    caregiver well-being and, 48
    depression and, 303
    health disparities and, 487

heart rate variability and, 58
  See also Anger; Cardiac rehabilitation; Cardiovascular
    disease (CVD); Heart disease-dietary factors;
    Heart disease-emotional distress; Heart disease-
    physical activity; Heart disease-tobacco use; Heart
    disease-type A behavior
Corticotropin-releasing hormone (CRH), 676, 680, 777
Cost-effectiveness analysis, 220-221
  accounting for costs, 224
  analysis perspective, 224
  behavioral health and, 226
  comparators in, 225
  cost-benefit analysis, 222-223
  cost-offset analysis, 222
  cost-utility analysis, 223
  discounting costs/outcomes, 225
  effectiveness measures, 224
  health-related quality of life approaches, 223
  historical significance of, 221-222
  practice considerations and, 224-225
  public policy and, 225
  quality-of-life analysis, 223-224
  sensitivity analysis and, 225
  time horizons, modeling of, 225
  traditional analysis, 223
  types of, 222-224, 222 (table)
  See also Health care costs
Council of Graduate Departments of Psychology
    (COGDOP), 380-381, 834-835
Crowding, 226
  measurement of, 226
  physical health and, 226-227
Cue reactivity, 277-278, 475, 735-736
Cultural consonance, 766-767
Cultural factors, 2, 3, 4, 228
  acculturation, language/communication and, 228-229
  cancer screening behaviors and, 134
  cultural stressors, 107-108
  health/illness, perceptions of, 229
  help-seeking behaviors, health decision-making and,
    229-230
  personality, stress/coping and, 229
Cytokines, 43, 678-679

Day-night/light-dark cycle, 41, 42
Death. *See* Bereavement; Mortality
Decade of Behavior, 381, 835
Defensive Pessimism Questionnaire (DPQ), 642
Dementia, 460, 816
  See also Alzheimer's disease (AD)
Demographic factors:
  access to health care, 3
  adherence prediction and, 7
  alcohol abuse and, 33-34

caregiver vulnerabilities and, 47
  demographic proxies and, 3
  diabetes mellitus and, 246
  gender, 3
  pain disability and, 15
  socioeconomic status, 3
Density. *See* Crowding
Dental care, 2
Depression, 3, 7
  allostatic overload and, 42
  arthritis and, 72
  autoimmune diseases and, 83
  brain function and, 78
  caregiving duties and, 46, 47-48
  chronic pain and, 15, 16
  comorbidity and, 207-209
  disease diagnosis and, 15
  functional status and, 234
  HIV/AIDS diagnosis and, 20
  lipids and, 584-585
  measurement of, 231-232
  morbidity/mortality and, 233-234, 303
  non-suicide mortality, 234
  pain experience and, 648-649
  suicide and, 234
  See also Antidepressant medication; Happiness;
    Loneliness
Depression Inventory for Youth, 232
Depression treatments, 235
  behavioral psychotherapy, 237
  biological treatment approaches, 237-239
  cognitive psychotherapy, 236
  current generation of, 238-239
  electroconvulsive therapy, 239
  evaluative comparisons of, 239-240
  interpersonal psychotherapy, 236-237
  monoamine oxidase inhibitors, 237-238
  psychological treatment approaches, 235-237
  selective serotonin reuptake inhibitors, 238
  tricyclic antidepressants, 238
Determinants of Myocardial Infarction Onset Study, 525
Detroit Community-Academic Urban Research Center, 202
  accomplishments/benefits of, 203
  challenges/barriers to, 203
  mission of, 202-203
Developing nations, 650-651
DHEA (dehydroepiandrosterone), 43
Diabetes mellitus (DM), 241
  activity/exercise levels and, 243
  adults and, 246-248
  biofeedback-assisted relaxation and, 243-244
  children/adolescents and, 245-246
  cognitive-behavioral therapy and, 243
  cognitive functioning and, 199

complementary/integrated medicine therapies and, 244
diet prescriptions in, 242
family involvement and, 243, 246
genetic influence on, 88
health disparities and, 488
hostility and, 525
management of, 241, 478
meal planning and, 242-243
mind-body therapies and, 243-244
neurocognitive functioning and, 245-246, 247
psychological adjustment and, 241-243, 245, 247, 248
psychosocial interventions and, 246, 248
quality of life and, 246, 247
self-care issues, 241-242
social supports and, 243
stress/coping and, 246, 247
See also Metabolic syndrome
Diagnostic Interview Schedule (DIS), 177
*Diagnostic and Statistical Manual of Mental Disorders
(DSM-IV)*, 0
alcohol abuse/dependence definition, 32-33
Alzheimer's disease, 45
depressive disorders, symptom criteria, 232
drug craving, 278
eating disorders, 279, 280-281 (table)
loneliness, mental health and, 586
Structured Clinical Interview, 177
Dialectical behavior therapy (DBT), 116
Dietary habits:
Asian/Pacific Islander practices, 74
children/adolescents, 113-114
diabetes mellitus and, 242
health disparities and, 490-491
healthy eating index, 504
westernization of traditional practice, 74
See also Cancer-diet relationship; Eating disorders; 5 A
Day For Better Health! Program; Heart disease-
dietary factors
Diet Quality Index (DQI), 504
Diet and Reinfarction Trial (DART), 502
Diffusion of innovation model, 248-249
communication processes/channels, 250
drug abuse prevention programs and, 272-273
factors in, 249-250
innovation characteristics, 249
social system contexts of, 250-251
time element in, 250
Disaster events, 251
mental/physical health outcomes and, 252-254
natural disasters, 252
technological disasters, 252
Discriminatory practices, 2, 254
accurate measurement of, 257-258
comprehensive measures of, 256-257

health disparities and, 492
low birth weight infants and, 591
mental health and, 255-256
pathogenic stressor of, 255
perceptions of, health effects and, 258-259
persistence of, 254-255
physical health and, 256
residential segregation, 591
scientific studies of, 255
See also Minority experience
Disease distribution. *See* Ecosocial theory
Disease prevention. *See* Health promotion
Disease risk:
allostatic overload and, 44
stress and, 107
See also Fundamental social causation of
disease/mortality
Disparities. *See* Health disparities
Division of Health Psychology (Div. 38), 381, 473,
498, 835
Divorce, 259-260
emotional health and, 260
physical health/longevity and, 260-261
Doctor-patient communication, 261
active listening and, 263
contextual factors and, 262
improvement of, 263-264
instrumental vs. affective communication, 262
patient reports and, 263-264
positive outcomes of, 262-263
problems with, 262
treatment outcomes/patient satisfaction and, 264-265
See also Health communication
Dominant culture, 1-2, 4
racial distinctions and, 12-13
racial equality, 13
See also Discriminatory practices; Minority experience
Drug abuse, 2
adherence to treatment and, 22
drug craving, 277-278
endogenous opioids and, 315
erectile dysfunction and, 316-317
HIV/AIDS transmission and, 19, 20, 25
loneliness and, 587
Drug abuse-behavioral treatment, 265-266
behavioral counseling/skills training and, 266
behavioral marital therapy and, 267-268
community reinforcement approach, 268
community reinforcement/family training approach, 269
contingency management and, 266-267
learning model vs. disease model and, 265-266
multimodal treatments, 268-269
relapse prevention and, 268
Drug abuse prevention, 269-270

behavior change theories and, 271
community programs, 274-275
comprehensive/multicomponent programs, 274-275
diffusion, effective programs and, 272-273
effectiveness in, 270-271
environmental-level factors, 272
future of, 275
intrapersonal factors, 271
issues in, 275
mass media programs, 274
meaning of, 270-271
parent programs, 273-274
policy programs, 274
program delivery settings, 273
program implementation/impact, 272
risk/protective factors and, 271-272
school programs, 273
social influence factors, 271-272
types of, 270
youth and, 272, 274
Drug craving, 277
cognitive explanations for, 278
cue-reactivity and, 277-278
implications of, 278
Drug-resistant disease, 6, 21, 28
Dysthymic Disorder (DD), 235

Eating disorder not-otherwise-specified (ED-NOS),
    281, 281 (table)
Eating disorders, 279
acculturation process and, 2
anorexia nervosa, 279, 283-284, 286
binge eating disorder, 281, 284-286, 287
body dissatisfaction and, 2, 283
bulimia nervosa, 114-117, 279, 281, 283-284, 286
cognitive risks of, 284
definition/diagnosis of, 279, 280-281 (table)
depression/anxiety and, 283
dieting activities and, 285
eating disorder not otherwise specified, 281
endogenous opioids and, 315
epidemiology of, 281-282
familial factors in, 284, 285
genetic risk factors in, 284
life event stress and, 285-286
loneliness and, 587
obesity and, 285
personality disorders/substance abuse and, 283
psychological factors in, 283-284, 285
psychological/medical consequences of, 282-283
puberty and, 284
sociocultural factors in, 283
treatments for, 286-287
weight cycling and, 285

Eat for Life, 196
Ecological models, 288
behavioral/health sciences applications, 288-289
behavior change and, 288, 290
non-health applications, 289-290
Ecological momentary assessment (EMA), 291-292
Economic factors. See Income inequality; Socioeconomic
    status (SES)
Ecosocial theory, 292
constructs of, 293-294
epidemiological research/practice and, 292-293
fractal metaphor in, 293
social determinants of health, 293
Educational interventions, 0
adherence-promotion interventions, 22
arthritis, 68-69
asthma, 76
bulimia nervosa and, 115
cancer treatment, 130
fibromyalgia syndrome and, 334
health behavior change and, 10-11
injury prevention and, 549-550
needle exchange programs, 25
sexual dysfunction and, 317
smoking education, 732, 746-747
social norm modification and, 11
See also Health literacy; Health promotion
Effect modification, 294-295
Effexor, 238
Effort-reward imbalance model, 295
aging and, 298
demand-control model and, 296-297
equity theory and, 297
health/disease studies and, 297-298
high cost/low gain experiences and, 296
intervention/policy implications of, 299
measurements of, 297
predictions and, 296
reward transmitter systems, 296
social exchange, role salience and, 295
theoretical foundation of, 295-296
work role and, 296
See also Job strain
Elder population:
cancer screening and, 134
gerotranscendence and, 785
physical activity interventions, 662-663
self-reported health measures and, 716, 717
stress response and, 779
successful aging and, 784-785
Electroconvulsive therapy (ECT), 239
Electromyography, 100
Electronic event monitors, 8, 22
Emerson-Tufts Health Communication Program, 483

Emotional abuse, 160
Emotional states:
    autoimmune disease and, 82-83
    cancer interventions and, 130-131
    chronic pain management and, 15-16
    HIV/AIDS diagnosis and, 20-21
    marriage and, 260
    motivation to change and, 11
    negative emotions, 300-306
    positive emotions, 306-309
    vagal reactivity, bronchoconstriction and, 78-79
    See also Anger; Anxiety
Endocrine system:
    autoimmune disease, 81
    neuroendocrine axis, 676
    psychological stress and, 78
    shift work effects and, 821
    See also Endogenous opioids
Endogenous opioids, 312
    anatomic distribution/functional significance of, 312-314
    cardiovascular disease, opioid dysfunction in, 314
    chronic pain and, 314
    classification of, 312
    clinical implications for, 314-315
    pain regulatory systems and, 313
    pituitary function and, 313
    post-traumatic stress disorder and, 314-315
    sympathetic nervous system and, 313-314
    treatment/prevention and, 315
Endometrial cancer, 125, 731
English language proficiency, 535, 579, 582
Environmental Protection Agency, 768
Environmental tobacco smoke (ETS), 746
Environmental variables:
    alcohol abuse and, 33
    asthma and, 80
    binge drinking and, 96-97
    cancer risk and, 129
    cardiovascular reactivity, situational determinants of, 156-157
    physical activity interventions and, 664
    stressful living, 107
    See also Behavioral genetics; Personality variables
Epidemiologic Catchment Area Study, 303
Epidemiologic paradox, 3, 213, 489, 580
Epidemiology Program Office (EPO), 164
Epstein-Barr virus (EBV), 327, 539
EQ-5D instrument, 687
Erectile dysfunction, 316
    behavioral treatment of, 317, 319
    cognitive restructuring and, 318-319
    communication training and, 319
    education and, 317
    etiology of, 316-317

prevalence of, 316
    psychological factors in, 317
    relationship difficulties and, 317
    sensate focus exercises and, 317-318
    stimulus control/scheduling and, 318
Esophageal cancer, 122
Ethical, Legal, and Social Implications (ELSI) program, 373
Ethnicity, 4, 12
    alcohol abuse and, 34
    caregiver vulnerabilities and, 47
    hypertension, factors in, 108
    low birth weight infants and, 591
    pain experience and, 72
    See also Discriminatory practices; Health disparities;
        Minority experience
Everyday Discrimination Scale, 257
Evidence-based behavioral medicine (EBBM), 319-320
    CONSORT guidelines and, 321, 322, 696
    development of, 320-321
    future of, 322
    limitations of, 321-322
    policy implications of, 322
    rationale for, 320
    RE-AIM framework and, 321-322
    utility of, 320
Exercise activities:
    Asian Americans/Pacific Islanders and, 75
    blood pressure and, 104-106
    cancer risk and, 121-122, 128
    chronic obstructive pulmonary disease and, 186-187
    diabetes mellitus and, 243
    ecological models and, 288-290
    health disparities and, 490-491
    hypertension prevention, 106
    progressive muscle relaxation and, 111
    See also Cancer-physical activity relationship; Cardiac
        rehabilitation; Heart disease-physical activity;
        Obesity in children; Physical activity; Physical
        activity interventions; Physical activity-mood
Exhaustion. See Vital exhaustion
Expanded Attributional Style Questionnaire (EASQ), 642
Expectancy theory, 271, 669, 709
Expectancy-value models, 474, 638, 793
Experience Sampling Method (ESM), 291
Explanatory style, 323
    cognitive personality variable of, 323
    measurement of, 323-324
    optimism/pessimism and, 323, 324-325
    physical health and, 324-325
    prevention/treatment implications of, 325
Expressive writing, 326
    beneficiaries of, 327
    effective task structure in, 327
    effects of, 326-327

therapeutic talk, comparison with, 327-328
typical exercise in, 326
utility of, 328
Extended Life Orientation Test (E-LOT), 641

Factitious disorder by proxy, 168
Fagerstrom Test for Nicotine Dependence (FTND), 738
Family influences, 2, 4
adolescent pregnancy and, 673
cancer caregiving, 131
cancer screening and, 134
cardiovascular reactivity and, 155
childhood obesity and, 634
chronic disease management, 171, 171 (figure), 172-173
diabetes mellitus and, 243, 246
eating disorders and, 284, 285
fibromyalgia syndrome and, 337
genetic counseling/testing and, 372-373
parenting beliefs, 2
Fatigue. See Chronic fatigue syndrome (CFS)
Fats. See Cholesterol counts; Heart disease-dietary factors;
    Lipids; Obesity
Fear. See Anxiety
Fecal occult blood testing (FOBT), 133, 134
Federation of Behavioral, Psychological and Cognitive
    Sciences, 381, 835
Feedback loops, 9, 680
triadic influence theory and, 802
See also Biofeedback; Motivational interviewing
Fee-for-service care, 478
Fetal alcohol effects (FAEs), 37
Fetal alcohol syndrome (FAS), 37
Fibromyalgia syndrome (FMS):
cognitive-behavioral approaches to, 334-336, 337
cognitive dysfunction and, 335
diagnosis/prevalence of, 329, 333-334
education and, 334
fibro fog and, 329, 333
function vs. cure focus in, 334
goal setting and, 334
hormone patterns/functions and, 330-331
imagery strategy, 335
interpersonal problems in, 337
life strain/emotional distress and, 329-330, 332
maladaptive thought patterns and, 335
pacing activities and, 335, 336
pain tolerance and, 331-332
patient heterogeneity in, 336-337, 336 (table)
physical symptoms, stress factors and, 330-332, 335
relapse prevention and, 336
relaxation and, 334
sleep sufficiency and, 335
Fight-or-flight response, 330, 599
Finnish Cancer Registry, 572

Finnish National Death Registry, 572
5 A Day For Better Health! Program, 338-339
components of, 340-342
diet-disease link and, 339
international applications of, 340
mass media/communications and, 340-341
outcomes of, 342
point-of-sale/produce industry initiatives, 341
research/evaluation and, 342
state/community programs, 341-342
structure of, 339-340, 339 (figure)
theory/research, practice and, 340
Folk medicine. See Traditional health practices
Food Frequency Questionnaire (FFQ), 504
Food Guide Pyramid, 504
Framingham Anger Scale, 49
Framingham Heart Study, 49, 343-344, 519
Framingham Type A Scale, 49, 344, 519
Fundamental social causation of disease/mortality, 344
basic causes concept and, 345
components of, 345
evidence of, 345-346
proximal risk factors and, 344
resource availability and, 345, 346
socioeconomic status and, 344-345

Gastric bypass surgery, 634
Gastric ulcers, 349
controllability and, 351
disorder spectrum of, 349-350
future research on, 354
helicobacter pylori bacteria and, 349, 353-354
perpetuating factors in, 353
precipitating factors in, 352-353
predictability and, 352
predisposing factors in, 351-352
psychological science, stress-causation and, 350-351
psychosomatic causation and, 349
stress and, 349
stress-diathesis approaches to, 351-353
Gastrointestinal system, 81, 778-779
Gate control theory, 355
body-self experience and, 357
central nervous system and, 355
modulation of inputs and, 355
neuromatrix theory of pain and, 356-375
pain, integrated model of, 646
paraplegics, pain experience of, 356
propositions in, 355
tonic inhibitory effect and, 355-356
Gender, 358
acculturation effects and, 3
autoimmune diseases and, 81, 815
behavioral differences and, 362-363

cardiovascular disease and, 155, 814
contextual aspects of, 362
gender construction/stratification, 360
gender roles, 360-361
health care access/utilization and, 359-360
HIV/AIDS infection and, 18
kidney cancer and, 122
macro-level differences, 360-362
marital status, longevity and, 260-261
micro-level differences, 362-364
morbidity rates and, 358-359
mortality rates and, 359
pain management and, 189
physical activity interventions and, 664
physiological responses and, 364
policy approaches and, 362
resources, access/control issues and, 361-362
self-reported health, survival and, 718
social supports and, 363-364
structural societal relations and, 362
type A behavior personality and, 156
widows/widowers, bereavement outcomes and, 92-93
workplace hazards/injury and, 636
General adaptation syndrome, 366
cognitive-transactional model of stress and, 367-368
phases of, 367, 367 (figure)
threat, physiological responses to, 366-367
Generalized anxiety disorder (GAD), 500
Genetics. *See* Behavioral genetics; Genetic testing;
Human genome project
Genetic testing, 368-369
access issues, 370-371
availability of, 369-370
family communication and, 372-373
future genetic interventions and, 373
predisposition inheritance, 369
psychiatric genetics, 372
results utilization, 368, 370
risk information, impact of, 371
social risks in, 372
uninformative results and, 370
Geriatric Depression Scale (GDS), 231
Geriatrics. *See* Elder population
Gerontological Society of America (GSA), 381, 835
Gerotranscendence, 785
GISSI-Prevenzione trial, 501
Giving-up response, 638-639
Globalization processes, 362
Glucocorticoid response, 42-43
Glycemic index (GI), 502-503
God-Locus-of-Control subscale, 218
Go Girls, 196
Graduate Ready for Activity Daily (Project GRAD),
661-662

Grave's disease, 81
Great American Smokeout, 143
Grief. *See* Bereavement
Group therapy, 83, 131
Guided imagery, 130-131, 335

Habitual behaviors, 9, 31-32
Hamilton Psychiatric Rating Scale for Depression
(HRSD), 231, 232
Happiness, 459
causal influences and, 460, 461-462
coping/adaptation and, 461
future research on, 462
health behaviors and, 462
immune function and, 461-462
longevity and, 462
mental health, subjective well-being and, 459-460
negative health conditions and, 460-461
physical health, subjective well-being and, 460-462
subjective vs. objective health and, 461
HardiAttitudes measure, 463-464
Hardiness, 463
health beliefs and, 463
research on, 463-464
HardiSkills, 463
HardiSurvey III-R, 464
HardiTraining workbook, 464
Harlem Health Connection, 195, 196 (table)
Harm reduction approach, 25
HARP, 196
Harvard Alumni Health Study, 464
cancer rates study, 466
findings of, 465
health benefits of activity, 466
longevity focus of, 465-466
physical activity recommendations and, 465
purpose of, 465
stroke rate study, 465
subject selection in, 464-465
Harvard School of Public Health College Alcohol Study
(CAS), 95
Headaches:
behavioral interventions, 468
biofeedback training and, 469, 470
cognitive-behavioral therapy and, 469, 470
comorbid psychiatric disorders and, 468
diagnosis of, 466-467
drug/psychological combined therapy and, 470
epidemiology of, 466
integrated treatment techniques and, 469
medical management of, 468
medication overuse and, 467-468
migraines, 467, 468, 469-470
precipitants of, 467

psychological management of, 468-469
psychosocial complications and, 467-468
relaxation training and, 468-469
tension-type headaches, 467, 468, 470
treatment efficacy evaluations, 469-470
treatment formats in, 469
Health Behavior News Service (HBNS), 163
Health and behavior organizations:
    American Psychological Association, 473
    American Psychosomatic Society, 473-474
    Division of Health Psychology (Div. 38), 473
    International Society of Behavioral Medicine, 472-473
    Society of Behavioral Medicine, 471-472
Health behaviors, 9
    biological determinants of, 11
    change process and, 9-10
    educational interventions, 10
    functional feedback loops in, 9
    habituation and, 9, 31-32
    happiness and, 462
    health disparities and, 489-491
    interpersonal environment and, 9
    personal goals and, 10
    readiness to change and, 11
    relational competence and, 10
    self-efficacy and, 10
    social environment and, 10-11
    See also Applied behavior analysis; Health and behavior
        organizations; Health belief model; Risk behaviors
Health belief model, 474
    cues to action and, 475
    demographic/sociocultural variables and, 475
    empirical evaluation of, 475-477
    history of, 474
    injury prevention and, 549
    perceived barriers and, 475
    perceived benefits and, 474-475
    perceived threat and, 474
    principles of, 474-475
    self-efficacy and, 475
    value-expectancy theory and, 474
Health beliefs/attitudes, 2
    cancer-related expectancies/beliefs, 134
    hardiness and, 463
    health behavior change and, 9-10
    John Henryism and, 16-17
    life stress and, 81
    pain experience and, 15-16, 648
    See also Control beliefs; Hopelessness; Self-efficacy;
        Spirituality
Health Care for All, 536
Health care costs, 477
    adherence problems and, 6
    allocation of resources, 478-479

consumer preferences and, 479
cost-effectiveness analysis and, 477-478
intervention planning and, 478
quality of adjusted life year measure, 477
relative costs, 477
resources, opportunity costs of, 477
uninsured workers and, 479, 479 (figure)
utilization rates and, 480
See also Cost-effectiveness analysis
Health care organizations/systems, 174
Health care service utilization, 479-480
    appropriateness of utilization and, 482
    behavioral risk factors and, 481
    cost-offset and, 482
    determinants of, 480-481
    intervention impact, time delay of, 481-482
    issues in, 481-482
    measurement methods of, 481
    out-of-system costs and, 482
    personal/clinical history factors and, 481
    sociodemographic factors and, 480-481
Health care workers. See Doctor-patient communication;
    Occupational safety
Health communication, 482, 760
    academic discipline of, 483
    behavior change and, 483, 484
    campaign framework, 484-485
    evolution of, 483-484
    future of, new technologies and, 485-486
    knowledge gap hypothesis and, 485
    mass media/social marketing campaigns, 482
    media strategies, health professionals and, 484-485
    multidisciplinarity in, 483
    pre-television era, 483
    public health initiatives and, 483
    types of, 484
    See also Doctor-patient communication; Tailored
        communications
Health disparities, 486-487
    access to health care resources and, 492
    alcohol consumption and, 490
    cancer and, 488
    cardiovascular diseases and, 487
    cerebrovascular disease and, 487
    diabetes and, 488
    dietary practices/exercise levels and, 490-491
    discrimination and, 492
    health behaviors and, 489-491
    HIV/AIDS infection and, 488
    hypertension and, 487
    immunizations and, 488-489
    infant mortality and, 488
    social/behavioral determinants of, 489-492
    social supports and, 491

socioeconomic position and, 489
stress and, 491
tobacco use and, 490
See also Metabolic syndrome
Healthfinder, 381, 835
Health insurance coverage, 2, 3, 175
    Child Health Insurance Plan, 536
    fee-for-service insurance, 478
Health literacy, 493
    chronic disease management and, 495
    functional literacy, 493-494
    health materials, literacy demands of, 494
    health status and, 494
    literacy skills, context specificity of, 495
    oral language skills/comprehension abilities and, 495
    research on, 494-495
Health maintenance organizations (HMOs), 769
Health Perception Questionnaire (HPQ), 714
Health Professionals' Follow-Up Study, 502, 503, 506
Health promotion, 9, 496
    adherence-promoting interventions, 22
    educational principles in, 496
    effort-reward imbalance model and, 299
    international efforts in, 496
    intervention classification in, 496
    lifestyle/environmental factors and, 495-496
    See also Doctor-patient communication; Health
        communication; School-based health promotion;
        Worksite health promotion
Health psychology, 497
    academic programs in, 497-498
    content of the field, 497
    history of, 498
    somatization, 558
Health Psychology, Division 38 of the American
    Psychological Association, 381, 835
Health Utilities Index, 223
Healthy Body/Healthy Spirit, 196
Healthy Eating Index (HEI), 504
Healthy Lifestyle and Tobacco-Related Disease Prevention
    Fund, 90
Healthy People 2010, 493, 582, 705
Healthy People 2000, 616
Healthy Youth Places Project, 661
Heart, Body and Soul, 196
Heart disease. *See* Bogalusa Heart Study; Cardiovascular
    disease (CVD); Coronary heart disease (CHD);
    Framingham Heart Study
Heart disease-dietary factors, 501
    alcohol consumption and, 504
    antioxidants and, 503
    carbohydrate-containing foods and, 502-503
    cholesterol and, 502
    dietary fats, types of, 501-502

dietary pattern analysis and, 504
    fiber and, 503
    folate and, 503-504
    glycemic index and, 502-503
    N-3 fatty acids and, 502, 525
    whole-grain products and, 503
    See also Lipids
Heart disease-emotional distress, 498-499
    anger and, 498-499
    anxiety and, 500
    depression and, 498-499
    diagnosis of, 499-500
    non-fear panic attacks and, 499
    organic causes of depression, 500
    psychophysiological pathways in, 499
    treatments of, 500
Heart disease-physical activity, 505, 509
    adherence to exercise, 508-509
    benefits, mechanisms of, 508
    motivation strategies, 509
    primary prevention strategy, 505-506
    recommended levels of exercise, 507
    resistance exercise, 507
    risks of exercise, 507
    secondary prevention strategy, 506-507
    transtheoretical model of behavior change and, 509
Heart disease-reactivity, 510
    cardiovascular reactivity to stress, 510-515
    coronary heart disease and, 513-515
    essential hypertension and, 512-513
    future research on, 515-516
    gene/environment modulated reactivity hypothesis, 516
    hemodynamic assessment, technological advances in, 511
    psychosocial factors and, 510
    reactivity-heart disease relationship, 511-512
    response measurement methods, 515-516
    trait stability/heritability and, 511
Heart disease-tobacco use, 517, 731
    causal mechanisms in, 517-518
    passive smoking/second-hand exposure and, 518
    smoking cessation, benefits of, 518
Heart disease-type A behavior, 518-519
    assessment methodology, 519
    behavior modification and, 520-521
    contradictory findings on, 519-520
    disease mechanisms, 520
    early research on, 519
    research contributions, 521
Heart rate variability (HRV), 58, 99, 149, 150, 530
Helicobacter pylori (Hp), 349, 353-354, 653-654, 779
Hepatitis infection, 35, 74, 128
Herpes viruses, 539
High-density lipoprotein (HDL) cholesterol, 343, 503,
    517, 583

Highly active antiretroviral treatment (HAART),
    19, 21-23
Hispanic Health and Nutrition Examination Survey
    (HHANES), 4
Hispanics, 1, 2
    acculturation hypothesis and, 3
    epidemiological paradox, 3, 489, 580
    sickle cell disease and, 15
    See also Health disparities; Latino health/behavior
HIV/AIDS, 6, 17-18
    adherence to treatment, 19, 20
    African American population and, 13-15
    cognitive functioning and, 199
    coping styles and, 15
    health disparities and, 488
    highly active antiretroviral treatment, 19, 21
    loneliness and, 588
    opportunistic infections in, 19
    prevention strategies, 19-20
    psychological response to, 20-21
    psychoneuroimmunology and, 680
    punishment concept and, 14
    stages of, 18
    suicide incidence and, 20-21
    transmission mechanisms of, 18
    treatment strategies, 18-19
HIV/AIDS prevention, 19-20, 21, 24
    blood supply protection, 24
    infected persons, risk reduction for, 27-28
    intervention program design, 27
    intravenous drug use, needle sharing and, 25
    maternal-child transmission reduction, 25
    occupational/accidental exposure and, 24-25
    postexposure prophylaxis, 25
    Project RESPECT, 165
    sexual transmission and, 25-28
    universal precautions procedures, 24
    vaccines, 28
HIV/AIDS stress management, 29
    bereavement stress, 30
    coping strategies and, 31
    cortisol levels and, 31
    disease progression, 29-30
    immune compromise, lifetime trauma and, 30
    social stress and, 30
HIV/AIDS treatment adherence:
    adherence-promotion interventions, 22
    antiretroviral therapy, patient commitment to, 21
    behavioral research and, 23
    clinical practice perspective and, 23
    factors associated with, 21-22
    health outcomes and, 22-23
Homeostasis, 41, 42
Home Visitation Program, 808

Homosexuals:
    disenfranchised grief and, 92
    See also HIV/AIDS
Hopelessness, 521, 640
    etiology of, 522-523
    health recovery and, 522
    hope, health maintenance and, 521-522
    instilling hope and, 523
    survival rates and, 522
    See also Optimism/pessimism
Hormone replacement therapy (HRT), 817
Ho Scale, 49, 53, 524, 528
Hospital Anxiety and Depression Scale (HADS), 232, 499
Hostility:
    anger, heart disease and, 524-525
    definition/measurement of, 524
    future research on, 525-526
    health links with, 523-524
    heart disease, physiological mechanisms, 524
    non-coronary disease outcomes and, 525
    type A behavior pattern and, 524
Hostility measurement, 526-527
    behavioral measurement of, 527
    self-report measures of, 527-528
Hostility psychophysiology, 529
    acute effects, 532
    anger and, 530-531
    anger-in/anger-out and, 531-532
    blood pressure/heart rate, 529-530, 531
    chronic physiological reactivity, 529-532
    coronary heart disease mechanisms and, 529
    heart rate variability, 530
    stress hormones, 530, 531-532
Human Factors and Ergonomics Society, 381, 835
Human genome project, 13, 88, 373
Human papillomavirus (HPV), 128-129
Huntington's disease (HD), 369-370
Hypertension, 49
    anger/hostility and, 50-52, 53, 54
    anger-suppression hypothesis and, 51
    anxiety and, 58
    behavioral genetics and, 88
    behavioral treatments of, 110-111
    biobehavioral stress reactivity and, 108-110
    biofeedback-assisted relaxation and, 111
    cardiovascular morbidity/mortality and, 102, 140
    clinical assessment of, 103
    cognitive functioning and, 199
    cultural stressors, 107-108
    discrimination/racism and, 108
    environmental stressors, 107
    etiology of, 106-107
    health disparities and, 487
    lifestyle incongruity and, 108

neurotic individuals and, 51
occupational stressors, 108
physical activity and, 106
progressive muscle relaxation and, 111
research on, 51-52, 111-112
stress appraisal, coping and, 108
stress models and, 107-110
transcendental meditation and, 111
white coat effect and, 51-52, 103
See also Anger measurement; Blood pressure;
    Cardiovascular reactivity
Hypertension in African Americans Working Group, 103
Hypnotherapy, 554-555
Hypothalamic-pituitary-adrenal (HPA) axis, 41-42, 44
asthma and, 78
autoimmune diseases and, 82
chronic fatigue syndrome and, 178
endogenous opioids and, 313-314
fibromyalgia syndrome and, 330-331
immune system and, 538, 675, 678
negative emotions and, 302
rheumatoid arthritis and, 699
stress response and, 777
Hypothalamic-sympatho-adrenomedullary (SAM) axis,
    313-314
Hysterectomy, 816

Illegal Immigration Reform and Immigrant Responsibility
    Act of 1996, 536
Illicit drug use. *See* Drug abuse
Illinois Bell Telephone (IBT) study, 463, 821
Immigrant populations, 1-2, 533
    access to health care and, 535
    acculturation hypotheses and, 3, 534
    definition of, 534
    demographic patterns, 533
    English proficiency and, 535
    gendered acculturation and, 3
    policy issues and, 535-536
    psychosocial issues and, 536-537
    self-reported health levels, 717
    tuberculosis prevalence and, 534-535
    See also Asian Americans/Pacific Islanders (AAPIs)
Immigration and Nationality Act of 1965, 533
Immune function:
    alcohol abuse and, 35
    anxiety and, 58
    compromise factors in, 30, 31
    coping strategies and, 31
    cytokines and, 43
    psychosocial interventions and, 131-132
    stress and, 79, 537-539, 778
    See also Autoimmune diseases;
        Psychoneuroimmunology

Immunizations, 2
    adherence failure and, 6
    cancer vaccines, 128-129
    health disparities and, 488-489
    HIV infections and, 28
    socioeconomic status and, 3
Income inequality:
    absolute income hypothesis, 539-540, 540 (figure)
    empirical evidence, health-income link, 542-543
    health status and, 539-541, 542
    health theory and, 541-543
    income inequality hypothesis, 540-541
    Lorenz Curve, 541, 541 (figure)
    measurement of, 541
    relative income hypothesis, 540
    relative rank hypothesis, 540
Infant health, 2
    maternal-child HIV transmission, 25
    See also Child health; Low birth weight
Infant mortality, 2
    health disparities and, 488
    low birth weight and, 589, 592
    See also Low birth weight
Infectious disease:
    crowding and, 227
    psychological stress and, 537-539
    psychoneuroimmunology and, 679-680
    See also Sexually transmitted diseases (STDs)
Infertility:
    assisted reproduction treatments, 544-547
    causes of, 543-544
    cognitive-behavioral interventions, 546
    coping responses and, 544-545
    grief response to, 544
    individual response to intervention and, 546-547
    interpersonal relationships and, 545
    intracytoplasmic sperm injection, 544
    psychophysiological interventions and, 546-547
    psychosocial impact of, 544
    social infertility, 544
    treatment failure, 545
    treatment outcomes, psychosocial factors in, 545-546
    in vitro fertilization, 544, 545-546
Inflammatory bowel disease, 81
Injuries:
    alcohol abuse and, 35
    wound healing, stress and, 826-828
Injury prevention, 547-548
    childhood injuries, epidemiology of, 548
    classification of approaches to, 549-551
    community-based strategies, 550
    decision making, strategy selection, 551-552, 552 (table)
    educational approaches to, 549-550
    environmental approaches to, 550

historical efforts of, 548-549
implementation of, 552-553
policy approaches to, 550-551
Innovations. *See* Diffusion of innovation model
Insomnia, 727-729
Institute for the Advancement of Human Behavior
  (HAHB), 381-382, 835-836
Institute for the Advancement of Social Work Research
  (IASWR), 382, 836
Institute of Medicine (IOM), 382, 483, 696, 706, 836
Instrumental activities of daily living (IADLs),
  159, 717, 785
Insulin-like growth factor (IGF), 122
Insulin resistance syndrome, 594
Insurance. *See* Health insurance coverage
Integrated worldview, 74
Intercultural Cancer Council (ICC), 382, 836
International Agency for Research on Cancer (IARC),
  123, 126
International Association for the Study of Pain (IASP),
  645, 648
International Classification of Sleep Disorders, 726
International Headache Society (IHS), 466-467
International Psycho-Oncology Society (IPOS), 382, 836
International Social Science Council (ISSC), 382, 836
International Society of Behavioral Medicine (ISBM),
  383, 472-473, 837
International Society for Developmental
  Psychobiology836-837, 382-383
Internet use:
  disease prevention role of, 20
  psychosocial health promotion programs and,
    712-713
Interpersonal analogue assessment, 54
Interpersonal psychotherapy (IPT):
  depression, 236-237
  eating disorders and, 115-116, 286-287
Interview Hostility Assessment Technique (IHAT), 527
Intracytoplasmic sperm injection (ICSI), 544
Intrapersonal influences, 27
Intravenous drug users (IDUs), 20, 25
Inventory of Depressive Symptomatology, 232
In Vitro fertilization (IVF), 544, 545-546
Iowa Women's Health Study, 506
IPAT 8-Parallel Form Anxiety Scale, 60
Irritable bowel syndrome (IBS), 554, 558
  abuse history and, 559
  brief psychodynamic psychotherapy and, 555
  cognitive/behavioral therapies and, 555-556, 557
  coping strategies and, 558-559
  hypnotherapy and, 554-555
  individual behavioral/cognitive treatments and, 556-557
  life stress and, 558-559
  progressive muscle relaxation and, 555

psychological state and, 558
pure cognitive therapy and, 556-557
See also Fibromyalgia syndrome (FMS)

Jenkins Activity Survey (JAS), 156, 519, 520
JH Scale of Active Coping (JHAC12), 565, 567-568
Job Content Questionnaire (JCQ), 562-563
Job strain, 108, 561
  demand-control model and, 562-564, 562 (figure)
  illness/disease mechanisms and, 562
  job decision latitude and, 561-562
  job demands and, 561
  skill discretion and, 561
  working life job strain, 564, 564 (figure)
  work systems and, 561
  See also Effort-reward imbalance model;
    Work-related stress
John Henryism (JH), 16-17, 229, 565
  assessment instrument in, 565, 567-568
  biological mechanisms, clinical outcomes and, 567
  empirical investigations of, 565-567
  gender and, 567
  job status, workplace factors and, 567
Johns Hopkins Precursors Study, 49-50
Joint Commission on Accreditation of Healthcare
  Organizations (JCAHO), 189
Joint Committee on National Health Education
  Standards, 493

Kaposi's sarcoma, 19, 30
Ketterer Stress Symptom Frequency Checklist-Revised
  (KSSFCR), 500
Key informants, 569
  characteristics of, 570
  ethnographic research, knowing and, 569
  gatekeeper position and, 570
  information, depth/breadth of, 570
  information limitations and, 571
  open-ended interview questions and, 570-571
  outside researchers and, 570
  rapport-building, personal relationships and, 569-570
Kidney cancer, 122, 125
Knowledge gap hypothesis, 485
Korotkoff sounds, 103, 147
Kuopio Ischemic Heart Disease Risk Factor (KIHD)
  study, 515, 571-572
  background on, 572
  health outcomes, 572-573
  key findings of, 573
  study population/protocol, 572

Lalonde Report, 496
LAMP, 196
Language acquisition, 1, 2

access to health care and, 3, 535
  acculturation research and, 4
  health outcomes and, 579
  See also Health literacy
Latino health/behavior, 575
  access to health care, 576, 577
  chronic health conditions and, 576-577
  death, causes of, 576
  epidemiological paradox and, 3, 489, 580
  future research on, 582-583
  health behavior-outcome framework, 580-582,
      581 (figure)
  health status and, 576
  individual factors and, 581-582
  poverty and, 580-581, 582
  risk/preventive health behaviors and, 577-579,
      577-578 (tables)
  self-care behaviors and, 578-579
  social/demographic profile and, 575-576
  sociocultural protective behaviors, 579-580
Laxative abuse, 115, 279
Learned helplessness, 114, 218-219, 351, 352
Left ventricular mass (LVM), 154, 514
Life expectancy, 539-540, 540 (figure)
Life Orientation Test (LOT), 640-642
Life satisfaction, 159, 459-460
Life Skills Training (LST), 808
Life stress, 77
  asthma incidence and, 80, 81
  bereavement and, 91, 94
  eating disorders and, 285-286
  fibromyalgia syndrome and, 329-330
  hypertension and, 107
  irritable bowel syndrome and, 558-559
  lifestyle incongruity and, 108, 766
  See also Explanatory style
Lifestyle incongruity hypothesis, 766
LIGHT Way, 196
Limited English Proficient (LEP) classification, 535, 579
Lipids, 140, 583
  Alzheimer's disease and, 596
  determinants of, 583-584
  mood states and, 584-585
  psychosocial mechanisms and, 585
  See also Metabolic syndrome
Listeria infection, 539
Literacy. *See* Health literacy
Liver disease:
  alcohol abuse and, 35, 36-37, 121
  cancer, 128
Locus-of-control (LOC), 217-218
Loneliness, 585-586
  anxiety/mood and, 586
  causal issues and, 588

eating disorders and, 587
  mental health and, 586-587
  mortality rates and, 587, 588
  personality characteristics and, 586
  physical health and, 587-588
  preventive health behaviors and, 588
  professional interventions, 588-589
  psychosis and, 587
  sleep disturbances and, 587
  social integration and, 587
  substance abuse and, 587
Longevity, 260-261, 462, 465-466
Longitudinal Study of Aging, 506
Long-term care facilities, 159
Lorenz Curve, 541, 541 (figure)
Low birth weight (LBW), 2, 589
  infant mortality and, 589, 592
  maternal context and, 590-591
  neighborhood context and, 591-592
  political/economic context and, 592
  preterm delivery and, 669-671
  psychosocial stress and, 590
  race/ethnicity and, 590
  racial discrimination and, 591
  residential segregation and, 591
  social context of, 591-592
  social supports and, 590
  socioeconomic status/social class and, 590-591
Low density lipoprotein (LDL) cholesterol, 502, 503,
    517, 583
Lubar protocol, 101
Lung cancer, 125, 127, 133, 137-138, 522, 731
Lupus. *See* Autoimmune diseases; Systemic
    lupus erythematosus
Luvox, 238
Lymphoma, 125

Maastricht Interview for Vital Exhaustion, 810
Maastricht Questionnaire (MQ), 809-810
MacArthur Foundation Research Network on
    Socioeconomic Status and Health, 40, 43
McGill Pain Questionnaire, 190
McMaster-Toronto Arthritis patient Function Preference
    Questionnaire (MACTAR), 687
Magnetic resonance imaging (MRI), 646
Major Depressive Disorder (MDD), 235
Malingering, 647
Mammography, 133, 134
Marital therapy, 267-268
Marlowe-Crowne Social Desirability Scale, 53
Marriage, 259-261
Massachusetts Male Aging Study, 363
Massachusetts Women's Health Study, 363
Mass media. *See* Media effects

Maternal-child disease transmission, 25
Meaning-focused coping, 775
Media effects:
    cancer screening and, 134
    dietary behavior change programs and, 340-341
    drug abuse prevention, 273, 274
    eating disorders and, 283
    social linking function of, 712-713
    tobacco advertising, 732, 747-748
    See also Health communication; Television viewing
Medicaid, 478, 536, 732
Medical psychology, 593
    See also Health psychology
Medicare, 478
Medications. *See* Antidepressant medications
Meditation, 111
MEDLINEplus, 383, 837
MEDLINE/PubMed, 383, 837
Menopause, 155, 817
Menstrual cycle, 155
Mental health, 2
    alcohol abuse and, 33
    cardiovascular physiologic responses and, 49
    child abuse and, 169-170
    comorbidity and, 207-209
    crowding effects and, 227
    dialectical behavior therapy and, 116
    disaster events and, 252-254
    discriminatory practices and, 255-256
    loneliness and, 586-587
    nicotine dependence and, 736
    self-reported health levels and, 717
    subjective well-being and, 459-460
    support groups and, 787-788
    See also Eating disorders; Happiness
Meridia, 634
Metabolic syndrome, 593-594
    clinical/biochemical tests for, 594, 596 (table)
    disease linkages and, 596
    food abundance, low physical activity and, 598-599
    modern society, psychosocial stress and, 599
    nature of, 594-596
    population-based/epidemiological studies and, 594-596, 595 (table)
    social inequalities and, 597, 598 (figure)
    stress factors and, 597-600
The Metanexus Institute, 383, 837
Mexican Americans, 2, 3
    acculturation scales for, 3-4
    low birth weight infants and, 591
    See also Health disparities; Latino health/behavior
Midwestern Prevention Project (MPP), 808
Migraine headaches, 467, 468, 469-470
Mind-body relations, 83, 655

diabetes therapy, 243-244
    gastric ulcers and, 349
    hostility-health links, 523-524
    neuromatrix theory of pain and, 356-357
Minimal Contact Education for Cholesterol Change, 196
Minimum Legal Drinking Age (MLDA) law, 97
Minnesota Heart Health Program (MHHP), 142-145
Minnesota Multiphasic Personality Inventory (MMPI/MMPI-2), 49, 60, 232, 524, 528
    medical/behavioral health settings, 601
    psychopathology screening, 601
    restandardization of, 601
    validity scales in, 600
Minority experience, 1-2
    disease prevention efforts and, 13-14
    doctor-patient relationship and, 15
    race construct and, 12-13
    See also Health disparities; Immigrant populations
Moderation Management (MM), 38
MONICA project, 572
Monitoring the Future Study, 95
Monitoring of Trends and Determinants of Cardiovascular Disease (MONICA), 572
Monoamine oxidase inhibitors (MAOIs), 237-238
Montgomery-Asberg Depression Rating Scale, 231
Mood states, 11, 20
    child abuse and, 169
    crowding effects and, 227
    headaches and, 468
    lipids and, 584-585
    loneliness and, 586
    neurofeedback and, 101
    See also Happiness; Loneliness; Physical activity-mood
Morbidity:
    asthma and, 78, 80
    cardiovascular disease and, 154
    crowding and, 226-227
    drug abuse and, 269
    gender differences in, 358-359
    hypertension and, 102, 103
    negative emotions and, 302-304
    occupational morbidity, 637
Mortality:
    anxiety and, 57-58
    cancer mortality rates, 127, 129, 133
    cardiovascular disease and, 154
    child abuse and, 168
    depression and, 233-234
    drug abuse and, 269
    eating disorders and, 283
    gender differences in, 359
    hypertension and, 102, 103, 106
    Latinos, 576
    loneliness and, 587, 588

marital status, longevity and, 260-261
negative emotions and, 302-304
obesity and, 628
occupational mortality, 637
pessimism and, 325, 640
self-reported health and, 718
suicide, 20-21, 24, 117, 234
widows/widowers and, 92-93
See also Fundamental social causation of
disease/mortality
Motivational interviewing (MI), 602
Motivation enhancement therapy (MET), 40
Multidimensional Anger Inventory, 524
Multidimensional Health Locus of Control (MHLC)
Scales, 218
Multilevel analysis, 604
contextual heterogeneity, description of, 604-605
cross-level interaction models, contextual effects and, 607
general issues in, 608
multilevel model, characteristics of, 606-607
multilevel statistical models, 605-608
nonlinear multilevel models, 607-608
random coefficients/random slopes models, 606
relationships, level-contingency and, 608
variance components/random intercepts model, 605-606
variance structures and, 608
variation, compositional and/or contextual sources, 604
Multilevel methods/theory, 602
clustered data in, 603
multilevel data structures, typology of, 603-604
multilevel designs, 603
nested structure and, 602-603
Multiple Affect Adjective Check List, 232
Multiple Risk Factor Intervention Trial (MRFIT), 520,
609-610
Multiple sclerosis, 81, 83, 460, 611
cognitive-behavioral therapy/antidepressant
medications, 612
depression and, 612
effects of depression treatment, 612
injection anxiety and, 612
neuropsychological symptoms of, 611
psychological symptoms of, 611-612
stress effects and, 613
suicide and, 611
Munchausen by proxy, 168
Musculoskeletal system, 100
Myocardial infarction (MI), 49, 139, 140, 199, 499, 500,
502, 525

Narcolepsy, 727, 729
Narcotics Anonymous (NA), 265
National Academy of Neuropsychology, 383, 837
National Academy of Sciences (NAS), 383, 837

National Adult Literacy Survey (NALS), 493, 494
National Cancer Institute (NCI), 340, 342, 373, 383, 837
National Center on Birth Defects and Developmental
Disabilities (NCBDDD), 165
National Center for Chronic Disease Prevention and
Health Promotion (NCCDPHP), 164
National Center for Complementary and Alternative
Medicine (NCCA), 383-384, 837-838
National Center for Environmental Health (NCEH), 164
National Center for Health Statistics (NCHS), 164, 548, 627
National Center for HIV, STD, and, TB Prevention
(NCHSTP), 164, 165
National Center for Infectious Diseases (NCID), 164
National Center for Injury Prevention and Control
(NCIPC), 164, 548
National Center on Minority Health and Health Disparities
(NCMHD), 384, 838
National Center for Research Resources (NCRR),
384, 838
National Cholesterol Education Program (NCEP), 143, 615
clinical practice guidelines, 615-616
community-level burden of disease and, 616
dietary fat intake data, 617
disease prevention/management and, 616
monitoring/management choices, 617
prevalence data, 616-617
primary prevention focus, 616
risk factors, treatment goal modification, 616
variable treatment strategies, 617
National Coalition of Health Professional Education in
Genetics (NCHPEG), 373
National College Health Risk Behavior Survey, 95
National Committee for Injury Prevention and Control, 548
National Guidelines Clearinghouse, 697
National Health Care Expenditures (NHE), 478
National Health Interview Survey (NHIS), 4, 576
National Health and Nutrition Examination Survey
(NHANES), 576, 595, 617, 653
National Heart, Lung, and Blood Institute (NHLBI), 384,
519, 520, 615, 627, 838
National High Blood Pressure Education Program, 102, 143
National Household Survey on Drug Abuse, 95
National Human Genome Research Institute (NHGRI),
88, 373, 384, 838
National Immunization Program (NIP), 164
National Institute on Aging (NIA), 386, 840
National Institute on Alcohol Abuse and Alcoholism
(NIAAA), 386, 840
National Institute of Allergy and Infectious Diseases
(NIAID), 384, 838
National Institute of Arthritis and Musculoskeletal and
Skin Diseases (NIAMS), 384, 838
National Institute of Child Health and Human
Development (NICHD), 384-385, 838-839

National Institute on Deafness and Other Communication Disorders (NIDCD), 386, 840

National Institute of Dental and Craniofacial Research (NIDCR), 385, 839

National Institute of Diabetes and Digestive and Kidney Diseases (NIDDK), 74, 395, 839

National Institute on Drug Abuse (NIDA), 386, 840

National Institute of Mental Health (NIMH), 239, 303, 385, 720, 839

National Institute of Mental Health Multisite Study, 27

National Institute of Neurological Disorders and Stroke (NINDS), 385, 839

National Institute of Nursing Research (NINR), 385, 839

National Institute for Occupational Safety and Health (NIOSH), 164

National Institutes of Health (NIH), 395, 487, 618, 839
    basic research areas, 619
    behavioral/social processes research, 619
    behavioral/social risk and protective factors, 619
    behavior/social science research history in, 618-619
    biopsychosocial processes research, 619
    clinical research, 619-620
    illness/physical condition effects, 619-620
    measurement/analysis/classification procedures, 619
    treatment outcomes research, 620
    women's health and, 819

National League for Nursing, 384, 838

National Library of Medicine (NLM), 386, 840

National Literacy Act of 1991, 493

National Longitudinal Mortality Study, 346

National Occupational Research Agenda (NORA), 637

National Opinion Research Center's General Social Surveys, 752

National origin groups, 4

National Origins Act of 1924, 533

National School Lunch Act, 704

National Science Foundation (NSF), 386, 840

National Sleep Foundation, 727

National Traumatic Occupational Fatalities data, 636

Native Americans, 1
    alcohol abuse and, 34
    caregiving coping strategies, 159
    sickle cell disease and, 15
    See also Health disparities

Needle exchange programs, 19, 25

Needle-sharing practices, 25

Negative emotions, 300
    anger, 304
    anxiety, 303-304
    depression, 303
    emotions vs. moods, definitions of, 301
    future research on, 305
    health effects of, 301-302
    historical perspective on, 300-301

    morbidity/mortality rates and, 302-304
    repressive coping and, 694
    reserve capacity of resources and, 305

Neglect in childhood, 169

Neighborhood influences, 2, 4, 620
    context vs. composition effects and, 621
    cross-sectional/longitudinal study designs and, 623-624
    crowding, 226-228
    effects research, challenges to, 621-624
    experimental study designs and, 624
    health behavior change and, 10-11, 19
    health outcomes, modeling weaknesses, 621
    immigrant populations and, 536
    individual-level effects and, 623
    injury prevention measures, 550
    investigative research approaches, 620-621
    localized research, 621
    low birth weight infants and, 591-592
    neighborhood characteristics, measurement of, 622-623
    neighborhood, definition of, 621-622
    spatial dependencies and, 624
    walkable neighborhoods, 289-290

Nervous systems. See Autonomic nervous system (ANS); Central nervous system (CNS); Parasympathetic nervous system (PSNS); Sympathetic nervous system (SNS)

Neurobehavioral Teratology Society (NBTS), 386, 840

Neuroendocrine axis, 676

Neurofeedback (NF), 100-101

Neuromatrix theory of pain, 356-357

New York Heart Association (NYHA), 499

Nicotine replacement therapy (NRT), 736, 738

Nicotine. See Smoking; Smoking/nicotine dependence

Nociception, 645

Non-insulin-dependent diabetes mellitus (NIDDM), 88

Nonsteriodal anti-inflammatory drugs (NSAIDs), 191, 468, 654, 655

Normative Aging Study, 49, 525

Normative lifestyles, 11

North Carolina Black Churches United for Better Health, 196

NOT Program, 749

Nottingham Health Profile (NHP), 686

Novaco Anger Inventory, 524

Nurses' Health Study, 501, 502, 503, 506

Obesity, 627
    applied behavior analysis and, 64
    behavioral genetics and, 88
    body mass index, 627
    cancer risk and, 122, 128
    definition of, 627
    determinants of, 627-628
    eating disorders and, 285
    environmental factors and, 628

genetics and, 627-628
health disparities and, 490-491
health risk factors, 628
insulin resistance and, 122
psychological effects/consequences and, 628-6209
social effects/consequences and, 629
television viewing and, 792
well-being and, 628-629
See also Body weight; Eating disorders; Metabolic syndrome
Obesity in children, 629-630
energy intake-expenditure relationship, 630
lifestyle education and, 630
nutrition interventions, 630-631
physical activity interventions, 630
prevention strategies, 631-632
Obesity prevention/treatment, 632-633
behavioral treatments, 633-634
childhood obesity, family involvement, 634
goals of treatment, 633
pharmacological treatments, 634
prevention efforts, 634-635
self-help/commercial programs, 633
surgical treatments, 634
treatment matching strategy, 633
Obsessive-compulsive disorder (OCD), 208
Obstructive sleep apnea syndrome, 199, 500, 727, 729
Occupational health and safety, 635
carcinogens, exposure to, 129
costs of illness/injury, 637
federal government involvement in, 636-637
HIV transmission and, 24-25
job strain, hypertension and, 108
occupational medicine specialty, 636
worker populations and, 636
workplace-specific hazards, 635-636
work-site physical activity interventions, 662
See also Job strain; Work-related stress; Worksite health promotion
Occupational Safety and Health Act of 1970, 637
Occupational Safety and Health Administration (OSHA), 636-637
Office of Behavioral and Social Sciences Research (OBSSR), 386, 618-619, 840
Office of Disease Prevention and Health Promotion (ODPHP), 386-387, 840-841
Office of Research on Women's Health (ORWH), 819
ONSET study, 49
Operant conditioning, 62-63, 130
Operant learning paradigm, 647
Opioids. See Chronic pain management; Endogenous opioids
Optimism/pessimism, 323-325, 637
behavioral responses and, 638
blood pressure regulation and, 639

disease management success and, 639-640
giving-up response, 638-639
health-related behaviors and, 638
mortality rates and, 640
physiological pathways, attitudes and, 639-640
theoretical foundation of, 638
well-being measures and, 639
Optimism-Pessimism Instrument (OP), 642
Optimism/pessimism measurement, 640
Attributional Style Questionnaire and, 641-642
Content Analysis of Verbatim Explanations and, 642
Defensive Pessimism Questionnaire and, 642-643
Life Orientation Test and, 641
Optimism-Pessimism Instrument and, 642
Optimism-Pessimism Test Instrument and, 643
unrealistic optimism measure, 642
Optimism-Pessimism Test Instrument (OPTI), 643
Oral cancer, 137
Organizational development and process theories, 273
Organizations. See Health and behavior organizations; Health care organizations/systems
Osteoarthritis, 71, 72
See also Arthritis; Rheumatoid arthritis
Ovarian cancer, 125, 133

PACE+ (Patient-Centered Assessment and Counseling for Exercise Plus Ntrition), 661
Pacific Rim Cancer Screening Awareness Through Churches, 196
Pain, 645
affective factors and, 648-649
biopsychosocial model, chronic pain, 646
cancer and, 130
cognitive factors and, 647-648
conceptualizations of, 645-646
depression and, 648-649
fibromyalgia syndrome and, 331-332
gate control model of, 646
HIV/AIDS and, 21
learning factors and, 647
malingering and, 647
nociception and, 645
psychogenic perspectives on, 646
psychological contributors to, 646-649
repressive coping and, 695
rheumatoid arthritis and, 698-699
self-regulation of, 648
sensory model of, 645-646
sickle cell disease and, 15-16, 724
subjective experience of, 649
See also Chronic pain; Chronic pain management; Gate control theory
Pain Disability Index, 190
Pancreatic cancer, 125

Pap smears, 129, 133, 134
   follow-up care, 136
   See also Women's health issues
Paradoxical findings, 3, 213, 489, 580
Parasympathetic nervous system (PSNS):
   asthma and, 78-79
   heart rate variability and, 530
   stress, cardiovascular response to, 148-149
Parenting beliefs, 2
Participatory research, 650
   applications of, 651
   degrees of participation, 651-652
   developing nations and, 650-651
   expanded application of, 652
   native communities, external researchers and, 651
   origins/development of, 650-651
   participants in, 651
   utility of, 652
   See also Community-based participatory research
Passive smoking, 731, 746
Patient-Centered Assessment and Counseling for Exercise
   Plus Nutrition (PACE+), 661
Patient compliance. *See* Adherence
Pawtucket Heart Health Program (PHHP), 142-145
Paxil, 238, 634
Peptic ulcers, 653-654, 779
   behavioral patterns and, 655
   development of, 654
   helicobacter pylori bacteria and, 653-654, 655
   history of, 655
   medical therapy for, 655
   nonsteroidal anti-inflammatory drugs and,
     654, 655
   stress and, 653, 654-655
Personality variables:
   breast cancer and, 525
   hypertensive personality, 51
   loneliness and, 586
   stress/coping mechanisms, cultural factors and, 229
   type A behavior, 49, 50, 114, 156, 344
   See also Explanatory style; Expressive writing; Heart
     disease-type A behavior
Personal Responsibility and Work Opportunity
   Reconciliation Act (PRWORA) of 1996, 535
Personal Views Survey III-R, 464
Persuasion marketing theory, 273
Pessimism. *See* Optimism/pessimism;
   Optimism/pessimism measurement
Pharmacotherapies:
   alcohol abuse treatments, 39
   nicotine addiction, 740, 741-742 (table)
   rheumatoid arthritis and, 700
   See also Antidepressant medications
Phenylketonuria (PKU), 368

Physical abuse:
   child physical abuse, 168
   intimate partner abuse, 808-809, 819
   irritable bowel syndrome and, 559
Physical activity, 656-675
   endurance exercise, 657, 658
   exercise prescriptions, 657-658, 659
   mental health and, 658-659
   physical health and, 657-658
   physiological adaptations and, 657
   psychophysiology and, 658-659
   strength training, 657
   See also Exercise activities
Physical activity interventions, 659
   adolescents/young adults and, 661-662
   child-centered interventions, 660-661
   environmental intervention, 664
   epidemiological research and, 660
   future research in, 663-664
   gender differences and, 664
   intergenerationl designs, 664
   measurement of activity and, 664
   middle-aged adults and, 662
   older adults and, 662-663
   work-site interventions, 662
Physical activity-mood, 665
   acute physical activity and, 666
   depression studies, 666
   experimental intervention studies on, 666-667
   mechanisms of, 667
   population studies on, 665-666
Physical functioning:
   allostatic overload and, 44
   Alzheimer's disease and, 46-47
   arthritis and, 72
   caregiving, resultant illness in, 46
   See also Exercise activities
Physical health:
   crowding effects and, 226-227
   disaster events and, 252-254
   discriminatory practices and, 256
   effort-reward imbalance and, 299
   explanatory style and, 324
   loneliness and, 587-588
   marital status, longevity and, 260-261
   subjective well-being and, 460-462
   support groups and, 788
Physiological variables, 22
   chronic stress/bereavement and, 46
   pathophysiological changes, 44
   See also Allostasis/allostatic load
Pituitary function, 313
Placebos, 668
   conditioning theory and, 668-669

effects magnitude, 668
response expectancy theory and, 669
Planned behavior. *See* Theory of planned behavior (TPB)
Policy:
 clean air legislation, 749
 cost-effectiveness and, 225
 drug abuse prevention and, 274
 effort-reward imbalance model and, 299
 evidence-based behavioral medicine and, 322
 injury prevention strategies, 550-551
 low birth weight infants and, 592
 research participants, gender of, 819
Population Information Program, 485
Positive emotions, 306
 broaden-and-build theory and, 306, 307-308
 coping strategies and, 307
 negative emotions and, 308
 optimism, 307
 physical/psychological health benefits of, 306-307
 resilience and, 308-309
 well-being, psychological resources and, 309
 written emotional disclosure, 307
 See also Happiness
Postexposure prophylaxis (PEP), 25
Post-traumatic stress disorder (PTSD), 30, 252
 brain function and, 78
 chronic pain and, 188
 endogenous opioids and, 314-315
Potential for Hostility (PH), 527
Poverty. *See* Socioeconomic status (SES)
Practice. *See* Clinical practice
Prader-Willi syndrome (PWS), 372
PRAISE!, 196
Precaution adoption process model, 549
Precede-proceed model, 549, 802
Pregnancy:
 alcohol abuse, unintended pregnancy and, 35
 individual resources and, 670
 infertility treatment and, 545
 preterm delivery/low birth weight, 669-671
 stress, early labor and, 670
 television influences and, 792-793
 See also Infertility; Low birth weight; Women's
  health issues
Pregnancy prevention-adolescents:
 adolescent birth rates, 672, 792
 adolescent pregnancy, current statistics on, 671-672
 effective interventions for, 674
 family factors and, 673
 health factors and, 673
 individual psychological factors and, 673
 peer group factors and, 673
 problem of, 672
 public policies/focus on, 672-673

religious factors and, 673
social support factors and, 673
socioeconomic factors and, 673
unmarried adolescents, birth increases, 672
Prenatal care, 2
Prescription drugs, 478
Preterm delivery (PTD), 669-671
Preventive health care, 2
 intervention sustainability, 27
 minority populations and, 13-14
 perceived susceptibility and, 476
 postexposure prophylaxis and, 25
 universal precautions procedures, 24
 See also Health promotion
Problem behavior theory, 271
Problem-solving therapy, 130, 131
Pro-Children Act of 1994, 749
Progressive muscle relaxation (PMR), 111, 130, 555
Project GRAD (Graduate Ready for Activity Daily),
  661-662
Project Joy, 196
Project MATCH (Matching Alcohol Treatments to Client
  Heterogeneity), 40
Project RESPECT, 165
Promoting Alternative THinking Strategies (PATHS),
  807-808
Proposition 187, 536
Proposition 99, 749
Prostate cancer, 122, 124-125, 133, 134
Prostate specific antigen (PSA), 133, 134
Prozac, 238, 634
Psychiatric genetics, 372
Psychological maltreatment, 160, 169
Psychological variables, 20, 22
 alcohol abuse and, 33
 crowding and, 227-228
 endocrine system, stress and, 78
 oxidative stress and, 80
 See also Anger; Anxiety; Behavioral genetics; Health
  psychology
Psychology.info, 387, 841
Psychoneuroimmunology, 21, 675
 acute stress-immunity in humans, 677
 autonomic nervous system and, 675-676
 behavioral change, cytokines and, 679
 behavioral/psychological influences and, 676-678
 cancer and, 680-681
 cardiovascular disease and, 679
 central modulation of immunity, 676
 central nervous system, cytokine influence on, 678-679
 chronic stress, depression and, 677
 clinical implications of, 679-681
 conditioning processes and, 676
 HIV/AIDS and, 680

immune system and, 675, 676
infectious disease risk and, 679-680
moderating variables and, 677-678
neuroendocrine axis and, 676
neurotransmitters and, 675
rheumatoid arthritis, stress/depression and, 680
sleep loss, cytokine expression and, 678
stress-immunity in animals, 677
PsychoNeuroImmunology Research Society (PNIRS), 387, 841
Psychonomic Society, 387, 841
Psychophysiological Investigations of Myocardial Ischemia (PIMI) study, 514
Psychophysiology, 681
ambulatory research methods and, 682-683
behavioral medicine and, 681-682
noninvasive measurement in, 683
positive/negative emotional states and, 683
psychological disposition and, 683
research strategies in, 682-683
well-being-behavior interactions, 682
whole-person focus in, 681
Psychosocial factors, 16
arthritis and, 71-72
asthma management, 76
autoimmune diseases and, 81-83
cancer screening/follow-up care and, 135-136
cardiac rehabilitation and, 141
caregivers of Alzheimer's patients, 45-48
cerebrovascular disease and, 166-167
child/adolescent cardiovascular risk and, 114
diabetes mellitus and, 245-248
hypertension and, 106-107
learned helplessness, 114
See also Cancer-psychosocial treatment
Psychosomatics. See American Psychosomatic Society; Health psychology; Mind-body relations
Psychotherapeutic interventions, 16
arthritis and, 69
autoimmune diseases and, 83
behavioral therapy, 237
bulimia nervosa and, 115-116
cognitive therapy, 236
depression treatments, 235-237
infertility treatment and, 546-547
interpersonal therapy, 236-237
Psychotropic medications:
alcohol abuse treatment and, 39
See also Antidepressant medications
Psych web, 387, 841
Public Health Institute (PHI), 387, 841
Public Health Practice Program Office (PHPPO), 164
Public health programs:
intervention dissemination, 27

needle exchange programs, 19, 25
self-efficacy and, 712-713
social epidemiology study, 31-32
See also Behavioral Risk Factor Surveillance System (BRFSS); Cancer prevention; Church-based interventions; Community-based participatory research (CBPR); Ecosocial theory; Health literacy
Public health research. See Community-based participatory research (CBPR); Participatory research
Public policy. See Policy
Puerto Ricans. See Health disparities; Hispanics; Latino health/behavior
Pulmonary disease. See Chronic obstructive pulmonary disease (COPD)

Quality of adjusted life year (QALY), 477
Quality of life:
adherence to treatment and, 22-23
analysis of, 223-224
diabetes mellitus and, 246, 247
Quality of life measurement, 685
disease-specific instruments, 686-687
feasibility of, 689
future use of, 689
generic measure, 686, 687
individualized instruments, 687
properties of measures, 688-689
reliability of, 688
responsiveness of, 688
transition measures and, 689
types of measurement, 686-688
utility of, 685-686
utility/preference-based measure, 687-688
validity of, 688
Quality of Well-Being (QWB) Scale, 223, 224
Quota Law of 1921, 533

Race, 12-13
asthma incidence and, 80
binge eating disorder and, 281-282
cardiovascular reactivity and, 155-156
discrimination/racism, hypertension and, 108
low birth weight infants and, 591
pain experience and, 72
See also Ethnicity
Raynaud's disease, 99, 691
behavioral treatment of, 692
peripheral blood flow, behavioral control of, 691-692
Reactive oxygen species (ROS), 80
Readiness state, 11, 21
RE-AIM framework, 321-322
Reasoned action. See Theory of reasoned action (TRA)
Reaven's syndrome X, 594

Recovery process, 522
Rectal cancer, 124, 128, 133
Recurrent Coronary Prevention Project (RCPP), 520
Reference group theory, 716
Referrals, 193
Relational competence, 10, 11
Relaxation therapy, 111, 243-244, 334, 468-469, 772
Religious practice. *See* Church-based interventions;
    Spirituality
Remeron, 238
Repressive coping, 693
    asthma incidence and, 695
    cancer and, 694
    childhood memories and, 694
    health outcomes and, 694-695
    heart disease and, 695
    negative emotions, avoidance of, 694
    pain perception and, 695
    physiological arousal and, 695
    research history on, 693
    seminal study on, 693-694
Reproductive function:
    alcohol abuse and, 35, 37
    stress response and, 779
    tobacco use and, 731
    See also Infertility; Pregnancy; Women's health issues
Research:
    acculturation research, 4
    adherence-promotion, 23
    adherence studies, 7-8
    clinical trials, 6
    discrimination studies, 256-259
    racial/ethnic representation in, 13
    See also Clinical practice; Community-based
        participatory research; Confounding; Key
        informants
Research Society on Alcoholism (RSA), 387, 841
Resiliency, 308-309, 463-464, 590
Respiratory function:
    biofeedback and, 99-100
    See also Lung cancer
Response expectancy theory, 669
Reynolds Adolescent Depression Scale, 232
Rheumatoid arthritis (RA), 71, 72, 81, 698
    biopsychosocial factors in, 698
    cognitive-behavioral therapies and, 700-701
    cognitive/coping factors in, 699-700
    fatigue and, 699
    negative affect and, 699
    pain in, 698-699
    pharmacological management of, 700
    stress and, 699
    stress/depression, neuroimmune mechanisms and, 680
    treatment, biopsychosocial considerations and, 700-701

work disability and, 700
    See also Arthritis
Risk behaviors, 2
    African Americans, HIV/AIDS and, 13-15
    assessment technology, 20
    binge drinking, 94-98
    intervention program design, 27
    reduction of, sustainability concerns, 27
    See also Alcohol abuse; Behavioral Risk Factor
        Surveillance System (BRFSS); Behavioral
        treatment models; Disease risk; Health behaviors;
        HIV/AIDS prevention
Ritalin, 101
Robert Wood Johnson Foundation, 387, 841
Role transition, 91, 116, 298

Safe Kids/Healthy Neighborhoods Coalition, 550
Safer-sex programs/practices, 26, 28
Sandwich generation, 46
Save Our Sons and Daughters Program, 808
Schizophrenia, 208, 459, 587
School-based health promotion, 703
    Child and Adolescent Trial for Cardiovascular Health,
        145, 660, 706-708
    definition of, 706
    effectiveness of, 707-708
    elements of, 705-706
    evolution of, 703-705
    family component in, 707
    financial resources for, 706
    food service personnel and, 707
    health curriculum, 706-707
    smoking interventions, 732, 746-747
Science.gov, 387-388, 841-842
Screening. *See* Cancer screening; Genetic testing; Health
    care costs
Second-hand smoke exposure, 731, 746
Seduction theory, 168
Segmented assimilation theory, 1, 4
Seizures. *See* Convulsive disorders
Selected Cities Project, 90
Selective serotonin reuptake inhibitors (SSRIs), 237, 238,
    500, 634
Self-efficacy, 10, 22, 229, 708-709, 793
    arthritis treatments and, 70
    causal structure, health behaviors and, 709, 710 (figure)
    chronic disease adjustments and, 182
    control beliefs and, 218
    diabetes mellitus and, 244
    health beliefs and, 475
    outcome expectation and, 709
    public health campaigns and, 712-713
    self-management model and, 709-712, 711 (figure)
    social cognitive theory and, 709

socially oriented approaches to health and, 713
social roles and, 298
subgoal attainments and, 710
transtheoretical model of behavior change and, 806
Self-esteem, 3, 283
Self-management:
arthritis treatment, 66-67
assertiveness, communication and, 67
cancer screening and, 135
chronic disease and, 172
endogenous opioids and, 315
fibromyalgia syndrome and, 334-336
pacing/goal-setting and, 66
problem-solving and, 66
relaxation/biofeedback strategies, 67
stepwise implementation model and, 711
See also Effort-reward imbalance model;
Self-efficacy
Self-protective action, 11
Self-Rating Depression Scale (SDS), 231
Self-regulation. *See* Self-management
Self-reported health, 714
adverse health outcomes and, 718-719
biomedical issues and, 715-716
cultural/environmental contexts and, 716, 717
demographic/socioeconomic factors and, 716
determinants of, 716-717
development of, 714-715
feelings of health, 715
functional issues and, 716-717
future of, 719
mental health and, 717
predictive value of, 717-719
scoring methods in, 715
sociological reference group theory and, 716
subjective evaluation of health and, 715-716
wording of the measure, 715
working conditions and, 716
Sensate focus exercises, 317-318
Serum lipids. *See* Lipids
Serzone, 238
Seven Countries Study, 501, 502
Sex practices, 2
abstinence programs, 25-26
alcohol abuse and, 35
condom use, 26
monogamous partnering, 26
multiple partners, 26
negotiated safety in, 26
safer-sex programs, 26
unprotected sex, 19, 28
See also HIV/AIDS; HIV/AIDS prevention; Pregnancy
prevention-adolescents; School-based health
promotion

Sex therapy, 317-318
Sexual abuse:
child sexual abuse, 168-169
intimate partner sexual violence, 808-809, 819
irritable bowel syndrome and, 559
Sexually transmitted disease prevention, 719
abstinence/delay of sexual initiation, 721
barriers to treatment success, 722
behavioral interventions, 721
behavior change theories and, 720
clinical care screening, 721-722
early treatment and, 722
epidemiology in, 719-720
infectiousness model, 720
partner notification/treatment, 722
prophylaxis and, 721
strategies in, 720-721
Sexually transmitted diseases (STDs), 19, 26
alcohol abuse, risk behaviors and, 35
HIV infection and, 28
intervention programs for, 27
Project RESPECT, 165
Shattuck report, 703
Short-Form 36-Item Health Survey (SF-36), 686
Sickle cell disease (SCD), 15-16, 368, 723
academic/psychosocial sequelae of, 725
acute complications of, 724
clinical severity of, 723-724
disability and, 725
medical treatment of, 724-725
work life and, 725
Sickness Impact Profile (SIP), 686
Signoidoscopy, 133, 134
Simpson's paradox, 213
SisterTalk Hartford, 196
Sjogren's syndrome, 66
Skin cancer, 125, 128
Sleep apnea, 199, 500, 727, 729
Sleep disorders, 678, 726
adherence to treatment and, 729
classification of, 726-727
clinical treatment of, 727
daytime sleepiness, treatments for, 729
insomnia, behavioral treatment for, 727-729
pediatric sleep disorders, 729
prevalence of, 727
sleep hygiene habits, 727, 728 (table)
Sleep rhythms, 41, 42, 587
Smart Recovery (SR), 38
Smoking, 730
cigarette composition, 731, 732-733
clinical interventions, 732
compensatory smoking, 731
damage reduction, 732-733

disease risk, interactions and, 732
educational interventions, 732
health effects of, 731-732
marketing efforts, 732, 748
passive smoking, 731
prevalence statistics, 73-731
pricing effects, 733
psychiatric disorders and, 736, 743
reproductive function and, 731
supply restriction, 732
workplace restrictions and, 733
See also Heart disease-tobacco use; Smoking/nicotine
    dependence; Tobacco use
Smoking cessation, 138, 186, 195, 267, 518, 732
adolescent smokers and, 749
alcohol abuse and, 743
clean air legislation, 749
psychiatric disorders and, 743
weight gain and, 740, 743
Smoking/nicotine dependence, 733-734
abuse liability and, 734
drug delivery system in, 735
individual differences in, 736
nicotine, addictive nature of, 734-735, 737
nicotine effects, 735
nicotine replacement therapy, 736
nicotine, use comparison studies, 734-735
reinforcement cues and, 735-736
self-administration and, 734
treatment implications, 736
withdrawal symptoms, 735
Smoking/nicotine dependence interventions, 737
alcohol abuse and, 743
cognitive/behavioral interventions and, 740
intensive treatment programs, 738
intervention delivery modes, 738-740, 739 (table)
motivation/readiness assessment, 737-738
nicotine fading strategy, 739-740
nicotine replacement therapy, 738
pharmacotherapy, 740, 741-742 (table)
physiological dependence, 738
professional treatment, 738-740
psychiatric disorders and, 736, 743
psychological dependence, 740
relapse prevention/change maintenance, 740
weight gain and, 740, 743
Smoking prevention-adolescents, 732, 744-745
advertising restrictions and, 747-748
community interventions, 747
direct restrictions and, 749
future efforts in, 749-750
influential variables and, 745-746
media campaigns and, 748
pricing/tax impediments, 748-749

sales restrictions and, 748
school-based education interventions, 746-747
school policies/penalties and, 747
smoking cessation interventions, 749
youth-specific smoking consequences, 745
Social behaviors, 11
alcohol abuse and, 33
See also Behavioral genetics; Fundamental social
    causation of disease/mortality
Social capital, 299, 536, 750-751
health outcomes, linking mechanisms and, 753
limitations of, 753
measurement of, 751-752
population health and, 752-753
social connectedness and, 753
trust perceptions and, 752-753
Social class, 590-591
Social cognitive theory, 27, 549, 709
Social development theory, 271
Social diffusion theory, 27
Social epidemiology study, 31-32
Social integration, 754
health, social networks/integration and, 755
health-social networks model, 756-758
material resources, access to, 758
neurosis, development of, 754
person-to-person contact and, 758
social engagement and, 757
social influence and, 757
social networks, behavioral aspects and, 756
social network theory and, 755
social relationship assessment, 756-757
social supports and, 757
theoretical orientations and, 754-755
Social learning theory, 271, 647
Social marketing, 759, 763
applications outcomes, 762-763
audience segmentation and, 761
commercial social marketing, 760
definitions of, 759-760
development/implementation/evaluation process, 761
effectiveness measures of, 763-764
health communication, 760
history/importance of, 760
integrated theory/framework in, 762
marketing mix in, 762
place elements, 762
price categories, 762
product in, 761-762
promotion activities, 762
reach of, 763
Social networks. See Social supports
Social network theory, 755
Social Sciences Institute (SSI), 388, 842

Social status incongruence, 764-766
Social supports, 2
    adherence practices and, 7, 22
    adolescent pregnancy and, 673
    allostatic overload and, 44
    autoimmune disease and, 82
    bereavement stress and, 93
    caregiving coping strategy, 160
    connectedness, stress and, 80
    crowding effects and, 227
    diabetes mellitus and, 243
    disease-related coping and, 15, 182
    gender differences in, 363-364
    health behavior change and, 9-11
    health disparities and, 491
    health outcomes and, 32
    immune compromise and, 30
    intervention dissemination and, 27
    low birth weight infants and, 590
    See also Loneliness; Social integration; Support groups
Society of Behavioral Medicine (SBM), 388, 471-472,
    696, 842
Society for Behavioral Neuroendocrinology (SBN), 388, 842
Society for Medical Decision Making, 388, 842
Society for Neuroscience (SfN), 388, 842
Society of Pediatric Psychology (SPP), 388-389, 842-843
Society for Prevention Research (SPR), 389, 843
Society for Psychophysiological Research, 389, 843
Society for Public Health Education (SOPHE), 389, 843
Society for Research in Child Development, 389, 843
Society for Research on Nicotine and Tobacco (SRNT),
    389, 843
Society for Stimulus Properties of Drugs (SSPD), 389, 843
Socioeconomic position (SEP), 489, 490-492
Socioeconomic status (SES), 2, 3, 768
    access to health care and, 769
    acculturation research and, 4
    adolescent pregnancy rate and, 672, 673
    alcohol abuse and, 34
    allostatic overload and, 44
    asthma incidence and, 80
    cancer mortality rates and, 129
    caregiver well-being and, 48
    crowding and, 226-227
    disease/mortality causation and, 344-346
    gender and, 770
    health association with, 768
    health behavior change and, 10-11
    health behaviors and, 769
    health effects on, 769
    low birth weight infants and, 590-591
    negative emotions and, 305
    physical conditions and, 768
    psychosocial responses and, 769

    race/ethnicity and, 769-770
    See also Income inequality
Sociological reference group theory, 716
Somatization, 558
    See also American Psychosomatic Society (APS);
        Health psychology; Mind-body relations
Specialized Center of Research-Arteriosclerosis
    (SCOR-A), 112
Spielberger Multidimensonal Anger Inventory, 49
Spielberger Trait Anger Scale, 53, 525
Spiral computed tomography, 133
Spirituality, 770-771
    adolescent pregnancy and, 673
    caregiving coping strategy, 160
    disease-related coping and, 15
    empirical links, spirituality/health, 771-772
    gerotranscendence, 785
    God-Locus-of-Health-Control scale, 218
    harmful role of, 772, 773
    health care services and, 773
    health outcomes and, 32, 74, 772-773
    healthy behaviors and, 772
    loving-God beliefs and, 771-772
    meaning of, 771
    prayer/meditation practices, 771
    relaxation response and, 772
    service attendance, 771
    social supports and, 772
    spiritual coping methods, 773
    spiritual struggles and, 772
    transcendental meditation, 111
    See also Church-based interventions
Sports, Play and Active Recreation for Kids (SPARK), 660
Stanford Adolescent Heart Health Program, 661
Stanford Heart Disease Prevention Program (SHDPP),
    142-145
State-Trait Anxiety Inventory (STAI), 60-61
Status incongruence. *See* Cultural consonance; Social
    status incongruence
Stockholm Heart Epidemiology Program (SHEEP),
    525, 564
Stomach cancer, 74, 125
Stress, 774
    acculturation process and, 2
    appraisal and, 774, 776
    arthritis and, 69
    asthma and, 77-81
    autoimmune diseases and, 82-83
    bereavement and, 93
    biobehavioral stress reactivity, 108-110
    caregiving duties and, 46
    coping and, 774-776
    cortisol levels and, 31
    crowding and, 226

definition of, 41-42
effort-reward imbalance and, 299
health care seeking and, 776
health disparities and, 491
HIV infection, stress management and, 28, 29-31
hormone activity in, 42-43
immune function and, 79, 537-539
oxidative stress, 80
social inequities and, 16
stress-disease models, 107
See also Allostasis/allostatic load; Coping strategies;
    Endogenous opioids; Gastric ulcers; Hypertension;
    Work-related stress
Stress-buffering hypothesis, 780-781
Stress-related growth, 779, 783
development of, 783
health/well-being and, 784
types of, 783
Stress response, 777
behavioral stress management techniques, 780
cardiovascular system and, 778
gastrointestinal system and, 778-779
growth and, 779
immune system and, 778
individual variability in, 779
metabolism and, 778
nervous system and, 777
reproductive system and, 779
Stroke. *See* Cerebrovascular disease
Structural equation modeling (SEM), 86
Structured Clinical Interview for DSM-IV (SCID), 177, 232
Structured interview (SI), 49, 54, 55, 527
Student health:
examination stress, 538-539
loneliness and, 587
physical activity interventions, 661-662
See also Binge drinking; School-based health promotion
Subjective well-being (SWB), 459-462
Substance Abuse and Mental Health Services Agency
    (SAMHSA), 98, 389-390, 843-844
Substance abuse. *See* Alcohol abuse; Drug abuse;
    Smoking
Successful aging, 784
gerotranscendence and, 785
model of, 784-785
predictors of, 785
Suicide:
bereavement and, 94
depression and, 234
eating disorders and, 283
HIV/AIDS diagnosis and, 20-21
inpatient treatment and, 117
multiple sclerosis and, 611
prevention programs, 808

Support groups, 786
characteristics of, 786-787
group format/structure of, 787
leadership in, 787
mental health effects of, 787-788
physical health effects of, 788
target population of, 786-787
See also Social support
Supportive-expressive group therapy (SEG), 83, 131
Surface electromyography (SEMG), 100
Survival, 42, 522, 718
Symar Amendment of 1991, 748
Sympathetic-adrenal medullary (SAM) axis, 302, 538, 699
Sympathetic nervous system (SNS), 42, 58
asthma and, 78-79
cardiovascular responses, stress and, 148-149
endogenous opioids and, 313-314
fibromyalgia syndrome and, 330
immune system function and, 675, 676, 678
stress response and, 779
Symptom Check List-90-R, 232
Systematic desensitization, 130
Systemic lupus erythematosus, 83, 199
Systemic vascular resistance, 148

Tailored communications, 789
algorithms in, 789-790
group-level cultural tailoring, 790-791
individualized information delivery and, 789, 791
psychologically-based interventions and, 791
targeted interventions and, 791
target health practice context and, 790
technology for, 789
terminology of, 790
The Taking Charge curriculum, 674
Taylor Manifest Anxiety Scale (TMAS), 60
Technology:
adherence to treatment and, 20
risk behavior assessment and, 20
Teen pregnancy. *See* Pregnancy prevention-adolescents
Television viewing, 791-792
advertising, food selection and, 792
health impacts of, 793
information source, 792
obesity and, 792
physical activity and, 792
sexual health and, 792-793
substance abuse and, 792
Temporomandibular disorders (TMDs). *See* Fibromyalgia
    syndrome (FMS)
Tension-type headaches, 467, 468, 470
Testicular cancer, 125
Theory of planned behavior (TPB), 793
application of, 794

beliefs and, 793, 794
change model, transtheoretical stages of, 795
criticisms of, 795-796
empirical support for, 794-795
human social behavior, considerations in, 793-794
intention and, 794, 795
intention-behavior relation and, 795
predictive validity of, 795
self-regulation, failures in, 795
Theory of reasoned action (TRA), 549, 796-797
application process of, 798-799
intentions, prediction of, 797-798
Theory of triadic influence (TTI), 799, 800 (figure)
causes of behavior, 799-802
dynamic system of causation and, 802
feedback influence and, 802
interpersonal/social causes of behavior, 801
interstream influences and, 801-802
levels/tiers of influence and, 799, 801
prevention/treatment design and, 802-803
related behaviors, role of, 802
sociocultural causes of behavior, 801
streams of influence and, 801
Therapeutic talk, 327-328
Threats, 366-367, 474
Three-Area Severity of Depression Scale, 231
Three Mile Island Nuclear Power Station (TMI), 253
Thyroid cancer, 731
Title VI, Civil Rights Act of 1964, 535
Tobacco use, 2
Asian Americans, 74-75
behavioral genetics and, 88
cancer risk and, 127, 137-138
cardiovascular risk and, 140
cessation of, 138, 186, 195
child/adolescent use, 113
gender and, 3
health disparities and, 490
oxidative toxins and, 80
See also Heart disease-tobacco use; Smoking
Traditional health practices, 75
Trait Anger Scale, 53, 525
Transactional theories, 271
Transcendental meditation (TM), 111
Transfusions. See Blood supply
Transtheoretical model (TTM) of behavior change, 509, 803-804
construct integration in, 806
decisional balance, pros/cons of change, 805-806
intermediate outcome variables, 804
processes of change in, 805
self-efficacy component of, 806
stages of change in, 804-805
stage-tailored interventions and, 803

Transvaginal ultrasound, 133
Treatment of Depression Collaborative Research Program, 239
Treatment regimens:
behavioral models of, 15
See also Adherence
Treatment-resistant organisms, 6, 21, 28
Triadic influence. See Theory of triadic influence (TTI)
Tricyclic antidepressants (TCAs), 238, 500
Tuberculosis (TB), 6
Asian Americans and, 74
HIV/AIDS infection and, 19
immigrant populations and, 534-535
Tuskegee Syphilis Study, 14
12-step facilitation therapy (TSF), 40
Twin studies, 86-87, 87 (figure), 155, 511
Type A behavior pattern (TABP), 49, 50, 114, 156, 344
evaluation of, 527
hostility and, 524
See also Heart disease-type A behavior

Ulcers. See Gastric ulcers; Peptic ulcers
Ultrasound imaging:
cardiovascular psychophysiological evaluation and, 149
transvaginal ultrasound, 133
United Nations Development Programme (UNDP), 361
Universal precautions procedures, 24
U. S. Department of Agriculture (USDA), 339, 504
U. S. Department of Health and Human Services, 493, 705
U. S. Guide to Community Prevention Services, 129
U. S. National Cholesterol Education Program, 594, 595
U. S. National Committee of the International Union of Psychological Science, 390, 844
U. S. Physicians' Health Study, 502
U. S. Preventive Services Task Force (USPSTF), 129, 320
U. S. Quality of Employment Surveys, 562, 563
Utilization of care. See Health care service utilization

Vaccines. See Immunizations
Value-expectancy theory, 474, 638
Vertical banded gastroplasty (VBG), 634
Violence prevention, 807
child maltreatment, 808
intimate partner sexual violence, 808-809
suicide, 808
youth violence, 807-808
Violent behavior, 34-35
Vital exhaustion, 809
assessment of, 809-810
biological correlates of, 811, 811 (table)
components of, 812
etiology/theoretical foundation of, 810

health risks of, 811, 811 (figure)
prevalence of, 810
treatment strategies for, 811-812

Waking activities, 41, 42
Ways of Coping, 775
Weight. *See* Body weight; Obesity
Western Collaborative Group Study (WCGS),
    49, 519, 520
Western Electric Study, 502
Western Ontario and McMaster Universities Arthritis
    Index (WOMAC), 686-687
West Haven-Yale Multidimensional Pain Inventory, 190, 336
White coat effect, 51-52, 103
Whitehall studies, 597
Women's Health Initiative (WHI), 390, 506, 844
Women's health issues, 813
    arthritis, 815
    autoimmune diseases, 815
    cancer mortality, 814
    cardiovascular disease, 814
    Cesarean sections, 817
    childbirth, 817
    death, primary causes of, 814
    dementia, 816
    demographic patterns and, 813-814
    diabetes mellitus, 815
    drug addictions, 817-818
    eating disorders, 814
    gynecological health, 816
    health risks, gender influences on, 817-818
    hormone replacement therapy, 817
    hysterectomy, 816
    measures/variables, gender specificity of, 819
    menopause, 817
    mental health, 814-815
    osteoporosis, 815-816
    physical activity and, 818
    pregnancy/infertility/contraception, 816-817
    research participants, health care policy and, 819
    societal influences on, 818
    urinary incontinence, 815
    violence, 818-819
    See also Breast cancer; Infertility
Work-related stress:
    cardiovascular disease and, 821
    long working hours and, 821-822
    professional driving and, 822
    shift work and, 820-821
    See also Job strain; Occupational health and safety
Worksite health promotion, 662, 823
    comprehensive programming and, 823-824
    development of, 823
    environmental/organizational-level interventions,
        824-825
    high-risk employees and, 823
    individual-level interventions, 824
    interpersonal-level interventions, 824
    labor-management relationships and, 825
    tailored approaches to, 824
    worker planning of, 825
World Health Organization (WHO), 17, 126, 358, 359,
    390, 572, 627, 844
Wound healing, 826
    behavioral stress and, 827
    inflammatory phase and, 826-827
    proliferative phase and, 827
    psychological stress and, 827-828
    remodeling phase and, 827
Writing. *See* Expressive writing

Xenical, 634

YMCA/YWCA, 747
Youth Risk Behavior Survey (YRBS), 704

Zoloft, 238, 500, 634
Zung Self-Rating Depression Scale (SDS), 231